OLYMPIC TEXTBOOK OF SCIENCE IN SPORT

OLYMPIC TEXTBOOK OF SCIENCE IN SPORT

VOLUME XV OF THE ENCYCLOPAEDIA OF SPORTS MEDICINE

AN IOC MEDICAL COMMISSION PUBLICATION

EDITED BY

RONALD J. MAUGHAN, PhD

WILEY-BLACKWELL

A John Wiley & Sons, Ltd., Publication

This edition first published 2009, © 2009 International Olympic Committee
Published by Blackwell Publishing Ltd

Blackwell Publishing was acquired by John Wiley & Sons in February 2007. Blackwell's publishing program has been merged with Wiley's global Scientific, Technical and Medical business to form Wiley-Blackwell.

Registered office: John Wiley & Sons Ltd, The Atrium, Southern Gate, Chichester, West Sussex, PO19 8SQ, UK

Editorial offices: 9600 Garsington Road, Oxford, OX4 2DQ, UK
The Atrium, Southern Gate, Chichester, West Sussex, PO19 8SQ, UK
111 River Street, Hoboken, NJ 07030-5774, USA

For details of our global editorial offices, for customer services and for information about how to apply for permission to reuse the copyright material in this book please see our website at www.wiley.com/wiley-blackwell

Library of Congress Cataloging-in-Publication Data
The Olympic textbook of science in sport / edited by Ron J. Maughan.
    p. ; cm. – (Encyclopaedia of sports medicine ; v. 15)
    "An IOC Medical Commission publication."
    Includes bibliographical references and index.
    ISBN 978-1-4051-5638-7
    1. Sports–Physiological aspects.   2. Physical fitness–Physiological aspects.   3. Human mechanics.
I. Maughan, Ron J., 1951-   II. IOC Medical Commission.   III. Series.
    [DNLM: 1. Sports–physiology.   2. Athletic Performance.   3. Biomechanics.   4. Exercise.
5. Nutrition Physiology.   6. Sports Medicine–methods. QT 13 E527 1988 v.15]
    RC1235.O59 2008
    613.7′11–dc22
                                                                    2008024090

ISBNs: 978-1-4051-5638-7
         978-1-4051-9257-6 (leather bound)

A catalogue record for this book is available from the British Library.

Set in 9/12 pt Palatino by Graphicraft Limited, Hong Kong
Printed and bound in Malaysia by Vivar Printing Sdn Bhd

1   2009

Contents

List of Contributors

SUSAN H. BACKHOUSE PhD, *Carnegie Research Institute, Leeds Metropolitan University, Leeds, UK*

VASILIOS BALTZOPOULOS PhD, *Institute for Biomedical Research into Human Movement and Health, Manchester Metropolitan University, Manchester, UK*

FRANK W. BOOTH PhD, *Department of Biomedical Sciences, Medical Pharmacology, and Physiology, University of Missouri, Columbia, MO, USA*

CLAUDE BOUCHARD PhD, *Pennington Biomedical Research Center, Baton Rouge, LA, USA*

LOUISE M. BURKE PhD, APD, *Department of Sports Nutrition, Australian Institute of Sport, Bruce, ACT, Australia, and Deakin University, Melbourne, Victoria, Australia*

FRANK CERNY PhD, *Department of Exercise and Nutrition Science, School of Public Health and Health Professions, State University of New York at Buffalo, Buffalo, NY, USA*

HELEN CREWE BSc (Hons), *UCT/MRC Research Unit for Exercise Science and Sports Medicine, Department of Human Biology, University of Cape Town, Newlands, South Africa*

PANTELEIMON EKKEKAKIS PhD, *Department of Kinesiology, Iowa State University, Ames, IA, USA*

MARTIN J. GIBALA PhD, *Exercise Metabolism Research Group, Department of Kinesiology, McMaster University, Hamilton, Ontario, Canada*

MICHAEL GLEESON PhD, *School of Sport and Exercise Sciences, Loughborough University, Loughborough, UK*

PAUL L. GREENHAFF PhD, *Centre for Integrated Systems Biology and Medicine, School of Biomedical Sciences, University of Nottingham Medical School, Queen's Medical Centre, Nottingham, UK*

GRAHAM P. HOLLOWAY PhD, *Department of Human Health and Nutritional Sciences, University of Guelph, Guelph, Ontario, Canada*

MASAKI ISHIKAWA PhD, *Department of Health and Sport Management, Osaka University of Health and Sport Sciences, Osaka, Japan*

ANDREW M. JONES PhD, *School of Sport and Health Sciences, University of Exeter, Exeter, UK*

PAAVO V. KOMI PhD, *Department of the Biology of Physical Activity, University of Jyväskylä, Jyväskylä, Finland*

KARL F. KOZLOWSKI EdM, *Department of Exercise and Nutrition Science, School of Public Health and Health Professions, State University of New York at Buffalo, Buffalo, NY, USA*

MICHAEL J. LAMONTE PhD, *Department of Social and Preventive Medicine, School of Public Health and Health Professions, State University of New York at Buffalo, Buffalo, NY, USA*

ADRIAN LEES PhD, *Research Institute for Sport and Exercise Sciences, Liverpool John Moores University, Henry Cotton Campus, Liverpool, UK*

CONSTANTINOS N. MAGANARIS PhD, *Institute for Biomedical Research into Human Movement and Health, Manchester Metropolitan University, Manchester, UK*

RONALD J. MAUGHAN PhD, *School of Sport and Exercise Sciences, Loughborough University, Loughborough, UK*

LYLE J. MICHELI MD, *Harvard Medical School, and Division of Sports Medicine, Children's Hospital Boston, Boston, MA, USA*

MARGO MOUNTJOY MD, *Health & Performance Centre, University of Guelph, Guelph, Ontario, Canada*

P. DARRELL NEUFER PhD, *Department of Exercise and Sports Sciences, and Department of Physiology, East Carolina University, Greenville, NC, USA*

MYRA A. NIMMO PhD, *School of Sport and Exercise Sciences, Loughborough University, Loughborough, UK*

TIMOTHY D. NOAKES MBChB, MD, DSc, *UCT/MRC Research Unit for Exercise Science and Sports Medicine, Department of Human Biology, University of Cape Town, Newlands, South Africa*

TIMOTHY OLDS PhD, *Nutritional Physiology Research Centre, University of South Australia, Adelaide, Australia*

BENTE K. PEDERSEN MD, DMSc, *Centre of Inflammation and Metabolism, Rigshospitalet 7641, Copenhagen, Denmark*

DAVID C. POOLE PhD, DSc, *School of Sport and Health Sciences, University of Exeter, Exeter, UK, and Departments of Kinesiology, Anatomy and Physiology, Kansas State University, Manhattan, KS, USA*

JOHN S. RAGLIN PhD, *Department of Kinesiology, Indiana University, Bloomington, IN, USA*

MARK RAKOBOWCHUK MSc, *Exercise Metabolism Research Group, Department of Kinesiology, McMaster University, Hamilton, Ontario, Canada*

TUOMO RANKINEN PhD, *Pennington Biomedical Research Center, Baton Rouge, LA, USA*

THOMAS REILLY DSc, *Research Institute for Sport and Exercise Sciences, Liverpool John Moores University, Henry Cotton Campus, Liverpool, UK*

WILHELM SCHÄNZER PhD, *Center for Preventive Doping Research, Institute of Biochemistry, German Sport University, Cologne, Germany*

NIELS H. SECHER MD, DMSc, *Department of Anaesthesia, Rigshospitalet, University of Copenhagen, Copenhagen, Denmark*

SUSAN M. SHIRREFFS PhD, *School of Sport and Exercise Sciences, Loughborough University, Loughborough, UK*

LAWRENCE L. SPRIET PhD, *Department of Human Health and Nutritional Sciences, University of Guelph, Guelph, Ontario, Canada*

FRANCIS B. STEPHENS PhD, *Centre for Integrated Systems Biology and Medicine, School of Biomedical Sciences, University of Nottingham Medical School, Queen's Medical Centre, Nottingham, UK*

MARIO THEVIS PhD, *Center for Preventive Doping Research, Institute of Biochemistry, German Sport University, Cologne, Germany*

ROSS TUCKER PhD, *UCT/MRC Research Unit for Exercise Science and Sports Medicine, Department of Human Biology, University of Cape Town, Newlands, South Africa*

CLYDE WILLIAMS PhD, *School of Sport and Exercise Sciences, Loughborough University, Loughborough, UK*

GREGORY WILSON PED, *Department of Exercise and Sport Science, University of Evansville, Evansville, IN, USA*

Foreword

The general aim of all volumes in the series, *Encyclopaedia of Sports Medicine*, is the enhancement of the health and welfare of athletes at all levels of competition in all parts of the world.

The most respected scientific investigators and clinicians have collaborated to produce each volume of the collection which contains reference texts that are both comprehensive for the topics and representative of the leading edge of knowledge.

Volume XV, *The Olympic Textbook of Science in Sport*, reexamines the biochemical, physiological, and biomechanical issues that were included in the original Volume I in 1988 and synthesizes the new research information that has been published during the last 20 years. I wish to congratulate Professor Ronald Maughan and all of the Contributing Authors on the excellent quality of their efforts and welcome this volume to the Encyclopaedia series.

Dr Jacques Rogge
President of the International Olympic Committee

Preface

As the standards of sporting excellence continue to rise to ever higher levels, so the scientific study of sport also continues to evolve. The Medical Commission of the International Olympic Committee has recognised that science is not parochial or nationalistic, but rather that scientific knowledge should be available to all athletes. As part of its mission to support athletes and those sports scientists from many different disciplines who, in turn, support them, the IOC Medical Commission decided to commission a *Textbook of Science in Sport*. The concept was of an encyclopaedia of sports science. An encyclopaedia should be a book or set of books giving information on many subjects or on many aspects of one subject: it should be both comprehensive and authoritative. The aim of this encyclopaedia therefore is to provide reviews of the many disciplines that comprise the sports sciences. To do so, a cast of leading experts from many countries was recruited as authors. These authors have given generously of their time and expertise and to them the credit is due for this volume.

I would like to extend special thanks to Howard "Skip" Knuttgen for his unfailing support in driving this project to its conclusion. His vast experience as Coordinator of Scientific Publications for the IOC Medical Commission has been an enormous asset at every stage of the process.

I am also deeply grateful to Victoria Pittman and Cathryn Gates, Development Editors at Wiley-Blackwell in Oxford, and to Alice Nelson who was production manager. All did an excellent job and ensured that the project remained on track.

Ronald J. Maughan, PhD

Introduction: Sport, Science and Sports Science

RONALD J. MAUGHAN

Sport occupies a prominent place in modern society and successful athletes enjoy a high level of financial and social reward, so there are considerable incentives to succeed. There are also many obstacles to success: the sportsman or woman who succeeds at the highest level faces bigger challenges than ever before. Although the falling rate of participation in sport and physical activity has been a major factor in the epidemic of obesity and related lifestyle diseases that has afflicted many countries in the last couple of decades, more people than ever before are participating in organized sport. This has brought a greater part of the human gene pool into play than was the case a century ago when the luxury of participating in sport was open to only a privileged few from a small number of countries. In many sports, the participation of women on a competitive basis is a recent phenomenon and female standards continue to rise rapidly as women catch up with their male counterparts.

There are many different factors that may contribute to success in sport, and the components of success will vary depending on the particular sport. Scientists, coaches, and athletes may argue about the terminology used, but some of the key characteristics that contribute to success in all sports are:

1 Talent;
2 Training;
3 Trainability;
4 Physical dimensions and body composition;

The Olympic Textbook of Science in Sport, 1st edition. Edited by R.J. Maughan. Published 2009 by Blackwell Publishing. ISBN: 978-1-4051-5638-7.

5 Motivation, tactical awareness, and other psychological characteristics;
6 Resistance to injury;
7 Nutritional status; and
8 Skill, technique, and related motor control and biomechanical considerations.

Of these, talent – which is determined entirely by genetic endowment – is undoubtedly the key, but many talented athletes fail to succeed at the highest level. Genetically gifted athletes who lack the motivtion to train consistently and intensively will not realize their genetic potential. Some of the components listed above are only conditional requirements; for example, a good selection of foods alone will not improve fitness in the absence of training. Likewise, the talented athlete who trains hard but who makes poor food choices is unlikely to be as successful as they could be.

Why should scientists study sport?

For some, especially perhaps those engaged in the study of the social sciences, the study of sport is an end in itself, an attempt to understand the mutual interactions between sport and society. For those interested in the biological sciences, the study of elite athletes offers an opportunity to study individuals at the extremes of the human gene pool who have subjected themselves to extremes of training over prolonged periods of time. By studying these extremes, new insights can be gained into normal human function.

Needless to say, many scientists study the science of athletic endeavor because of a strong personal

1

commitment to sport and exercise. It is not often appreciated that A.V. Hill, whose pioneering work on muscle physiology earned him a share (with Otto Meyerhof) of the 1922 Nobel Prize in Physiology or Medicine, was himself an accomplished athlete. His reported times of approximately 53 s for 440 yards (401 m) and 2 min 3 s for 880 yards (802 m; Hill & Lupton 1923) indicate a considerable degree of sporting talent, bearing in mind that limited training was the norm at that time. A generation later, Roger Bannister, the first man to break the 4-min mile barrier in 1954 and later a successful neurologist, spent time working in Cunningham's physiology laboratory in Oxford and, in that same year, published a paper on the respiratory and performance effects of breathing hyperoxic mixtures during exercise (Bannister & Cunningham 1954). Another holder of the World Mile Record and triple Olympic Gold medalist, Peter Snell, has also pursued a highly successful career as an exercise physiologist.

Many exercise scientists also have considerable experience of participation as experimental subjects in their own investigations. Indeed, this is perhaps the norm rather than the exception. J.B.S. Haldane was perhaps the most reckless of self-experimenters, and almost died on a number of occasions while researching underwater physiology for the British Admiralty during the Second World War. The two subjects whose muscle glycogen responses to exercise and subsequent carbohydrate feeding were reported in a classic paper published in Nature in 1966 were in fact the authors, Jonas Bergstrom and Eric Hultman (Bergstrom & Hultman 1966). Phil Gollnick, whose cardiac problems led to the fitting of a heart pacemaker, experimented on himself to establish his own cardiovascular responses to exercise of different intensities at fixed heart rates. Paavo Komi was the first volunteer for a series of studies measuring the forces generated in the human tendon using a transducer implanted around the Achilles tendon (Komi *et al.* 1987). This personal dimension can, of course, be a two-edged sword. On the one hand, the personal experience of exercise can provide insights that would not arise from mere observation alone. On the other hand, however, there is the danger that personal experience, with all

the beliefs and prejudices that accompany it, will intrude on the scientific method and will bias the observer.

It is also true, of course, that a significant number of exercise physiologists have little interest in sport. Rather, they use exercise as a tool to study normal physiology. Often, these studies provide insights that can benefit the sports community, but this is a by-product of the research rather than an end in itself. The functional characteristics of many tissues are fully revealed only when the body is engaged in exercise. Resting skeletal muscle has some unique metabolic properties, but only when the responses of muscle to differing exercise challenges are studied do these characteristics become apparent.

The normal heart at rest can cope comfortably with the demands of the organism for the supply of oxygen. This is achieved with a cardiac output of about 5 $L\cdot min^{-1}$, which in turn is met by a heart rate of about 70 beats$\cdot min^{-1}$ and a stroke volume of about 70 mL. During exercise, both heart rate and stroke volume increase to meet the increased oxygen demands, but there is an upper limit to the levels of both that can be achieved. For 'normal' adults, this is reached at a heart rate of approximately 200 beats$\cdot min^{-1}$ and a stroke volume of approximately 100–125 mL, giving a maximum cardiac output in the region of 20–25 $L\cdot min^{-1}$. The elite male endurance athlete, however, can achieve cardiac outputs in excess of 40 $L\cdot min^{-1}$, even though the maximum heart rate remains unchanged or may even be decreased, meaning that the maximum stroke volume is in excess of 200 mL (Ekblom & Hermansen 1968). Such values are never seen in sedentary individuals. Accompanying changes in the capacity of the heart to deliver blood to the periphery are local changes within the muscle; for example, a greatly increased capillary network allows the blood much closer contact with each individual muscle fiber (Andersen 1975) and the muscles themselves have a greatly increased capacity for oxidative metabolism (Holloszy 1967).

These physical and metabolic adaptations can go a long way towards explaining the incredible exercise performance of the elite athlete. In the exercise physiology laboratory, healthy and recreationally active young males can sustain a power output of perhaps 150 W for an hour; the cyclist who wants to break the 1-hour World Track Record must sustain a power output in excess of about 460 W. Likewise, the elite male marathon runner who wants to break Haile Gebreselassie's current World Record of 2 h 4 min 26 s must run at an average speed of 5.65 m·s^{-1}, or 20.3 km·h^{-1}; while the woman seeking to break Paula Radcliffe's record of 2 h 15 min 25 s must run only slightly slower than this. Even those who consider themselves to be very fit cannot run at these speeds for more than a few minutes.

In part these performances reflect the genetic endowment of the elite athlete and considerable effort is being devoted to identifying the possible genetic mutations that are associated with outstanding performance. However, many people who do have the genetic make-up either do not have the opportunity to be involved in sport because of socio-cultural limitations or because they simply choose not to participate. An understanding of the motivations of athletes and the factors that predispose participation in sport may help our understanding of why so many in the general population shun exercise at every opportunity, even though they are well aware of the health risks that accompany a sedentary life. There are good animal models to show that there is a strong genetic component to the predisposition to participation, and some inbred strains of rats show compulsive running behaviors, similar to those of some athletes (Makatsori *et al.* 2003). An understanding of the neurochemical processes involved may help to determine why some people choose to be active in their spare time while others avoid all unnecessary exercise.

Sports science support

As the rewards in sport have increased, an industry has grown up to provide support for participants. The elite athlete is only one member of a team that will include a coach, fitness specialists, advisers on tactics and technique, a medical doctor, and a physiotherapist, and perhaps also a physiologist, psychologist, nutritionist/dietitian, biomechanist, and a performance analyst, as well as several others. Each

of these professionals plays – or at least should play – a vital role in ensuring that the athlete can undertake the rigorous training that is a prerequisite of success. They will also ensure that the athlete is prepared for competition by addressing all of the problems that may prevent optimum performance. One challenge facing those who seek to apply science to sports performance is the fact that essentially all of the published research is based on non-elite athletes. Indeed, most published studies in areas such as exercise physiology and biochemistry have used subjects that were not athletes at all. This is usually because athletes are not prepared to disrupt training or preparation for competition by participating in experiments. They are also understandably reluctant to take part in invasive studies that involve repeated blood sampling, muscle biopsies, or other invasive procedures, although the introduction of non-invasive techniques for the analysis of muscle function, such as magnetic resonance spectroscopy, has made it possible to study the effects of interventions on national level athletes (e.g., Derave *et al.* 2007).

It is also important to recognize that statistical significance, as described in most experimental investigations, may have little relevance in the world of elite sport where the margin between victory and defeat can be vanishingly small. Most laboratory studies are not designed for this purpose and a more useful concept may be the "smallest worthwhile effect", as described by Hopkins (2006). An important element of this concept is to recognize the existence of individual differences in responses that make population estimates irrelevant to the individual athlete. This is perhaps the key difference between the sports scientist and the scientist who studies sport: the former is concerned with optimizing the health and performance of the individual athlete, while the latter is focused on the population as a whole. In the study by Derave *et al.* (2007) cited above, there was no beneficial effect of supplementation with β-alanine on 400-m running performance in well-trained runners, even though this supplement is used widely by athletes.

Both of these approaches are perfectly valid, and the scientist with an interest in sport will switch between these approaches. It is this combination of deep insight and practical relevance that makes the sports sciences so rewarding for all who work in this area.

Sport, exercise and health

It is easy to forget that the common perception, not so long ago, was that participation in sport was likely to shorten, rather than prolong, life (Polednak 1979). Even very recently, the focus of a UK government intervention aimed at reducing the prevalence of coronary disease was on smoking cessation and diet, with no mention of physical activity (DHSS 1987). Today, as a large part of the world confronts the consequences of the obesity epidemic, this seems hardly credible. The role of exercise as a crucial element in any lifestyle intervention targeted at non-communicable diseases has gained widespread, though still not universal, acceptance. Translating this into practice, however, remains a formidable challenge. Today, many who take regular exercise at health clubs have no desire to participate in organized sports, but their commitment to exercise is no less for that. The sports sciences today embrace the study of physical activity and health as an important area. Even those whose primary concern is with the performance of athletes recognize that they also need to stay healthy, both while they are competing and in the years after retirement from serious competition. Many exercise scientists have emerged, however, with little interest in sport but with a strong desire to understand the consequences of active or sedentary lifestyles.

Sports science is therefore different things to different people. No-one should doubt, though, that new developments in this dynamic area of science affect all our lives.

This book aims to provide an introduction to the core disciplines that comprise the sports sciences. It includes reviews by recognized experts who bring a wealth of experience to bear on the fundamental sciences and on their application to elite sport.

References

Andersen, P. (1975) Capillary density in skeletal muscle of man. *Acta Physiologica Scandinavica* **95**, 203–205.

Bannister, R.G. & Cunningham, D.J.C. (1954) The effects on the respiration and performance during exercise of adding oxygen to the inspired air. *Journal of Physiology* **125**, 118–137.

Bergstrom, J. & Hultman, E. (1966) Muscle glycogen synthesis after exercise: an enhancing factor localised to the muscle cells in man. *Nature* **210**, 309–310.

Derave, W., Ozdemir, M.S., Harris, R.C., Potter, A. Reyngoudt, H., Koppo, K., *et al.* (2007) β-Alanine supplementation augments muscle carnosine content and attenuates fatigue during repeated isokinetic contraction bouts in trained sprinters. *Journal of Applied Physiology* **103**, 1736–1743.

DHSS (1987) *On the state of the public health for the year 1986.* HMSO, London.

Ekblom, B. & Hermansen, L. (1968) Cardiac output in athletes. *Journal of Applied Physiology* **25**, 619–625.

Hill, A.V. & Lupton, H. (1923) Muscular exercise, lactic acid, and the supply and utilization of oxygen. *Queen's Journal of Medicine* **16**, 137–171.

Holloszy, J.O. (1967) Biochemical adaptations in muscle. *Journal of Biological Chemistry* **242**, 2278–2282.

Hopkins, W.G. (2006) Estimating sample size for magnitude-based inferences. *Sportscience* **10**, 63–67.

Komi, P.V., Salonen, M., Jarvinen, M. & Kokko, O. (1987) *In vivo* registration of Achilles tendon forces in man. *International Journal of Sports Medicine* **8** (suppl.), 3–8.

Makatsori, A., Duncko, R., Schwendt, M., Moncek, F., Johansson, B.B. & Jezova, D. (2003) Voluntary wheel running modulates glutamate receptor subunit gene expression and stress hormone release in Lewis rats. *Psychoneuroendocrinology* **28**, 702–714.

Polednak, A.P. (1979) *The Longevity of Athletes* CC Thomas, Springfield: vii–ix.

Part 1

Physiology and Biochemistry

Chapter 1

Muscle: Producing Force and Movement

PAAVO V. KOMI AND MASAKI ISHIKAWA

The central nervous system (CNS) naturally plays a very important role in the initiation of force and movement. It also coordinates the final action, together with the information coming from the various receptors residing in skeletal muscles, joints, ears, eyes, etc. Skeletal muscle contains all of the elements needed for force and movement production, but without nervous control it is incapable of generating any force above that of passive tension. This may be due to the structural elements of skeletal muscle, which offer resistance to stretch. Nonetheless, the muscle can be activated by impulses coming along the final common pathway, the alpha motor neuron. Upon activation it then has a special ability to generate force, resulting in either shortening (concentric action) or resistance to external loads (lengthening contraction or eccentric action). A complex integrative process involving the three components – the nervous system, skeletal muscle, and the external load – determines the final direction of movement as well as its velocity (or rate) and magnitude. It is the purpose of this chapter to characterize the factors that are important in understanding the basic interaction between the elements mentioned above. Greater emphasis will, however, be given to the important concepts of muscle mechanics as well as to the interaction between the contractile structures and tensile elements in the process of force production under varying movement conditions.

The Olympic Textbook of Science in Sport, 1st edition. Edited by R.J. Maughan. Published 2009 by Blackwell Publishing. ISBN: 978-1-4051-5638-7.

The motor unit and its functional significance

It is usually believed that human skeletal muscle fibers are innervated by only one motor neuron branch, but this branch may be one from between 10 and 1000 similar branches, all having the same axon. Therefore, one axon innervates a number of muscle fibers and this functional unit is called a motor unit. Consequently, a motor unit is defined as a combination of an alpha motor neuron and all the muscle fibers innervated by that neuron. Motor unit size (muscle fibers per alpha motor neuron) varies within a muscle, and the number of motor units varies between muscles. As illustrated in Fig. 1.1, the motor units have different structural and functional characteristics, which result in their differences with regard to rate of force development, peak force production, and maintenance of force level without loss of tension (fatigue). The fast fatigable (FF) unit develops tension quickly, but is also very easily fatigued. At the opposite end, the slow oxidative (SO) unit has a slow rate of force production but can produce the same tension (force) repeatedly for longer periods of time without signs of fatigue; it is therefore also called a fatigue-resistant motor unit. In addition to the events described in Fig. 1.1, there are also other functional differences between motor unit types. One particular feature that illustrates such differences is the response of the motor units to tetanic stimulation. The FF type unit requires a high stimulation frequency to reach a state of tetanus. In contrast, the slower unit requires a much lower fusion frequency. When subjected to repetitive tetanic

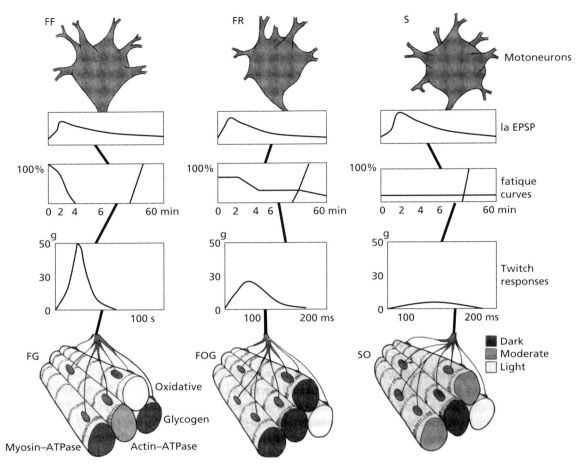

Fig. 1.1 An illustrative example of the functional interrelationship between a motor neuron and its muscle fibers within different types of motor units. Motor neurons may be phasic (fire rapidly but with sort bursts) or tonic (slow and continuous). Axon diameter size is directly related to conduction velocity. The muscle fibers have been stained to show: myosin-ATPase, acid-ATPase, succinate dehydrogenase (an oxidative enzyme), and glycogen. Note the differences in twitch tension for each motor unit. EPSP, excitatory post-synaptic potential; FF, fast-twitch and fatigable; FG, fast-twitch and glycolytic; FOG, fast-twitch oxidative and glycolytic; FR, fast-twitch and fatigue resistant; S, slow-twitch; SO, slow-twitch oxidative. (Reproduced with permission from Edington & Edgerton 1976.)

stimulation, the resulting difference in mechanical response between the two extreme types of motor units is remarkable. One important feature must be emphasized here: the type of alpha motor neuron determines the histochemical profile and biochemical performance of the individual muscle fibers in a motor unit. Consequently, all of the fibers in the same unit have a similar chemical profile. It is well known in the literature that muscles differ in their fiber composition (and thus in their motor unit pro-

files), and that there can be great variation among athletes with regard to the fiber structure in a specific muscle. For example, in the vastus lateralis (VL) muscle, sprinters may have a motor unit composition that causes most of the fibers in that muscle to be of a fast type, and thus capable of producing force at a high rate, but with low fatigue resistance. Endurance runners, on the other hand, have primarily slow type fibers in the same muscle for the purpose of high resistance to fatigue, but at the same time the rate of force production is lower than in their sprinter counterparts. It has been reported from studies with monozygotic twins that genetic factors strongly influence the variation observed among individuals in muscle fiber composition of a specific muscle (e.g., see Komi *et al*. 1977). This raises the question of whether the fiber composition of an individual athlete is an acquired phenomenon or is due to a genetically-determined code. There is naturally no direct answer to this problem and further discussion of this particular topic is beyond the scope of this chapter.

Basic muscle mechanics

Types of muscle action

In order to understand the way that skeletal muscle functions during normal locomotion, the relation between stimulus and response needs to be examined in more isolated forms of muscle actions: isometric, concentric and eccentric. The term "contraction" may be thought of as the state of a muscle when it is activated via its alpha motor neurons, which generates tension across a number of actin and myosin filaments. Depending on the external load, the direction and magnitude of action is different, as shown in Table 1.1. In a concentric action the muscle shortens (i.e., the net muscle moment is in the same direction as the change in joint angle and mechanical work is positive). In an eccentric action the muscle actively resists while it is being lengthened by some external force, such as gravity. In this case the resulting muscle moment is in the opposite direction to the change in joint angle, and the mechanical work is negative. The use of the term muscle contraction is therefore sometimes confusing, and we would prefer to follow a suggestion made by Cavanagh (1988) that "contraction" should be replaced by "action."

The muscle action most frequently used to characterize the performance of human skeletal muscle is isometric action, which by definition refers to the "activation of muscle (force production) while the length of the entire muscle-tendon unit (MTU) remains the same, and the mechanical work is zero." The use of isometric action in locomotion is not, however, meaningless; it plays a very important role in pre-activation of the muscle before other actions take place (Komi 2000).

Force production in all types of muscle actions can be seen in the internal rearrangements in length between the contractile and elastic elements. Figure 1.2 depicts these events for isometric and concentric actions. For the isometric action, the simplest muscle model, force is generated through the action of the contractile component (CC) on the series elastic component (SEC), which is stretched. The resulting S-shaped force-time (F-T) curve is shown on the right side of Fig. 1.2. Concentric action, where the load is attached to the end of the muscle, is always preceded by an isometric phase with a concomitant rearrangement in the lengths of CC and SEC. The final movement begins when the pulling force of CC on the SEC equals, or slightly exceeds, that of the load. In eccentric action some external force, for example gravity and antagonist muscles, forces the activated muscle to lengthen.

Of the two "dynamic" forms, eccentric action plays perhaps a more important role in locomotion. When the active MTU is lengthening – after the pre-activation (isometric) phase – it forms the basis of a stretch-shortening cycle (SSC), the natural form of muscle function in sports and normal daily life involving movement of the joints or the whole body. Before considering the SSC in more detail, the main mechanical attributes of muscle function need some consideration. This will help the reader

Table 1.1 Classification of muscle action or exercise types.

Type of action	Function	External mechanical work*
Concentric	Acceleration	Positive (W = F(+D))
Isometric	Fixation	Zero (no change in length)
Eccentric	Deceleration	Negative (W = F(–D))

*D, distance; F, force; W, work.

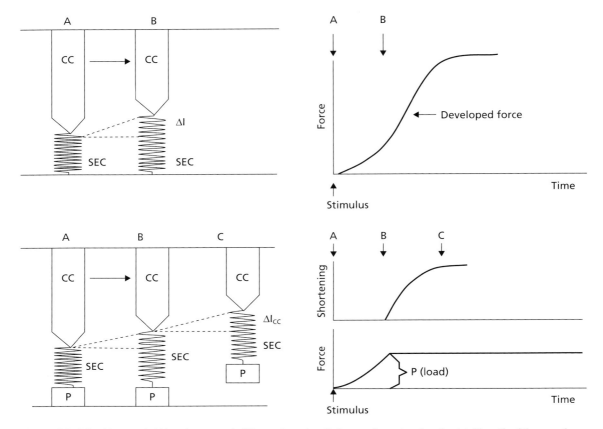

Fig. 1.2 Models of isometric (A) and concentric (B) muscle action. In isometric contraction the total length of the muscle does not change, but activation (A–B) causes the contractile component (CC) to shorten and hence stretch the series elastic component (SEC). Concentric action is then begun with a similar isometric phase as above (A→B), where CC first shortens and stretches SEC (A–B). Actual movement occurs when the pulling force of CC on SEC equals or slightly exceeds that of the load P (B–C). (Adapted with permission from Sonnenblick 1966.)

to understand why the SSC has such an important role in force and power production.

Force-time (F-T) characteristics

As is evident from Fig. 1.2, to perform movement at a joint requires time, which is calculated from the first intentional "command" either from the CNS or via reflexes from, for example, proprioceptive feedback. This time delay has several components, including both neuronal conduction delays such as synaptic transmission, events for excitation-contraction coupling, as well as mechanical charac-

teristics of the muscle fibers that receive the command signal. In this regard, isometric action is a very convenient model for describing the stimulus-response characteristics of human skeletal muscle. The first principle of muscle mechanics, the "F-T" relationship, varies as a function of stimulus strength as well as between muscles and different species. The size of a single twitch response depends on the stimulus strength: a single shock, if sufficiently strong, will produce only a small twitch; a second repetitive shock adds to the force of the first stimulus when it is given before complete recovery from the first response. If one imagines a real movement situation in which the load is fixed to the end of the muscle, that load does not begin to move before the stimulus strength to the contractile component to pull the elastic component of the muscle equals or exceeds the total load. When stimulus frequency is increased, the force gradually reaches a tetanic state that ultimately describes the maximum F-T characteristics of a muscle in isometric action. As already referred to, the isometric F-T relationships are different between muscles and species. The most fundamental feature for human locomotion is the difference between the fast-type and endurance-type muscles: muscles consisting of a majority of fast-twitch fibers (and consequently innervated more heavily by fast conducting alpha motor neurons) have a faster rate of force development compared to muscles possessing a majority of slow (endurance)-type fibers (e.g., Komi 1984).

In spite of this clear difference, the existing experimental evidence in humans does not always support the interrelationships (structure vs. function) found in isolated muscle preparations. For example, some studies (Viitasalo & Komi 1978; Viitasalo & Bosco 1982) have demonstrated a significant relationship between structure and function in the case of isometric force production, while the same authors (e.g., Viitasalo & Komi 1981) failed to do so in another study. Similar contradictions have been observed for the vertical jump test. Consequently F-T characteristics of either isometric or dynamic origin seem to be under strong environmental influence. Effects of training, for example, on the F-T curve are probably of greater importance than the muscle structure itself. Voluntary explosive force production requires a well-controlled, synchronized activation process. Thus, the experimental situation is very different from that of isolated preparations, which utilize constant electrical stimulation either on the muscle or its nerve. In normal human locomotion, the movement is seldom, if at all, initiated from zero activation. Pre-activation is a natural way to prepare the muscle for fast force (and movement) production; to set zero electromyographic (EMG) activity as a required condition may not be successful in all individuals. The important role of pre-activation will be discussed later.

The ability to modify the F-T curve for a specific muscle or muscle group has important implications for athlete training. In sporting activities the time to develop force is crucial, because the total action times for a specific muscle may vary between less than 100 ms to a few hundred ms. Thus, if the F-T curve is measured, for example for the leg extensor muscles, the peak force is sometimes reached after 1000 ms, implying that a specific movement in a real life situation would already be over before these force values were reached. Consequently, training studies have recently concentrated on examining the F-T curve in its early rising phase. Several methods have been used in the literature to assess the rate of force development. As recently examined by Mirkov et al. (2004), most of these methods may be considered as fairly reliable but their "external validity," in terms of evaluating the ability to perform rapid movements, remains questionable. The F-T curve also reveals that if the movement begins at point zero EMG activity (the force is also zero) then the practical consequences would be catastrophic. This is naturally corrected by pre-activating the muscles appropriately before the intended movement begins. Pre-activation is pre-programmed (Melvill-Jones & Watt 1977) and is introduced to take up all of the slack within the muscle before the initiation of fast movements. This pre-activation corresponds usually, but not always, to the isometric phase before the other forms of action take place. Its EMG magnitude is a function of an expected load to move or an impact load to receive, such as in running (Komi et al. 1987). This pre-activity corresponds to the initial stimulation, which is a necessary component in the measurement of concentric and isometric actions. This requirement is in agreement with the measurement techniques applied in isolated preparations (Hill 1938; Edman et al. 1978).

Force-length (F-L) relationship

It is not a surprise that resting muscle is elastic and able to resist the force that stretches it. During this stretching, however, the muscle becomes more and more inextensible; i.e., the force curve becomes steeper with larger stretches (Fig. 1.3). This curve represents a passive force-length (F-L) relationship

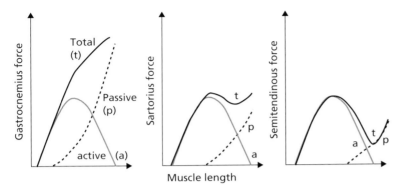

Fig. 1.3 Active (a), passive (p), and total (t) force-length relationships for tree frog muscles. Note that the passive force comes into play at distinctly different regions of the active force-length relationship.

that is determined largely by the connective tissue structures such as endomysium, perimysium, epimysium, and tendon. The active curve in Fig. 1.3 constitutes the contractile component, whose form represents the contribution of the contractile material (fascicle or muscle fibers) to the total force curve, which is the sum of the active and passive forces at given muscle lengths. It must be emphasized that the active curve is not a continuous one. Rather, it represents discrete data points observed when the muscle is held at different lengths and then stimulated maximally (or supramaximally) in each length position. The total F-L relationship differs between the muscles, and for this reason no definite F-L relationship can be described that would be applicable to all skeletal muscles. The active component of these curves (Fig. 1.3) has received significantly more attention as it resembles the F-L curve of individual sarcomeres. As will be discussed later, the working range of the sarcomere F-L curve seems to be different depending on the activity. The form of the active F-L curve depends upon the number of cross-bridges that are formed at different sarcomere lengths. The sarcomere number is not fixed, even in adult muscles, being capable of either increasing or decreasing (for details see Goldspink & Harridge 2003). For the entire MTU, however, exhaustive fatigue has been shown to shift the total F-L and torque-angle curve to the right (Komi & Rusko 1974; Whitehead *et al.* 2001), and in severe eccentric exercise this shift has been considered to reliably indicate the degree of muscle damage (Jones *et al.* 1997). In addition to differences between muscles, the type of muscular exercise seems to determine

the portion of the F-L curve (descending limb, plateau phase, or ascending limb) in which a particular muscle operates during locomotion (see "Task (movement) specificity").

It should be mentioned that until recently it was very difficult to obtain anything other than a measure of the torque-angle relationship in humans, leading to an estimate of the F-L changes. At present, accurate tensile force calculations can be performed *in vivo* by applying devices such as buckle transducers (Komi 1990) or the optic fiber method (Komi *et al.* 1996) directly to human tendons. With the development of real-time ultrasonography it is now possible to examine, both non-invasively and *in vivo*, the respective length changes of the fascicles and tendinous tissues (TT: aponeuroses and the free length of the in-series tendon) during exercise. In general, the obtained results highlight the complexity of interaction between fascicle and TT components (see "Task (movement) specificity").

Force-velocity (F-V) relationship

Hill's classic paper (1938) describes the force-velocity (F-V) relationship of an isolated muscle preparation. This curve can be obtained with constant electrical stimulation against different mechanical loads. The muscle is maximally (or supramaximally) stimulated and when the isometric F-T curve reaches its maximum, the muscle is suddenly released and, depending on the magnitude of the extra load, the resulting shortening speed can be determined. In this relationship the maximum force decreases in the concentric mode in a curvilinear fashion, and

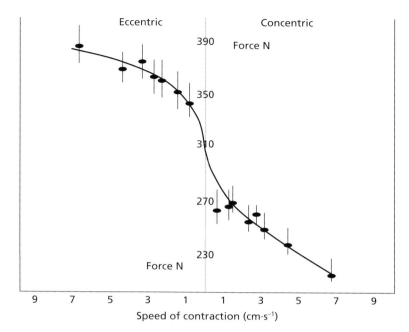

Fig. 1.4 A force-velocity relationship in eccentric and concentric muscle action for elbow flexor muscle. The measurements were preformed with an electromechanical dynamometer, which was designed to apply a constant velocity of shortening or lengthening for the biceps brachii muscle. (Reproduced with permission from Komi 1973 courtesy of S. Karger AG, Basel.)

as a function of the shortening speed. It must be emphasized that the obtained curve is not a continuous one, but a discrete relationship between distinct data points. This classic curve demonstrates the fundamental properties of the skeletal muscle, and its form has also been confirmed in human experiments with maximal efforts against different loads (Wilkie 1949) or with maximal efforts at different constant angular velocities (Komi 1973). When the F-V measurements are extended to the eccentric side by allowing the muscle to actively resist the imposed stretch that begins after the maximum (isometric) force level has been reached, maximum force increases as a function of stretching velocity, as shown in Fig. 1.4. An important prerequisite in the measurements of eccentric and concentric F-V curves is the strict control of the maximum pre-activation before the movement begins. When human experiments have followed the methods of isolated models (Hill 1938; Edman 1978), the voluntary concentric and eccentric F-V relationships were similar to those obtained using isolated preparations (Wilkie 1949; Komi 1973; Linnamo et al. 2006). This includes the finding of similar maximal EMG activities across all contraction modes (eccen-

tric, isometric, and concentric) and velocities (e.g., Komi 1973). The observation that voluntary eccentric force can sometimes be less than isometric force (Westing et al. 1991) may well be explained by the fundamental differences between experiments, especially when the pre-activation was not maximal before recording the concentric and eccentric forces at different velocities of shortening and stretch, respectively. This possible reduction in eccentric force as compared to isometric force has also been suggested to be due to the inhibition of EMG activity. Again the differences in protocols between these experiments and those of the classical model could be considered as a possible source of reduced EMG and respective force level in eccentric action. Consequently, it is quite clear that force and power characteristics of skeletal muscle are greatest in the eccentric mode. Figure 1.5 makes an additional note of the measurement of maximum eccentric force, and demonstrates force enhancement above the isometric level during the lengthening phase.

Although the Hill curve was not introduced to describe the instantaneous F-V relationship (see "Instantaneous F-V relationship during SSC"), it has been used successfully to follow specific training

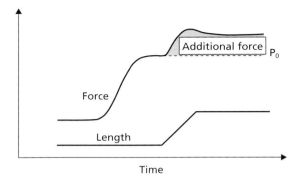

Fig. 1.5 A schematic presentation to show that if human skeletal muscle is stretched (eccentric action) after maximal isometric force (P_0) has been attained, then the force increases considerably. A similar phenomenon is seen in isolated sarcomeres.

adaptations of human skeletal muscle. These adaptations deal with the concept of power training, especially for sporting activities requiring high levels of force and speed. From the Hill curve, it can be calculated that muscle mechanical power (the product of force and velocity) usually reaches its peak when the speed and forces that are involved represent about one-third to one-half of the discrete points in the F-V relationship. The peak power is very sensitive to differences in muscle fiber composition. Faulkner (1986), among others, demonstrated that the peak power output of fast-twitch fibers in human skeletal muscle was four-times that of slow-twitch fibers due to a greater velocity of shortening for a given afterload. In mixed muscle the fast-twitch fibers may contribute 2.5-times more to the total power production than the slow-twitch fibers. In human experiments it is difficult to utilize shortening (and also eccentric) velocities that can load the muscles with a suitable protocol (as described above) across the entire range of physiological speeds. The maximum speed of most commercially available instruments can cover only 20–30% of the different physiological maxima. As Goldspink (1978) has demonstrated, the peak efficiencies of isolated fast- and slow-twitch fibers occur at completely different contraction speeds. Therefore, it is possible that in measurements of the F-V curve in humans, when

the maximum angular velocity reaches a value of 3–4 rad·s^{-1}, only the efficient contraction speeds of slow-twitch fibers will be reached. The peak power of fast-twitch fibers may occur at angular velocities more than three-times greater than our present measurement systems allow. Notwithstanding, Tihanyi *et al.* (1982) were able to show clear differences in F-V and power-velocity (P-V) curves for leg extension movements between subject groups that differed in the fiber composition of their VL muscle.

If the F-V (and P-V) curve demonstrates the primary differences between concentric and eccentric actions, there are some additional features that stress the importance of the performance potential between these isolated forms of exercise. As already mentioned, the maximum EMG activity between concentric and eccentric actions should be approximately the same. However, it is well documented that the slopes representing EMG and force relationships are different in these two forms of exercise (Bigland & Lippold 1954; Komi 1973; Fig. 1.6). To attain a certain force level requires much less motor unit activation in eccentric than in concentric action. Logically then, oxygen consumption is much lower during eccentric exercise than in comparable concentric exercise (Asmussen 1953; Knuttgen 1986). Furthermore, in relation to movement in general these earlier findings, including the important reference to Margaria (1938), emphasize that mechanical efficiency can be very high during eccentric exercise as compared to concentric exercise (Fig. 1.6c).

One additional and particularly relevant question is "what happens to the fascicle length (magnitude and change of length) during different muscle actions?" In our recent studies we were able to demonstrate that during pure concentric actions the fascicles show normal shortening (Finni *et al.* 1998), the magnitude of which may be intensity dependent (Reeves *et al.* 2003). In pure eccentric actions, fascicle lengthening (resistance to stretch while muscle fibers are active) should be expected and has indeed been well demonstrated by Finni *et al.* (2003) for the VL muscle. In this study, the fascicle lengths remained constant during eccentric action at all measured isokinetic speeds, but they were also shorter than those measured at higher concentric velocities.

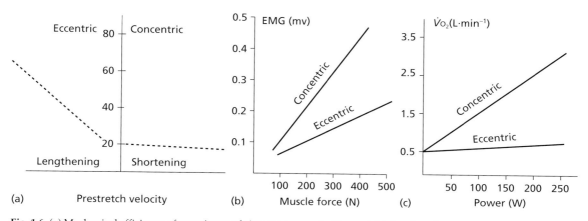

Fig. 1.6 (a) Mechanical efficiency of negative work (eccentric exercise) is much higher than that on positive work (concentric exercise). The drawing in (a) is based on the EMG-force relationship (b) and the $\dot{V}o_2$-power relationship (c). Important references: (a) Aura and Komi 1987; (b): Asmussen 1953, Komi 1973; (c): Asmussen 1953.

Although the latter finding does not directly imply the magnitude or even direction of shortening/lengthening, it may indicate an important point; i.e., the fascicle length change may be dependent on the muscle and also on the specific movement. This notion becomes even more important when the fascicle-tendon interaction is studied under conditions of different intensity SSC exercise.

Stretch-shortening cycle (SSC) of muscle function

When the different isolated muscle actions were explained in the previous paragraphs, indications were given that they are often used successfully in describing the force transmission and related metabolic events in well-controlled experimental situations. In natural situations and environments, human (and animal in general) skeletal muscle produces force and movement by utilizing a combination of eccentric and concentric actions, and the isometric action plays more of a role in pre-activation; i.e., to prepare the muscle to take up the expected load. The function of the triceps surae muscle during the ground contact phase in running, hopping, and even walking can be used as a typical example to describe normal muscle action – the SSC. Before ground contact the muscle is pre-activated, the level

of which is a function of the expected impact load (or running velocity, for example; Komi *et al.* 1987). The pre-activated triceps surae muscle begins its eccentric action upon the initial ground contact, when the MTU lengthens and receives activation signals from the nervous system. This eccentric or braking phase is then followed, without much delay, by the shortening (concentric) action which, depending on the intensity of effort, can take place in many cases as a recoil phenomenon with relatively low EMG activity. Consequently, SSC has important functions in locomotion: (i) to minimize unnecessary delays in the F-T relationship by matching the pre-activated force level to the level required to meet the expected eccentric loading; and (ii) to make the final concentric action (push-off phase in running, for example) more powerful (in maximal effort) or to generate force more economically (submaximal conditions), as compared to the corresponding isolated concentric actions. Cavagna *et al.* (1965, 1968) were among the first to describe the mechanisms underlying this performance potentiation in SSC by using elegant control situations of force and stimulus in a device designed for the group's first experiments with isolated frog sartorius muscle (Cavagna *et al.* 1965), and later also with human forearm flexors (Cavagna *et al.* 1968). Based on these findings and some others (e.g., Aura & Komi 1986),

SSC power production is very likely to be dependent not only on the stretch velocity, but also on the time delay (coupling time) between the stretch (eccentric) and shortening (concentric) phases; performance enhancement of the force (and power) output takes place in the final concentric phase of SSC. Economy has subsequently been shown to improve in SSC movements with a shorter coupling time between the braking and push-off phase in more natural types of hopping movements (Aura & Komi 1986). The mechanisms of this performance potentiation involve the important parts of the entire MTU; i.e., the fascicles and TT.

Instantaneous F-V relationship during SSC

The F-V relationship of the isolated muscle actions (Hill 1938) describes the fundamental mechanical properties of human ske letal muscle. However, its direct application to natural locomotion, such as SSC, is difficult to ascertain as the *in situ* preparations utilize constant electrical stimulation. The techniques available for measuring the instantaneous F-V relationship in human muscle include the buckle transducer and fine optic fiber (for details, see Komi 2000). When these techniques have been applied in human Achilles tendon (AT) and patella tendon during SSC movements, the F-V curve during the functional contact phase of running was completely different from the classic F-V relationship (Komi *et al.* 1992; Fig. 1.7a). Characteristic of the natural instantaneous F-V curve is the considerable force potentiation in the final push-off (concentric) phase of ground contact. Figure 1.7b demonstrates two important aspects of human skeletal muscle function: first, in short-contact hopping the triceps surae muscle behaves in a bouncing ball type of fashion; second, when the hopping intensity is increased or changed from a hopping type of movement, the contribution of the patella tendon force increases and that of the AT may decrease (Finni *et al.* 2001). The classic type of curve obtained for concentric action with constant maximal activation is superimposed on Fig. 1.7b. The shaded area denotes remarkable performance potentiation, although the hopping effort was submaximal (Finni *et al.* 2001). Animal experiments performed by Gregor *et al.* (1988) have produced similar results. Such a difference between the instantaneous curve and the classic curve is partly due to a natural difference in muscle activation levels between the two conditions.

Natural locomotion utilizes primarily SSC actions and involves controlled release of high forces caused mainly by the eccentric action of the cycle. This high force favors the storage of elastic strain energy in MTU. A portion of this energy can be recovered during the subsequent shortening phase and used for performance potentiation. Thus, natural locomotion

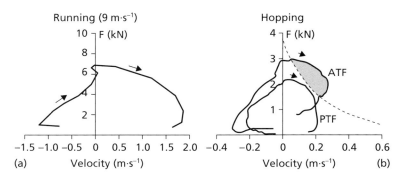

Fig. 1.7 Examples of instantaneous force-velocity curves measured in human running (a) and hopping (b). The records in (a) were obtained with a buckle transducer (reproduced with permission from Komi 1990) and those in (b) with an optic fiber (reproduced with permission from Finni 2001). Each record is for a functional (contact) phase on the ground. A record (b) demonstrates greater loading of the Achilles tendon (ATF) as compared to the patellar tendon (PTF). The left side of both figures represents eccentric action and the right side concentric action. The dashed line (b) signifies the force-velocity curve for plantar flexors, as measured in the classical way.

with SSC actions may produce efficient muscle outputs, which can be very different from the conditions of isolated preparations (where activation levels are kept constant and the storage of strain energy is limited). Another important point needs to be emphasized here: in SSC activity performed without fatigue, the muscle EMG activity usually peaks before the eccentric phase ends, thus confirming the important role that the eccentric part plays in the SSC action.

SSC muscle function has one additional, but very important characteristic. Due to the high stretch loads, it can efficiently utilize stretch reflex contributions to enhance force production. This has been clearly demonstrated in many studies (for a review see Komi & Gollhofer 1997), although its exact magnitude is almost impossible to quantify from global EMG measurements. Its role is also to make the impact in running, for example, take place smoothly. In marathon running, there is a parallelism between the changes in the amplitude of the short-latency stretch reflex component (SLC) and the impact force peak. When the fatigue progresses, the impact peak and subsequent immediate force reduction increase while the SLC decreases (Avela & Komi 1998), indicating a loss of reflex contribution to the force production of the respective muscles. The occurrence of the stretch reflex during running and hopping is easier to record in the soleus (SOL) than gastrocnemius (GA) muscle, although recent high speed ultrasound measurements have demonstrated a clear short duration stretching of the GA fascicles during the very early phase of ground contact (Ishikawa *et al.* 2006). In addition to the obvious role of gamma activation, stretching of the fascicles (extrafusal fibers) must be considered as a prerequisite for initiation of muscle spindle activation.

Force potentiation

As has become evident from the previous discussions, SSC is intended to enhance the force or power output of the muscle over the pure concentric action. This additional force output can be called pre-stretch-induced force enhancement, which results in greater performance of the final push-off (concentric action) phase. This performance potentiation

naturally has several mechanisms, which are sometimes very complicated and remain contentious among researchers (e.g., see van Ingen Schenau *et al.* 1997). In the following discussion we make no attempt to illustrate all of the possibilities for force potentiation in SSC, but merely concentrate on the most obvious ones.

In addition to the reflex-induced force potentiation discussed above, the mechanical aspects associated with optimal coupling between stretch and shortening play an important role in increasing force, velocity, and power production during the final concentric phase. This is in contrast to the situation in which a pure concentric action is produced without pre-stretch of a pre-activated muscle; where the muscle performs normal shortening (concentric action), the potential to increase power or movement velocity in a step-like sequence of cross-bridge attachment, detachment, and reattachment is very limited. To overcome this limitation some sort of spring must be employed in order to store elastic energy and to utilize this energy to transform muscle action into movement more efficiency. The role of the whole MTU can be considered in this particular phenomenon. During human movements the energy stored during lengthening can amplify force production in the subsequent shortening phase and/or reduce the metabolic consumptions due to the decreased work of muscle fibers (Cavagna *et al.* 1968; Asmussen & Bonde-Petersen 1974; Komi & Bosco 1978). This ability of muscle to store and utilize elastic energy could be dependent on such factors as stretch velocity, muscle length, the force attained at the end of the pre-stretch, as well as the coupling time during the SSC action (Cavagna *et al.* 1965; Bosco *et al.* 1982). The elastic properties of MTU seem to be located mainly in TT, although muscle fibers also possess elastic properties in the cross-bridges (Huxley & Simmons 1971) and in the giant cytoskeletal protein called titin (Maruyama *et al.* 1977). Stretched tendons can recoil elastically much faster than any muscle can shorten. Alexander and Bennet-Clark (1977) proposed that tendon elasticity may be much more important than muscle elasticity and estimated the elastic strain energy stored in tendons to be 5–10-times higher than that stored in the muscle. This return of elastic energy in tendons has

Normal action   Concerted action

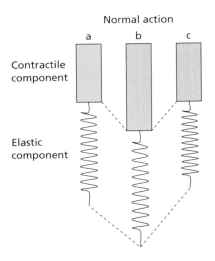
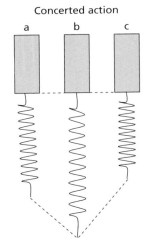

Contractile component

Elastic component

Fig. 1.8 A schematic diagram of a two-component Hill muscle model during a stretch (a → b)-shortening (b → c) cycle. During concerted action (right) the contractile component remains the same length when muscles are stretched and the elastic component can stretch more than during normal action (left). (Adapted with permission from Hof *et al.* 1983.)

been reported as approximately 93% of the work previously done during stretching it and as 7% of heat dissipation (Bennet *et al.* 1986). The work done during the recoil phase is almost independent of shortening velocity over a wide range of speeds.

The idea of concerted action plays an important role in the utilization of tendon elasticity (Hof *et al.* 1983). In this concept, muscle activation is matched to maintain a constant length of the contractile components or even cause shortening of the muscle when the MTU is forced to lengthen during the braking phase of the SSC (Fig. 1.8). The negative work done on the muscle fibers, where the length is close to the optimum of the F-L relationship, can be converted into tendon elastic energy. Several studies have confirmed this behavior in GA muscle during human SSC movements (Fukunaga *et al.* 2001; Kawakami *et al.* 2002; Ishikawa *et al.* 2005a). Another concept is "catapult action," in which the spring stretches slowly and recoils rapidly. In this action, power output can be amplified by the rapid positive work against the negative work done during the slow stretch, as demonstrated by an insect jumping (Bennet-Clark & Lucey 1967; Bennet-Clark 1975; Alexander & Bennet-Clark 1977). Ishikawa *et al.* (2005b) also reported this behavior during human walking. One may therefore ask which mechanism would be responsible for causing utilization of elastic energy during activities that involve different stretch and recoil patterns of the TT, such as

the ground contact phases of walking and running, which differ in terms of contact duration.

Behavior of fascicle-tendon interactions during SSC movements

The role of muscle fibers and MTU in producing force and movement in experimental conditions seems clear. However, the manner in which fascicle-tendon interaction occurs during human SSC movements is not well recognized. The traditional geometric approximation treats the muscle fibers and tendons as an array of parallelograms. Non-invasive ultrasonographic techniques measure fascicle and tendon length changes directly during movements (Fukunaga *et al.* 2002; Fig. 1.9). This dynamic condition can reveal how the interaction between muscle fibers and tendons can be modified to utilize the tendon elasticity, for example. This modification is dependent on variable EMG activity including pre-activation and stretch reflex EMG. The final objective would be to capture the fascicle-tendon interaction in such a way that the roles of both tendon elasticity and the reflex contribution can be clarified to explain the power output and mechanical efficiency in SSC types of locomotion. This cannot be achieved with any available approximation methods, but the direct measurement approach utilizing moderate-speed ultrasound has revealed that the behavior of the overall MTU is not the same

Fig. 1.9 A schematic model of the gastrocnemius muscle fascicle and tendon length measurements. This model requires that the total muscle-tendon unit (MTU) length is recorded continuously (e.g., kinematically) during locomotion. The rest of the measurements are calculated using continuous ultrasound records. (Important methodological references: Fukunaga *et al.* 2001; Zajac 1989.)

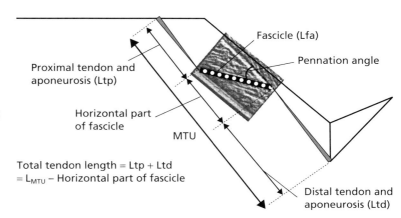

Proximal tendon and aponeurosis (Ltp)

Horizontal part of fascicle

Fascicle (Lfa)

Pennation angle

MTU

Total tendon length = Ltp + Ltd
= L_{MTU} – Horizontal part of fascicle

Distal tendon and aponeurosis (Ltd)

as that of the muscle fibers (Fukunaga *et al.* 2002). In fact, recent studies have indicated that the entire fascicle-tendon interaction is very complex and subject to adaptation including muscle, intensity, and task (movement) specificities.

Muscle specificity

There are arguments in the literature suggesting that the fascicles can maintain a constant length (Fukunaga *et al.* 2001; Kawakami *et al.* 2002), shorten (Ishikawa *et al.* 2005a, 2006), or lengthen (Ishikawa & Komi 2004; Ishikawa *et al.* 2003, 2005a) during the braking phase of the ground contact of SSC exercises. These observations have come from conditions utilizing a single muscle method only. As the mechanical behavior of muscles may vary, these patterns may not apply when the muscles have different basic functions. For example, in contrast to the SOL muscle, the GA muscle is clearly bi-articular and has unique functions in conserving energy and power flow from one joint to another during locomotion. In addition, the force sharing (Herzog *et al.* 1994) and motor unit recruitment (Moritani *et al.* 1990) between synergistic muscles (GA and SOL) may occur differently. The GA muscle activity can also play an important role in generating forward propulsion in walking, whereas the SOL functions in stabilization and load bearing during the early stance phase (Gottschall & Kram 2003). Consequently, it is not surprising that fascicle-tendon interaction does not occur in a same manner in these two muscles in this particular movement condition. As already mentioned, the GA

fascicles can remain the same length, shorten, or be lengthened during the braking phase of SSC movements. In contrast, during the same movement, the VL and SOL fascicles are continuously lengthened prior to shortening (Ishikawa *et al.* 2005a; Sousa *et al.* 2007). The differences in fascicle behavior between GA and SOL support the idea that a bi-articular muscle can be involved in the fine regulation of the distribution of net torques over two joints, whereas mono-articular muscles may act mainly as force generators or load bearers (van Ingen Schenau *et al.* 1987).

Intensity specificity

As referred to earlier, the GA fascicles also behave differently from the SOL fascicles during drop jumps (DJ). In this activity, the GA shortening continues during the braking phase until the optimal stretch load condition has been achieved. When the dropping height exceeds the optimal stretch load, the GA fascicles shorten only initially but are suddenly stretched during the rest of the braking phase. In this extreme drop intensity condition, the estimated AT force (ATF) values were 10–12-times body weight. Consequently, the stretch load upon impact was so high that GA fascicles could only maintain a constant length during the initial braking phase. Thereafter they were forced to lengthen suddenly at 30–50 ms after contact. Thus, it appears that fascicle behavior in the GA muscle is, as an overall concept, dependent on the stretch load intensity. If we draw the length changes of the GA fascicle

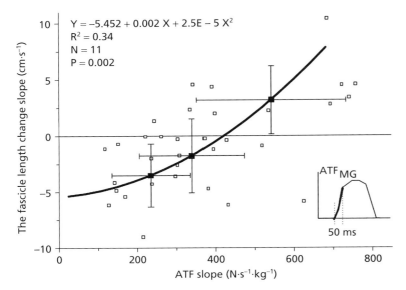

Fig. 1.10 Correlation between the slope of medial gastrocnemius (MG) fascicle length changes from 30 ms after contact to the end of the braking phase, and the averaged slope of Achilles tendon force (ATF) according to body weight. (Used with permission from Ishikawa *et al.* 2005a.)

against the ATF slope measured during the braking phase of DJ, we obtain the relationship shown in Fig. 1.10. This quadratic relationship may be indicative of the critical stretch load for the GA (*y* axis = 0; Fig. 1.10) to maintain the concerted action effectively in the fascicle-TT interaction before being suddenly overstretched. On the other hand, in the SOL and VL muscles rapid stretching of the fascicles was not observed. Consequently, these muscles were still able to function "normally" without any additional rapid fascicle length changes (Ishikawa *et al.* 2005a; Sousa *et al.* 2007). These results clearly indicate the existence of intensity-specific interactions between fascicles and TT in a given muscle.

Task (movement) specificity

One question that may arise is whether the differences in movement types influence fascicle-tendon interactions. This problem has recently been investigated by comparing high intensity SSC exercises with different contact times. The rationale behind this comparison was that the contact time in the rapid SSC movements (cf. sprint running < 100 ms) may not be enough for the efficient storage and recoil of elastic energy. This is because the resonant oscillating frequency of the elastic component in the

ankle extensors (3.33 ± 0.15 Hz; Bach *et al.* 1983) has a range of 2.6–4.3 Hz. This corresponds to a ground contact time between 233 and 385 ms (300 ms is 3.33 Hz). These values are well above those observed for running and hopping, for example. However, despite the strict theoretical oscillating frequencies for elastic components, TT can show lengthening before shortening during the contact phase of running (Ishikawa *et al.* 2006; Fig. 1.11). The same is true in the short contact DJ (Ishikawa *et al.* 2005a). One possible explanation for the elastic behavior during rapid movements is that the shortening of GA fascicles due to high muscle activation during pre-activation and braking phases of rapid SSC movements can increase TT strain rates. Viscoelastic material is stronger and becomes stiffer at increasing strain rates (Arnold 1974; Welsh *et al.* 1971). Consequently, during short-contact SSC movements, increased TT strain rates make the TT stiffer due to fascicle length regulation. This would not apply to walking where muscle activation during the pre-activation and braking phases is low and fascicles are lengthened during the long (> 500 ms) contact phase (Fig. 1.11). Consequently, it is very likely that differences in movements, especially in the contact times during running, hopping, and walking, are involved in fascicle and TT interactions, and in determining how TT viscoelasticity can be utilized.

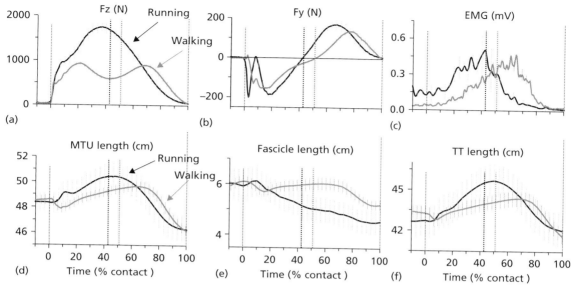

Fig. 1.11 Records of the measured and calculated parameters during the contact phase of running and walking showing: vertical (a; Fz) and horizontal (b; Fy) ground reaction forces; electromyographic (EMG) activities of the medial gastrocnemius (c; MG); and lengths of the muscle-tendon unit (d; MTU), fascicle (e) and tendinous tissues (f; TT). The contact period was normalized to 100%. Bars show SE values. The vertical lines denote the contact point, transition point from braking to push-off phases, and the take-off. (Used with permission from Ishikawa *et al.* 2006.)

In human movements the fascicles play an important role, not only to produce force by themselves but to regulate force and power production for TT. At the sarcomere level, fascicle contraction occurs around the plateau region of the F-L curve (Hof *et al.* 1983; Fukunaga *et al.* 2002). It is very likely that utilization of the specific points in the sarcomere F-L curve may vary depending on the type of movement. For example, the working range of active muscle fibers in the F-L relationship can shift more to a plateau (optimal) phase at normal walking speed (1.5 ± 0.1 m·s^{-1}) as compared to slow walking (0.8 m·s^{-1}, Fig. 1.12; Fukunaga *et al.* 2002). This would effectively favor the relatively larger force generation. This is not the case for rapid SSC movements; when the movement changes from walking to running the working range of muscle fibers can shift more towards an ascending limb (shorter length). This shift in running is suggested to make efficient use of greater TT stretching (Ishikawa *et al.* 2006). These assumptions further suggest that modulation of GA fascicle-TT interactions takes place in response to changes in mechanical demands

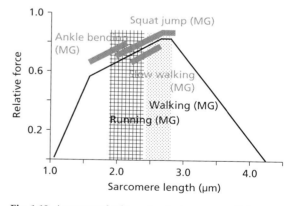

Fig. 1.12 A proposed scheme for the human medial gastrocnemius (MG) muscle to utilize the various parts of the sarcomere force-length relationship during human movements. The shaded and meshed ranges for sarcomere length are shown during the contact phase of walking and running with same subject group, respectively. Please note that working length of sarcomeres shifts to the ascending limb when the activity changes from walking to running. (For further details see Fukunaga *et al.* 2002; Ishikawa *et al.* 2006.) (Used with permission from Ishikawa *et al.* 2006.)

associated with locomotor tasks in order to utilize the elasticity of TT effectively.

Conclusion

In conclusion, nervous control is essential for force and power production in human movement. This activation is nicely integrated with the mechanical structure and function of the human skeletal muscle. The mechanical characteristics, such as F-T, F-L, and F-V relationships, are different depending on the motor unit make-up of the neuromuscular system. A skeletal muscle containing primarily fast motor units can produce greater force and power than the slower-type muscle whose motor unit composition has a greater proportion of slow motor units (and corresponding slow-type muscle fibers), which are meant to maintain force and power for a longer period of time.

In natural locomotion, some of these mechanical features cannot be applied directly. For example, the F-V relationships of MTU measured in isolated conditions are not applicable to natural locomotion where the F-V relationships is characterized by the so-called instantaneous F-V curve whose form is completely different to the classical one. This difference is due to the ability of the human neuromuscular system to activate muscle in proper correspondence with external load and intended velocity of movement. A specific feature of this interaction is a well-controlled variability of the nervous input to the muscle as well as purposeful proprioceptive feedback. This makes force and movement production not only more difficult to understand but also more challenging to explore. In this regard, especially relevant is a recent new finding that the external load is not the only factor that determines the fascicle-TT interaction during human movement. When the measurements are performed during natural movements, called SSC action, movement specificity is complemented with differences in the fascicle-TT interactions that are also muscle, movement and intensity specific.

Consequently, it is not possible to understand the complexity of the mechanisms that contribute to the production of force and movement by human skeletal muscles by extrapolation from well-controlled studies of individual muscle actions or measurements made using isolated muscle preparations. This complexity also applies to the mechanisms of force and power potentiation that characterize natural SSC movements.

References

Alexander, R.M. & Bennet-Clark, H. (1977) Storage of elastic strain energy in muscle and other tissues. *Nature* **265**, 114–117.

Arnold, G. (1974) Biomechanische und rheologische Eigenschaften menschlicher Sehnen. *Zeitschrift der Anatomischen Entwicklungsgeschichte* **143**, 262–300.

Asmussen, E. (1953) Positive and negative muscular work. *Acta Physiologica Scandinavica* **28**, 364–382.

Asmussen, E. & Bonde-Petersen, F. (1974) Apparent efficiency and storage of elastic energy in human muscles during exercise. *Acta Physiologica Scandinavica* **92**, 537–545.

Aura, O. & Komi, P.V. (1986) Effects of prestretch intensity on mechanical efficiency of positive work and on elastic behavior of skeletal muscle in stretch-shortening cycle exercise. *International Journal of Sports Medicine* **7**, 137–143.

Aura, O. & Komi, P.V. (1987) The mechanical efficiency of human locomotion in different work intensity level. In: *International Series on Biomechanics, Biomechnics XI-A* (Groot, G., Hollander, A.P., Huijing, P.A. & Van Ingen Schenau, G., eds.) Amsterdam, Free Uni. Press: 48–51.

Avela, J. & Komi, P.V. (1998) Interaction between muscle stiffness and stretch reflex sensitivity after long-term stretch-shortening cycle exercise. *Muscle and Nerve* **21**, 1224–1227.

Bach, T.M., Chapman, A.E. & Calvert, T.W. (1983) Mechanical resonance of the human body during voluntary oscillations about the ankle joint. *Journal of Biomechanics* **16**, 85–90.

Bennet-Clark, H.C. (1975) The energetics of the jump of the locust *Schistocerca gregaria*. *Journal of Experimental Biology* **63**, 53–83.

Bennet-Clark, H.C. & Lucey, E.C. (1967) The jump of the flea: a study of the energetics and a model of the mechanism. *Journal of Experimental Biology* **47**, 59–76.

Bennett, M.B., Ker, R.F., Dimery, N.J. & Alexander, R.M. (1986) Mechanical properties of various mammalian tendons. *Journal of Zoology. Series A* **209**, 537–548.

Bigland, B. & Lippold, O.C. (1954) The relation between force, velocity and integrated electrical activity in human muscles. *Journal of Physiology* **123**, 214–224.

Bosco, C., Viitasalo, J.T., Komi, P.V. & Luhtanen, P. (1982) Combined effect of elastic energy and myoelectrical potentiation during stretch-shortening cycle exercise. *Acta Physiologica Scandinavica* **114**, 557–565.

Cavagna, G.A., Saibene, F.P. & Margaria, R. (1965) Effect of negative work on the amount of positive work performed by an isolated muscle. *Journal of Applied Physiology* **20**, 157–158.

Cavagna, G.A., Dusman, B. & Margaria, R. (1968) Positive work done by a previously stretched muscle. *Journal of Applied Physiology* **24**, 21–32.

Cavanagh, P.R. (1988) On 'muscle action' vs. 'muscle contraction'. *Journal of Biomechanics* **22**, 69.

Edington, D.W. & Edgerton, V.R. (1976) *The Biology of Physical Activity*. Houghton Mifflin Co., Boston.

Edman, K.P.A., Elzinga, G. & Noble, M.I.M. (1978) Enhancement of mechanical performance by stretch during tetanic contractions of vertebrate skeletal muscle fibres. *Journal of Physiology* **281**, 139–155.

Faulkner, J.A. (1986) Power output of the human diaphragm. *American Review of Respiratory Disease* **134**, 1081–1083.

Finni, T. (2001) Muscle mechanics during human movement revealed by *in vivo* measurements of tendon force and muscle length. PhD Thesis. University of Jyväskylä, Finland.

Finni, T., Komi, P.V. & Lepola, V. (1998) *In vivo* muscle dynamics during jumping. In: *Third Annual Congress of the European College of Sport Science*, 15–18 July 1998. Manchester, UK.

Finni, T., Komi, P.V. & Lepola, V. (2001) *In vivo* muscle mechanics during normal locomotion is dependent on movement amplitude and contraction intensity. *European Journal of Applied Physiology* **85**, 170–176.

Finni, T., Ikegawa, S., Lepola, V. & Komi, P.V. (2003) Comparison of force-velocity relationships of vastus lateralis muscle in isokinetic and in stretch-shortening cycle exercises. *Acta Physiologica Scandinavica* **177**, 483–491.

Fukunaga, T., Kubo, K., Kawakami, Y., Fukashiro, S., Kanehisa, H. & Maganaris, C.N. (2001) *In vivo* behavior of human muscle tendon during walking. *Proceedings of the Royal Society of London B* **268**, 229–233.

Fukunaga, T., Kawakami, Y., Kubo, K. & Kanehisa, H. (2002) Muscle and tendon interaction during human movements. *Exercise and Sport Sciences Reviews* **30**, 106–110.

Gregor, R.J., Roy, R.R., Whiting, W.C., Lovely, R.G., Hodgson, J.A. & Edgerton, V.R. (1988) Mechanical output of the cat soleus during treadmill locomotion: *in vivo* vs. *in situ* characteristics. *Journal of Biomechanics* **21**, 721–732.

Goldspink, G. (1978) Energy turnover during contraction of different types of muscles. In: *Biomechanics VI-A* (Asmussen, E. & Joergensen, K., eds.) University Park Press, Baltimore: 27–29.

Goldspink, G. & Harridge, S. (2003) Cellular and molecular aspects of adaptation in skeletal muscle. In: *Strength and Power in Sport*, 2nd edition (Komi, P.V., ed.) Blackwell, Oxford: 231–251.

Gottschall, J.S. & Kram, R. (2003) Energy cost and muscular activity required for propulsion during walking. *Journal of Applied Physiology* **94**, 1766–1772.

Herzog, W., Zatsiorsky, V., Prilutsky, B.I. & Leonard, T.R. (1994) Variations in force-time histories of cat gastrocnemius, soleus and plantaris muscles for consecutive walking steps. *Journal of Experimental Biology* **191**, 19–36.

Hill, A.V. (1938) The heat of shortening and the dynamic constants of muscle. *Proceedings of the Royal Society B* **126**, 136–195.

Hof, A.L., Geelen, B.A. & Van den Berg, J.W. (1983) Calf muscle moment, work and efficiency in level walking; role of series elasticity. *Journal of Biomechanics* **16**, 523–537.

Huxley, A.F. & Simmons, R.M. (1971) Mechanical properties of the cross-bridges of frog striated muscle. *Journal of Physiology* **218**, 59P–60P.

Ishikawa, M. & Komi, P.V. (2004) Effects of the different dropping intensities on fascicle and tendinous tissue behavior during stretch-shortening cycle exercise. *Journal of Applied Physiology* **96**, 848–852.

Ishikawa, M., Finni, T., & Komi, P.V. (2003) Behaviour of vastus lateralis muscle-tendon during high intensity SSC exercises *in vivo*. *Acta Physiologica Scandinavica* **178**, 205–213.

Ishikawa, M., Niemela, E. & Komi, P.V. (2005a) Interaction between fascicle and tendinous tissues in short-contact stretch-shortening cycle exercise with varying eccentric intensities. *Journal of Applied Physiology* **99**, 217–223.

Ishikawa, M., Komi, P.V., Grey, M.J., Lepola, V. & Bruggemann, G.P. (2005b) Muscle-tendon interaction and elastic energy usage in human walking. *Journal of Applied Physiology* **99**, 603–608.

Ishikawa, M., Pakaslahti, J. & Komi, P.V. (2006) Medial gastrocnemius muscle behavior during human running and walking. *Gait and Posture* **25**, 380–384.

Jones, C., Allen, T. & Talbot, J. (1997) Changes in the mechanical properties of human and amphibian muscle after eccentric exercise. *European Journal of Applied Physiology* **76**, 21–31.

Kawakami, Y., Muraoka, T., Ito, S., Kanehisa, H. & Fukunaga, T. (2002) *In vivo* muscle fibre behaviour during counter-movement exercise in humans reveals a significant role for tendon elasticity. *Journal of Physiology* **540**, 635–646.

Knuttgen, H.G. (1986) Human performance in high-intensity exercise with concentric and eccentric muscle contractions. *International Journal of Sports Medicine* **7** (Suppl. 1), 6–9.

Komi, P.V. (1973) Relationship between muscle tension, EMG and velocity of contraction under concentric and eccentric work. In: *New Developments in Electromyography and Clinical Nerophysiology* (Desmedt, J.E., ed.) Karger, Basel: 596–606.

Komi, P.V. (1984) Biomechanics and neuromuscular performance. *Medicine and Science in Sports and Exercise* **16**, 26–28.

Komi, P.V. (1990) Relevance of *in vivo* force measurements to human biomechanics. *Journal of Biomechanics* **23**, 23–34.

Komi, P.V. (2000) Stretch-shortening cycle: a powerful model to study normal and fatigue muscle. *Journal of Biomechanics* **33**, 1197–1206.

Komi, P.V. & Bosco, C. (1978) Utilization of stored elastic energy in leg extensor muscles by men and women. *Medicine and Science in Sports and Exercise* **10**, 261–265.

Komi, P.V. & Gollhofer, A. (1997) Stretch reflexes can have an important role in force enhancement during SSC exercise. *Journal of Applied Biomechanics* **13**, 451–460.

Komi, P.V. & Rusko, H. (1974) Quantitative evaluation of mechanical and electrical changes during fatigue loading of eccentric and concentric work. *Scandinavian Journal of Rehabilitation Medicine Supplement* **3**, 121–126.

Komi, P.V., Viitasalo, J.H., Havu, M., Thorstensson, A., Sjodin, B. & Karlsson, J. (1977) Skeletal muscle fibres and muscle enzyme activities in monozygous and dizygous twins of both sexes. *Acta Physiologica Scandinavica* **100**, 385–392.

Komi, P.V., Gollhofer, A., Schmidtbleicher, D. & Frick, U. (1987) Interaction between man and shoe in running: considerations for a more comprehensive measurement approach. *International Journal of Sports Medicine* **19**, 196–202.

Komi, P.V., Fukashiro, S. & Järvinen, M. (1992) Biomechanical loading of Achilles tendon during normal locomotion. *Clinics in Sports Medicine* **11**, 521–531.

Komi, P.V., Belli, A., Huttunen, V., Bonnefoy, R., Geyssant, A. & Lacour, J.R. (1996) Optic fibre as a transducer of tendomuscular forces. *European Journal of Applied Physiology* **72**, 278–280.

Linnamo, V., Strojnik, V., Komi, P.V. (2006) Maximal force during eccentric and isometric actions at different elbow angles. *European Journal of Applied Physiology* **96**, 672–678.

Margaria, R. (1938) Physiology and energy expenditure during walking and running at different speeds and slopes of the ground. *Atti della Reale Accademia Nazionale dei Lincei* **7**, 277–283.

Maruyama, K., Matsubara, S., Natori, R., Nonomura, Y. & Kimura, S. (1977) Connectin, an elastic protein of muscle. Characterization and function. *Journal of Biochemistry* **82**, 317–337.

Mevill-Jones, G. & Watt, D.G.D. (1977) Observations on the control of stepping and hopping movements in man. *Journal of Physiology* **219**, 709–727.

Mirkov, D.M., Nedeljkovic, A., Milanovic, S. (2004) Muscle strength testing: evaluation of tests of explosive force production. *European Journal of Applied Physiology* **91**, 147–154.

Moritani, T., Oddson, L. & Thorstensson, A. (1990) Electromyographic evidence of selective fatigue during the eccentric phase of stretch/shortening cycles in man. *European Journal of Applied Physiology* **60**, 425–429.

Reeves, N.D., Narici, M.V. & Maganaris, C.N. (2003) Behavior of human muscle fascicles during shortening and lengthening contractions in vivo. *Journal of Applied Physiology* **95**, 1090–1096.

Sonnenblick, E.H. (1966) Mechanics of myocardial contraction. In: *The Myocardial Cell: Structure, Function, and Modification* (Briller, S.A. & Conn, H.L., eds.) University of Pennsylvania Press, Philadelphia: 173–250.

Sousa, F., Ishikawa, M., Vilas-Boas, J.P., Komi, P.V. (2007) Intensity- and muscle-specific fascicle behavior during human drop jumps. *Journal of Applied Physiology* **102**, 382–389.

Tihanyi, J., Apor, P. & Fekete, G. (1982) Force-velocity-power characteristics and fibre composition in human knee extensor muscles. *European Journal of Applied Physiology* **48**, 331–343.

van Ingen Schenau, G.J., Bobbert, M.F. & Rozendal, R.H. (1987) The unique action of bi-articular muscles in complex movements. *Journal of Anatomy* **155**, 1–5.

van Ingen Schenau, G.J., Bobbert, M.F. & de Haan, A. (1997) Does elastic energy enhance work and efficiency in the stretch-shortening cycle? *Journal of Applied Biomechanics* **13**, 389–415.

Viitasalo, J.T. & Bosco, C. (1982) Electromechanical behaviour of human muscles in vertical jumps. *European Journal of Applied Physiology* **48**, 253–261.

Viitasalo, J.T. & Komi, P.V. (1978) Force-time characteristics and fibre composition in human leg extensor muscles. *European Journal of Applied Physiology* **40**, 7–15.

Viitasalo, J.T. & Komi, P.V. (1981) Interrelationships between electromyographic, mechanical, muscle structure and reflex time measurements in man. *Acta Physiologica Scandinavica* **111**, 97–103.

Welsh, R.P., McNab, I. & Riley, P. (1971) Biomechanical studies of rabbit tendon. *Clinical Orthopedics and Related Research* **81**, 171–177.

Westing, S.H., Cresswell, A.G. & Thorstensson, A. (1991) Muscle activation during maximal voluntary eccentirc and concentric knee extension. *European Journal of Applied Physiology* **62**, 104–108.

Whitehead, N.P., Weerakkody, N.S. & Gregory, J.E. (2001) Changes in passive tension of muscle in humans and animals after eccentric exercise. *Journal of Physiology* **533**, 593–604.

Wilkie, D.R. (1949) The relation between force and velocity in human muscle. *Journal of Physiology* **110**, 249–280.

Zajac, F.E. (1989) Muscle and tendon: properties, models, scaling, and application to biomechanics and motor control. *Critical Reviews in Biomedical Engineering* **17**, 359–411.

Chapter 2

Physiological Demands of Sprinting and Multiple-Sprint Sports

CLYDE WILLIAMS

Sprinting is simply running at maximum speed, irrespective of the absolute speed of the runner or the distance. Sprinting speed is influenced by a wide range of factors both internal and external: age, gender, size, and experience are some of the internal influences; whereas running surface and environmental conditions such as altitude and wind speed are some of the external influences. The ability to run at maximum speed is part of the evolutionary survival physiology, as was the ability of our ancestors to walk long distances in search of food. The ability to be able to sprint, albeit over short distances, enabled our ancestors to catch small animals for food and also to avoid becoming the prey of larger predators. In summary, it appears, from close examination of the capacity for energy production in human skeletal muscles, that our ancestors were long-distance walkers with the ability to sprint for brief periods as and when necessary.

To the public at large, sprinting is an activity that takes place in athletics competitions and is the centre piece of track races. However, when pressed to take a broader view of this activity it is recognized as a core activity in many sports, such as football (soccer), basketball, rugby, field hockey, tennis, and badminton, all of which are played recreationally as well as professionally. Although there are several studies on the physiology of 100 m sprinters, there is relatively little equivalent information on sprinters taking part in team sports. This is largely because

sprinting in these sports and games is, unlike the 100-m sprint, unstructured and unpredictable in duration, distance, and timing.

To be able to out-sprint an opponent in team sports has obvious advantages that include moving quickly into "tactically right positions." Those players who combine their ability to move quickly and have tactical experience of their sport always appear to have much more time to play shots or receive a pass than slower and less experienced players. However, while speed provides players with clear advantages, it is the ability to sprint repeatedly with little recovery time that often separates the successful players from those who are simply fast on the track. Therefore, it is difficult to even document sprinting "*in situ*" let alone study the physiological demands of sprinting on players.

The aim of this chapter is therefore to present an overview of the available information on sprinting, first as the traditional "100-m event" that is the centre-piece of track and field competitions, and second within the context of sports such as football, basketball, rugby, field hockey, and tennis.

Sprinting: 100 m

Sprinting holds such a central place in sport that it is not surprising that the earliest records of the ancient Olympic Games give prominence to an outstanding sprinter. Coroebus won the sprint event in the ancient Olympics of 776 BC. The sprinters ran the length of the stadium, called a stade, which was about 192 m. There were two other races in the ancient Olympic Games, the *diaulos,* which was two lengths

The Olympic Textbook of Science in Sport, 1st edition. Edited by R.J. Maughan. Published 2009 by Blackwell Publishing. ISBN: 978-1-4051-5638-7.

of the stadium (384 m), and a longer race over about 24 stades (4615 m; Durant 1961).

Of course, even if the length of the stadium was not exactly the same in each of the city states of ancient Greece, this was of little concern because the prize went to the fastest runner. In this one respect the modern Olympic Games shares the same principle with the games of Greek antiquity: it is the fastest athlete on the day who wins the prize and not necessarily the athlete who sets a new World Record during periods between the Games. This is one reason why the Olympic gold medal holds such a unique place in the minds of spectators and athletes alike. World Records punctuate the progress of the event, but it is with a gold medal that sprinters earn lasting recognition as well as their place in the record books.

Records are a relatively new phenomenon. They emerged when accurate and reliable forms of time-keeping became available. Electronic timing was introduced in 1968 and has since become the standard method of timekeeping in all major sprint championships. A claim for a new World Record is scrutinized rigorously, and competitors are aware that they should ensure that the competition and conditions are acceptable to the International Amateur Athletics Federation (IAAF) before attempting to set new records. The IAAF not only establishes a strict set of conditions for timing an event, but also considers the nature of the track before recognizing new records. The current World Records for the 100-m sprint are shown in Tables 2.1 and 2.2.

Multiple-sprint sports

In contrast to the number of studies on 100-m sprinting, there is relatively little information on sprinting as an integral part of many sports, such as football, rugby football, and field hockey. The activity patterns of the players in these sports consist of various combinations of walking, jogging, running, and sprinting. Although the distance covered in a single sprint is always less than 100 m, the total distance sprinted during a game is significantly greater. Identifying the distance covered and the duration of each sprint in these sports is technically more demanding because a wide range of extraneous variables influence

Table 2.1 World Record breakers for the men's 100-m sprint.

Name	Time (s)	Country	Year
Usain Bolt	9.72	Jamaica	2008
Asafa Powell	9.74	Jamaica	2007
Asafa Powell	9.77	Jamaica	2005
Tim Montgomery	9.78[d]	USA	2002
Maurice Greene	9.79	USA	1999
Donavon Bailey	9.84	Canada	1996
Leroy Burrell	9.85	USA	1994
Carl Lewis	9.86	USA	1991*
Leroy Burrell	9.90	USA	1991*
Carl Lewis	9.92	USA	1988
Ben Johnson	9.79[d]	Canada	1988
Calvin Smith	9.93	USA	1983*
Jim Hines	9.95	USA	1968
Armin Hary	10.0	Germany	1960
Willie Williams	10.1	USA	1956
Jesse Owens	10.2	USA	1936
Percy Williams	10.6	Canada	1930
Charles Paddock	10.4	USA	1921
Donald Lippincott	10.6	USA	1912

*Records set at non-Olympic events; [d]record disallowed.

Table 2.2 World Record breakers for the women's 100-m sprint.

Name	Time (s)	Country	Year
Florence Griffiths-Joiner	10.49	USA	1988
Evelyn Ashford	10.76	USA	1983
Lyudmila Kondratyeva	10.87	USSR	1980
Marlies Oelsner	10.88	DDR	1977
Renate Stecher	10.9	DDR	1973
Wyomia Tyus	11.0	USA	1968
Irene Kirzenstein	11.1	Poland	1965
Wilma Rudolph	11.2	USA	1961
Shirley Strickland	11.3	AUS	1955
Marjorie Jackson	11.4	AUS	1952
Helen Stephens	11.5	USA	1936
Helen Stephens	11.6	USA	1935
Tollien Schuuman	11.9	Netherlands	1932
Betty Roberts	12.0	USA	1928
Leni Junker	12.2	Germany	1925
Lenie Junker	12.4	Germany	1925
Marie Mejzlikova	12.8	Czech Republic	1923
Emmy Haux (110 yards)	12.7	Germany	1923
Mary Lines	12.8	UK	1922

performance. For example, players are either "drib-bling," "carrying," or "chasing" a ball, and in some situations they are trying to achieve all three. Further-more, these activities are made even more difficult by the presence of the opposition who attempt to prevent a player's progress. The sprint perform-ances are also influenced by the nature of surface on which the games are played. Even though football, rugby and, at a recreational level, field hockey, are played on grass the conditions of the surface can vary not only from day-to-day but also between the beginning and end of the competition.

The activity patterns of players in these multiple-sprint sports have been obtained by "time and motion" studies, which are also described as "match analyses." Match analyses range from simple obser-vation and manual recording of players' positions on the field of play, through to multiple video camera recordings and computer digitization or GPS mon-itoring that can provide moment-by-moment move-ment records for all players. In many of the earlier studies information on sprinting per se was not documented because "fast running and sprinting" were simply reported as high-intensity running.

Most of the information on sprinting in sports has been provided by match analyses of football (soccer). Even so, it is only possible to provide broad generalizations about the sprint performances of soccer players because of the wide range of condi-tions that dictate the game, even in premier divi-sion (elite) matches. For example, the total distance covered by elite outfield players in top division matches is between 9 and 12 km. These distances are covered by a combination of activities that include mainly walking, jogging, and cruising with inter-mittent periods of high-speed running and sprint-ing (Reilly 2000). However, the "position" of players determines the duration and distance of their sprints. Nevertheless, information from several match ana-lysis studies of elite soccer players suggests that they rarely sprint for more than about 2 to 3 s, cover-ing a total distance of approximately 10 to 20 m each time; players are engaged in high-speed running about every 30 s and perform maximal sprints about every 90 s (Spencer et al. 2005). When attempting to compare the results of match analyses of earlier and more recent studies there is the issue of whether or not the wide range in reported results is due simply to differences in methodology, fitness status, play-ing surface, and level of competition, or to actual performance differences.

Although there are fewer studies on field hockey, the available evidence for elite players suggest that the average duration of each sprint is also about 2 s, but maximum sprint durations of up to 4 s were also recorded (Spencer et al. 2004). In rugby football, the average duration of sprints ranges from about 1.8 to 3.0 s, with the average sprint duration being longer for the backs than for the forwards (Docherty et al. 1988; Duthie et al. 2005; Deutsch et al. 2007). A recent report on the demands of basketball matches played by elite young players, showed that the duration of each sprint is about 2 s in duration ,with an average time between sprints of about 39 s (Abdelkrim et al. 2007). There were positional differences in the fre-quency of sprints performed by guards, centers, and forwards, as is the case in other team sports.

In comparison to the team sports mentioned above, tennis is very much a multiple-sprint sport because there is little low level activity between points. No more than 20 s is allowed between games and only 90 s between each change of ends. In a singles tennis match the mean distance covered per shot has been estimated to be about 3 m and the dis-tance run per point is about 8–12 m, which might include rallies that take between 3 and 8 s (Ferrauti et al. 2001).

Even though players in these sports sprint for no more than about 3 s and cover a distance of approx-imately 10–20 m, they do so repeatedly and therein lies the challenge. It has been estimated that in elite soccer, rugby, and field hockey matches players per-form about 20–30 sprints, covering a total distance of approximately 700–1000 m (Spencer et al. 2005). One of the main determinants of how many sprints a player can perform is the recovery period between sprints. Balsom and colleagues (1992) demonstrated quite clearly the impact of the recovery duration on subsequent sprint performance. They reported that when their subjects performed 15 sprints of 40 m with a 120-s recovery period they were able to complete 11 sprints without a decrement in speed. However, when the recovery period was reduced to 60 s and then 30 s, the decrement in sprint speed occurred after seven and three sprints, respectively (Balsom *et al.* 1992). Of course, in most of the multiple-sprint sports considered in this chapter, repeated 40-m sprinting occurs only rarely. Therefore it is of interest that Balsom and colleagues (1992) also reported the influences of the different recovery periods on speeds for the first 15 m of the 40-m sprints. They found that the acceleration time over the first 15 m of the sprint was slower only when the recovery period was reduced to 30 s. The mean time for 0–15 m in the first sprint was 2.58 s, compared with 2.78 s for the last of the 40-m sprints. Although this difference in speed does not appear to be large, it can make the difference between success and failure in, for example, challenging for a ball, running past an opponent, or executing a skill or change of direction rapidly.

When the period between sprints is too short for optimum recovery then the consequences are not simply a slight reduction in speed in subsequent sprints. For example, it is not uncommon in football for a period of high-intensity running, which includes sprinting, to be followed immediately by a longer period of self-selected lower-intensity activity (Mohr *et al.* 2005). It appears that the players experience a "temporary fatigue" that is overcome by a reduced activity level for several minutes during a match.

The detrimental influence of short recovery periods on subsequent sprint performance is almost entirely the consequence of the finite time required to rapidly replace the energy stores of phosphocreatine (PCr) and possibly also the restoration of ionic balances within active muscles (see Chapters 5 and 20).

Characteristics of elite sprinters

Aerobic power

The maximal oxygen uptakes ($\dot{V}_{O_{2max}}$) of sprinters and strength athletes are generally not different from those of sedentary people, when corrected for body mass (Neuman 1988). Values for sprinters range from about 48 to 55 mL·kg body mass^{-1}·min^{-1} for men and 43 to 50 mL·kg body mass^{-1}·min^{-1} for women. However, in absolute terms (L·min^{-1}), $\dot{V}_{O_{2max}}$ may be larger for sprinters because they have greater muscle and body mass than sedentary people (Barnes 1981). The nature of sprint training for the track athlete is such that it does not promote as large an increase in $\dot{V}_{O_{2max}}$ as endurance training. Furthermore, the genetic factors that contribute to a higher proportion of fast twitch fibers in elite sprinters are not, in general, accompanied by the potential to develop an exceptionally large capacity for oxygen transport. However, sprinters in team sports often have higher $\dot{V}_{O_{2max}}$ values than those of track sprinters. There are advantages to having a high aerobic capacity in sports that demand frequent sprinting with only short recovery periods. As the number of sprints in a game increases so there is an ever greater reliance on aerobic metabolism for energy production (Balsom *et al.* 1994). There is also some evidence to suggest that the rate of recovery of PCr is faster in those players who have a high aerobic capacity (Bogdanis *et al.* 1996).

Body composition

Sprinters are generally heavier and more muscular than other runners. The benchmark study by Tanner (1964) of the physique of the Olympic athlete was one of the first to document the anthropometric differences between track and field athletes. Follow-up studies by Koshla (1978) reported that male sprinters have heights ranging from 1.57 to 1.90 m and body mass which range from about 63 to 90 kg. It was later reported that female track sprinters are generally shorter and lighter, with a height range of 1.57 to 1.78 m and weights of 51 to 71 kg (Koshla & McBroome 1984).

The anthropometric characteristics of participants in sports that demand multiple-sprints, such as football (Davis *et al.* 1992), basketball (Ostojic *et al.* 2006), rugby (Nicholas 1997), field hockey (Lawrence & Polglaze 2000), and tennis (Weber *et al.* 2007), are similar to those of the track sprinters. Of course, in sports such as basketball the average height of these sportsmen and women is generally greater than sprinters in other sports. There are also differences in the anthropometric characteristics of players depending on the position they play, such as the forwards and backs in rugby (Nicholas 1997).

Table 2.3 Mean (± SD) stride rate, stride length, and reaction times for the four fastest sprinters in the 100-m final at the 1991 World Athletics Championships in Tokyo. (Reproduced with permission from Ae *et al*. 1992.)

Variable	Lewis	Burrell	Mitchell	Christie
Stride rate (strides·s^{-1})	4.51 (0.3)	4.40 (0.33)	4.70 (0.21)	4.55 (0.32)
Stride length (m)	2.37 (0.41)	2.41 (0.38)	2.25 (0.38)	2.33 (0.38)
Reaction time (s)	0.14	0.12	0.09	0.126

Height or, more importantly, leg length, has an obvious influence on stride length of sprinters during track races. During a 100-m race, elite sprinters (both men and women) take between 44 and 53 strides to cover the distance (Moravec *et al*. 1988). This amounts to stride rates of about 4.23 to 5.05 m·s^{-1}. For example, in the 1987 World Athletics Championships in Rome the eight men in the 100-m final averaged 45.7 strides to complete the race at a stride frequency of 4.6 strides·s^{-1} (Moravec *et al*. 1988). The average values for stride rates and stride lengths for the four fastest sprinters in the 100-m final of the 1991 Tokyo World Athletics Championships are shown in Table 2.3.

As might be expected, tall sprinters have longer stride lengths and slower stride rates than shorter sprinters, who have smaller stride lengths but faster stride rates. However, it is interesting to note that female sprinters of the same height, leg length, and stride length as male sprinters record times for the 100 m that are about 1 s slower than the performance of men. The difference is attributed to the slightly slower stride frequency of the female sprinters (Hoffman 1972).

In team games the distance sprinted is rarely more than about 20 m and so speed over the first few meters is all important; those sprinters who can accelerate rapidly over the first few meters may be more successful than faster sprinters who take longer to achieve their maximum speeds. Therefore, it seems that short and fast stride rates are the characteristics of successful sprinters in team sports and individual sports such as tennis.

Muscle fiber composition

The early muscle biopsy studies on elite athletes showed that sprinters tend to have large proportions of the fast-contracting, fast-fatiguing type of fibers (type 2b) than the slow-contracting, slow-fatiguing fibers (type 1) that are characteristic of endurance runners. The ratio of fast- to slow-twitch muscle fibers is also greater for sprinters than it is for the general population of men and women of similar ages (Costill *et al*. 1976). In this respect sprinters share these characteristics with power athletes (Thorstensson *et al*. 1977; Tesch and Karlsson 1985). Although the skeletal muscles of elite power athletes and sprinters have characteristically high proportions of fast-twitch fibers, it is unlikely that this fiber composition is a result of strength training per se. However, strength training in preparation for sprinting may cause a change in the composition of the sub-populations of type 2 fibers (Tesch 1992) but probably not a conversion of slow to fast fibers (i.e., type 1 to type 2). Esbjornsson and colleagues (1993) reported that the power output during cycling was directly related to the percentage of type 2 fibers in the vastus lateralis muscles of their subjects and to the potential for anaerobic metabolism (as reflected by the activity of the enzymes lactate dehydrogenase and phosphofructokinase), with the authors stating that there were "no sex differences in this relationship." Of course, it is not only the fiber composition that influences sprinting speed, but also the number of fibers and their recruitment during exercise.

Muscle strength

The large muscle mass that is characteristic of elite sprinters contributes to their running success because it allows them to generate large forces quickly. The generation of high forces is essential during the start of a race, and it is particularly important during the section of the race when sprinters reach their maximum speeds and have only the briefest contact with the track. The leg strength of sprinters is greater than that of distance runners (Maughan *et al.* 1983; Hakkinen & Keskinen 1989) and of the general population (Barnes 1981). The relationship between leg strength and sprint performance was examined in a group of sprinters using isokinetic dynamometry. An isotonic strength profile was developed for each runner by recording his or her responses to a progressive isotonic load using a Lido dynamometer. Each runner performed a series of leg extensions against progressively higher loads. Peak power was calculated along with average peak velocity for quadriceps and hamstring muscles (Mahler *et al.* 1992). The isotonic peak power output thresholds for these muscles were derived from plotting peak power output against a range of workloads. The strongest correlation was between 100-m performance times and the isotonic peak power output threshold ($r = 0.957$) for the hamstrings. It was concluded that this result was consistent with the fact that the hamstrings are the limiting muscle group during sprinting.

However, many of the strength-testing methods are, unfortunately, non-specific for athletes in general and sprinters in particular. Therefore, it is not surprising that strong correlations are not always reported between various measures of strength and sprinting performance (Farrar & Thorland 1987). Ideally, strength measurements on sprinters should be made while these athletes are performing movements that are part of the running action, but this has not yet been accomplished because of the technical difficulties involved. Of course, another view is that while a certain level of strength is essential for successful sprinting, strength alone is not a determinant of sprinting success (Farrar & Thorland 1987).

Movement speed

Sprinters, by definition, move quickly. The world's elite male and female sprinters achieve maximal running velocities of at least 11.0 and 10.0 m·s^{-1}, respectively. It would therefore be reasonable to assume that elite sprinters have nerve conduction velocities that are faster than those of non-sprinters.

For example, in the 1999 World Athletics Championships (Spain) the reaction time for the winner of the 100 m – Maurice Green (9.80 s) – was recorded as 0.132 s, whereas the reaction time for the last to finish the race (10.24 s) was 0.173 s. Casabona and colleagues (1990) used surface electrodes and electrical stimulation to assess neural conduction velocities in sprinters; they concluded that these athletes have faster conduction velocities than strength-trained athletes (Casabona *et al.* 1990). There also appears to be a good correlation between neural conduction velocity and the relative area of type 2 muscle fibers (i.e., the greater the relative type 2 fiber area, the greater the conduction velocity; Sadoyama *et al.* 1988).

A comparison of the patellar tendon reflex characteristics of endurance-trained and sprint-trained athletes showed that the sprinters exhibited greater peak force, faster time to peak force, and faster reflex latency following stimulation than endurance athletes (Koceja & Kamen 1988). These differences may reflect differences in muscle-tendon stiffness, but they may also reflect differences in neural organization. Circumstantial evidence suggests that the functional organization of the neuromuscular system in sprinters may be different from that of endurance athletes and sedentary people.

In the 100-m sprint, reaction time is clearly important because it is essential that runners respond rapidly to the starter's pistol. Nevertheless, athletes will often record different reaction times, even in the same competition, depending upon whether they are running in heats or in finals. The reaction times become slower as the distances are extended from 100 to 400 m. Generally, the overall performances of sprinters are affected very little, if at all, by slight changes in their speeds of reaction to the starter's signal (Atwater 1982; Moravec *et al.* 1988); however, this may not be true for the world's elite sprinters.

Knowing the fastest reaction times of World Class sprinters allows manufacturers of timing systems to electronically program the starting blocks to the starter's gun. Therefore, a false start will register if a runner moves before 100 ms has elapsed. But this value is an arbitrary one, and the final decision about a false start rests with the official starter. For example a recent study reported that sprinters responded much faster to an audio signal than the lower limit of 100 ms that is imposed as a "false start" in international athletics championships. Pain and Hibbs (2007) reported that the reaction times of their sprinters were under 85 ms.

The introduction of electronic timing has also helped in deciding the outcome of races that would have been difficult to confirm with confidence using manual timing. Even so the advance in timing systems does not always confirm the winner of the 100-m sprint race. This is especially true when the races are between the world's elite sprinters. In some of these elite races the differences in finishing times are so close that they are unmeasurable, even with the best technology. An example of this phenomenon occurred at the 2007 World Athletics Championships in Osaka where two athletes recorded the same time of 11.01 s for the women's 100-m final. On this occasion the winner, Campbell of Jamaica, could only be decided on the basis of a photo finish.

Being able to run fast is only a precondition for successful sprinting; it is not the determinant of success during competition among athletes of a similar standard. The 100-m sprint is made up of several sections, and is not, as the casual observer might conclude, a simple race between gun and tape (Table 2.4; Radford 1990). Sprinters have different strengths: some may be slow starters but have the ability to sustain their maximal speeds to the finish line, whereas others may be fast starters and fade toward the end of the race. Nevertheless, the elite sprinter must be able to achieve maximal efficiency over each section of the race if he or she seeks to cross the finishing line ahead of the competition.

Table 2.4 Approximate times (s) for phases of a 100-m sprint. (Reproduced with permission from Radford 1990.)

Phase	Men (10 s)	Women (11 s)
Reaction to the gun	0.1–0.3	0.1–0.3
Drive off the blocks	0.3–0.4	0.3–0.4
Acceleration	5.5–7.0	5.0–6.0
Maximum speed	1.5–3.0	1.5–2.5
Deceleration	1.0–1.5	1.5–2.5

Sprinters must be able to generate large forces rapidly against their starting blocks to accelerate effectively. This requires considerable strength, flexibility, and coordination. Acceleration is the longest stage of the 100-m sprint; thereafter, the sprinter tries to maintain maximum speed for as long as possible. The traditional view of the kinetics of sprinting over 100 m is that maximum speed is normally achieved about 40 to 60 m into the race. This may be the reason why in indoor athletics competitions the sprint race is over a distance of 60 m. The times for the 60-m sprint are between 6 and 7 s, whereas the current World Record achieved by Maurice Greene (USA) is 6.39 s. Athletes in the 60-m sprint achieve their maximum speeds towards the end of the race. In the 100-m sprint the challenge is to maintain this peak speed for the remainder of the race.

In the 1987 World Athletic Championships in Rome the finalists in the men's 100-m sprint reached their maximum speeds at distances of between 50 and 60 m, and they were able to maintain those speeds for the remainder of the race. In the women's 100-m final the sprinters achieved their maximum velocities at about the same distances as the men, but appeared unable to sustain their running speeds for the rest of the race. An analysis of the performances of the two fastest men in the race, namely Johnson (9.83 s) and Lewis (9.93 s), shows that Johnson had a faster average stride rate while Lewis had a longer average stride length. It seems that Johnson won the race in the first 20 m when his contact time with the ground and his flight phase were less than those of Lewis, because after 20 m these factors were the same for both athletes, as were their average running velocities (Moravec et al. 1988).

In contrast, the peak velocities of the four fastest men in the 100-m final of the 1991 Tokyo World Athletic Championships were achieved between 70 and 80 m into the race, which is unique in top class sprinting (Table 2.5). They also appeared to be able to increase their running speeds over the last 10 m of the race. Therefore, one of the distinguishing features of the world's best sprinters is that they are not only able to run fast, but they are also to maintain these speeds throughout the latter part of a 100-m race (Table 2.6).

Table 2.5 Speeds (m·s⁻¹) over 10-m sections of the 100-m final for the four fastest sprinters at the 1991 World Athletics Championships in Tokyo. (Reproduced with permission from Ae *et al.* 1992.)

Distance (m)	Lewis	Burrell	Mitchell	Christie
10	5.31	5.46	5.56	5.41
20	9.26	9.43	9.35	9.43
30	10.87	10.99	10.75	10.87
40	11.24	11.36	11.36	11.24
50	11.90	11.49	11.49	11.76
60	11.76	11.63	11.49	11.63
70	11.90	11.49	11.63	11.63
80	12.05	11.90	11.63	11.76
90	11.49	11.24	11.36	11.11
100	11.63	11.49	11.24	11.36
Finishing times (s)	9.86	9.88	9.91	9.92

Table 2.6 Speeds (m·s⁻¹), over 10-m sections of the 100-m final for the three fastest sprinters at the 1999 World Athletics Championships in Seville.

Distance (m)	Green	Surin	Chambers
10	5.37	5.32	5.35
20	9.71	10.0	9.80
30	10.89	10.99	10.87
40	11.36	10.99	11.11
50	11.63	11.76	11.63
60	11.91	11.76	11.90
70	11.76	11.63	11.36
80	11.76	11.63	11.11
90	11.76	11.63	11.24
100	11.63	11.36	11.11
Finishing times (s)	9.80	9.84	9.97

Mechanical limitations

An increase in running speed is achieved by an increase in both stride length and frequency. In the 100-m sprint races the ability to increase stride length is progressively limited as runners approach maximum speeds; eventually an increase in speed can only be achieved by increasing stride frequency (Hay 1985). Furthermore, the contact time with the track is reduced as maximum speed is achieved and so the opportunity to develop greater driving force to improve or maintain forward velocity diminishes.

These mechanical factors may be as limiting as the biochemical process required to generate energy to support rapid contractions of the musculature engaged in sprinting.

Running with or against the wind can influence the outcome of a race. The legal wind speed limit is +2 m·s⁻¹, but this has relevance only when sprint times are approaching Championship and/or World Records. World Class sprinters in a race in which there is a tail wind of 2 m·s⁻¹ may have an advantage of about 0.1 s compared to when there is a head-wind of 2 m·s⁻¹ (Mureika 2001).

Air resistance also contributes to the sprinter's inability to sustain maximal velocity throughout a race. Therefore, sprinting on tracks located at high altitude give the athlete a significant advantage (Davies 1980). It has been estimated that World Class sprinters gain an advantage of about 0.03 to 0.04 s for every 1000 m of altitude for the 100 m (Mureika 2001).

The nature of the running track is another factor that can influence sprinting speed. Comparisons of contemporary sprint times with those established prior to the 1970s must take into account the fact that some early records were set on cinder tracks. Not only did the quality of such tracks change with weather conditions, but the number of races that preceded a given sprint also influenced the times achieved during the competition. For example, the sprint relays are traditionally held at the end of the track races; thus, in the days before synthetic tracks, the relay team frequently had to contend with a running surface that was rutted and slippery. It is remarkable therefore, that in the final of the 4 × 100 m relay race in the 1964 Tokyo Olympics, Bob Hayes recorded a world best time of 8.86 s for the last 100 m on a cinder track. There also appear to be fast tracks around the world on which sprinters frequently record their best times. Very hard tracks favor the sprinters but may disadvantage 10 000 m runners because of their potential to cause injury.

The IAAF has laid down clear guidelines for track surfaces, and only approved tracks are normally considered as venues for International and World Championships. The IAAF-approved tracks must be designed to be suitable for range of races and therefore should not favor one type over another.

Table 2.7 Performance times of sprinters who competed in the 100-m finals at both the 1991 World Athletics Championships in Tokyo and in the 1992 Olympic Games in Barcelona. (Reproduced with permission from Tempe 1993.)

Sprinter (Country)	Times (s)	
	Tokyo 1991	Barcelona 1992
L. Burrell (USA)	9.88	10.10
D. Mitchell (USA)	9.91	10.04
L. Christie (UK)	9.92	9.96
F. Fredericks (Nam.)	9.95	10.02
R. Stewart (Jam.)	9.96	10.22
B. Surin (Can.)	10.14	10.09

In the 1991 World Athletics Championship in Tokyo the fast times achieved have been attributed to the track in the Japanese National Stadium. Six men ran the 100 m in less than 10 s, and two sprinters beat the former World Record of 9.90 s: Carl Lewis and Leroy Burrell ran the 100 m in 9.86 and 9.88 s, respectively; the previous record was 9.9 s. It has been reported that the Tokyo track did not conform to the specifications stipulated by the IAAF, so the performances of these sprinters both in the 100 m and in the long jump may be partly explained by the hard track on which they were achieved. The difference in track surfaces is offered as one explanation for the poorer performances of the same six runners when competing in the 1992 Olympics in Barcelona (Table 2.7).

Bearing in mind the IAAF regulations that tracks should be designed to provide an appropriate surface for all running events, organizers of the 2007 World Athletic Championships in Osaka commissioned the construction of a unique track to comply with these regulations. The track in the Nagi stadium was promoted as one of the fastest in the world because a hard surface was laid over a softer surface containing floating ceramic balloons; the grain of the track surface was laid so that it ran from side to side, which provides the athlete with more purchase from each foot contact. Furthermore, the track was "cooler" than other tracks, and so these unique characteristics should benefit the sprinters as well as the 10 000 m athletes. However, even though

the athletes competed on the most technologically advanced track, no World Records were set in either the men's or the women's 100-m events. The women's 100 m was won in a disappointing time of 11.01 s, which was first achieved 40 years earlier (see Table 2.2). These observations serve to highlight the multiplicity of factors that can influence the outcome of competitions in which the sprinters are closely matched.

In many team sports the quality and type of playing surface may vary from match to match. For example, the quality of playing surface is rarely uniform when matches are played on grass pitches. Furthermore, playing football matches in the rain results in the grass surface changing as the match progresses and so sprinting becomes harder towards the end of the game. The nature of the surface also influences the "bounce of the ball" adding to the difficulty of executing relevant skills while running at high speed.

In tennis, different types of playing surfaces may be used for different tournaments and so it is not surprising that some players become successful only on one type of surface. The Australian and US Open Tournaments are played on hard courts, whereas the French Open is played on clay and the Wimbledon Tournament is played on grass. Only the world's best players develop the ability to successfully switch from playing tournaments on different surfaces. The type of surface has a profound influence on the way that the game is played. For example, the average time per point is longer on clay (~10 s) than on hard courts (~5 s), which in turn is longer than on grass (~3 s). These examples also help raise awareness of some of the factors that influence sprinting performance in some of the most popular sports.

Environmental influences

In 100-m track competitions the sprinter has to perform no more than two or three times day, i.e., heats. Therefore, high temperatures and humidity probably do not have a detrimental influence on the sprinting performance per se. However, in multiple-sprint sports in which the competitions last for at least 60 min, fatigue occurs earlier when performing in the heat than when performing in a more temperate environment. For example, the performances of male and female games players was shown to be reduced by half when they performed prolonged intermittent high-intensity shuttle running at 30°C compared to their performances at 17°C (Morris *et al.* 2000, 2005). Their 15-m sprint times were also slower in the heat compared with their performances in the cooler environment. Furthermore, Morris and colleagues found strong correlations between the total distance covered and the rate of rise in rectal temperatures during prolonged intermittent exercise in the heat (30°C) for male and female games players (r = −0.90 and r = −0.94, respectively; Morris *et al.* 2000, 2005). The combination of dehydration and a subsequent rapid rise in core temperature to "critical levels" appears to be the main cause of the early onset of fatigue rather than differences in metabolic responses to exercise (Morris *et al.* 2005). Given the link between a rapid rise in core temperature and onset of fatigue, it is not surprising that some attempts have been made to pre-cool players before competition. However, this appeared to have no physiological benefits during a subseqnet 90-min soccer-specific intermittent running test on a non-motorized treadmill (Drust *et al.* 2000).

Power output during sprinting

Sprinters are generally regarded as the power athletes in sport because of their ability to generate large forces rapidly in their pursuit of maximum running speeds. Therefore, it is not surprising that several methods have been developed for measuring the maximum power output of these athletes (Bar-Or *et al.* 1977; Bouchard *et al.* 1982; Lakomy 1987). Currently the method of choice involves cycling at maximum speed against a predetermined external resistive load for 30–40 s. This test of maximal power output is generally referred to as the Wingate Anaerobic Test (WAnT; Bar-Or 1987). Values for peak power, mean power, and end power output can be determined during maximal exercise by simply using a mechanically braked cycle ergometer linked to a computer (Lakomy 1986). A fatigue index can also be calculated from the differences between peak and end power outputs (Fig. 2.1).

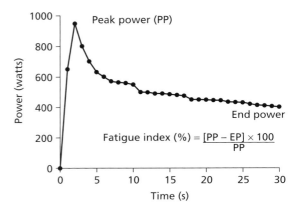

Fig. 2.1 Power output during a 30-s Wingate Anaerobic Test (WAnT) on a cycle ergometer.

There are clear differences between the power outputs of sprinters and endurance runners when they complete the WAnT procedure (Fig. 2.2; G. Bogdanis, Loughborough University, Loughborough, UK, pers. comm.). Sprinters and power athletes generate greater peak power, but they also have a more marked onset of fatigue than endurance athletes. Thus, this test can be used to study the power outputs of different populations of athletes in an attempt to describe more precisely their physiological characteristics. For example, Denis and colleagues (1992) compared the peak power outputs of 100-m sprinters and 800-m runners using the WAnT procedure during cycling. Twelve runners cycled for 45 s: the

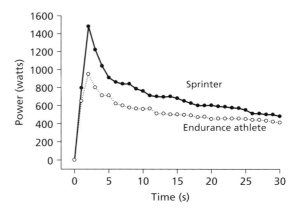

Fig. 2.2 Power output of a sprinter and an endurance athlete during a 30-s Wingate Anaerobic Test (WAnT) on a cycle ergometer.

peak power outputs of the sprinters and middle-distance runners were 1006 W (14.8 ± 1.4 W·kg^{-1}) and 796 W (11.9 ± 1.6 W·kg^{-1}), respectively. As might be expected, the average peak power outputs of the sprinters were significantly higher than the values obtained for the middle-distance runners. The mean peak power output achieved by the sprinters was also greater than those achieved by the middle-distance runners. However, there was no difference between the total work done by the two groups of runners. The reason for this lack of difference is that the initial high peak power outputs of the sprinters decreased rapidly towards the end of the test and so the total work was not different between the two groups. Nevertheless, it is the peak power output that is of interest when studying the characteristics of sprinters, and so in this respect the WAnT test is another useful research tool.

A more relevant method of assessing the power output of sprinters is based on the use of a non-motorized treadmill that is instrumented with a load-cell and linked to a computer. Using this system the running speed and horizontal component of force can be captured and the power output of the sprinter calculated (Fig. 2.3; Lakomy 1987). Peak, mean, and end power outputs, as well as a fatigue index, can be calculated for runners during this sprint version of the WAnT procedure. Using this system the power outputs of sprinters and sprint-trained sportsmen and sportswomen have been

determined (Cheetham *et al.* 1985). However, the power output values obtained for trained athletes during sprint running for 30 s are about 150–200 W lower than those obtained during sprint cycling, using the same WAnT procedure (Cheetham *et al.* 1987). The reason for this difference is that during sprint running only the horizontal component of force is used to calculate power output. Furthermore, peak and mean speeds achieved on the sprint treadmill are approximately 80 and 75% of those achieved during 30 s of free running on a track, respectively (Lakomy 1987). What is interesting is that sprinters with the highest peak power outputs in relation to body mass also experience the fastest onset of fatigue (Cheetham *et al.* 1987). Even though the absolute speeds are lower than those achieved during free running, the method provides the opportunity to study the physiological responses to sprinting in a controlled environment (Cheetham *et al.* 1985).

Energy metabolism during sprinting

Because sprinting requires a maximum rate of energy expenditure it must be matched by a rapid rate of energy resynthesis. The terms "anaerobic power" and "anaerobic capacity" are commonly used to describe exercise performances of maximum intensity and brief duration that, of necessity, rely mainly on anaerobic biochemical events to generate energy rapidly.

In biochemical terms, anaerobic power describes the rate of ATP resynthesis by a series of non-oxidative reactions in skeletal muscle. The two principal anaerobic sources for ATP resynthesis are: (i) PCr; and (ii) non-oxidative degradation of glycogen to lactate (anaerobic glycogenolysis). In theory, the maximal anaerobic capacity can be calculated from the size of PCr and glycogen stores in active muscles. In practice, however, not all of the available PCr and glycogen can be used to replace ATP. Nevertheless, biopsy samples taken from quadriceps muscle before and after brief high-intensity exercise provide data for the calculation of the rate of ATP resynthesis; i.e., anaerobic power (Sahlin & Henriksson 1984). For example, when a 6-s maximum sprint was performed on a mechanically-braked

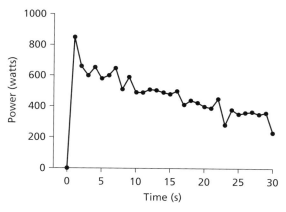

Fig. 2.3 Power output of an athlete during a 30-s maximal sprint on a non-motorized treadmill. (Reproduced with permission from Lakomy 1987.)

cycle ergometer, the rate of ATP resynthesis was calculated to be between 10.4 and 13.4 mmol·kg dry material (dm) $^{-1}$·s^{-1} (Boobis 1987; Gaitanos *et al.* 1993). These values are close to the predicted maximal value of 17 mmol·kg dm^{-1}·s^{-1} for ATP resynthesis in human skeletal muscle (McGilvery 1975). Similarly, estimates of anaerobic capacity can also be made from an analysis of PCr and glycogen stores before and after maximal exercise. Values ranging from 258 to 387 mmol ATP·kg dm^{-1} [60–90 mmol ATP·kg wet weight (ww)$^{-1}$] have been reported in studies using electrical stimulation of skeletal muscle (Spriet *et al.* 1987), single leg exercise (Bangsbo *et al.* 1993), or two leg cycling (Medbo & Tabata 1993).

There are only a few studies on the metabolic responses to 100-m sprinting and even fewer on the responses in multiple-sprint sports. In one study on 100-m sprinting, Hirvonen *et al.* (1987) clearly showed the essential contribution of PCr to energy production. Muscle biopsy samples were obtained from a group of seven sprinters before and after running 100 m as fast as possible, and also before and after completing runs of 40, 60, and 80 m. Half of the resting PCr concentration (21.7 mmol·kg ww^{-1} or 94.3 mmol·kg dm^{-1}) was used during the vigorous warm-up before each race over the intermediate distances. Nevertheless, taken as a whole, the PCr values show that most of this substrate was used during the first 5–6 s of the race (Fig. 2.4).

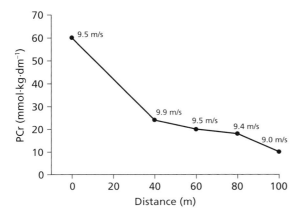

Fig. 2.4 Phosphocreatine (PCr) concentrations in muscle at various running speeds during a simulated 100-m track race. (Reproduced with permission from Hirvonen *et al.* 1987.)

The authors concluded from the constant rate of lactate accumulation that the contribution of glycogenolysis was constant throughout the sprint and that the fall in PCr concentrations was the reason the sprinters were unable to maintain their maximal running speeds for the latter part of the race (Hirvonen *et al.* 1987).

In the absence of additional studies on the metabolic responses to track sprinting, some insight into the metabolic events taking place in skeletal muscles can be obtained from laboratory studies. Using a non-motorized treadmill, Cheetham and colleagues reported that when female games players completed a 30-s sprint, glycolysis contributed 63%, PCr degradation 32%, and ATP depletion 5% to the total ATP production (183.8 mmol·kg dm^{-1}) (Cheetham *et al.* 1986). Muscle lactate increased from 2.7 to 78.0 mmol·kg dm^{-1} and muscle pH decreased from 7.05 to 6.73, whereas blood pH decreased from 7.40 to 7.16. Accompanying these metabolic changes was a four-fold increase in the concentration of plasma catecholamines. Interestingly, the changes in catecholamine concentrations were even higher when a group of ten men performed the same 30-s sprint on a non-motorized treadmill. The men recorded a peak power output of 653 W, whereas the value for the women was 534 W. Plasma norepinephrine and epinephrine concentrations increased from resting values of 2.2 to 13.4 nmol·L^{-1} and 0.2 to 1.4 nmol·L^{-1}, respectively. There was also a two-fold increase in the opioid β-endorphin in response to the 30-s maximal sprint (Brooks *et al.* 1988). Similar metabolic and catecholamine responses to a 30-s sprint were also reported for male and female games players prior to an eight-week sprint training program (Fig. 2.5; Nevill *et al.*, 1989). Another indication of metabolic perturbations during a single 30-s sprint is the significant increase in levels of growth hormone that persist for an hour after this short bout of exercise (Nevill *et al.* 1996). It is important to note that the average distance covered during a 30-s sprint on a non-motorized treadmill is about 160 to 170 m, and so closer to a 200-m rather than a 100-m track race. Nevertheless, the information obtained from these studies provides an insight into the magnitude of the metabolic responses to maximum sprinting.

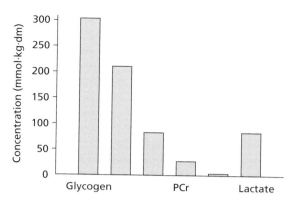

Fig. 2.5 Changes in the concentrations of muscle glycogen, phosphocreatine, and lactate after a 30-s sprint on a non-motorized treadmill. (Reproduced with permission from Nevill *et al.* 1989.)

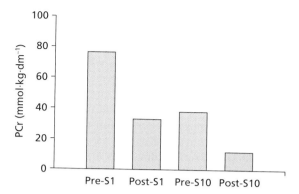

Fig. 2.6 Phosphocreatine concentrations before and after the first and 10th sprint of 6 s duration in a series of 10 sprints. (Reproduced with permission from Gaitanos *et al.* 1993.)

Energy metabolism during multiple sprints

Assessing the metabolic demands during multiple-sprint sports is very difficult because of the obvious practical problems of intervening during match play. At best, information on the metabolic responses of players can only be obtained in "friendly matches" between lower rather than premier division teams (Krustrup *et al.* 2006). In field studies blood lactate measurements are commonly used to give some indication of the contribution of glycogenolysis to energy metabolism during training and competition. However, blood lactate values are only a reflection of the most recent activity. Therefore, in sports where participants perform a range of activities, blood lactate values probably do not provide a true picture of the metabolic events taking place in skeletal muscles (Bangsbo *et al.* 2006). Therefore, in order to gain a better insight into the metabolic events underlying the performance of multiple-sprints we have to rely largely on laboratory studies.

For example, in one such study the changes in power output and muscle metabolites were monitored during ten 6-s maximum sprints on a cycle ergometer, with a 30-s recovery period between sprints. The power output gradually decreased such that during the last sprint it was 33% lower than during the first sprint (Fig. 2.6). There was a significant reduction in the contribution of glycogenolysis and glycolysis to energy production during the

last of the ten sprints. During the last sprint the contribution of PCr was about 80% compared to 50% during the first sprint, but in absolute terms this contribution was significantly smaller (i.e., 25 mmol·kg dm^{-1} vs. 44 mmol·kg dm^{-1}), as was the power output. What was also clear from this study was that the PCr stores were not being replaced during the 30-s recovery between each sprint. The remaining 20% of energy production was provided largely by aerobic metabolism of available carbohydrate and probably also muscle lactate (Gaitanos *et al.* 1993). It is clear from subsequent studies that as the number of sprints increases there is an ever greater contribution from aerobic metabolism to energy production (Balsom *et al.* 1994). Furthermore, there is some evidence to suggest a positive link between aerobic power and the rate of recovery of PCr stores (Bogdanis *et al.* 1996).

Using the same 6-s sprint protocol, the power outputs of sprint-trained sportsmen and women were compared whilst running on a non-motorized treadmill. As might be predicted, the values for the men were significantly greater than for the women. It would be reasonable to suggest that this difference was mainly the result of the greater body mass of the men. However, when the peak power output values were corrected for body mass there were still significant differences between the men and women, but they had similar values for blood lactate, pH, and also for rates of decline in power output, i.e., fatigue index. Interestingly, plasma epinephrine concentrations increased to maximal values after five sprints and were significantly higher for the men (9.2 nmol·L^{-1}) than for the women (3.7 nmol·L^{-1}). In contrast, peak plasma norepinephrine concentrations occurred after ten sprints for the men (31.6 nmol·L^{-1}) and after only five sprints for the women (27.4 nmol·L^{-1}). This information suggests that there are gender differences in the physiological responses to sprinting as there are to prolonged submaximal exercise.

These laboratory studies isolate only segments of the activity patterns that are common in multiple-sprint sports; nevertheless, they help provide some insight into the maximum metabolic demands on the athlete. However, their obvious short-coming is that they do not mimic the actual activity patterns that occur in sport. In an attempt to redress this situation, Nicholas et al. (2000) developed a shuttle running protocol that included many of the activity patterns that are common in sports such as football, rugby, and field hockey. The Loughborough Intermittent Shuttle Running Test (LIST) is based on shuttle running between two lines 20 m apart. The 90-min LIST is composed of six 15-min blocks of activity, with 3-min rest periods between each block. In each 15-min block the participants jog (55% $\dot{V}o_{2max}$), cruise (95% $\dot{V}o_{2max}$), walk, and sprint; this pattern is repeated approximately 11 times. Therefore, in the 90-min LIST each participant completes 66 maximum sprints and each sprint is timed over 15 m. In this test the sub-maximal running speeds are calculated for each participant based on estimated $\dot{V}o_{2max}$ values and are dictated by a computer-generated audio signal; whereas each sprint is performed maximally and timed electronically. The demands of the LIST for acceleration, sprinting, deceleration, and repeated changes of direction have close similarities to the patterns of activity that are common to many team sports.

The distance covered and the physiological responses of sportsmen performing the LIST are similar to the values reported from time and motion analyses of football matches (Nicholas et al. 2000; Krustrup et al. 2006). For example, during the LIST the glycogen concentration decreased from 410 mmol·kg dm^{-1} to 165 mmol·kg dm^{-1} in samples of mixed muscle; however, the decrease measured in type 2 fibers was greater than that in type 1 fibers (Nicholas et al. 1999). The decrease in muscle glycogen concentration recorded for mixed muscle samples was 60% by the end of 90 min. In a study of the metabolic responses of football players during a friendly match, muscle glycogen decreased by 42% (Krustrup et al. 2006). The smaller amount of glycogen used by the football players may be a consequence of the lower exercise intensity and smaller distance covered during the "friendly match." However, the values for muscle and blood lactate concentrations, as well as blood glucose, plasma free fatty acids, and glycerol, were almost identical between the two studies. Collectively these field studies provide an insight into the physiological and metabolic demands of football as one example of a multiple-sprint sport.

Metabolic limitations in sprinting

The inability to maintain speed during the 100-m sprint may be a consequence of a reduction in PCr stores to such low levels that they are unable to replace ATP fast enough to support the high energy expenditure (Hirvonen et al. 1987). Although this substrate depletion probably makes a significant contribution to the fatigue process, there is also a mechanical limitation: the contact time of the foot with the track becomes less as the sprinter reaches maximum speed and so presents a mechanical limitation to sprinting. Therefore, it is even more remarkable that the world's best sprinters are able to maintain their running speed through to the end of the 100-m race.

In longer sprint races, e.g., 400 m, fatigue is more closely associated with a reduction in skeletal muscle PCr stores to critically low concentrations. In one of the few track studies on the metabolic responses to sprinting, Hirvonen et al. (1992) reported PCr concentrations of 1.7 mmol·kg ww^{-1} of muscle (7.3 mmol·kg dm^{-1}) at the end of a 400-m race. These values for mixed muscle samples are similar to those obtained following a 30-s sprint on a non-motorized treadmill. Furthermore, at the end of the 30-s sprint the PCr concentrations in type 1 and type 2 fibers were 12.2 and 5.0 mmol·kg dm^{-1},

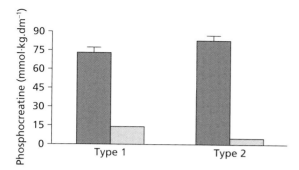

Fig. 2.7 Phosphocreatine concentrations in type 1 and in type 2 muscle fibers before (dark bars) and after (light bars) a 30-s sprint on a non-motorized treadmill. (Reproduced with permission from Greenhaff *et al.* 1992.)

respectively (Fig. 2.7). Muscle glycogen concentration decreased by 27% in the type 2 fibers and by only 20% in type 1 fibers, whereas the ATP content of muscle fibers decreased by only 20% (Greenhaff *et al.* 1992). These values are similar to those obtained following histochemical analysis of glycogen depletion in different muscle fiber populations during 30 s of maximal cycling exercise (Vollestad *et al.* 1992). Therefore, even at the point of fatigue there appears to be sufficient glycogen in both populations of fibers to support energy production during one 30-s bout of maximum exercise.

The explanation for the inability of skeletal muscles to exploit the available substrate for energy production in a single sprint has yet to be established. However, Hultman *et al.* (1987) suggested that when the PCr stores are exhausted, muscle is prevented from generating force by the increasing amounts of hydrogen (H^+), inorganic phosphate (P_i), and even free magnesium (Mg^{2+}) ions – all products of the high rates of energy metabolism in the working muscles (Hultman *et al.* 1987). The authors suggest that the accumulation of these products inhibits cross-bridge recycling between actin and myosin filaments and hence suppresses activation of the contractile system. Therefore, once the PCr stores are insufficient for rapid resynthesis of ATP, the continuing high rate of anaerobic glycogenolysis generates byproducts that not only inhibit glycolysis but, more importantly, prevent the use of the available ATP by impairing the excitation-contraction process.

Regardless of the precise mechanism, it seems clear that when there is a marked reduction in intramuscular PCr stores, even though glycogen is readily available, the glycogen cannot be used quickly enough to sustain the high rates of ATP utilization required for maximum exercise.

Furthermore, low concentrations of PCr and ATP may also induce an increased activity of the purine cycle, leading to a further decrease in the available pool of adenine nucleotides and an increase in ammonia concentrations, first in muscle and later in plasma (Schlicht *et al.* 1990; Tullson & Terjung 1990). It has been postulated that high concentrations of plasma ammonia may contribute to the onset of fatigue by adversely affecting the central nervous system (Banister & Cameron 1990). This may be the case during 400 m running and during repeated shorter sprints in training, but it is probably not a factor during a 100-m race.

In multiple-sprint sports the underlying mechanism for the onset of fatigue is also difficult to explain. At one level there is evidence that inadequate glycogen stores will result in a reduction in the exercise capacity of, for example, football players (Saltin 1973; Krustrup *et al.* 2006). In laboratory studies it appears that the reduction in PCr stores following repeated sprints with inadequate recovery may be a precipitating influence on the process of fatigue. However, in the study of the metabolic responses of football players in a friendly football match Krustrup and colleagues (2006) provided evidence to suggest that the cause of fatigue, i.e., the decrease in sprint speed, may not be low PCr concentrations, high concentrations of ammonia, or an energy crisis in skeletal muscle fibers. Rather, they suggest that greater attention should be directed at the changes in interstitial potassium concentrations (see Chapter 20). Nevertheless, they concluded that the very low concentration of muscle glycogen, and total depletion in some fibers, probably makes the most significant contribution to the onset of fatigue during football matches. Whereas depletion of muscle glycogen stores appears to contribute to overall fatigue during a football match, it does not appear to be the cause of episodes of "transient fatigue" that occur following periods of high-intensity activity (Krustrup *et al.* 2006). Players recover quite quickly from these brief episodes of fatigue, but only when they are followed by a period of low-intensity activity. However, the mechanisms responsible for this phenomenon have yet to be elucidated.

Summary

To the casual observer the 100-m sprint appears to involve only minimal skill, but in reality it is a complex activity involving a host of finely tuned biochemical, neurological, mechanical, and psychological events. Sprinting challenges energy metabolism to replenish ATP in working muscle at the highest possible rates. Limitations to this process are manifest as a reduction in running speed towards the end of the race. The limited available evidence suggests that when the concentrations of PCr in skeletal muscle are reduced during sprinting, then speed also begins to decline because glycogenolysis cannot generate ATP fast enough to cover the energy needs of working muscles. At the elite level, the ability to run at high speeds is an obvious precondition for successful sprinting, but it is not necessarily a determinant of a winning performance. Starting technique and the ability to control form, acceleration, and speed in discrete portions of the race are all important considerations to winning races.

The repeated short sprints that are part of many sports and team games rely heavily on the ability to regenerate PCr rapidly. Failure to repeatedly regenerate PCr in such sports as football, rugby, field hockey, basketball, and tennis leads to underperformance of essential skills and often the difference between winning and losing. A significant reduction in muscle glycogen also contributes to the onset of fatigue during multiple-sprint sports and maybe the most influential contributor to this phenomenon.

References

Abdelkrim, N., El Fazaa, S. & El Ati, J. (2007) Time-motion analysis and physiological data of elite under-19 year old basketball players during competition. *British Journal of Sports Medicine* **41**, 69–75.

Ae, M., Ito, A. & Suzuki, M. (1992) The men's 100 metres. *New Studies in Athletics* **7**, 47–52.

Atwater, A.E. (1982) Kinematic analyses of sprinting. *Track and Field Quarterly Review* **82**, 12–16.

Balsom, P., Seger, J., Sjodin, B. & Ekblom, B. (1992) Maximal-intensity intermittent exercise: effect of recovery duration. *International Journal of Sports Medicine* **13**(7), 528–533.

Balsom, P., Gaitanos, G. & Sjodin, B. (1994) Reduced oxygen availability during high intensity intermittent exercise impairs performance. *Acta Physiologica Scandinavica* **152**, 279–285.

Bangsbo, J., Johansen, L., Graham, T. & Saltin, B. (1993) Lactate and H$^+$ effluxes from human skeletal muscles during intense, dynamic exercise. *Journal of Physiology* **462**, 115–133.

Bangsbo, J., Mohr, M. & Krustrup, P. (2006) Physical and metabolic demands of training and match play in the elite soccer player. *Journal of Sports Science* **24**(7), 665–674.

Banister, E.W. & Cameron, B J.C. (1990) Exercise-induced hyperammonemia: peripheral and central effects. *International Journal of Sports Medicine* **11**(suppl.2), S129–S142.

Bar-Or, O. (1987) The Wingate anaerobic test. An update on methodology, reliability and validity. *Sports Medicine* **4**, 381–394.

Bar-Or, O., Dotan, R. & Inbar, O. (1977) A 30 sec. all out ergometer test-its reliability and validity for anaerobic capacity. *Israel Journal of Medical Sciences* **13**, 126–130.

Barnes, W.S. (1981) Selected physiological characteristics of elite male sprint athletes. *Journal of Sports Medicine and Physical Fitness* **21**, 49–54.

Bogdanis, G., Nevill, M., Boobis, L. & Lakomy, H. (1996) Contribution of phosphocreatine and aerobic metabolism to energy supply during repeated sprint exercise. *Journal of Applied Physiology* **80**, 876–884.

Boobis, L. (1987) Metabolic aspects of fatigue during sprinting. In: *Exercise, Benefits, Limitations and Adaptations* (Macleod, D., Maughan, R., Nimmo, M., Reilly, T. & Williams, C., eds.) E. & F.N. Spon, London: 116–140.

Bouchard, C., Taylor, A. & Dulac, S. (1982) Testing maximal anaerobic power and capacity. In: *Physiological Testing of the Elite Athlete* (MacDougal, J.D., Wenger, H.A. & Green, J.H., eds.) Mutual Press Ltd., Ottawa: 61–74 .

Brooks, S., Burrin, J., Cheetham, M.E., Hall, G.M., Yeo, T. & Williams, C. (1988) The responses of the catecholamines and β-endorphin to brief maximal exercise in man. *European Journal of Applied Physiology* **57**, 230–234.

Casabona, A., Polizzi, M.C. & Perciavalle, V. (1990) Differences in H-reflex between athletes trained for explosive contractions and non-trained subjects. *European Journal of Applied Physiology* **61**, 26–32.

Cheetham, M., Williams, C. & Lakomy, H.K. (1985) A laboratory running test: metabolic responses of sprint and endurance trained athletes. *British Journal of Sports Medicine* **19**, 81–84.

Cheetham, M., Boobis, L., Brooks, S. & Williams, C. (1986) Human muscle metabolism during sprint running. *Journal of Applied Physiology* **61**, 54–60.

Cheetham, M.E., Hazeldine, R.J., Robinson, A. & Williams, C. (1987) Power output of rugby forwards during maximal treadmill sprinting. In: *Science and Football* (Reilly, T., Lees, A., Davids, K. & Murphy, W., eds.) E. & F.N. Spon, London: 206–210.

Costill, D.L., Daniels, J., Evans, W., Fink, W., Krehenbuhl, G. & Saltin, B. (1976) Skeletal muscle enzymes and fiber composition in male and female track athletes. *Journal of Applied Physiology* **40**, 149–154.

Davies, C. (1980) The effects of wind assistance and resistance on the forward motion of a runner. *Journal of Applied Physiology* **48**, 702–709.

Davis, J., Brewer, J. & Atkin, D. (1992) Pre-season physiological characteristics of English first and second division soccer players. *Journal of Sports Science* **10**, 541–547.

Deutsch, M., Kearney, G. & Rehrer, N. (2007) Time-motion analysis of professional rugby union players during match-play. *Journal of Sports Science* **25**, 461–472.

Docherty, D., Wenger, H. & Neary, P. (1988) Time-motion analysis related to the physiological demands of rugby. *Journal of Human Movement Studies* **14**, 269–277.

Drust, B., Cable, N. & Reilly, T. (2000) Investigation of the effects of the pre-cooling on the physiological responses to soccer-specific intermittent exercise. *European Journal of Applied Physiology* **81**, 11–17.

Durant, J. (1961) *Highlights of the Olympics: From Ancient Times to the Present* Arco Publications, London

Duthie, G., Pyne, D. & Hooper, S. (2005) Time motion analysis of 2001 and 2002 Super 12 rugby. *Journal of Sports Science* **23**, 523–530.

Esbjornsson, M., Sylven, C., Holm, I. & Jansson, E. (1993) Fast-twitch fibres may predict anaerobic performance in both females and males. *International Journal of Sports Medicine* **14**, 257–263.

Farrar, M. & Thorland, W. (1987) Relationship between isokinetic strength and sprint times in college age men. *Journal of Sports Medicine and Physical Fitness* **27**, 368–372.

Ferrauti, A., Pluim, B. & Weber, K. (2001) The effect of recovery duration on running speed and stroke quality during intermittent training drills in elite tennis players. *Journal of Sports Science* **19**, 235–242.

Gaitanos, G.C., Williams, C., Boobis, L. & Brooks, S. (1993) Human muscle metabolism during intermittent maximal exercise. *Journal of Applied Physiology* **75**, 712–719.

Greenhaff, P.L., Nevill, M.E., Soderlund, K., Boobis, L., Williams, C. & Hultman, E. (1992) Energy metabolism in single muscle fibres during maximal sprint exercise in man. *Journal of Physiology* **446**, 528P.

Hakkinen, K. & Keskinen, K.L. (1989) Muscle cross-sectional area and voluntary force production characteristics in elite strength and endurance trained athletes and sprinters. *European Journal of Applied Physiology* **59**, 215–220.

Hay, J.G. (1985) *The Biomechanics of Sports* Prentice-Hall, New Jersey.

Hirvonen, J., Rehunen, S., Rusko, H. & Harkonen, M. (1987) Breakdown of high-energy phosphate compounds and lactate accumulation during short supramaximal exercise. *European Journal of Applied Physiology* **56**, 253–259.

Hirvonen, J., Nummela, A., Rusko, H., Rehunen, S. & Harkonen, M. (1992) Fatigue and changes of ATP, creatine phosphate, and lactate during the 400-m sprint. *Canadian Journal of Sport Science* **17**, 141–144.

Hoffman, K. (1972) Stride length and frequency of female sprinters. *Track Technique* **48**, 1522–1524.

Hultman, E., Spriet, L.L. & Sodelund, K. (1987) Energy metabolism and fatigue in working muscle. In: *Exercise, Benefits, Limitations and Adaptations* (Macleod, D., Maughan, R., Nimmo, M., Reilly, T. & Williams, C., eds.) E. & F.N. Spon, London: 63–80.

Koceja, D.M. & Kamen, G. (1988) Conditioned patellar tendon reflexes in sprint and endurance trained athletes. *Medicine and Science in Sports and Exercise* **20**, 172–177.

Khosla, T. (1978) Standards of age, height and weight in Olympic running events for men. *British Journal of Sports Medicine* **12**, 97–101.

Khosla, T. & McBroom, V.C. (1984) The Physique of Female Olympic Finalists: Standards on Age, Height and Weight of 824 Finalists from 47 Events Welsh National School of Medicine, Cardiff.

Krustrup, P., Mohr, M., Steensberg, A., Bencke, J., Kjaer, M. & Bangsbo, J. (2006) Muscle and blood metabolites during a soccer game: implications for sprint performance. *Medicine and Science in Sports and Exercise* **38**, 1165–1174.

Lakomy, H.K.A. (1986) Measurement of work and power output using friction-loaded cycle ergometers. *Ergonomics* **29**, 509–517.

Lakomy, H.K.A. (1987) The use of a non-motorized treadmill for analysing sprint performance. *Ergonomics* **30**, 627–637.

Lawrence, S. & Polglaze, T. (2000) Protocols for the physiological assessment of male and female field hockey players. In: *Physiological Tests for Elite Athletes* (Gore, J., ed.) Human Kinetics, Illinois.

Mahler, P., Mora, C., Gremion, G. & Chantraine, A. (1992) Isotonic muscle evaluation and sprint performance. *Excel* **8**, 139–145.

Maughan, R.J., Watson, J.S. & Weir, J. (1983) Relationship between muscle strength and muscle cross-sectional area in male sprinters and endurance runners. *European Journal of Applied Physiology* **50**, 309–318.

McGilvery, R. (1975) The use of fuels for muscular work. In: *Metabolic Adaptation to Prolonged Physical Exercise* (Howald, H. & Poortmans, J., eds.) Birkhauser Verlag, Basel: 119–126.

Medbo, J. & Tabata, I. (1993) Anaerobic energy release in working muscle during 30 s to 3 min of exhausting bicycling. *Journal of Applied Physiology* **75**(4), 1654–1660.

Mohr, M., Krustrup, P. & Bangsbo, J. (2005) Fatigue in soccer: A brief review. *Journal of Sports Sciences* **23**, 593–599.

Moravec, P., Ruzicka, J., Susanka, P., Dostal, M., Kodejs, M. & Norsek, M. (1988) The 1987 International Athletic Foundation/IAAF scientific project report: time analysis of the 100 metres events at the II World Championships in Athletics. *New Studies in Athletics* **3**, 61–96.

Morris, J., Nevill, M. & Williams, C. (2000) Physiological and metabolic responses of female games and endurance athletes to prolonged, intermittent, high intensity running at 30°C and 16°C ambient temperatures. *European Journal of Applied Physiology* **81**, 84–92.

Morris, J., Nevill, M., Boobis, L., MacDonald, I. & Williams, C. (2005) Muscle metabolism, temperature, and function during prolonged intermittent high intensity running in air temperatures of 33°C and 17°C. *International Journal of Sports Medicine* **26**, 805–814.

Mureika, J. (2001) A realistic quasi-physical model for the 100 m dash. *Canadian Journal of Physiology* **79**, 697–713.

Neuman, G. (1988) Special performance capacity. In: *The Olympic Book of Sports Medicine* (Dirix, A., Knuttgen, H.G. & Tittel, K., eds.) Blackwell Scientific Publications, Oxford.

Nevill, M., Boobis, L., Brooks, S. & Williams, C. (1989) Effect of training on muscle metabolism during treadmill sprinting. *Journal of Applied Physiology* **67**, 2376–2382.

Nevill, M., Homyard, D., Hall, G., Allsop, P., van Oosterhout, A., Burrin, J. *et al.* (1996) Growth hormone responses to treadmill sprinting in sprint- and endurance trained athletes. *European Journal of Applied Physiology* **72**, 460–467.

Nicholas, C. (1997) Anthropometric and physiological characteristics of rugby union fooball players. *Sports Medicine* **23**, 375–396.

Nicholas, C., Nuttall, F. & Williams, C. (2000) The Loughborough Intermittent Shuttle Test: A field test that simulates the activity pattern of soccer. *Journal of Sports Science* **18**, 97–104.

Nicholas, C., Williams, C., Boobis, L. & Little, N. (1999) Effect of ingesting a carbohydrate-electrolyte beverage on muscle glycogen utilisation during high intensity, intermittent shuttle running. *Medicine and Science in Sports and Exercise* **31**, 1280–1286.

Ostojic, S., Mazic, S. & Dikic, N. (2006) Profiling in basketball: physical and physiological characteristics of elite players. *Journal of Strength and Conditioning Research* **20**, 740–744.

Pain, M. & Hibbs, A. (2007) Sprint starts and the minimum auditory reaction time. *Journal of Sports Sciences* **25**, 79–86.

Radford, P.F. (1990) Sprinting. In: *Physiology of Sports* (Reilly, T., Secher, N., Snell, P. & Williams, C., eds.) E. & F.N. Spon, London: 71–99.

Reilly, T. (2000) The physiological demands of soccer. In: *Soccer and Science* (Bangsbo, J., ed.) Munksgaard, Denmark: 91–106.

Sadoyama, T., Masuda, T., Miyata, H. & Katsuta, S. (1988) Fibre conduction velocity and fibre composition in human vastus lateralis. *European Journal of Applied Physiology* **57**, 767–771.

Sahlin, K. & Henriksson, J. (1984) Buffer capacity and lactate accumulation in skeletal muscle of trained and untrained men. *Acta Physiologica Scandinavica* **122**, 331–339.

Saltin, B. (1973) Metabolic fundamentals of exercise. *Medicine and Science in Sports and Exercise* **15**, 366–369.

Schlicht, W., Naretz, W., Witt, D. & Rieckert, H. (1990) Ammonia and lactate: differential information on monitoring training load in sprint events. *International Journal of Sports Medicine* **11**(suppl.2), S85–S90.

Spencer, M., Lawrence, S., Rechichi, C., Bishop, D., Dawson, B. & Goodman, C. (2004) Time-motion analysis of elite field hockey, with special reference to repeated-sprint activity. *Journal of Sports Sciences* **22**, 843–850.

Spencer, M., Bishop, D., Dawson, B. & Goodman, C. (2005) Physiological and metabolic responses of repeated-sprint activities. *Sports Medicine* **35**, 1025–1044.

Spriet, L.L., Soderlund, K., Bergstrom, K. & Hultman, E. (1987) Anaerobic energy release in skeletal muscle during electrical stimulation in men. *Journal of Applied Physiology* **62**, 611–615.

Tanner, J. (1964) *The Physique of the Olympic Athlete* George Allen and Unwin Ltd., London.

Tesch, P.A. (1992) Short and long term histochemical and biochemical adaptations in muscle. In: *Strength and Power in Sport* (Komi, P.V., ed.) Blackwell Scientific Publications, Oxford: 239–248.

Tesch, P. & Karlsson, J. (1985) Muscle fibre types and size in trained and untrained muscles of elite athletes. *Journal of Applied Physiology* **59**, 1716–1720.

Thorstensson, A., Larsson, L., Tesch, P.A. & Karlsson, J. (1977) Muscle strength and fibre composition in elite athletes and sedentary men. *Medicine and Science in Sports and Exercise* **9**, 26–30.

Tullson, P.C. & Terjung, R.L. (1990) Adenine nucleotide degradation in striated muscle. *International Journal of Sports Medicine* **11**(suppl.2), S47–S55.

Vollestad, N.K., Tabata, I. & Medbo, J.I. (1992) Glycogen breakdown in different human muscle fiber types during exhaustive exercise of short duration. *Acta Physiologica Scandinavica* **144**, 135–141.

Weber, K., Pieper, S. & Exler, T. (2007) Characteristics and significance of running speed at the Australian Open 2006 for training and injury prevention. *Medicine and Science in Tennis* **12**, 14–17.

Chapter 3

Physiological Demands of Endurance Exercise

ANDREW M. JONES AND DAVID C. POOLE

Exactly what constitutes "endurance exercise" eludes simple definition but incorporates "staying power," "continuance," and "suffering patiently without sinking" (Chambers 1965). In athletics, all the track events including and beyond the 800 m race are typically referred to as endurance events, and yet the "type" of endurance required for 800 m running is quite clearly very different from that required for marathon running. It might be suggested that endurance exercise encompasses all those (usually continuous) sports events or physical activities that rely predominantly on oxidative metabolism for energy supply, provided that they are sustained for a "sufficiently" long period of time (e.g., ≥90 s during high intensity exercise, and ≥10 min during submaximal exercise).

It is now widely accepted that endurance performance is associated with a number of "parameters" of aerobic fitness including the maximal oxygen uptake ($\dot{V}O_{2max}$), the economy or efficiency with which submaximal exercise can be performed, and the fraction of the $\dot{V}O_{2max}$ that can be sustained for different durations (Coyle 1995). The last is associated with the degree of blood lactate accumulation during exercise, for which a plethora of terms exists including lactate threshold, lactate turn-point, maximal lactate steady state, onset of blood lactate accumulation, gas exchange threshold, and ventilatory threshold (Jones & Doust 2001). The relative "weighting" of these (and other) factors in the determination of

endurance performance will, of course, depend upon the distance or duration of the event or activity. Shorter events, which will be performed at a higher average intensity, will typically depend more upon the $\dot{V}O_{2max}$ as well as other factors perhaps including the so-called "anaerobic capacity," whereas in longer events, performed at a lower average intensity, the exercise economy and fractional utilization of the $\dot{V}O_{2max}$ become increasingly important. The speed with which $\dot{V}O_2$ rises towards the steady state ($\dot{V}O_2$ kinetics) will determine, in part, the magnitude of the O_2 deficit and the degree to which non-oxidative metabolic processes are activated, and this is likely another important physiological determinant of endurance exercise performance (Jones & Poole 2005). Ultimately, it is the interaction of these factors that will determine the success with which the event or activity can be performed (Coyle 1995; Jones & Doust 2001).

This chapter attempts to provide a fresh approach to an established topic by focusing on the physiological demands of endurance exercise from an oxygen (O_2) transport and utilization perspective. Specifically, within the relevant exercise-intensity domain(s), those factors that determine the oxygen requirement (i.e., the running velocity or power output, oxygen uptake [$\dot{V}O_2$] kinetics, and economy) will be balanced with the structural and functional requirements for achieving and sustaining the prodigious O_2 fluxes demanded by superlative endurance performance. Novel discoveries regarding microvascular regulation among different muscle fiber types are introduced to complement and extend more established aspects of cardiovascular and metabolic

The Olympic Textbook of Science in Sport, 1st edition. Edited by R.J. Maughan. Published 2009 by Blackwell Publishing. ISBN: 978-1-4051-5638-7.

control within the context of the elite endurance athlete.

Progressing logically through three sections, this chapter builds upon basic physiological principles and novel experimental findings to construct a comprehensive picture of the endurance athlete as follows:

1 *Requirements:* frames conceptually the so-called exercise intensity "domains" and the pertinent fatigue mechanisms that form an upper limit to human energy expenditure;

2 *Physiological responses:* presents the coordinated response of the pulmonary–cardiovascular–muscular systems required to fulfill these energetic demands by moving O_2 to the muscle capillary and addresses the challenges faced at the final frontier (i.e., the movement of O_2 from the red blood cell to the mitochondria);

3 *World's best:* examines the physiology of Paula Radcliffe (PR), World Record holder in the women's marathon, and addresses how her unique physiology enables her to achieve the pinnacle of endurance performance.

Requirements

The relationship between running speed or power output and time-to-fatigue is characterized by a rectangular hyperbola as depicted in Fig. 3.1. This figure is useful because it conflates physical performance with the underlying physiological determinants of that performance. The curve itself comprises two components that define the sustainable limit of exercise tolerance at severe intensities (Poole *et al.* 1988; Jones & Carter 2000; Smith & Jones 2001). Thus, for fatiguing exercise, the time-to-fatigue (t_{lim}) will be set by the proximity of running velocity (V) to the asymptote (the critical velocity [CV], or critical power [CP]) and the absolute size of the energy store component (W′) within the exercising muscles, such that $t_{lim} = W'/(V–CV)$. The CV component represents the highest rate of energy expenditure sustainable without drawing continuously on W′, and hence exercise at this velocity can be continued for a prolonged period until, for example, muscle glycogen stores are depleted (Hultman & Greenhaff 1991; Schulman & Rothman 2001). In contrast, veloc-

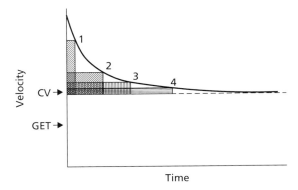

Fig. 3.1 Velocity–time (V–t) relationship for high intensity fatiguing running in non-highly trained individuals. The curve is constructed by having the individual run on four or more occasions (1–4, each separated by at least 1 day) at a constant speed to reach exhaustion within 2–20 min. The asymptote parameter of the relationship is critical velocity (CV, which denotes the maximum velocity that can be sustained for a prolonged period) and the curvature parameter is termed W′, which represents a finite and constant intramuscular energy store. Fatigue ensues when that store is depleted. Notice that, for each bout, the area of the rectangle – which denotes energy – is the same. GET denotes the gas exchange threshold as determined during separate ramp or incremental exercise testing and occurs at a speed and $\dot{V}o_2$ substantially below CV.

ities above CV result in inexorable depletion of W′ at a rate proportional to V–CV. Notice that in Fig. 3.1, which represents data from healthy but not highly trained individuals, the CV is located considerably above (i.e., at a higher running velocity) the gas exchange threshold (GET). The range of metabolic rates bounded by the GET at the lower end and the CV at the upper end constitutes the domain of heavy exercise, whereas that below the GET has been termed moderate exercise. With endurance training, the $\dot{V}o_{2max}$ increases and the GET and CV (or CP) are both elevated but disproportionately to one another and also to $\dot{V}o_{2max}$ such that the range of running velocities (and thus metabolic rates) in the heavy and severe domains becomes reduced (Poole *et al.* 1990; Jones & Carter 2000).

CV thus represents a demarcation between the domains of heavy and severe intensity exercise, each of which elicit distinctive metabolic responses (gas exchange, acid–base) (Fig. 3.2; Poole *et al.* 1988).

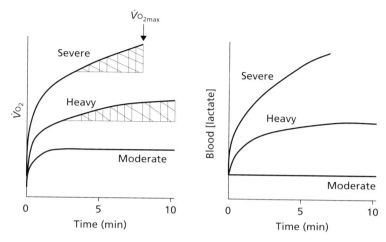

Fig. 3.2 Metabolic ($\dot{V}o_2$ and blood lactate) responses to constant-load exercise performed in the moderate, heavy, and severe intensity domains. Moderate exercise is characterized by a mono-exponential $\dot{V}o_2$ response that reaches an asymptote within 2–3 min, and blood lactate remains close to resting values. Heavy exercise evinces a slow component of the $\dot{V}o_2$ response that is superimposed upon the rapid exponential response seen at exercise onset (hatched area). The slow component delays attainment of a steady state (at submaximal $\dot{V}o_2$) and elevates $\dot{V}o_2$ above that predicted from the $\dot{V}o_{2m}$–velocity or $\dot{V}o_{2m}$–power relationship determined during ramp or incremental ergometry. Blood lactate increases substantially above resting values but reaches steady, but elevated, levels at approximately the same time as $\dot{V}o_2$ reaches its steady state – for most individuals. Severe exercise causes both $\dot{V}o_2$ and blood lactate to increase inexorably towards their maximum values which may be attained before ($\dot{V}o_{2max}$) or after (lactate) fatigue ensues. Arrow denotes both $\dot{V}o_2$ and the point of fatigue for this example. Note that there is a substantial slow component that drives $\dot{V}o_{2max}$ to $\dot{V}o_{2max}$. Thus, the severe exercise intensity domain constitutes a broad range of exercise challenges that will all engender $\dot{V}o_{2max}$ if sustained for sufficient time.

Fatigue at exercise intensities above CV is characterized by low intramuscular pH and creatine phosphate concentration (PCr) and high levels of diprotonated inorganic phosphate ($H_2PO_4^-$) – all of which have been implicated in the fatigue process (Wilson *et al.* 1988; Hultman & Greenhaff 1991; Karatzaferi *et al.* 2001; for CP, Jones *et al.* 2008). The W' component expended in the severe (but not heavy) intensity domain is comprised of energy derived from intramuscular PCr stores and anaerobic glycolysis as well as a small contribution from oxygen stores and is closely analogous to the "anaerobic work capacity" (Poole *et al.* 1988). The magnitude of W' will be strongly influenced by the muscle mass recruited and also the predominant fiber type because the latter determines the size of the PCr stores, the glycolytic potential, and the O_2 stores. As illustrated in Fig. 3.2, severe exercise is characterized by the absence of a $\dot{V}o_2$ or blood lactate steady state. Rather, $\dot{V}o_2$ proceeds inexorably to $\dot{V}o_{2max}$ and blood lactate

increases until exercise is terminated (Poole *et al.* 1988). These profiles contrast sharply with those for exercise in the heavy intensity domain where both $\dot{V}o_2$ and blood lactate can achieve delayed steady state conditions. Consequently, CV also approximates the so-called maximal lactate steady state (Poole *et al.* 1988; Jones & Carter 2000).

From Fig. 3.1 it is evident that one of the energetic challenges facing the endurance athlete is how to maximize running velocity without depleting W' to the extent that it causes premature fatigue during the race. The adenosine triphosphate (ATP) requirement for sustained exercise is so substantial that, if ATP were not reconstituted, the quantity expended during the course of the marathon would weigh more than the athletes themselves! Obviously, oxidative phosphorylation and energetic buffering of ATP turnover are essential to maintain intracellular ATP concentrations close to resting. Where excursions into the severe domain occur, the sum total of these must neither expend W' nor result in intracellular perturbations (i.e., $\uparrow H^+$, $\uparrow H_2PO_4^-$, $\downarrow PCr$) that compromise subsequent muscle function. From the American College of Sports Medicine (ACSM) guidelines (1991) for exercise testing and prescription, it can be calculated that running a 2 h 15 min 25 s marathon (PR's World Record time) on a flat surface, which entails maintaining an average pace of 311.6 $m \cdot min^{-1}$, would require a $\dot{V}o_2$ of 3.14 and 4.39 $L \cdot min^{-1}$ for a 50 and a 70 kg runner, respectively. These values may overestimate those for some elite distance runners because running economy would be expected to be greater in such individuals (see pp. 49–50). However, marathon courses deviate substantially from the level running considered in the ACSM guidelines and this in itself would incur an additional O_2 cost not apparent in the above calculations. The coordinated pattern of physiological responses that facilitate achievement and maintenance of these prodigious O_2 fluxes from atmosphere to mitochondria is discussed below.

Physiological responses

$\dot{V}o_2$ kinetics

At the immediate onset of exercise there is a coordinated pulmonary–cardiovascular–muscle response that serves to move O_2 from the atmosphere to the mitochondria of the exercising muscles (Fig. 3.3).

Heart rate and minute ventilation begin accelerating with minimal inertia (<1 s, 1 breath), elevating cardiac output and pulmonary gas exchange and supplying oxygenated blood to the contracting muscles (Jones & Poole 2005). Within contracting muscles, vasodilatation and muscle pump activity increase vascular conductance and provide the muscle fibers with at least sufficient O_2 to meet their needs. Indeed, there is evidence that muscle O_2 supply may exceed $\dot{V}o_2$ demands at least for the first few seconds of exercise (Grassi et al. 1996; Bangsbo et al. 2000; Behnke et al. 2002) and thus the $\dot{V}o_2$ kinetics are believed to be limited by an oxidative enzyme inertia and not O_2 supply (Jones & Poole 2005).

The effect of this coordinated function is that O_2 pressures ($Pmvo_2$) within the microcirculation of slow (but not fast; Behnke et al. 2003; McDonough et al. 2005) twitch fibers are maintained close to resting values for 10–20 s, allowing muscle $\dot{V}o_2$ to increase exponentially from exercise onset with essentially no delay. The speed or kinetics of that exponential increase is critical because, as ATP requirements are believed to be elevated as a step function, slower $\dot{V}o_2$ kinetics will elevate the muscle O_2 deficit and exacerbate intracellular perturbations (i.e., $\uparrow H^+$, $\uparrow H_2PO_4^-$, $\downarrow PCr$, $\uparrow ADP_{free}$). In turn, these perturbations act to accelerate glycolysis and the use of the finite glycogen stores with consequent negative implications for muscle function. It should also be appreciated that the effects of this phenomenon are

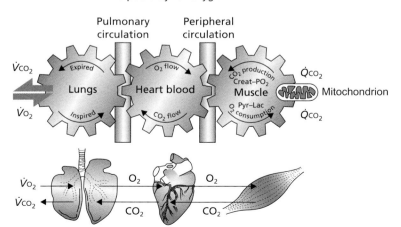

The pathway for oxygen

Fig. 3.3 Depiction of the O_2 transport pathway consisting of a series of interconnected cogs representing the respiratory–cardiovascular–muscle coupling that must occur to effectively support muscle oxidative metabolism during exercise. Given the complexity of the mechanisms involved it is remarkable that, at exercise onset, $\dot{V}o_2$ in endurance athletes increases with a time constant of as little as 8–10 s. In contrast, cardiopulmonary diseases such as chronic obstructive pulmonary disease (COPD) and heart failure as well as diabetes may slow the $\dot{V}o_2$ time constant to 70 s or more.

not restricted to the initial exercise period; they "set" the conditions that exist for the duration of exercise at a given $\dot{V}_{O_2}$. Accordingly, athletes with very fast $\dot{V}_{O_2}$ kinetics (see pp. 51–52) possess a distinct advantage over those with a more sluggish response. The O_2 deficit can be estimated as the product of the $\dot{V}_{O_2}$ time constant (τ) in minutes and the increased (i.e., Δ) $\dot{V}_{O_2}$ from baseline to steady state: O_2 deficit (L) $= \tau \times \Delta \dot{V}_{O_2}$ (i.e., in Fig. 3.2 the area encompassed by a horizontal line projected back to the Y-axis from the end-exercise $\dot{V}_{O_2}$ and the actual $\dot{V}_{O_2}$ profile). It is also pertinent that slower $\dot{V}_{O_2}$ kinetics and their intramuscular consequences may exacerbate the $\dot{V}_{O_2}$ slow component that attends heavy and severe exercise and thereby increase the $\dot{V}_{O_2}$ demands of exercise performed in these domains. There is thus the clear and compelling mandate for endurance athletes to possess very fast $\dot{V}_{O_2}$ kinetics.

O_2 delivery to the exercising muscles

Elite human endurance athletes who can achieve $\dot{V}_{O_{2max}}$ values of over 5–6 L·min^{-1} must achieve cardiac outputs well in excess of 30 L·min^{-1} to deliver the O_2 to the exercising muscles (Fig. 3.4). One consequence of a very high cardiac output is that, because the lung only has a finite (and small) capillary volume, the pulmonary capillary red blood cell transit time may become so short that O_2 loading is limited (diffusion limitation) and athletes,

in particular, experience exercise-induced arterial hypoxemia (EIAH; Powers *et al.* 1989). An extreme example of this phenomenon is the thoroughbred racehorse which has been subjected to many generations of selective breeding. Today the thoroughbred racehorse is endowed with a heart size in excess of 1% of its body mass and a maximum cardiac output approaching 1 L·kg^{-1}·min^{-1}. It is this enormous cardiac output that reduces pulmonary capillary red blood cell transit time and helps drive arterial P_{O_2} below 60 mmHg during maximal exercise (hemoglobin saturation <85%; Poole & Erickson 2004). Despite the greater tendency for individuals (particularly women) with high $\dot{V}_{O_{2max}}$ values to experience EIAH, the arterial O_2 content is relatively well maintained (hemoglobin saturation >85%; Powers *et al.* 1989; Harms *et al.* 1998). Notwithstanding the propensity for athletes to experience EIAH and therefore reduced muscle inflowing arterial O_2 pressures (P_{O_2}), which may lower muscle oxygenation (Legrand *et al.* 2005), it is the O_2 extraction by muscle (i.e., blood–myocyte O_2 flux) that fuels mitochondrial ATP regeneration and is thus the focus of our interest for this chapter.

O_2 extraction within the exercising muscles

As shown in Fig. 3.4(a), the rate of muscle blood flow increase above rest is 5–6 times that of $\dot{V}_{O_2}$ (Poole 1997). This relationship dictates that O_2 extraction

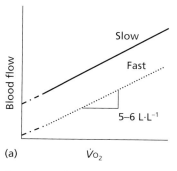
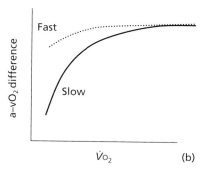

(a)   (b)

Fig. 3.4 (a) Quantitative relationship between blood flow (Q) and $\dot{V}_{O_2}$ from rest to maximal exercise. (b) Arterial minus venous O_2 content difference (a–vO_2 difference) as a function of $\dot{V}_{O_2}$. The hyperbolic nature of the a–vO_2 difference arises as a function of the positive *y*-intercept and the proportional subsequent increase in Q as a function of $\dot{V}_{O_2}$ (see text for more details). Note that the intercept is far lower for fast-twitch than slow-twitch fibers and this will result in a far greater a–vO_2 difference at rest and thus less room for a further increase with elevated $\dot{V}_{O_2}$. This behavior underlies the very low microvascular O_2 driving pressures present at the onset of contractions in the microvasculature of fast-twitch fibers (Fig. 3.5) and helps explain why such fibers would evince slow $\dot{V}_{O_2}$ kinetics and be disadvantageous to the endurance athlete.

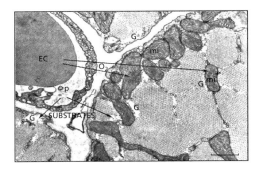

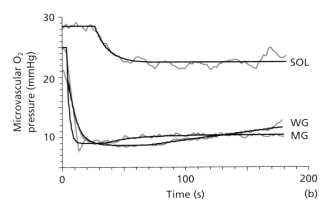

(a)

(b)

Fig. 3.5 (a) Anatomic perspective of blood–myocyte O_2 flux that is driven exclusively by the microvascular O_2 pressure (PmvO_2) from the erythrocyte (EC) to the mitochondria (mi) (Weibel 1984). (b) Microvascular O_2 pressures (PmvO_2) at the onset of 1 Hz contractions in rat soleus (slow-twitch) and medial (fast oxidative glycolytic) and white (fast glycolytic) gastrocnemius muscles measured by phosphorescence quenching (McDonough *et al*. 2005).

(arterial minus venous O_2 content, a–v$O_{2difference}$) must increase hyperbolically as a function of $\dot{V}o_2$ (in L·min^{-1}) according to the approximate equation: a–vO_2 difference (mL·100 mL^{-1}) = $(20 \times \dot{V}o_2)/(1 + \dot{V}o_2)$ (Fig. 3.4b). As demonstrated by Ferreira *et al*. (2006), this relationship is constant across fiber types but because resting blood flow is much higher in slow-twitch than fast-twitch muscle fibers, O_2 extraction is much higher at rest in fast-twitch fibers and therefore increases less with exercise compared with that observed for slow-twitch fibers. One consequence of this inter-fiber type behavior is that microvascular Po_2 is lower at rest and falls more rapidly in muscles or muscle parts comprised of fast-twitch fibers (Fig. 3.5b; Behnke *et al*. 2003; McDonough *et al*. 2005). Given that lower microvascular Po_2 dictates a decreased intracellular Po_2 and lowered energetic steady state, it is quite possible that the enhanced glycolysis characteristic of fast-twitch fibers results, in part, from the decreased microvascular Po_2 to which they are subjected. Notice from Fig. 3.4 that the higher the $\dot{V}o_2$, the greater will be the O_2 extraction and therefore the lower will be the microvascular Po_2. Hence, all else being equal, the fitter the athlete and the greater the $\dot{V}o_2$ achieved either at maximum or some percentage thereof (e.g., CV), the lower will be the microvascular Po_2 that they will have to endure.

In balancing the O_2 delivery vs. O_2 extraction capabilities of skeletal muscle, the insightful conflation

of the Fick principle with Fick's law as proposed initially by Peter Wagner is valuable. In Fig. 3.6 it is demonstrated that $\dot{V}o_{2max}$ occupies the unique inter-section between muscle conductive O_2 delivery (Fick principle) and a finite O_2 diffusing capacity (Fick's law) (Roca *et al*. 1992). This relationship helps explain the residual O_2 remaining in the venous blood by considering the finite diffusing capacity of muscle. For the athlete with a prodigious capacity to deliver O_2 to the working muscles, those muscles must possess an equivalently spectacular O_2 diffusing capacity or microvascular Po_2 will have to rise and fractional O_2 extraction fall (Fig. 3.6a; Roca *et al*. 1992). The microvascular determinants of O_2 delivery and muscle diffusing capacity are discussed briefly below.

Determinants of blood–myocyte O_2 flux

It is intuitive that the ability to deliver O_2 to muscle is the product of blood flow and O_2 content. What is not intuitive is how the individual red blood cells (RBCs) are distributed within the microcirculation and how their behavior affects muscle O_2 diffusing capacity. For example, the highly tortuous and branched capillaries of skeletal muscle are lined with a fuzzy coat of sugar moieties termed the glycocalyx. This glycocalyx retards plasma flow along the capillary walls such that, in resting muscle, the RBCs may have a mean velocity three or more times

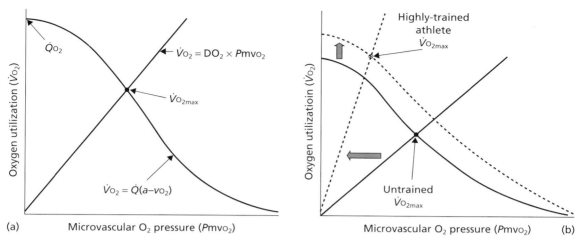

Fig. 3.6 (a) Schematic demonstrating the determination of maximal muscle O_2 uptake ($\dot{V}O_{2max}$) by muscle conductive ($\dot{Q}O_2$, upper y-axis intercept) and diffusive (DO_2) movement of O_2 by the cardiovascular and muscle microcirculatory systems. Curved line denotes mass balance according to the Fick principle ($\dot{V}O_2 = \dot{Q}(a - vo_{2difference})$) where $\dot{Q}$ is muscle blood flow and a and v are the arterial and venous O_2 concentrations, respectively, and the straight line from the origin (of slope DO_2, effective diffusing capacity) represents Fick's law of diffusion. Thus, $\dot{V}O_2 = DO_2 \times Pm vo_2$ (where intramyocyte Po_2 is assumed close to $0\,mmHg$ and ignored). $Pm vo_2$ is the mean O_2 partial pressure in the microvascular compartment. $\dot{V}O_{2max}$ occurs at the intersection of the two lines. For the purposes of this illustration $Pm vo_2$ is considered broadly analogous to venous values. (b) Note that the highly-trained athlete (dashed lines and hollow circle) has an elevated $\dot{V}O_{2max}$ compared to that of an untrained individual (solid line and circle). The elevation of $\dot{V}O_{2max}$ results from a combination of increased $\dot{Q}O_2$ and DO_2 and also note that $Pm vo_2$ falls to lower values as the athlete extracts a greater percentage of the O_2 delivered ($\dot{Q}O_2$).

that of the plasma. This effectively reduces the capillary hematocrit to less than one-third of systemic and, because plasma has a very low O_2 solubility, the muscle O_2 diffusing capacity is reduced in proportion to the number of RBCs adjacent to the myocytes at any given instant (Klitzman & Duling 1979). Hence, irrespective of the capillary : fiber ratio, capillary density or even the capillary–fiber surface contact, capillary hematocrit largely dictates muscle O_2 diffusing capacity (Federspiel & Popel 1986). During hyperemic states such as muscle contraction, animal investigations indicate that capillary hematocrit may rise towards systemic values. Unfortunately, current technology cannot resolve capillary hematocrit in human muscle. Moreover, it is commonly asserted that the muscle capillary neogenesis that accompanies endurance training is important for ensuring that capillary RBC transit time does not fall consequent to the elevated muscle blood flow found at high to maximal metabolic rates. Whether this is, in fact, true cannot at present be educed. It is pertinent that at the highest muscle blood flows yet measured in

humans ($\sim 4\,L \cdot kg^{-1} \cdot min^{-1}$), which produced estimated mean capillary RBC transit times $\leq 0.3\,s$ – thought at one time to be limiting for O_2 offloading – fractional O_2 extraction approached 85% (Richardson et al. 1994). This percentage extraction is close to that observed for maximal exercise conditions with much lower blood flows (Richardson et al. 1994), suggesting that very short capillary RBC transit times may not be as limiting to O_2 offloading as was once believed. However, short capillary RBC transit times will increase the rate of O_2 flux per RBC (i.e., O_2 flux density), which will mandate a greater fall in intramyocyte Po_2 and thus potentially stimulate glycolysis and accelerate glycogen depletion. Hence, all else being equal, at the same muscle blood flow and $\dot{V}O_2$, it would be advantageous to maximize capillary RBC transit time by either increasing capillary volume per volume of muscle (by growing new capillaries) and/or increasing capillary hematocrit. In this regard it is pertinent that endurance trained athletes have a substantially higher capillary : fiber ratio compared to their untrained counterparts (Ingjer & Brodal 1978).

As highlighted above, there are many uncertainties regarding what happens in the microcirculation of human athletes during heavy or severe intensity exercise. What is evident, however, is that very highly trained humans achieve and sustain high muscle conductive (blood flow >20 L·min^{-1}, O_2 delivery >4 L·min^{-1}) and diffusive O_2 fluxes during competition and that they do this without lowering the microvascular O_2 pressures to the extent that it constrains intracellular oxidative metabolism sufficiently to impair performance.

World's best

$\dot{V}o_{2max}$ and exercise economy

In most endurance sports events, the objective is to cover a certain distance in the shortest possible time (or in a shorter time than the other competitors). This will necessarily involve sustaining the highest possible average speed throughout the event. The higher the exercise speed, the higher is the metabolic rate (and hence $\dot{V}o_2$) required to sustain that speed. For this reason, a high $\dot{V}o_{2max}$ value (in L·min^{-1} in activities where the body weight is supported such as swimming, rowing, and cycling on flat terrain, and in mL·min^{-1}·kg^{-1} in activities where the body weight has to be carried such as in running and cycling on hilly terrain) is often considered to be a prerequisite for success in endurance sports. For example, in the laboratory, assuming a Δ efficiency value of 10 mL·min^{-1}·W^{-1} during cycle ergometry, a power output of 300 W will require, in the steady state, a $\dot{V}o_2$ of 3 L·min^{-1} above that measured during "unloaded" pedalling at the same cadence, whereas a power output of 400 W will require a $\dot{V}o_2$ of 4 L·min^{-1}, and so on. Clearly, in this example, a higher $\dot{V}o_{2max}$ would permit the attainment of a higher power output which, all else being equal including the aerodynamics of the bicycle and rider during outdoor cycling, should translate into a faster speed over the ground. The possession of a high $\dot{V}o_{2max}$ value would also mean that any absolute submaximal power output would require a lower fraction of the $\dot{V}o_{2max}$ relative to other competitors, which in itself could be beneficial. It is not surprising, therefore, that elite endurance athletes have remarkably high $\dot{V}o_{2max}$ values; values of ~6 L·min^{-1} in a World Class

male rower (Godfrey et al. 2005), ~90 mL·min^{-1}·kg^{-1} in a World Class male cyclist (Coyle 2005), and ~80 mL·min^{-1}·kg^{-1} in a World Class female distance runner (Jones 2006) have been reported.

From the above, it might be assumed that the athlete who can sustain the highest metabolic rate throughout an endurance sport event would inevitably be the winner. However, such an assumption is confounded by the fact that the energy (and hence O_2) cost of exercise at a certain speed or power output can exhibit considerable interindividual variability (i.e., some individuals are more economical than others). The extent of this variability in the O_2 cost of exercise is related to the "technicality" of the exercise mode. For example, interindividual variability in the O_2 cost of exercise is generally less during cycle ergometry than during more technically "complex" activities such as swimming or running. This reflects the fact that interindividual differences in economy are related to physiological, anatomic, biomechanical, and technical factors (Jones & Carter 2000). During treadmill running, the $\dot{V}o_2$ while running at a speed of 16 km·h^{-1} can range from as low as 44 mL·min^{-1}·kg^{-1} to as high as 58 mL·min^{-1}·kg^{-1} (i.e., a difference of around 30%) in well-trained runners. In cycle ergometry, the Δ efficiency can also vary, although usually within a more narrow range (i.e., between ~9 and ~11 mL·min^{-1}·W^{-1}). Notwithstanding this interindividual variability, economy and/or efficiency is generally better the higher the standard of the athlete (Morgan et al. 1995; cf. Moseley et al. 2004).

Although it is the interplay between an athlete's economy and/or efficiency characteristics and their $\dot{V}o_{2max}$ that will, in part, determine athletic performance, improved exercise economy and/or efficiency, per se, can be considered beneficial to the athlete. Biomechanical factors are likely to have a key role in determining the efficiency of locomotion. However, from a physiological perspective, improved economy and efficiency might reflect a reduction in the ATP turnover rate required to generate a given muscle power output, a reduction in the O_2 consumed for the same muscle ATP turnover rate (i.e., a higher P : O ratio), or both. Other factors such as a reduction in the resting metabolic rate or a reduced O_2 cost of cardiac or respiratory muscle work might also contribute to improvements in economy or efficiency.

At the muscle level, fiber type distribution and motor unit recruitment patterns during exercise have been speculated to have a role in the determination of individual economy characteristics because it is known that type 2 or "fast-twitch" muscle fibers have both a higher phosphate energy cost of muscle contraction and a lower P : O ratio compared with type 1 or "slow-twitch" fibers (Bottinelli & Reggiani 2000).

The available evidence suggests that enhancement of the efficiency of O_2 utilization during submaximal exercise has a key role in the improvement of endurance performance over the longer term in elite athletes, provided that $\dot{V}O_{2max}$ is at least maintained. For example, peak performances both in Lance Armstrong (the 6-times winner of cycling's Tour de France; Coyle 2005) and Paula Radcliffe (the World Record holder for the women's marathon; Jones 2006) have been reported to be closely linked with progressive improvements in cycling efficiency and running economy, respectively, because $\dot{V}O_{2max}$ appears to change relatively little with further training in already highly trained athletes. The cause(s) of the continued improvement in exercise economy with long-term training is obscure and certain to be multifactorial (and for running, at least, might well include [subtle] changes in running technique); however, one possibility is that chronic endurance training results in a gradual shift in muscle fiber type distribution towards the more efficient type 1 fiber profile.

Possession of excellent economy can be seen to be important for two (linked) reasons. First, a lower energy – and hence O_2 – cost for exercise at a particular speed or work rate will demand a lower rate of carbon-substrate utilization. Fatigue during longer term, and even mid-term (Newsholme et al. 1992), endurance exercise has been associated with the depletion of muscle glycogen stores to some critically low level (Gollnick et al. 1972; Vollestad et al. 1992), and therefore a lower energy turnover for a given exercise intensity will spare muscle glycogen and permit either an increased time-to-exhaustion at a fixed work rate or a faster time to cover a given distance. Glycogen sparing will also be facilitated by a greater propensity for β-oxidation in the trained state (Jeukendrup et al. 1998) although, interestingly, a shift from carbohydrate towards fatty acid utilization will simultaneously increase the O_2 cost

of exercise. Second, a lower O_2 cost of exercising at a certain work rate will require a smaller % of $\dot{V}O_{2max}$ and could result in an athlete moving from a higher to a lower exercise domain (i.e., from severe to heavy, or heavy to moderate) with consequent positive effects on pulmonary gas exchange kinetics, blood acid–base balance, and endurance. Fatigue during endurance events, at least those of ~2–60 min duration, is associated with the development of a significant metabolic acidosis. Whether this association is causal or merely coincidental is debated (Robergs et al. 2004; Cairns 2006). However, interventions (including training) that reduce the rate of lactate and H^+ accumulation during exercise result in improved endurance performance by enabling a higher fraction of the $\dot{V}O_{2max}$ to be sustained for longer periods (Costill et al. 1973).

Critical velocity and $\dot{V}O_2$ kinetics

Some aspects of the physiological responses to exercise in the world's best female marathon runner (PR) have been presented and discussed previously (Jones 1998; Jones 2006). These papers document the high $\dot{V}O_{2max}$ (consistently >70 mL·kg^{-1}·min^{-1}); the prodigious improvement in running economy caused by over a decade of endurance training culminating in a steady state $\dot{V}O_2$ at 16 km·h^{-1} and 1% treadmill grade of just 44–46 mL·kg^{-1}·min^{-1} (~15% lower than the expected value); and the high running speeds (and %$\dot{V}O_{2max}$) attained before the measurement of an appreciable increase in blood [lactate]. Figure 3.7 illustrates the relationship between $\dot{V}O_2$ and running speed for PR and for a representative age-matched untrained woman.

The CP/CV concept provides a useful framework with which to explore the limitations to endurance exercise performance. Figure 3.8 shows the relationship between running velocity and time-to-fatigue for PR based on personal best times for 800 m (2:05 in 1995), 1500 m (4:05 in 2001) and 3000 m (8:22 in 2002). Note the characteristic hyperbolic profile of the relationship. Based on these race times, PR's CV can be calculated to be 5.83 m·s^{-1} with a curvature constant (W') equivalent to 70 m. The running speed at the lactate threshold in 2003 (defined as the speed immediately before an increase in blood [lactate] above a baseline of ~1 mmol), which incidentally

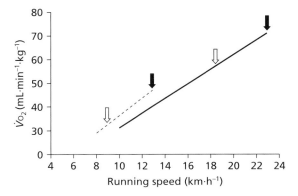

Fig. 3.7 Relationship between $\dot{V}o_2$ and treadmill running speed in Paula Radcliffe (PR) (solid line) and a hypothetical age-matched sedentary female (dashed line). Notice that the slope of the $\dot{V}o_2$–speed relationship, representative of running economy, is less steep in PR. Notice also that the $\dot{V}o_{2max}$ and the running speed corresponding to $\dot{V}o_{2max}$ (filled arrows) and the running speed corresponding to the lactate/gas exchange thresholds (open arrows) are much higher in PR.

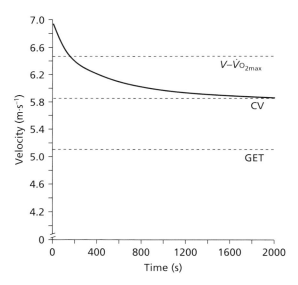

Fig. 3.8 Hyperbolic relationship of running speed to time-to-exhaustion in Paula Radcliffe (PR) based upon her personal best times for 800, 1500, 3000, and 5000 m. Note the narrow range of running speeds between the gas exchange threshold (GET) and the $\dot{V}o_{2max}$, a "compression" that is a characteristic effect of long-term endurance training. CV, critical velocity; GET, gas exchange threshold.

was very similar to the average speed sustained during the setting of the World Marathon Record of 2:15:25 in the same year, was 5.14 m·s^{-1}. The running speed at the lactate turn-point in 2003 (defined as the second, "sudden and sustained," increase in blood [lactate] at around 3 mmol) was 5.56 m·s^{-1}. Finally, the estimated running speed at the $\dot{V}o_{2max}$ (computed by solving the regression equation describing the submaximal $\dot{V}o_2$–running speed relationship for $\dot{V}o_{2max}$) in 2003 was approximately 6.47 m·s^{-1}. Therefore, the range of running speeds between the lactate threshold (LT) and $\dot{V}o_{2max}$ (covering the entire heavy and severe exercise intensity domains) is just 1.33 m·s^{-1}. This "compression" of the LT/CV/$\dot{V}o_{2max}$ appears to be a consequence of long-term endurance training and is characteristic of the physiology of elite endurance athletes (Coyle 2005; Jones 2006). This can be clearly seen when comparing and contrasting Figs 3.1 and 3.7 where the GET to CV separation is ~40% and ~10% of the CV in the non-highly trained individual and PR, respectively.

A high CV is important to endurance exercise performance because it represents the highest running speed that can be maintained without a continuous rise in blood [lactate] and $\dot{V}o_2$ with time. Fukuba and Whipp (1999) have suggested that what they have termed the "endurance parameter ratio" (W' : CV) might also be an important determinant of endurance performance in the sense that it will dictate the athlete's optimal pacing strategy during competition. That is, in endurance events lasting up to approximately 30 min, the W' : CV determines the flexibility in running speed that an athlete can tolerate around the optimal constant speed for the race without compromising performance. Naturally, an athlete with a high CV relative to their W' would be better suited to a high sustained pace throughout a race whereas an athlete with a lower CV and a large W' might prefer a slower average race pace and a fast finish. Ideally, athletes require both a high CV and a high W' but it is likely that possession of high values for CV and W' is, at least to some extent, mutually exclusive. For the same relative performance standard, and in comparison to longer distance specialists, middle-distance runners would be expected to have a larger W' both in absolute terms and relative to the CV (owing to their larger muscle mass and greater proportion of type 2 muscle fibers). Information contained in the relationship between running speed and time-to-fatigue is clearly valuable, not only in differentiating performance potential in different athletes competing in different events, but also in informing the race tactics that individual athletes might utilize to optimize their performance.

We contend that $\dot{V}_{O_2}$ kinetics is another important, and currently underappreciated, physiological parameter that can exert considerable influence over endurance exercise performance. Again, the data of PR can be used to illustrate this point. Figure 3.9 shows PR's $\dot{V}_{O_2}$ response in the abrupt transition from standing to running on a motorized treadmill for 4 min at 16 km·h^{-1} and 1% grade. It can be seen that $\dot{V}_{O_2}$ rises very quickly such that a complete steady state is attained within ~45 s. Of all the various parameters of aerobic fitness reported herein and previously for this great athlete (Jones 1998; Jones 2006), the speed of the $\dot{V}_{O_2}$ adaptation to exercise is perhaps the most remarkable. PR's τ value (which represents the time required for 63% of the increase in $\dot{V}_{O_2}$ above baseline to be reached) is 9 s. For comparison, the τ value for an age-matched sedentary but healthy woman would be ~30–35 s (Berger *et al.* 2006) while the τ value for a thoroughbred horse ($\dot{V}_{O_{2max}}$ of ~133 mL·kg^{-1}·min^{-1}) has been reported to be ~10 s (Langsetmo *et al.* 1997). As highlighted earlier, fast $\dot{V}_{O_2}$ kinetics minimize the magnitude of the O_2 deficit incurred in the transition to a higher metabolic rate, and thus enable higher work rates to be achieved with a reduced homeostatic

challenge (i.e., the fall in muscle high-energy phosphates (chiefly PCr) and the activation of glycolysis will be reduced, as will the rise in muscle lactate, H$^+$, and P$_i$), a concept termed "tighter metabolic control" (Hochachka & Matheson 1992).

For the same increment in external work rate, elite endurance athletes would be expected to have both faster $\dot{V}_{O_2}$ kinetics and a smaller increase in $\dot{V}_{O_2}$ in the steady state (i.e., better exercise economy). Both of these factors will interact to result in the incurrence of a small O_2 deficit. For example, for an increase of running speed of 10 km·h^{-1}, an elite endurance athlete such as PR might have a τ value of 10 s and an increase in $\dot{V}_{O_2}$ above that at rest of about 1.2 L·min^{-1}. An untrained woman of the same age (and a similar body mass of 55 kg) would have a τ value of 30 s and an increase in $\dot{V}_{O_2}$ above that at rest of about 1.7 L·min^{-1}. The difference in the O_2 deficit incurred in these two individuals is approximately fourfold: 0.2 L in PR (i.e., 10/60·1.2) and 0.85 L in the untrained woman (30/60·1.7). The importance of fast $\dot{V}_{O_2}$ kinetics can perhaps be most clearly visualized in the shorter endurance events in which the time during which $\dot{V}_{O_2}$ is rising towards the required (generally maximal) value constitutes a large fraction of the total race time. In these events, which are performed at considerably higher intensities than the CV, optimal performance will require the complete utilization of the W'. Fast $\dot{V}_{O_2}$ kinetics across the initial transition from rest to race pace will allow more of the available W' to remain intact; this remaining W' could subsequently be exploited by the maintenance of a higher average pace for the remainder of the race or by its rapid utilization in a fast finish. However, the importance of fast $\dot{V}_{O_2}$ kinetics to endurance performance should not be underestimated even in much longer endurance events where the transition to the steady state requires only a very small fraction of the total race time, such as in the marathon. This is because the initial O_2 deficit (and its metabolic corollaries) is not recovered once the steady state is attained, such that the muscle metabolic conditions prevailing over the first minute or two of exercise might influence physiological responses and performance capacity even during long-term exercise. For example, a low muscle [PCr] and correspondingly high [ADP$_{free}$]

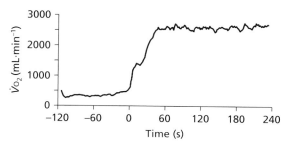

Fig. 3.9 $\dot{V}_{O_2}$ response of Paula Radcliffe (PR) following a step transition from standing rest to 4 min of treadmill running at 16 km·h^{-1} and 1% grade. Notice the very rapid kinetics resulting in the attainment of a complete steady state within 45 s.

and $[P_i]$ would provide a continued stimulus for glycolysis which could lead to earlier depletion of the finite muscle glycogen stores.

The physiological basis for the much faster $\dot{V}o_2$ kinetics observed in endurance athletes is unclear but is likely to involve both a greater capacity for rapid delivery of O_2 to contracting muscle following the onset of exercise and a greater capacity of the mitochondria to utilize the available O_2 (Tschakovsky & Hughson 1999; Jones & Poole 2005). Endurance training is known to result in faster muscle blood flow kinetics and an increase in the activity of (potentially rate-limiting) oxidative metabolic enzymes and thus both factors might contribute to the faster $\dot{V}o_2$ kinetics that are commonly observed (Jones & Carter 2000; Jones & Koppo 2005). Indeed, endurance training remains the most potent stimulus for an enhanced $\dot{V}o_2$ kinetic response to exercise (Jones & Koppo 2005). However, manipulation of the warm-up activities performed prior to a bout of high intensity exercise has the potential to facilitate the transient $\dot{V}o_2$ response and, in so doing, enhance performance (Jones *et al.* 2003a,b; Burnley *et al.* 2005). An appropriate warm-up (in terms of the intensity, volume, and recovery period elapsing before the competition begins) might be more effective in enhancing performance than a variety of putative ergogenic aids. Athletes and coaches might therefore be advised to give due consideration to the physiological effects of factors such as warm-up activities and pacing strategy on endurance performance.

In summary, endurance exercise mandates the efficient transport and utilization of O_2 by skeletal muscle. This involves a highly integrated response of the pulmonary, cardiovascular, and muscular systems, and is manifest in a range of measurable parameters of aerobic fitness: $\dot{V}o_{2max}$, exercise economy, lactate and gas exchange threshold, critical power/velocity, and $\dot{V}o_2$ kinetics. Science has provided the means to quantify these parameters – but it is coupling that science with the study of great athletes at the apogee of human performance that will bring us closer to understanding the physiological bases for truly extraordinary athletic ability.

References

American College of Sports Medicine (1991) *ACSM Guidelines for Exercise Testing and Prescription*, 4th edn. Lea & Febiger, London: 299.

Bangsbo, J., Krustrup, P., Gonzalez-Alonso, J., Boushel, R. & Saltin, B. (2000) Muscle oxygen kinetics at onset of intense dynamic exercise in humans. *American Journal of Physiology: Regulatory, Integrative and Comparative Physiology* **279**, R899–R906.

Behnke, B.J., Kindig, C.A., McDonough, P., Poole, D.C. & Sexton, W.L. (2002) Dynamics of microvascular oxygen pressure during rest-contraction transition in skeletal muscle of diabetic rats. *American Journal of Physiology: Heart and Circulatory Physiology* **283**, H926–H932.

Behnke, B.J., McDonough, P., Padilla, D.J., Musch, T.I. & Poole, D.C. (2003) Oxygen exchange profile in rat muscles of contrasting fibre types. *Journal of Physiology* **549**, 597–605.

Berger, N.J., Tolfrey, K., Williams, A.G. & Jones, A.M. (2006) Influence of continuous and interval training on oxygen uptake on-kinetics. *Medicine and Science in Sports and Exercise* **38**: 504–512.

Bottinelli, R. & Reggiani, C. (2000) Human skeletal muscle fibres: molecular and functional diversity. *Progress in Biophysics and Molecular Biology* **73**, 195–262.

Burnley, M., Doust, J.H. & Jones, A.M. (2005) Effects of prior warm-up regime on severe-intensity cycling performance. *Medicine and Science in Sports and Exercise* **37**, 838–845.

Cairns, S.P. (2006) Lactic acid and exercise performance: culprit or friend? *Sports Medicine* **36**, 279–291.

Chambers, W.R. (1965) *Chambers's Twentieth Century Dictionary*. Villafield Press, Glasgow.

Costill, D.L., Thomason, H. & Roberts, E. (1973) Fractional utilization of the aerobic capacity during distance running. *Medicine and Science in Sports* **5**, 248–252.

Coyle, E.F. (1995) Integration of the physiological factors determining endurance performance ability. *Exercise and Sport Sciences Reviews* **23**, 25–63.

Coyle, E.F. (2005) Improved muscular efficiency displayed as Tour de France champion matures. *Journal of Applied Physiology* **98**, 2191–2196.

Federspiel, W.J. & Popel, A.S. (1986) A theoretical analysis of the effect of the particulate nature of blood on oxygen release in capillaries. *Microvascular Research* **32**, 164–189.

Ferreira, L.F., McDonough, P., Behnke, B.J., Musch, T.I. & Poole, D.C. (2006) Blood flow and O_2 extraction as a function of O_2 uptake in muscles composed of different fiber types. *Respiration Physiology and Neurobiology* **153**, 237–249.

Fukuba, Y. & Whipp, B.J. (1999) A metabolic limit on the ability to make up for lost time in endurance events. *Journal of Applied Physiology* **87**, 853–861.

Godfrey, R.J., Ingham, S.A., Pedlar, C.R. & Whyte, G.P. (2005) The detraining and retraining of an elite rower: a case study. *Journal of Science and Medicine in Sport* **8**, 314–320.

Gollnick, P.D., Piehl, K., Saubert, C.W. 4th, Armstrong, R.B. & Saltin, B. (1972) Diet, exercise, and glycogen changes in human muscle fibers. *Journal of Applied Physiology* **33**, 421–425.

Grassi, B., Poole, D.C., Richardson, R.S., Knight, D.R., Erickson, B.K. & Wagner, P.D. (1996) Muscle O_2 uptake kinetics in humans: implications for metabolic control. *Journal of Applied Physiology* **80**, 988–998.

Harms, C.A., McClaran, S.R., Nickele, G.A., Pegelow, D.F., Nelson, W.B. & Dempsey, J.A. (1998) Exercise-induced arterial hypoxaemia in healthy young women. *Journal of Physiology* **507**, 619–628.

Hochachka, P.W. & Matheson, G.O. (1992) Regulating ATP turnover rates over broad dynamic work ranges in skeletal muscles. *Journal of Applied Physiology* **73**, 1697–1703.

Hultman, E. & Greenhaff, P.L. (1991) Skeletal muscle energy metabolism and fatigue during intense exercise in man. *Science Progress* **75**, 361–370.

Ingjer, F. & Brodal, P. (1978) Capillary supply of skeletal muscle fibers in untrained and endurance-trained women. *European Journal of Applied Physiology and Occupational Physiology* **38**, 291–299.

Jeukendrup, A.E., Saris, W.H. & Wagenmakers, A.J. (1998) Fat metabolism during exercise: a review. Part II: Regulation of metabolism and the effects of training. *International Journal of Sports Medicine* **19**, 293–302.

Jones, A.M. (1998) A five year physiological case study of an Olympic runner. *British Journal of Sports Medicine* **32**, 39–43.

Jones, A.M. (2006) The physiology of the world record holder for the women's marathon. *International Journal of Sports Science and Coaching* **2**, 101–116.

Jones, A.M. & Carter, H. (2000) The effect of endurance training on parameters of aerobic fitness. *Sports Medicine* **29**, 373–386.

Jones, A.M. & Doust, J.H. (2001) Limitations to submaximal exercise performance. In: *Exercise and Laboratory Test Manual*, 2nd edn. (Eston, R. & Reilly, T., eds.) E. & F.N. Spon London and New York: 235–262.

Jones, A.M. & Koppo, K. (2005) Effect of training on $\dot{V}o_2$ kinetics and performance. In: *Oxygen Uptake Kinetics in Sport, Exercise and Medicine* (Jones, A.M. & Poole, D.C., eds.) Routledge London and New York: 373–398.

Jones, A.M., Koppo, K. & Burnley, M. (2003a) Effects of prior exercise on metabolic and gas exchange responses to exercise. *Sports Medicine* **33**, 949–971.

Jones, A.M. & Poole, D.C. (2005) Oxygen uptake dynamics: from muscle to mouth: an introduction to the symposium. *Medicine and Science in Sports and Exercise* **37**, 1542–1550.

Jones, A.M., Wilkerson, D.P., Burnley, M. & Koppo, K. (2003b) Prior heavy exercise enhances performance during subsequent perimaximal exercise. *Medicine and Science in Sports and Exercise* **35**, 2085–2092.

Jones, A.M., Wilkerson, D.P., DiMenna, F., Fulford, J. & Poole, D.C. (2008) Muscle metabolic responses to exercise above and below the "critical power" assessed using 31P-MRS. *American Journal of Physiology: Regulatory, Integrative and Comparative Physiology* **294**, R585–93.

Karatzaferi, C., de Haan, A., Ferguson, R.A., van Mechelen, W. & Sargeant, A.J. (2001) Phosphocreatine and ATP content in human single muscle fibres before and after maximum dynamic exercise. *Pflugers Archiv* **442**, 467–474.

Klitzman, B. & Duling, B.R. (1979) Microvascular hematocrit and red cell flow in resting and contracting striated muscle. *American Journal of Physiology* **237**, H481–H490.

Langsetmo, I., Weigle, G.E., Fedde, M.R., Erickson, H.H., Barstow, T.J. & Poole, D.C. (1997) $\dot{V}o_2$ kinetics in the horse during moderate and heavy exercise. *Journal of Applied Physiology* **83**, 1235–1241.

Legrand, R., Ahmaidi, S., Moalla, W., et al. (2005) O_2 arterial desaturation in endurance athletes increases muscle deoxygenation. *Medicine and Science in Sports and Exercise* **37**, 782–788.

McDonough, P., Behnke, B.J., Padilla, D.J., Musch, T.I. & Poole, D.C. (2005) Control of microvascular oxygen pressures in rat muscles comprised of different fibre types. *Journal of Physiology* **563**, 903–913.

Morgan, D.W., Bransford, D.R., Costill, D.L., Daniels, J.T., Howley, E.T. & Krahenbuhl, G.S. (1995) Variation in the aerobic demand of running among trained and untrained subjects. *Medicine and Science in Sports and Exercise* **27**, 404–409.

Moseley, L., Achten, J., Martin, J.C. & Jeukendrup, A.E. (2004) No differences in cycling efficiency between world-class and recreational cyclists. *International Journal of Sports Medicine* **25**, 374–379.

Newsholme, E.A., Blomstrand, E. & Ekblom, B. (1992) Physical and mental fatigue: metabolic mechanisms and importance of plasma amino acids. *British Medicine Bulletin* **48**, 477–495.

Poole, D.C. (1997) Influence of exercise training on skeletal muscle oxygen delivery and utilization. In: *The Lung Scientific Foundations.* (Crystal, R.G., West, J.B., Weibel, E.R. & Barnes, P.J., eds.) Raven Press, New York: 1957–1967.

Poole, D.C. & Erickson, H.H. (2004) Heart and vessels: Function during exercise and response to training. In: *Equine Sports Medicine and Surgery* (Hinchcliff, K., Kaneps, A.J. & Geor, R.J., eds.) Elsevier Science: 699–727.

Poole, D.C., Ward, S.A., Gardner, G.W. & Whipp, B.J. (1988) Metabolic and respiratory profile of the upper limit for prolonged exercise in man. *Ergonomics* **31**, 1265–1279.

Poole, D.C., Ward, S.A. & Whipp, B.J. (1990) The effects of training on the metabolic and respiratory profile of high-intensity cycle ergometer exercise. *European Journal of Applied Physiology and Occupational Physiology* **59**, 421–429.

Powers, S.K., Lawler, J., Dempsey, J.A., Dodd, S. & Landry, G. (1989) Effects of incomplete gas exchange on $\dot{V}o_{2max}$. *Journal of Applied Physiology* **66**, 2491–2495.

Richardson, R.S., Poole, D.C., Knight, D.R. & Wagner, P.D. (1994) Red blood cell transit time in man: theoretical effects of capillary density. *Advances in Experimental Medicine and Biology* **361**, 521–532.

Robergs, R.A., Ghiasvand, F. & Parker, D. (2004) Biochemistry of exercise-induced metabolic acidosis. *American Journal of Physiology: Regulatory, Integrative and Comparative Physiology* **287**, R502–R516.

Roca, J., Agusti, A.G., Alonso, A., et al. (1992) Effects of training on muscle O_2 transport at $\dot{V}o_{2max}$. *Journal of Applied Physiology* **73**, 1067–1076.

Shulman, R.G. & Rothman, D.L. (2001) The "glycogen shunt" in exercising muscle: A role for glycogen in muscle energetics and fatigue. *Proceedings of the National Academy of Sciences, USA* **98**, 457–461.

Smith, C.G. & Jones, A.M. (2001) The relationship between critical velocity, maximal lactate steady-state velocity and lactate turnpoint velocity in runners. *European Journal of Applied Physiology* **85**, 19–26.

Tschakovsky, M.E. & Hughson, R.L. (1999) Interaction of factors determining oxygen uptake at the onset of exercise. *Journal of Applied Physiology* **86**, 1101–1113.

Vollestad, N.K., Tabata, I. & Medbo, J.I. (1992) Glycogen breakdown in different human muscle fibre types during exhaustive exercise of short duration. *Acta Physiologica Scandinavica* **144**, 135–141.

Weibel, E.R. *The Pathway for Oxygen.* Harvard University Press, London: 1984.

Wilson, J.R., McCully, K.K., Mancini, D.M., Boden, B. & Chance, B. (1988) Relationship of muscular fatigue to pH and diprotonated Pi in humans: a ^{31}P-NMR study. *Journal of Applied Physiology* **64**, 2333–2339.

Chapter 4

Physiological Adaptations to Training

MARTIN J. GIBALA AND MARK RAKOBOWCHUK

Physical training refers to repeated performance of acute exercise. Although there is no consensus regarding terminology, the trained state is typically associated with "adaptation" or a relatively stable change in one or more physiological variables compared to the pre-trained state (Tipton & Franklin 2006). In contrast to the immediate and relatively transient physiological disturbances associated with an acute bout of activity, chronic changes induced by training persist for an appreciable period of time and serve to minimize disruption of homeostasis during subsequent exercise (Booth & Thomason 1991). Less disruption of the "milieu interieur" permits the individual to perform exercise for a longer period of time at a given workload before fatigue. For the competitive athlete, a more important consideration is that training can increase the peak power that can be generated during a brief, maximal effort, or the average power or speed that can be sustained for a given period of time or over a fixed distance (i.e., a race).

Our current understanding of physiological adaptations to training in humans is based largely on longitudinal studies of previously sedentary or moderately fit individuals who performed a structured program of exercise for periods lasting from a few days up to several months. Subjects in these studies have tended to be young healthy men, although there is a growing appreciation for the manner in which training-induced changes are influenced by

The Olympic Textbook of Science in Sport, 1st edition. Edited by R.J. Maughan. Published 2009 by Blackwell Publishing. ISBN: 978-1-4051-5638-7.

sex, age, and disease conditions. Much less is known regarding the adaptive response in already highly-trained individuals, as it has proved difficult for scientists to persuade athletes to experiment with their habitual programs or to consent to invasive procedures (e.g., muscle biopsies) for elucidating potential mechanisms underlying performance adaptations (Hawley 2002). A limited number of studies have described changes in selected physiological markers after relatively short-term (usually ≤1 month) interventions in well-trained athletes (e.g., Weston et al. 1997). However, information regarding long-term training adaptations in humans has mainly been garnered from cross-sectional comparisons between individuals that were either untrained or that had trained regularly for many years (e.g., D'Antona et al. 2006), and from case studies of world-class athletes (e.g., Coyle 2005). An inherent limitation to these investigations is that one cannot discern to what extent the proposed adaptation resulted from, or was brought to, the habitually active lifestyle (Dempsey et al. 2006).

As noted by Hawley (2002), the capacity to perform work ultimately depends on the rate and efficiency at which chemical energy can be converted into mechanical energy for skeletal muscle contraction. Thus, from a physiological perspective, training can improve exercise capacity through several general mechanisms, including: (i) altering rates of energy provision from both non-oxidative and oxidative sources; (ii) maintaining tighter metabolic control through a closer matching between rates of ATP hydrolysis and synthesis; (iii) improving fatigue resistance; and (iv) increasing economy of motion

(Hawley 2002). These general mechanisms are in turn dependent on a complex array of adaptations within multiple physiological systems that act in an integrative manner to coordinate energy delivery and regulate force production.

The present chapter focuses on structural and functional remodeling of the musculoskeletal, cardiovascular, and respiratory systems in response to physical training in humans. Animal studies have contributed greatly to our basic understanding of the molecular and cellular adaptations induced by chronic changes in contractile activity (Booth & Thomason 1991); however, the models employed only simulate human physical activity to varying degrees and the present review therefore emphasizes adaptations demonstrated in humans. We do not consider training-induced changes in other systems, such as those involved with thermoregulatory, endocrine, and immune function; such topics are addressed in other sections of this book. Finally, while the present chapter highlights training-induced changes in the musculoskeletal system, the metabolic significance of these adaptations and underlying molecular signaling events are explored in greater detail in separate chapters dedicated to these two topics (see Chapters 5 & 13, respectively).

The training stimulus

Physiological disturbances induced by an acute bout of exercise are highly specific to the mode of exercise undertaken and corresponding pattern of motor unit recruitment (Saltin & Gollnick 1983), with subsequent adaptations largely dependent on the "training impulse" or the frequency, intensity, and volume of work performed (Hawley 2002). Training protocols are thus infinitely variable and the relatively simple interventions often employed in laboratory studies can be quite removed from the complex, periodized strategies normally practiced by competitive athletes. From a scientific perspective, relatively simple designs improve the likelihood of establishing cause and effect (i.e., the extent to which a specific, quantifiable perturbation causes a specific, measurable change in a given physiological variable). However, from a coaching perspective, complex training interventions are formulated to

elicit the greatest improvement in performance, regardless of the precise mechanism(s) involved, which can include variables (e.g., mood, motivation, perception of effort, etc.) that are not readily explained by physiological changes.

There are essentially three main types of exercise training stimuli that differ with respect to the nature of the load placed on skeletal muscle. In accordance with the classification scheme of Saltin & Gollnick (1983), the present chapter therefore employs the terms "endurance", "strength", and "sprint" to categorize training adaptations, with the general nature of each stimulus defined by the following examples. "Endurance training" refers to repeated sessions of continuous dynamic exercise (e.g., running, cycling) that is performed against a moderate workload usually defined as a percentage of peak oxygen uptake (e.g., 60–85% of $\dot{V}o_{2peak}$) for an extended period of time (e.g., from 10 min to up to several hours). "Strength training" refers to repeated sessions of very brief, intermittent exercise (e.g., squat, bench press, elbow flexor curl) performed against a heavy resistance (e.g., imposed by a weighted bar or weight stack) that is usually characterized as a relatively high percentage of the maximal workload that can be generated during a single, maximal effort (i.e., one-repetition maximum, 1RM). A single effort typically lasts for up to several seconds and this is repeated several times (e.g., 3–12) with minimal rest within a single set, and several sets (e.g., 3–4) are usually performed for a given exercise with a few minutes of rest between sets. Finally, "sprint training" refers to repeated sessions of relatively brief, intermittent exercise (e.g., running, cycling), often performed with an "all-out" effort or at an intensity close to that which elicits peak oxygen uptake (i.e., $\geq 90\%$ of $\dot{V}o_{2peak}$). A single effort typically lasts from a few seconds to up to several minutes, and this is repeated several times (e.g., 4–10) with a few minutes of either complete rest or low-intensity exercise performed during recovery between each effort.

While the general adaptive response to a given training impulse is relatively predictable, the rate and magnitude of change vary greatly between individuals and depend upon the initial physiological state and genetic predisposition for adaptation (Hawley 2002; Rankinen et al. 2006). Lack of consensus regarding terminology has also hampered the characterization of exercise-induced changes over time (Tipton & Franklin 2006). For example, the phrase "short-term training" has been used to describe changes that occur over a period ranging from a few days to up to several months. There is also growing appreciation for the paradigm that chronic training adaptations are generated by the cumulative effects of the transient events that occur during recovery from each acute exercise bout (Hawley et al. 2006). Thus, the answer to the question "when do repeated bouts of exercise become training" can vary depending on the specific variable of interest. In the follow sections we review the major physiological adaptations induced by the three main types of exercise training, and highlight recent findings that shed new light on well-established phenomenon or address controversial or emerging areas of research.

Adaptations to endurance training

Skeletal muscular system

One of the most prominent adaptations to endurance training is an increase in the oxidative capacity of skeletal muscle, as evidenced by morphological assessment of mitochondrial volume density or biochemical determination of the total protein content or maximal activity of various mitochondrial enzymes (Saltin & Gollnick 1983; Fluck & Hoppeler 2003). Mitochondrial volume density is increased relatively quickly by endurance training in the three muscle fiber types found in mixed human muscle, provided the intensity is sufficient to recruit all motor units. For example, Howald et al. (1985) reported increases of 35, 55 and 35% in type 1, 2a, and 2x fibers, respectively, after 6 weeks of cycle exercise training (30 min, 5 times·wk^{-1}, at ~80% $\dot{V}O_{2peak}$). Mitochondria located around the periphery of myofibers (i.e., subsarcolemmal mitochondria) tend to be increased to a greater extent after training as compared to those located closer to the centre of the fiber (i.e., intramyofibrillar mitochondria); however, the functional significance of this differential response remains to be elucidated (Fluck & Hoppeler 2003).

Increased mitochondrial content is an important factor responsible for the reduced rate of carbohydrate (CHO) utilization and increased capacity for lipid oxidation at a given absolute work intensity after training (Holloszy & Coyle 1984). Improved respiratory control sensitivity refers to the phenomenon whereby an increased mitochondrial content reduces the rate of oxygen and substrate flux per individual mitochondrion, and thus a lower concentration of free ADP is required to activate cellular respiration to achieve given rate of ATP formation (Holloszy & Coyle 1984). Since free ADP also activates enzymes that control glycogenolysis and glycolysis, the higher mitochondrial content provides a mechanism to reduce CHO utilization at a given absolute workload after training. Other skeletal muscular adaptations to training that influence the acute metabolic response to exercise, including changes in the regulation of specific enzymes and metabolite transport proteins, are discussed in detail in Chapter 5.

Recent studies in humans have addressed the issue of whether the specific activity of skeletal muscle mitochondria (i.e., activity expressed relative to mitochondrial mass) is altered by exercise training. Work by Tonkonogi & Sahlin (2002) showed that the increase in citrate synthase maximal activity after 6 weeks of endurance training was matched by similar increases in mitochondrial oxygen consumption in both isolated mitochondria and skinned fibers. This suggests that training-induced changes in mitochondrial respiration are attributable to the expansion of mitochondrial mass rather than to changes in specific activity. Interestingly, these researchers have also shown that the apparent Km for ADP is increased after training, which indicates the sensitivity of each individual mitochondrion is reduced (Walsh et al. 2001). A training-induced decrease in ADP sensitivity at the individual mitochondrion level seems to be paradoxical because it acts in the opposite direction to the increased ADP sensitivity associated with the increased total mitochondrial volume. However, the decreased ADP sensitivity appears to be counteracted by an enhanced stimulatory effect of creatine, and this may provide an advantage by increasing the overall efficiency of oxidative phosphorylation and reducing the formation of reactive oxygen species in endurance-trained muscle (Tonkonogi & Sahlin 2002).

Our understanding of the mechanisms underlying mitochondrial adaptation has also advanced rapidly over the past decade, although most of this work has been conducted using experimental models that do not involve exercise (e.g., transgenic animals or overexpression studies in cell culture; Hood & Irrcher 2006). Nonetheless, these studies provide valuable insight into the molecular signals that link acute changes in the energy status of the muscle cell to subsequent long-term increases in mitochondrial content. For example, increases in intracellular Ca^{2+} and ATP turnover are believed to activate specific enzymes (e.g., calcium/calmodulin-dependent protein kinase, CAMK; AMP-activated protein kinase, AMPK) that trigger signaling pathways leading to mitochondrial biogenesis, likely via the transcriptional coactivator peroxisome proliferator-activated receptor (PPAR) γ coactivator 1 α (PGC-1α); Hood & Irrcher 2006). Consistent with this hypothesis, there is a large transient increase in PGC-1α transcription and mRNA content in human skeletal muscle during recovery from an acute bout of prolonged exercise (Pilegaard et al. 2003). Chapter 13 provides a comprehensive discussion of molecular adaptations that facilitate training-induced adaptations in skeletal muscle.

Cardiovascular system

The principle cardiovascular adaptations to endurance training include an increase in maximal stroke volume (SV_{max}) and cardiac output with no change or a slight decrease in maximal heart rate, an increase in blood volume and remodeling of the vascular system (Blomqvist & Saltin 1983; Brown 2003; Prior et al. 2004; Moore 2006). The increased SV_{max} is almost always associated with a training-induced increase in maximal left ventricular (LV) end diastolic volume (EDV), due in part to myocardial growth that facilitates an increase in LV chamber dimension (Moore et al. 2006). In contrast to the situation observed in pathological states such as hypertension, physiological LV hypertrophy in endurance athletes permits an increased peak workload at the cost of only a small increase in basal myocardial oxygen consumption

(Kjaer et al. 2005). Training-induced changes in LV-EDV may also be attributable to alterations in intrinsic contractile function and higher filling pressures that result from blood volume expansion and increased myocardial compliance, which refers to the ability of the chamber to change its volume in response to a given change in pressure (Moore et al. 2006). The relative bradycardia observed during rest and exercise at a given absolute workload after training is also attributable to the same mechanisms that cause the increase in SV_{max}.

The process of vascular remodeling can occur at a number of different levels including large conduit arteries that regulate bulk flow delivery, smaller resistance vessels that regular flow within the microvascular network around cells, and the capillary network that regulates the exchange of gases and metabolites between blood and tissues. Two important but distinct processes involved in vascular remodeling are "arteriogenesis" and "angiogenesis". The former refers to enlargement of existing arterial vessels and is effective for increasing bulk flow to downstream elements, whereas the latter refers to de novo formation of new capillaries and facilitates exchange between blood and tissues (Prior et al. 2004). Potential stimuli involved in the process of vascular remodeling include growth factors such as vascular endothelial growth factor, physical forces such as shear stress, or mechanical stretch and hypoxia (Prior et al. 2004).

Evidence for vascular remodeling in humans includes the long recognized fact that endurance training increases the capillary density of exercised muscles (Blomqvist & Saltin 1983). An improved capillary network provides a greater surface area for diffusion, meaning that for a given blood flow into the muscle, the time available for exchange between blood and tissues is enhanced. Capillary proliferation also reduces the average diffusion distance from blood to any given myocyte, provided the degree of angiogenesis exceeds any potential increase in fiber cross-sectional area (i.e., muscle hypertrophy). Collectively these changes facilitate improved delivery of oxygen and substrates such as free fatty acids to mitochondria after training, and enhanced removal of carbon dioxide and metabolic intermediates such as lactate.

Training-induced changes in cardiac mass also increase myocardial need for oxygen and energy substrates, which increases the demand placed on the coronary vasculature. Cross-sectional studies using Doppler echocardiography have reported larger coronary arteries and greater peak vasodilatory capacity in endurance athletes compared to sedentary controls (Kozakova *et al.* 2000). While no longitudinal studies have been conducted in humans, investigations performed on monkeys and dogs have demonstrated increased cross-sectional areas of the left anterior descending and circumflex arteries after several months to years of running training (Brown 2003).

Respiratory system

In contrast to the cardiovascular and skeletal muscular systems, there is relatively little evidence to show that endurance training (or strength or sprint training) markedly alters the structure or function of the respiratory system in humans (Wagner 2005; Dempsey *et al.* 2006). Animal studies have demonstrated that respiratory muscles are metabolically plastic and that endurance training increases oxidative capacity and antioxidant enzyme activity in the diaphragm and accessory muscles (Powers *et al.* 1997). No comparable human data are available, although biopsy studies in patients with chronic obstructive pulmonary disease (COPD) have confirmed that chronic changes in respiratory muscle work are associated with alterations in mitochondrial content and fiber composition (Levine *et al.* 2001). Indirect evidence of a training effect in healthy humans comes from studies showing reduced diaphragm fatigue during heavy exercise, owing to a blunted hyperventilatory response at a given power output (Dempsey *et al.* 2006).

With respect to lung function, there are no major differences between endurance trained and healthy untrained individuals in terms of static lung volume, maximal flow-volume loops, or lung diffusion capacity at rest and during exercise (Dempsey *et al.* 2006). Swimmers may be the exception, and data from both cross-sectional and longitudinal studies suggests that intense swimming training induces small but significant changes in both static lung volume

and respiratory muscle function (Dempsey *et al.* 2006). Specific respiratory muscle training, which refers to several techniques including voluntary isocapnic hyperpnea, flow resistive loading, and pressure threshold loading, has been purported to improve lung function but the data are inconsistent and the potential mechanisms involved are unclear (McConnell & Romer 2004).

The relative unresponsiveness of the lung to exercise training is perplexing, given that the respiratory system may limit performance in certain exercise situations and this is particularly evident in highly-trained endurance athletes (Wagner 2005; Dempsey *et al.* 2006). Arterial oxygen content is maintained relatively constant during heavy exercise in most individuals, which suggests that the lung, airways, and respiratory muscles are "overbuilt" with respect to gas transport requirements. However, exercise-induced arterial hypoxemia (EIAH) has been observed to occur at or near maximal exercise in many fit subjects, and overcoming the condition by breathing hyperoxic gas leads to a measurable increase in performance (Wagner 2005). Women may be more susceptible to EIAH than men; however, recent data highlight the importance of absolute lung size or aerobic fitness in determining susceptibility to EIAH rather than gender *per se* (Olfert *et al.* 2004). The precise cause of EIAH has not been elucidated but potential mechanisms include relative hypoventilation, an oxygen diffusion limitation, ventilation/perfusion mismatching, or pulmonary shunts (Dempsey *et al.* 2006).

Adaptations to strength training

Skeletal muscular

The major morphological adaptation to strength training is an increased skeletal muscle mass and whole-muscle cross sectional area (CSA), as evidenced by scanning techniques such as magnetic resonance imaging (MRI) or computerized tomography (Folland & Williams 2007). Increased muscle CSA is generally attributable to hypertrophy or growth of existing muscle fibers as opposed to hyperplasia or the formation of new muscle fibers (MacDougall 1992). Fiber hypertrophy is in turn due to myofibrillar growth and proliferation with little change in the packing density of individual myofibrils (MacDougall 1992). Hypertrophy occurs in all three major fiber types in human muscle, with a tendency for greater relative hypertrophy in type 2 fibers, provided the training program is of sufficient intensity and duration (Fluck & Hoppler 2003). Most longitudinal studies report no major fiber type conversion in humans (i.e., between type 1 and type 2); however, more subtle shifts may occur, with a tendency for transition from type 2x to 2a fibers (Folland & Williams 2007). This trend is supported by studies that have classified muscle composition based on myosin heavy chain (MHC) isoforms, with a decrease in MHC 2x (predominant in type 2x fibers) and increase in MCH 2a (predominant in type 2a fibers) demonstrated after several months of strength training (Folland & Williams 2007). However, as noted by D'Antona *et al.* (2006), the shift in fiber type composition observed in most longitudinal strength training studies (i.e., 2x to 2a) is surprisingly similar to that observed after endurance training (Baumann *et al.* 1987). The precise relevance of training-induced adaptations in fiber type for muscle function remains unclear (Ingalls 2004), especially when considered relative to the pronounced bias in fiber type distribution observed in comparative studies of elite athletes (i.e., towards "fast" fibers in bodybuilders and sprinters, and towards "slow" fibers in marathon runners).

It remains controversial whether muscular enlargement as a result of strength training in humans is solely attributable to fiber hypertrophy. Hyperplasia – assessed using histochemical and biochemical methods that attempt to count total fibers – has been reported in animals after high-resistance training, with compensatory hypertrophy induced by synergist ablation and chronic stretch (Folland & Williams 2007). For ethical and technical reasons, hyperplasia can only be assessed indirectly in humans, by comparing whole muscle CSA (determined using imaging techniques) to fiber CSA (determined from a muscle biopsy) under conditions characterized by significant muscle hypertrophy. Longitudinal studies in humans have generally found no evidence of hyperplasia, such as work by McCall *et al.* (1996) that reported similar increases in muscle CSA (13%)

and mean fiber area (15%) in the biceps brachii of recreational weightlifters after 12 weeks of intensified heavy resistance training. However, D'Antona and colleagues (2006) recently concluded that the extreme hypertrophy of the vastus lateralis muscle found in elite bodybuilders as compared to healthy untrained controls could not be explained simply on the basis of muscle fiber hypertrophy. The CSA of the vastus lateralis measured by MRI was found to be 54% larger in the bodybuilders compared to controls, whereas the difference in mean fiber area was only 14%. In addition, these authors reported a markedly bias towards type 2x fibers in the bodybuilders, which would not be expected based on the shift from type 2x to 2a generally reported in longitudinal training studies (Folland & Williams 2007).

Muscle fiber hypertrophy after strength training occurs when the rate of skeletal muscle protein synthesis exceeds the rate of protein breakdown over a given period time, leading to net accretion of contractile protein (Rasmussen & Phillips 2003; Rennie *at al.* 2004). It is well established that an acute bout of heavy resistance exercise – the most common form of strength training – is a potent stimulator of mixed skeletal muscle protein synthesis and this effect may persist for up to 48 h (Phillips *et al.* 1997). Recent studies have confirmed the increased muscle protein synthesis is mainly due to synthesis of myofibrillar proteins (Hasten *et al.* 2000), as expected given the myofibrillar growth and proliferation observed in longitudinal training studies (MacDougall 1992). Muscle protein balance is also elevated after acute resistance exercise and net muscle protein balance actually remains negative in the fasted state (i.e., breakdown > synthesis; Phillips *et al.* 1997). However, acute resistance exercise combined with protein ingestion during recovery produces a net positive muscle protein balance (i.e., synthesis > breakdown), which favors muscle anabolism (Tipton & Wolfe 2004; Phillips *et al.* 2005). As discussed further in Chapter 13, our understanding of the molecular and cellular events involved in the response of skeletal muscle to strength training and nutritional manipulation has advanced rapidly over the past several years (Rennie *et al.* 2004; Deldicque *et al.* 2005). Much attention has focused on the mammalian target of rapomycin (mTOR), which is a central regulatory protein that integrates signals related to the energy status of the cell and environmental stimuli. Heavy resistance exercise and amino acids appear to employ different upstream pathways to activate mTOR, which in turn affects skeletal muscle growth by regulating the activity of several downstream targets linked to hypertrophy including p70 ribosomal protein S6 kinase (p70 S6K) and eukaryotic initiation factor 4E-binding protein (4E-BP1) (Deldicque *et al*. 2005).

Longitudinal studies have demonstrated that strength training attenuates the increase in muscle protein synthesis after an acute bout of resistance exercise, even when comparisons are made at the same relative work intensity (Kim *et al*. 2005). Muscle protein breakdown rate is also reduced after exercise (Phillips *et al*. 2002) and the blunted muscle protein turnover response may explain in part the reduced rate of muscle hypertrophy that is commonly observed after several months of strength training. Interestingly, cellular protein subfraction analyses performed by Kim *et al*. (2005) showed that the dampened mixed skeletal muscle synthesis response to exercise after training was mainly attributable to non-myofibrillar proteins, whereas the synthesis of myofibrillar proteins was preserved. The authors speculated that in the untrained state, resistance exercise serves as a relatively novel stimulus that stimulates a non-specific rise in the synthesis of all muscle proteins. However, signals that stimulate muscle protein synthesis in the untrained are "refined" after resistance training and preferentially directed towards the synthesis of myofibrillar proteins. Recent studies also suggest that the muscle adaptive response to strength training may be altered by nutritional manipulation. For example, Andersen *et al*. (2005) reported greater fiber hypertrophy in type 1 and type 2 fibers in vastus lateralis after 14 weeks of resistance training when subjects ingested a protein supplement immediately after each training session.

The marked increase in contractile protein that occurs with strength training has been reported to lead to a dilution of mitochondrial content, with volume densities as low as 2% noted in elite bodybuilders as compared to normal values of 4–5% in untrained healthy controls (Hoppler & Fluck 2003). Several other longitudinal and cross-sectional studies (reviewed in Tang *et al*. 2006) have shown reduced maximal activities of mitochondrial enzymes, suggesting that chronic strength training may impair the capacity for aerobic energy provision in skeletal muscle. However, a resent study by Tang *et al*. (2006) reported increased muscle oxidative capacity in the vastus lateralis muscle of previously untrained men after a 12 week strength training program that induced significant muscle hypertrophy. The maximal activities of citrate synthase and β-hydroxyacyl CoA dehydrogenase, expressed relative to total muscle protein content, increased by 24 and 22%, respectively, despite a mean increase of 12% in type 1, 2a, and 2x fiber areas. While a number of potential factors, including the degree of muscle hypertrophy, may explain the equivocal results between the study by Tang *et al*. (2006) and previous authors (Hoppler & Fluck 2003), the recent findings nonetheless indicate that heavy resistance training may provide a stimulus for mitochondrial biogenesis. Acute resistance exercise dramatically increases intracellular Ca^{2+} flux and ATP turnover and could therefore activate some of the same signaling cascades that are believe to induce mitochondrial biogenesis after endurance exercise (Hood & Irrcher 2006). As discussed in more detail in Chapter 13, there is "cross-talk" between the various molecular pathways activated by strength and endurance exercise (Baar 2006), and thus the potential for adaptations typically associated with one form of training to be affected (positively or negatively) by the other form of training.

Cardiovascular

Cardiovascular adaptations to strength training have long been a controversial topic. From reports of cardiac hypertrophy to potential conduit artery stiffening, the high arterial blood pressures experienced during heavy resistive-type exercise have often been associated with what are often characterized as "unfavorable" adaptations in the cardiovascular system. Cardiac hypertrophy, more specifically left ventricular "concentric hypertrophy" does occur with resistance training; however, the rate is similar to observations of unaltered cardiac mass in ~40% of athletes. Detrimental hypertrophy, similar to that which develops with disease states such as congestive heart failure, has not been observed to occur with resistance training (Haykowsky *et al.* 2002). Moreover, cardiac dimension adaptations appear to be modality-specific with eccentric hypertrophy developing in association with incorporation of high repetition, multiple-set resistance training methods, while concentric hypertrophy develops in association with Olympic style weightlifting training, involving brief maximal repetitions (Haykowsky *et al.* 2002). Although resistance exercise training may increase basal myocardial oxygen demand, this minor increase has little bearing on sport performance due to the limited reliance on oxidative metabolism. Conversely, from a cardiac performance perspective, tissue Doppler imaging and m-mode ultrasonography in resistance-trained individuals show enhanced contractile function that mirrors the cardiac performance of trained endurance athletes (Fisman *et al.* 2002). Indeed, increased stroke volume due to greater EDV and smaller end systolic volume at the end of exercise may reduce myocardial oxygen consumption both at rest and immediately following exhaustive aerobic exercise (Fisman *et al.* 2002).

Another potential negative effect of resistance exercise training is an increase in myocardial oxygen demand due to increased aortic impedance. Central artery stiffness, which has been noted in some (Miyachi *et al.* 2004; Kawano *et al.* 2006), but not all, resistance training studies (Rakobowchuk *et al.* 2005a; Poelkens *et al.* 2007) could increase myocardial oxygen consumption due to greater cardiac work resulting from increased wave reflection and afterload. Similar to the potential effect on cardiac hypertrophy (Haykowsky *et al.* 2002), vascular adaptations may depend upon the specific type of strength training performed (e.g., power lifting vs. body building). Although increases in central arterial stiffness have been observed in some resistance-training studies, to date there is no evidence that suggests that these vascular changes increase the risk of cardiac events or disease. Indeed, any stiffening of the vasculature that may occur with resistance training is likely a protective adaptation that serves to maintain arterial endothelial cell cohesion or wall structural integrity, rather than adversely impacting on cardiac systolic function (Fisman *et al.* 2002).

Arteriogenesis does occur with resistance training (Fig. 4.1), and increases in conduit vessel size

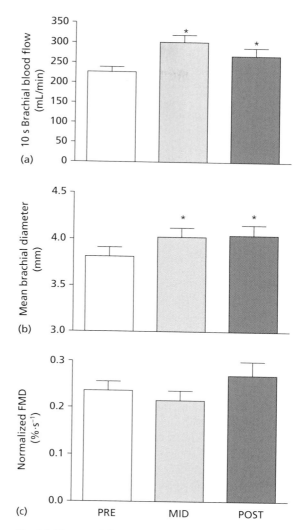

Fig. 4.1 Hyperemic brachial arterial blood flow (a), mean brachial artery diameter (b), and relative flow-mediated dilatation (FMD; c) before (PRE), during (MID), and after (POST) 6 and 12 weeks of elbow flexor strength training in young men. *$P < 0.05$ vs. Pre. (Adapted with permission from Rakobowchuk *et al.* 2005.)

similar to that noted with endurance exercise training have been observed (Rakobowchuk *et al.* 2005b). Though conduit artery vasodilatory capacity is unchanged, reactive hyperemic blood flow increases following resistance training (Fig. 4.2) as a result of angiogenesis or enhanced resistance vessel function (Rakobowchuk *et al.* 2005b). Furthermore,

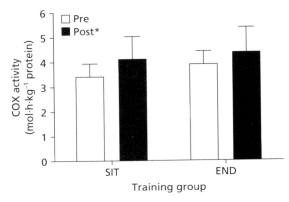

Fig. 4.2 Maximal activity of the mitochondrial marker cytochrome c oxidase (COX) measured in resting human skeletal muscle biopsy samples obtained before (open bars) and after (filled bars) six sessions of sprint interval training (SIT) or endurance training (END) over 2 weeks in young men. *$P < 0.05$ vs. pre-training (main effect for time). (Adapted with permission from Gibala *et al.* 2006.)

long-term resistance training maintains basal limb vascular conductance in middle-aged athletes compared to sedentary counterparts (Miyachi *et al.* 2005). These adaptive responses are likely to ensure rapid reperfusion following the occlusive nature of resistive movements, thus contributing to waste-product removal and tissue reoxygenation. In support of this at the microcirculatory level, maintenance of capillary density or the capillary-to-fiber ratio concurrent with fiber hypertrophy is expected, which would thus increase the total cross-sectional area of the microcirculation and the area for diffusion of substrates and products (Harris 2005).

Adaptations to sprint training

Skeletal muscular

Similar to endurance and strength training, the skeletal muscular adaptive response to sprint training is highly dependent on the precise nature of the training stimulus, i.e., the frequency, intensity and volume of work performed. However, unlike the other two forms of exercise which primarily rely on either oxidative (endurance) or non-oxidative (strength) energy to fuel ATP provision, the bioenergetics of sprint exercise can differ markedly

depending on the duration and intensity of each sprint bout, the number of intervals performed, and the duration of recovery between efforts (Ross & Leveritt 2001). While no form of exercise is purely "aerobic" or "anaerobic", sprinting is unique because cellular energy during a given exercise bout may be derived primarily from non-oxidative or oxidative metabolism. Consequently, sprint training can elicit a broad range of physiological adaptations, some of which resemble changes usually associated with traditional endurance or strength training (Ross & Leveritt 2001; Juel 2006).

Improved high-intensity exercise performance after sprint training appears related in part to increases in the maximal activities of enzymes that regulate non-oxidative energy provision (e.g., glycogen phosphorylase, phosphofructokinase) as well as an increased muscle buffering capacity (Ross & Leveritt 2001; Kubukeli *et al.* 2002). A number of ionic adaptations have also been reported after sprint training, including an increased content and function sodium-potassium ATPase (Na^+-K^+-ATPase) content, net Na^+ and K^+ uptake by contracting muscle, and reduced hyperkalemia during intense, matched-work exercise (Harmer *et al.* 2000; Neilsen *et al.* 2004). In terms of muscle fiber composition, several studies have reported a bidirectional shift to type 2a (i.e., from type 1 or type 2x to 2a), similar to the general trend observed after both endurance and strength training as previously discussed, although this is not a universal finding (Ross & Leveritt 2001; Kubukeli *et al.* 2002). Sprint training does not appear to have a major effect on muscle size, although a few studies have reported modest but significant hypertrophy of both type 1 and type 2 fibers after many months of training (Ross & Leveritt 2001).

It has long been recognized that sprint training has the potential to increase muscle oxidative capacity (Saltin & Gollnick 1983). However, until recently little was known regarding the effect of sprint training on skeletal muscle adaptations during aerobic-based exercise or the minimum volume of training necessary to elicit mitochondrial adaptations. Burgomaster *et al.* (2006) reported reduced rates of muscle glycogen utilization and lactate accumulation during a matched-work exercise challenge (10 min at 60% $\dot{V}o_{2peak}$ followed by 10 min at

90% of $\dot{V}o_{2peak}$) after only six sessions of brief, repeated "all-out" sprints ($4–6 \times 30$ sec efforts with 4 min of recovery between). The total volume of work performed in the study by Burgomaster *et al.* (2006) was surprising small and amounted to only 16 min of very intense exercise spread over a total time commitment of 2.5 h. The results also confirmed earlier findings by the same group (Burgomaster *et al.* 2005) that six sessions of sprint training over two weeks was sufficient to increase muscle oxidative capacity. The magnitude of the increase in citrate synthase maximal activity in these studies (Burgomaster *et al.* 2005, 2006) was comparable to that reported after several weeks of traditional endurance training, which suggested that sprint training was a very potent and time-efficient training strategy.

Surprisingly, only a few studies have directly compared changes in muscle oxidative capacity after interval versus continuous training in humans, with equivocal results (see references in Gibala *et al.* 2006). Moreover, every study that has examined this has used a matched-work design in which total work was similar between groups. Recently, we directly compared changes in muscle oxidative capacity and exercise performance after low-volume sprint training and traditional high-volume endurance training. The sprint protocol was based on other recent studies from our laboratory (Burgomaster *et al.* 2005, 2006) and consisted of six sessions of brief, repeated "all-out" 30 s cycling efforts, interspersed with a short recovery, over 14 days. The endurance protocol consisted of six sessions of 90–120 min of moderate-intensity cycling exercise, with 1–2 days of recovery interspersed between training sessions. As a result, subjects in both groups performed the same number of training sessions on the same days with the same number of recovery days; however, total training time commitment was 2.5 and 10.5 h, respectively, for the sprint and endurance group, and training volume differed by 90% (630 versus 6500 kJ). Biopsy samples obtained before and after training revealed similar increases in muscle oxidative capacity, as reflected by the maximal activity of cytochrome c oxidase (COX) and the protein content of COX subunits II and IV, as well as similar changes in cycling time-trial performance.

The potency of sprint training to elicit rapid changes in oxidative capacity comparable to endurance training is no doubt related to its high level of muscle fiber recruitment, and the potential to stress type 2 fibers in particular. As highlighted previously and discussed further in Chapter 13, contraction-induced metabolic disturbances in muscle activate several kinases involved in signal transduction, such as AMPK and CAMK, which are believed to play a role in promoting specific co-activators involved in mitochondrial biogenesis and metabolism (Hood & Irrcher 2006). Recently, Terada *et al.* (2005) reported similar increases in PGC-1 protein content after a single session of exercise that consisted of either high-intensity swimming (14×20 s intervals while carrying a load equivalent to 14% of body mass, with 10 s of rest between intervals) or low-intensity swimming (2×3 h with no load, separated by 45 min of rest), and concluded "high-intensity exercise is a potent tool to increase mitochondrial biogenesis, probably through enhancing PGC-1 expression." No studies have directly compared adaptations induced by different types of exercise training in humans; however, several groups have described changes in the expression of PGC-1 and other metabolic transcriptional co-activators and transcription factors after acute exercise (Pilegaard *et al.* 2003).

Cardiovascular

Relatively few studies have examined cardiovascular adaptations to sprint training in humans. For the most part, adaptations that benefit performance have been determined from measurements of blood flow and kinetic responses. These dynamic responses have been used to determine alteration in the flux of metabolic substrates and products such as lactate, potassium, or oxygen as a result of the sprint training. Thus, few insights regarding arterial structural, functional or microcirculatory alterations will be discussed. Myocardial adaptations that mirror those of endurance training occur in elite athletes with resultant positive relationships with enhanced performance and increased cardiac performance (enhanced ejection fraction; Legaz-Arrese *et al.* 2006). The timeline of these adaptations may be quite rapid in previously sedentary individuals, as evidenced by increased aortic cross-sectional areas with concomitant increases in left ventricular ejection fraction and reductions in resting heart rate after six weeks of intense sprint interval training (Rakobowchuk *et al.*, McMaster University, Hamilton, ON, unpublished observations). Heart rate is also reduced during a matched-work exercise challenge while cardiac output is maintained, suggesting enhanced stroke volume compensation similar to traditional endurance training (Rakobowchuk *et al.*, McMaster University, Hamilton, ON, unpublished observations).

In the only other study of its type that we are aware of, Warburton and colleagues (2004) examined mycocardial adaptations following 12 weeks of interval training (2 min intervals at 90% of $\dot{V}o_{2max}$ with recovery at 40% of $\dot{V}o_{2max}$) compared to a control endurance-trained group (~65% $\dot{V}o_{2max}$) who performed equal total work. Similar to the changes seen in the endurance-trained group, cardiac function at maximal exercise was enhanced in the interval-trained group with specific increases in EDV, stroke volume, cardiac output, and enhanced diastolic function yielding improved performance (Fig. 4.3). These adaptations likely contributed to the observed increase in $\dot{V}o_{2max}$ with an enhanced Frank-Starling mechanism likely playing a significant role independent of increases in blood volume, which were also measured in both groups (Warburton *et al.* 2004).

Bangsbo and colleagues have investigated both basal limb blood flow as well as blood flow responses at low, moderate, and high-intensity exercise after interval training in humans (Juel *et al.* 2004; Krustrup *et al.* 2004; Nielsen *et al.* 2004). These studies reported enhanced blood flow and vascular conductance at moderate and high intensities, which would serve to provide greater oxygen availability in trained limbs. This enhanced delivery promotes increased O_2 utilization, primarily at exercise onset (Krustrup *et al.* 2004), while concurrently limiting lactate accumulation (Juel *et al.* 2004) and reliance upon anaerobic metabolism during the initial phases of exercise, and may aid in recovery release of metabolic waste products as noted by the increased post-exercise blood flow following an incremental exercise to exhaustion (Juel *et al.* 2004). Mechanisms responsible for the enhanced blood flow are likely

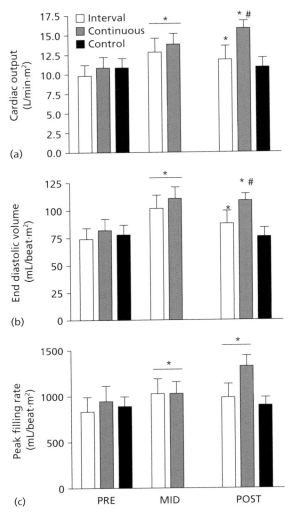

Fig. 4.3 Maximal exercise cardiac output (a) end diastolic volume (b) and peak filling rate (c) before (PRE) and after 6 (MID) and 12 weeks (POST) of either high-intensity interval or continuous endurance training, or equivalent period without training (control) in young men. (Adapted from Warburton *et al.* 2004 with permission.)

to involve both microvascular proliferation and conduit artery arteriogenesis/remodeling. Capillary density and capillary-to-fiber ratios are increased by four weeks of training, with greater capillary contacts per fiber in both type 1 and type 2 fibers (Jensen *et al.* 2004). Further mechanistic insight is noted by an increase in endothelial cell proliferation although the potent endothelial growth factor VEGF does not appear to be involved as protein content is unaltered with training (Jensen *et al.* 2004).

Conclusion

Physical training induces profound changes in the structure and function of the musculoskeletal and cardiovascular systems, whereas remodeling of the pulmonary system is less apparent. Training adaptations are highly dependent on the nature of the exercise performed (i.e., endurance, strength or sprint), however there is a surprising degree of overlap between specific stimuli, particularly early in the adaptive process. The mechanisms responsible for many training adaptations remain to be fully elucidated and this field continues to be a very fruitful area of study for those interested in human integrative physiology.

References

Andersen, L.L., Tufekovic, G., Zebis, M.K., Crameri, R.M., Verlaan, G., Kjaer, M., *et al.* (2005) The effect of resistance training combined with timed ingestion of protein on muscle fiber size and muscle strength. *Metabolism* **54**, 151–156.

Baar, K. (2006) Training for endurance and strength: lessons from cell signaling. *Medicine and Science in Sports and Exercise* **38**, 1939–1944.

Baumann, H., Jaggi, M., Soland, F., Howald, H. & Schaub, M.C. (1987) Exercise training induces transitions of myosin isoform subunits within histochemically typed human muscle fibers. *Pflugers Archives* **409**, 349–360.

Blomqvist, C.G. & Saltin, B. (1983) Cardiovascular adaptations to physical training. *Annual Review of Physiology* **45**, 169–189.

Booth, F.W. & Thomason, D.B. (1991) Molecular and cellular adaptation of muscle in response to exercise: perspectives of various models. *Physiologic Reviews* **71**, 541–585.

Brown, M.D. (2003) Exercise and coronary vascular remodelling in the healthy heart. *Experimental Physiology* **88**, 645–658.

Burgomaster, K.A., Hughes, S.C., Heigenhauser, G.J.F., Bradwell, S.N. & Gibala, M.J. (2005) Six sessions of sprint interval training increases muscle oxidative potential and cycle endurance capacity in humans. *Journal of Applied Physiology* **98**, 1985–1990.

Burgomaster, K.A., Heigenhauser, G.J. & Gibala, M.J. (2006) Effect of short-term sprint interval training on human skeletal muscle carbohydrate metabolism during exercise and time-trial performance. *Journal of Applied Physiology* **100**, 2041–2047.

Coyle, E.F. (2005) Improved muscular efficiency displayed as Tour de France champion matures. *Journal of Applied Physiology* **98**, 2191–2196.

D'Antona, G., Lanfranconi, F., Pellegrino, M.A., Brocca, L., Adami, R., Rossi, R., *et al.* (2006) Skeletal muscle hypertrophy and structure and function of skeletal muscle fibers in male body builders. *Journal of Physiology* **570**, 611–627.

Deldicque, L., Theisen, D. & Francaux, M. (2005) Regulation of mTOR by amino acids and resistance exercise in skeletal muscle. *European Journal of Applied Physiology* **94**, 1–10.

Dempsey, J.A., Miller, J.D. & Romer, L.M. (2006) The respiratory system. In: *ACSM's Advanced Exercise Physiology* (Tipton, C.M., ed.) Lippincott Williams & Wilkins, Philadelphia: 246–299.

Fisman, E.Z., Pelliccia, A., Motro, M., Auerbach, I., Frank, A.G. & Tenenbaum, A. (2002) Effect of intensive resistance training on isotonic exercise doppler indexes of left ventricular systolic function. *American Journal of Cardiology* **89**, 887–891.

Fluck, M. & Hoppeler, H. (2003) Molecular basis of skeletal muscle plasticity – from gene to form and function. *Review of Physiology, Biochemistry and Pharmacology* **146**, 159–216.

Folland, J.P. & Williams, A.G. (2007) The adaptations to strength training: morphological and neurological contributions to increased strength. *Sports Medicine* **37**, 145–168.

Gibala, M.J., Little, J.P., van Essen, M., Wilkin, G.P., Burgomaster, K.A., Safdar, A., *et al.* (2006) Short-term sprint interval versus traditional endurance training: similar initial adaptations in human skeletal muscle and exercise performance. *Journal of Physiology* **575**, 901–911.

Harmer, A.R., McKenna, M.J., Sutton, J.R., Snow, R.J., Ruell, P.A., Booth, J., *et al.* (2000) Skeletal muscle metabolic and ionic adaptations during intense exercise following sprint training in humans. *Journal of Applied Physiology* **89**, 1793–1803.

Harris, B.A. (2005) The influence of endurance and resistance exercise on muscle capillarization in the elderly: A review. *Acta Physiologica Scandinavica* **185**, 89–97.

Hasten, D.L., Pak-Loduca, J., Obert, K.A. & Yarasheski, K.E. (2000) Resistance exercise acutely increases MHC and mixed muscle protein synthesis rates in 78–84 and 23–32 yr olds. *American Journal of Physiology* **278**, E620–E626.

Hawley, J.A. (2002) Training for enhancement of sports performance. In: *Physiologic Bases of Sports Performance* (Hargreaves, M.A. & Hawley, J.A., eds) McGraw Hill, Sydney: 125–151.

Hawley, J.A., Tipton, K.D. & Millard-Stafford, M.L. (2006) Promoting training adaptations through nutritional interventions. *Journal of Sports Sciences* **24**, 709–721.

Haykowsky, M.J., Dressendorfer, R., Taylor, D., Mandic, S. & Humen, D. (2002) Resistance training and cardiac hypertrophy: Unravelling the training effect. *Sports Medicine* **32**, 837–849.

Holloszy, J.O. & Coyle, E.F. (1984) Adaptations of skeletal muscle to endurance exercise and their metabolic consequences. *Journal of Applied Physiology* **56**, 831–838.

Hood, D.A. & Irrcher, I. (2006) Mitochondrial biogenesis induced by endurance training. In: *ACSM's Advanced Exercise Physiology* (Tipton, C.M., ed.) Lippincott Williams & Wilkins, Philadelphia: 437–452.

Hoppeler, H. & Fluck, M. (2003) Plasticity of skeletal muscle mitochondria: structure and function. *Medicine and Science in Sports and Exercise* **35**, 95–104.

Howald, H., Hoppeler, H., Claassen, H., Mathieu, O. & Straub, R. (1985) Influences of endurance training on the ultrastructural composition of the different muscle fiber types in humans. *Pflugers Archives* **403**, 369–376.

Ingalls, C.P. (2004) Nature vs. nurture: can exercise really alter fiber type composition in human skeletal muscle? *Journal of Applied Physiology* **97**, 1591–1592.

Jensen, L., Bangsbo, J., & Hellsten, Y. (2004) Effect of high intensity training on capillarization and presence of angiogenic factors in human skeletal muscle. *Journal of Physiology* **557**, 571–582.

Juel, C. (2006) Training-induced changes in membrane transport proteins of human skeletal muscle. *European Journal of Applied Physiology* **96**, 627–635.

Juel, C., Klarskov, C., Nielsen, J.J., Krustrup, P., Mohr, M. & Bangsbo, J. (2004) Effect of high-intensity intermittent training on lactate and H^+ release from human skeletal muscle. *American Journal of Physiology* **286**, E245–E251.

Kawano, H., Tanaka, H. & Miyachi, M. (2006) Resistance training and arterial compliance: Keeping the benefits while minimizing the stiffening. *Journal of Hypertension* **24**, 1753–1759.

Kim, P.L., Staron, R.S. & Phillips, S.M. (2005) Fasted-state skeletal muscle protein synthesis after resistance exercise is altered with training. *Journal of Physiology* **568**, 283–290.

Kjaer, A., Meyer, C., Wachtell, K., Olsen, M.H., Ibsen, H., Opie, L., *et al.* (2005) Positron emission tomographic evaluation of regulation of myocardial perfusion in physiologic (elite athletes) and pathological (systemic hypertension) left ventricular hypertrophy. *American Journal of Cardiology* **96**, 1692–1698.

Kozakova, M., Galetta, F., Gregorini, L., Bigalli, G., Franzoni, F., Giusti, C., *et al.* (2000) Coronary vasodilator capacity and epicardial vessel remodeling in physiologic and hypertensive hypertrophy. *Hypertension* **36**, 343–349.

Krustrup, P., Hellsten, Y. & Bangsbo, J. (2004) Intense interval training enhances human skeletal muscle oxygen uptake in the initial phase of dynamic exercise at high but not at low intensities. *Journal of Physiology* **559**, 335–345.

Kubukeli, Z.N., Noakes, T.D. & Dennis, S.C. (2002) Training techniques to improve endurance exercise performances. *Sports Medicine* **32**, 489–509.

Legaz-Arrese, A., Gonzalez-Carretero, M. & Lacambra-Blasco, I. (2006) Adaptation of left ventricular morphology to long-term training in sprint- and endurance-trained elite runners. *European Journal of Applied Physiology* **96**, 740–746.

Levine, S., Nguyen, T., Shrager, J., Kaiser, L., Camasamudram, V. & Rubinstein, N. (2001) Diaphragm adaptations elicited by severe chronic obstructive pulmonary disease: lessons for sports science. *Exercise and Sport Sciences Reviews* **29**, 71–75.

MacDougall, J.D. (1992) Hypertrophy or hyperplasia. In: *Strength and Power in Sport* (Komi, P., ed.) Blackwell Scientific Publications, London: 230–238.

McCall, G.E., Byrnes, W.C., Dickinson, A., Pattany, P.M. & Fleck, S.J. (1996) Muscle fiber hypertrophy, hyperplasia, and capillary density in college men after resistance training. *Journal of Applied Physiology* **81**, 2004–2012.

McConnell, A.K. & Romer, L.M. (2004) Respiratory muscle training in healthy humans: resolving the controversy. *International Journal of Sports Medicine* **25**, 284–293.

Miyachi, M., Kawano, H., Sugawara, J., Takahashi, K., Hayashi, K., Yamazaki, *et al.* (2004) Unfavorable effects of resistance training on central arterial compliance: A randomized intervention study. *Circulation* **110**, 2858–2863.

Miyachi, M., Tanaka, H., Kawano, H., Okajima, M. & Tabata, I. (2005) Lack of age-related decreases in basal whole leg blood flow in resistance-trained men. *Journal of Applied Physiology* **99**, 1384–1390.

Moore, R.L. (2006) The cardiovascular system: cardiac function. In: *ACSM's Advanced Exercise Physiology* (Tipton, C.M., ed.) Lippincott Williams & Wilkins, Philadelphia: 326–342.

Nielsen, J.J., Mohr, M., Klarskov, C., Kristensen, M., Krustrup, P., Juel, C., *et al.* (2004) Effects of high-intensity intermittent training on potassium kinetics and performance in human skeletal muscle. *Journal of Physiology* **554**, 857–870.

Olfert, I.M., Balouch, J., Kleinsasser, A., Knapp, A., Wagner, H., Wagner, P.D., *et al.* (2004) Does gender affect human pulmonary gas exchange during exercise? *Journal of Physiology* **557**, 529–541.

Phillips, S.M., Tipton, K.D., Aarsland, A., Wolf, S.E. & Wolfe, R.R. (1997) Mixed muscle protein synthesis and breakdown following resistance

exercise in humans. *American Journal of Physiology* **273**, E99–E107.

Phillips, S.M., Parise, G., Roy, B.D., Tipton, K.D., Wolfe, R.R. & Tamopolsky, M.A. (2002) Resistance-training-induced adaptations in skeletal muscle protein turnover in the fed state. *Canadian Journal of Physiology and Pharmacology* **80**, 1045–1053.

Phillips, S.M., Hartman, J.W. & Wilkinson, S.B. (2005) Dietary protein to support anabolism with resistance exercise in young men. *Journal of the American College of Nutrition* **24**, 134S–139S.

Pilegaard, H., Saltin, B. & Neufer, P.D. (2003) Exercise induces transient transcriptional activation of the PGC-1alpha gene in human skeletal muscle. *Journal of Physiology* **546**, 851–858.

Poelkens, F., Rakobowchuk, M., Burgomaster, K.A., Hopman, M., Phillips, S.M. & MacDonald, M.J. (2007) Effect of unilateral resistance training on arterial compliance in elderly men. *Applied Physiology, Nutrition and Metabolism* **32**(4), 670–676.

Powers, S.K., Coombes, J. & Demirel, H. (1997) Exercise training-induced changes in respiratory muscles. *Sports Medicine* **24**, 120–131.

Prior, B.M., Yang, H.T. & Terjung, R.L. (2004) What makes vessels grow with exercise training? *Journal of Applied Physiology* **97**, 119–128.

Rakobowchuk, M., McGowan, C.L., de Groot, P.C., Bruinsma, D., Hartman, J.W., Phillips, S.M., *et al.* (2005a) Effect of whole body resistance training on arterial compliance in young healthy males. *Experimental Physiology* **90**, 645–51.

Rakobowchuk, M., McGowan, C.L., de Groot, P.C., Hartman, J.W., Phillips, S.M. & MacDonald, M.J. (2005b) Endothelial function of young healthy males following whole-body resistance training. *Journal of Applied Physiology* **98**, 2185–2190.

Rankinen, T., Bray, M.S., Hagberg, J.M., Perusse, L., Roth, S.M., Wolfarth, B., *et al.* (2006) The human gene map for performance and health-related fitness phenotypes: the 2005 update. *Medicine and Science in Sports and Exercise* **38**, 1863–1888.

Rasmussen, B.B. & Phillips, S.M. (2003) Contractile and nutritional regulation of human muscle growth. *Exercise and Sport Sciences Reviews* **31**, 127–131.

Rennie, M.J., Wackerhage, H., Spangenburg, E.E. & Booth, F.W. (2004)

Control of the size of the human muscle mass. *Annual Review of Physiology* **66**, 799–828.

Ross, A. & Leveritt, M. (2001) Long-term metabolic and skeletal muscle adaptations to short-sprint training: implications for sprint training and tapering. *Sports Medicine* **31**, 1063–1082.

Saltin, B. & Gollnick, P.D. (1983) Skeletal muscle adaptability: significance for metabolism and performance. In: *Handbook of Physiology – Skeletal Muscle* (Peachey, L.D., ed.) American Physiologic Society, Bethesda: 555–631.

Tang, J.E., Hartman, J.W. & Phillips, S.M. (2006) Increased muscle oxidative potential following resistance training induced fiber hypertrophy in young men. *Applied Physiology, Nutrition and Metabolism* **31**, 495–501.

Terada, S., Kawanaka, K., Goto, M., Shimokawa, T. & Tabata, I. (2005) Effects of high-intensity intermittent swimming on PGC-1 protein expression in rat skeletal muscle. *Acta Physiologica Scandinavica* **184**, 59–65.

Tipton, C.M. & Franklin, B.A. (2006) The language of exercise. In: *ACSM's Advanced Exercise Physiology* (Tipton, C.M., ed.) Lippincott Williams & Wilkins, Philadelphia: 3–10.

Tipton, K.D. & Wolfe, R.R. (2004) Protein and amino acids for athletes. *Journal of Sports Sciences* **22**, 65–79.

Tonkonogi, M. & Sahlin, K. (2002) Physical exercise and mitochondrial function in human skeletal muscle. *Exercise and Sport Sciences Reviews* **30**, 129–137.

Wagner, P.D. (2005) Why doesn't exercise grow the lungs when other factors do? *Exercise and Sports Sciences Reviews* **33**, 3–8.

Walsh, B., Tonkonogi, M. & Sahlin, K. (2001) Effect of endurance training on oxidative and antioxidative function in human permeabilized muscle fibers. *Pflugers Archives* **442**, 420–425.

Warburton, D.E., Haykowsky, M.J., Quinney, H.A., Blackmore, D., Teo, K.K., Taylor, D.A., *et al.* (2004) Blood volume expansion and cardiorespiratory function: Effects of training modality. *Medicine and Science in Sports and Exercise* **36**, 991–1000.

Weston, A.R., Myburgh, K.H., Lindsay, F.H., Dennis, S.C., Noakes, T.D. & Hawley, J.A. (1997) Skeletal muscle buffering capacity and endurance performance after high-intensity interval training by well-trained cyclists. *European Journal of Applied Physiology* **75**, 7–13.

Chapter 5

Skeletal Muscle Metabolic Adaptations to Training

GRAHAM P. HOLLOWAY AND LAWRENCE L. SPRIET

Strenuous exercise can increase the energy expenditure of skeletal muscle by 100-fold over resting basal metabolic conditions, placing an enormous challenge on the bioenergetic pathways in terms of maintaining homeostatic levels of adensine triphosphate (ATP), the basic unit of energy within cells (Saltin & Gollnick 1983; Spriet & Howlett 1999). The majority of the ATP requirement during exercise (~70%) is consumed by myosin ATPases to maintain cross-bridge cycling and the generation of force. Ion pumping also consumes ATP, with Ca^{2+} ATPases consuming ~25% of the required ATP and sodium-potassium (Na^+-K^+) ATPases consuming ~5% (Kushmerick 1983).

Skeletal muscle is well equipped to regenerate ATP as it has the ability to metabolize fuels in the form of carbohydrate and fat to produce reducing equivalents that can be used to resynthesize ATP from adensine diphosphate (ADP) and inorganic phosphate (P_i), during the process of oxidative phosphorylation within the mitochondria (Fig. 5.1). Importantly, there are two main sources of carbohydrate in the body, namely liver and skeletal muscle glycogen, and also two sources of fat in the body – adipose tissue and skeletal muscle triacylglycerol (TAG; Fig. 5.2). Thus, for each fuel source one depot is present within skeletal muscle and the other is located externally and has to be transported to the muscle when required (for a review see van Loon 2004). Each fuel source provides the necessary reducing equivalents, or electron donors [i.e.,

The Olympic Textbook of Science in Sport, 1st edition. Edited by R.J. Maughan. Published 2009 by Blackwell Publishing. ISBN: 978-1-4051-5638-7.

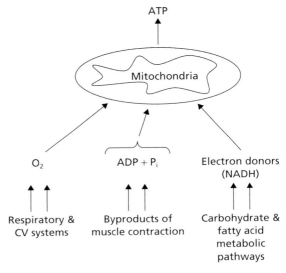

Fig. 5.1 Factors affecting aerobic respiration. ADP, adenosine diphosphate; ATP, adenosine triphosphate; CV, cardiovascular; O_2, oxygen; P_i, inorganic phosphate.

reduced nicotinamide adenine dinucleotide (NADH)] for aerobic respiration and the generation of ATP (Fig. 5.1). Both carbohydrate and fatty acids are important during varying exercise intensities and durations, and while carbohydrate can be used to make ATP at a faster rate, fatty acids represent an essentially limitless energy supply. The maximum rate of fatty acid oxidation occurs at about 65% of peak oxygen uptake ($\dot{V}o_{2peak}$); thereafter the rate of fatty acid oxidation declines and the fractional – as well as the absolute – rate of carbohydrate oxidation increases (Fig. 5.3). Additional fuels including amino

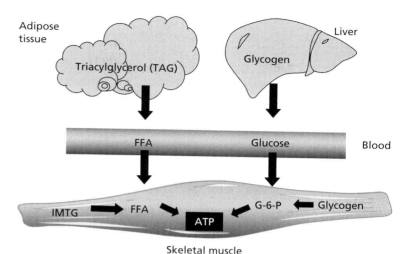

Fig. 5.2 Locations of fuel sources used during exercise. ATP, adenosine triphosphate; FFA, free fatty acid; G-6-P, glucose-6-phosphate; IMTG, intramuscular triacylglycerol; TAG, triacylglycerol.

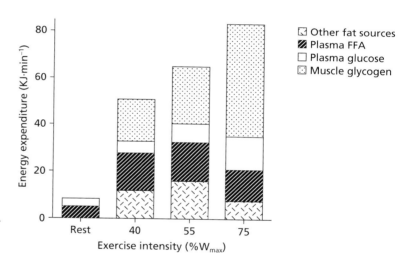

Fig. 5.3 Contribution of fuel sources at various intensities of exercise. FFA, free fatty acid. (Reproduced with permission from van Loon 2004.)

acids and ketone bodies can be oxidized when carbohydrate and fat are in short supply.

The muscle can also regenerate ATP in substrate phosphorylation reactions that do not require oxygen and which occur mainly in the cytoplasm (Spriet & Howlett 1999). The most notable of these are the breakdown of phosphocreatine (PCr) to produce ATP in the creatine kinase reaction and the reactions of the glyoclytic pathway. While aerobic metabolism dominates the production of ATP in most exercise situations, anaerobic metabolism contributes energy when: (i) transitioning from rest to exercise or from one power output to a higher power output;

(ii) exercising at power outputs that require energy at a faster rate than can be provided for aerobically; and (iii) oxygen availability is limiting. The aerobic and anaerobic systems work together to ensure that the required ATP for muscle contractions is provided at a rate that closely matches the demand, so that the muscle ATP concentration is held constant.

Skeletal muscle is a very adaptable organ as it responds to repeated bouts of exercise by enhancing the rates at which ATP can be synthesized, in some cases by increasing the mass of muscle involved in ATP production. A central adaptation to repeated exercise is an increase in mitochondrial volume per unit of muscle mass (for a review see Holloszy & Coyle 1984). Since mitochondria are the organelles responsible for aerobic ATP provision, an increase in mitochondrial volume would represent an increase in the maximum aerobic generation capacity. In addition, and as discussed later in this chapter, an increase in mitochondria also has profound effects on energy provision at submaximal exercise intensities. The remainder of this chapter is dedicated to reviewing recent literature in an attempt to understand how bioenergetic pathways in skeletal muscle are altered with training and how these alterations are beneficial with respect to ATP homeostasis.

The realization that skeletal muscles could be trained

It has long been known that sedentary individuals can improve their exercise endurance by performing regular exercise, such as long-distance running. However, in the early 1960s this improvement was believed to be solely the result of adaptations in the cardiovascular system resulting in greater oxygen delivery to the contracting muscles (Holloszy & Coyle 1984). The suggestion was that the muscles did not adapt and that muscle mitochondrial content was largely a function of genetics. Although a suitable genetic endowment is an obvious requirement for elite athletic ability, research by Holloszy and colleagues in the late 1960s and early 1970s demonstrated the remarkable plasticity of skeletal muscle, and the power of training with respect to its ability to alter muscle characteristics (Holloszy & Coyle 1984). Earlier training studies using rats failed to show changes in muscle characteristics following a 30-min chronic swim-training protocol (Hearn & Wainio 1956; Gould & Rawlinson 1959). Holloszy reasoned that the intensity of the training was not sufficient to induce metabolic changes within skeletal muscle, because pilot work in his laboratory showed that rats could swim continuously for 6 h. Therefore, Holloszy proceeded with a 15-week treadmill running program that continuously increased in duration and intensity until week 12, and thereafter was maintained at 2 h of running a day at $32 \text{ m} \cdot \text{min}^{-1}$, with short sprints (1 min) at $42 \text{ m} \cdot \text{min}^{-1}$ every 10 min. This training program resulted in

remarkable improvements in run time to exhaustion tests (Holloszy 1967). This concept of overload is now regarded as fundamental to all forms of training, but 40 years ago this was a major step forward. Research over the next 10 years focused on unraveling what was responsible for the improved performance following training and also examined the responses in human skeletal muscle. However, to this day the understanding of what causes the training-induced changes in muscle continue to evolve, especially with the advent of molecular biology techniques. It should be noted however, that the focus of this chapter is not to examine the molecular mechanisms responsible for increasing mitochondrial content (biogenesis). This area is covered in detail in Chapter 13, and in recent reviews (e.g., Hood & Saleem 2007).

Several important concepts emerged from Holloszy's landmark studies, but the most important was the concept of mitochondrial biogenesis (Holloszy 1967; Holloszy & Oscai 1969; Holloszy et al. 1970; Mole & Holloszy 1970; Oscai & Holloszy 1971). Oxidative metabolism of both carbohydrate and fatty acid fuel sources occurs within the mitochondria. While adequate supplies of oxygen, ADP, P_i, and NADH are required for mitochondrial ATP production, the mitochondrial volume or machinery available for generating it is also important. Therefore, a greater mitochondrial volume following training provides the means for a greater capacity to produce NADH from carbohydrate and fat, and hence more ATP in the electron transport chain (ETC). These alterations also place a greater stress on the other metabolic pathways to increase provision and availability of carbohydrate and fatty acids.

This chapter will examine how training affects the sites of regulation in carbohydrate and fatty acid metabolism. Each bioenergetic pathway will be examined in a sequential fashion, starting with fuel delivery and subsequently each purported site of metabolic regulation. The focus will be on understanding how training alters the regulation and production of mitochondrial ATP, including the interactions between the various metabolic pathways, and why a greater reliance on fatty acids is observed at the same absolute exercise intensity following training.

Mitochondrial biogenesis with training

Mitochondria, unlike other organelles, contain two membranes: an outer and an inner (for a review see McGarry & Brown 1997). The outer membrane allows some biochemical compounds to diffuse through and is therefore considered semi-permeable. The inner membrane does not allow compounds to diffuse through in any measurable quantity and is considered non-permeable. Classically, mitochondrial content has been determined biochemically by measuring "marker" enzymes and proteins located in the various mitochondrial pathways [transport proteins, pyruvate dehydrogenase (PDH), tricarboxylic acid (TCA) cycle, beta-oxidation pathway, electron shuttle enzymes, ETC]; more recently molecular techniques have enabled researchers to quantify the amount of mitochondrial DNA. Histochemical and electron microscope techniques have also been used to assess mitochondrial volume changes. Regardless of the measurement techniques implemented to study mitochondrial proliferation following classic aerobic training (1–2 h·day^{-1} at ~60% $\dot{V}o_{2peak}$), a repeatable observation is an increase of approximately 30% in mitochondrial content in human skeletal muscle (Henriksson & Reitman 1977; Green *et al.* 1995; Chesley *et al.* 1996; Phillips *et al.* 1996b; Spina *et al.* 1996). It should be mentioned that training consisting of repeated bouts of short duration (30–240 s), intense exercise (90–150% $\dot{V}o_{2peak}$) has recently been shown to elicit similar adaptations in mitochondrial content with much lower volumes of training (MacDougall *et al.* 1998; Burgomaster *et al.* 2005; Perry *et al.* 2007; Talanian *et al.* 2007). Since the inner mitochondrial membrane does not allow glucose or fatty acids to diffuse into the mitochondria at sufficient rates, both require a transport system to gain access to the mitochondrial matrix – the site of aerobic respiration. Carbohydrate metabolism (either glucose or glycogen) is initiated in the cytoplasm, and the end product is two molecules of pyruvate, two or three of ATP (from glucose and glycogen, respectively), and two of NADH. The pyruvate is transported into mitochondria and metabolized by PDH to produce acetyl-CoA, carbon dioxide (CO_2) and NADH (for reviews see Peters 2003; Spriet & Watt 2003; Fig. 5.4). Acetyl-CoA is the "starting

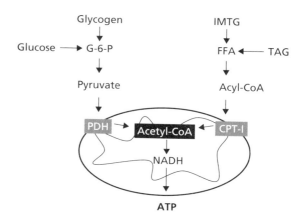

Fig. 5.4 Merging enzymatic pathways involved in aerobic respiration. ATP, adenosine triphosphate; CPT-I, carnitine palmitoyltransferase-I ; G-6-P, glucose-6-phosphate; IMTG, intramuscular triacylglycerol; PDH, pyruvate dehydrogenase; TAG, triacylglycerol.

point" of the TCA cycle, going through several enzymatic reactions (including reactions controlled by citrate synthase, isocitrate dehydrogenase and α-ketoglutarate dehydrogenase) creating more NADH for the ETC. The NADH generated in the cytoplasm during the production of pyruvate is also transported into the mitochondria by two independent mechanisms. The first, known as the glycerol-phosphate, shuttle is not altered with training (Holloszy & Oscai 1969), while the second, known as the malate aspartate shuttle, has a higher capacity in aerobically-trained individuals (Schantz *et al.* 1986; Perry *et al.* 2007).

Fatty acids are transported by the carnitine shuttle, and the rate-limiting enzyme in this pathway is carnitine palmitoyltransferase-I (CPT-I; for review see McGarry & Brown 1997). Aerobically-trained individuals have a higher maximal CPT-I activity indicating a greater capacity to transport fatty acids into mitochondria (Starritt *et al.* 2000). Fatty acids are also metabolized by dehydrogenase reactions (e.g., via acyl-CoA dehydrogenase) in the beta-oxidation pathway within mitochondria creating acetyl-CoA, which enters the TCA cycle in a similar fashion to carbohydrate (Fig. 5.4).

Holloszy demonstrated that endurance training increased the mitochondrial protein and content and ability of rat skeletal muscle to oxidize various lipid species (palmitate, oleate, palmitoyl-CoA, palmitoyl-carnitine) and pyruvate by ~60% (Mole & Holloszy 1970; Mole et al. 1971). Subsequent work reported that the activities of the enzymes involved in the TCA cycle (citrate synthase, isocitrate dehydrogenase, α-ketoglutarate dehydrogenase, succinate dehydrogenase, and malate dydrogenase), the ETC (complexes I, II, IV, and cytochrome C), and pathways specific to fatty acid oxidation (acyl-CoA synthetase, CPT-I, and acyl-CoA dehydrogenase), all increased by between 50 and 100% (Holloszy & Coyle 1984; Henriksson et al. 1986). Importantly, isolated mitochondria also displayed an increased ability to oxidize these substrates, even when normalized to mitochondrial protein (Holloszy 1967). These measurements showed for the first time that not only did the mitochondrial content within skeletal muscle increase following training, but that the mitochondrial machinery required for ATP production increased in concert such that the capacity for ATP production from fat and carbohydrate was enhanced. In addition, it appeared that the increase in mitochondria was energetically important, as the phosphate-to-oxygen (P/O) coupling ratios were stoichiometrically relevant at ~2.5 (indicating the generation of ATP).

The general findings of these studies have been replicated several times, although the magnitudes of the changes are much smaller in human skeletal muscle (~30%) compared to adaptations in rodents (~100%). Classic endurance training (2 h·day^{-1} at ~60% $\dot{V}o_{2peak}$), sprint interval training, and high-intensity intermittent training, all increased mitochondrial enzymes by ~30%, despite variations in intensity, frequency, and total exercise time. This potential difference between rodents and humans may be related to the low activity levels of rats housed in small cages, as severely untrained humans also experience larger adaptations to training (Bruce et al. 2006). Since the TCA cycle and the ETC are common pathways in carbohydrate and fatty acid metabolism, the importance of these alterations with respect to performance may not be apparent at first. However, the mitochondrial volume has a large influence on fuel selection, both at the onset and during sustained exercise.

Fatty acid metabolism

Originally, fatty acid oxidation was believed to be entirely regulated by substrate delivery from peripheral adipose tissue, and the passive diffusion of fatty acids across the plasma membrane. This concept was largely derived from a lack of known regulation and from the observation that providing more fatty acids, as during lipid infusion studies, increased fatty acid oxidation. However, it has become apparent over the last decade that fatty acid metabolism has several sites of regulation, including lipolysis and release from adipose tissue, transport in the plasma, plasma membrane transport, lipolysis in the muscle, and transport into mitochondria (for a review see Spriet 2006). One of the most reproducible findings of training is an enhanced reliance on fatty acids as a fuel source during submaximal exercise (Chesley et al. 1996; Phillips et al. 1996a; Putman et al. 1998; Talanian et al. 2007). The focus of this chapter is on skeletal muscle adaptations to training, and therefore a detailed assessment of how adipose tissue is altered with training will not be undertaken. However, peripheral lipolysis of TAG within adipose tissue has been suggested to be either unaltered with training, or slightly decreased (Martin et al. 1993; Phillips et al. 1996a). Once TAG are degraded into the constituent three free fatty acids (FFA) and glycerol, some of the FFA are released into the circulation and bound to albumin.

The transport of fatty acids across the muscle membrane is no longer viewed as an entirely passive diffusion event (Bonen et al. 1998; Bonen et al. 2007). Studies of plasma membrane transport protein activity and saturation kinetics suggested that fatty acid transport proteins are involved in the transport of FFA into muscle cells (Bonen et al. 1998; Turcotte et al. 2000). In addition, a correlation exists between the abundance of transport proteins and fatty acid transport, such that more transport proteins on the plasma membrane means more FFA transport into the muscle (Bonen et al. 2004; Koonen et al. 2004). Two important fatty acid transport proteins have been shown to exist on the muscle membrane and intracellularly, including fatty acid translocase (FAT/CD36; Bonen et al. 2000; Koonen et al. 2005; Chabowski et al. 2005) and fatty acid-binding protein

(FABPpm; Koonen *et al.* 2004; Han *et al.* 2007). Training studies have shown that both FAT/CD36 mRNA and protein expression increase in whole skeletal muscle samples (Tunstall *et al.* 2002; Talanian *et al.* 2007). However, this does not indicate that transport is increased, as these measurements do not provide information regarding subcellular locations. Future work in humans is required to determine if the levels of plasma membrane transport proteins are elevated following training, and if plasma membrane FFA transport into the muscle increases in parallel. While the issue of peripheral FFA oxidation following training remains controversial, the increased role of TAG hydrolysis now appears clear (Phillips *et al.* 1996a; van Loon *et al.* 2004; Stellingwerff *et al.* 2007). Training has been shown to increase the amount of fat stored within muscle (Phillips *et al.* 1996b; Lee *et al.* 2007), and chronically trained individuals have higher TAG contents (Goodpaster *et al.* 2001; Thamer *et al.* 2003), as well as higher rates of fatty acid oxidation. Phillips and colleagues (1996a) have shown that classic aerobic training (2 h·day^{-1} for 31 days at ~60% $\dot{V}o_{2peak}$) increased the amount of fat oxidized by 70% during a 90 min standardized cycling test as a result of an increase in TAG utilization, while reporting a concomitant decrease in adipose tissue lipolysis. Hormone sensitive lipase (HSL) has been considered the rate-limiting enzyme in TAG lipolysis in both adipose tissue and skeletal muscle. HSL is regulated through phosphorylation at several serine/threonine sites by epinephrine (EPI), calcium, and several downstream signaling intermediates, including extracellular signal-regulated kinase (ERK) and mitogen-activated protein kinase (MAPK) (for a review see Watt and Spriet 2004). Phosphorylation can activate and/or inhibit HSL activity, and ultimately the activity of HSL will be determined by the sum of all regulators. Studies examining the maximum activity of HSL following training, as well as the various phosphorylated sites, have not reported differences and yet TAG utilization is increased (Enevoldsen *et al.* 2001). It has previously been suggested that HSL must be translocated to perilipin, a protective covering around TAG, to be fully activated (for a review see Tansey *et al.* 2004). The measurements employed in training studies to measure maximal HSL activity do not provide an insight into the location of HSL before and after training, which may explain the discrepancies. Alternatively, a "new" enzyme called adipose tissue triacylglycerol lipase (ATGL), named because it was originally found in adipose tissue, has been found to preferentially breakdown TAG within skeletal muscle; but this enzyme has not been studied following training (Zimmermann *et al.* 2004; Jocken *et al.* 2007). Following training, circulating EPI levels are reduced at the same absolute intensity (Phillips *et al.* 1996a), which would contribute to decreased HSL activity. However, TAG use is increased and this may be due to additional contraction-related signals (e.g., calcium) that activate HSL within muscle. Although the exact mechanisms remain unclear, it appears that TAG provides a greater proportion of energy following training (Phillips *et al.* 1996a).

Regardless of the source, once FFA are in the cytosol they must be bound to a cytosolic FABP (FABPc) to solubilize the fat in an aqueous environment (Glatz *et al.* 2003). FABPc appears to be present in excess and is not believed to be rate-limiting in any respect, as genetic modifications with rodents have shown that a reduction of more than 50% in levels of this protein does not have any detrimental effects on fatty acid metabolism (Luiken *et al.* 2003). However, it should be pointed out that complete ablation of this protein compromised fatty acid oxidation by ~70%, indicating that FABPc are necessary (Luiken *et al.* 2003). In addition, training has been shown to increase this protein in skeletal muscle by ~50% (Lee *et al.* 2007). Prior to either storage or oxidation, fatty acids must be activated to a CoA thioester, and bound to another cytosolic protein – acyl-CoA binding protein. The subsequent fatty acyl-CoA is a substrate for CPT-I, the enzyme that has traditionally been considered a rate-limiting step in fatty acid oxidation transport into mitochondria (for a review see McGarry & Brown 1997). CPT-I has been shown to be upregulated following training (Mole *et al.* 1971; Bruce *et al.* 2006), and therefore the mitochondrial capacity to transport acyl-CoA is increased. The subsequent oxidation of acyl-CoA through beta oxidation, the TCA cycle, and the ETC is mainly regulated through *de novo* expression of the respective enzymes. Since training increases mitochondrial biogenesis (Holloszy & Coyle 1984), these combined effects increase the rate of fatty acid oxidation. As previously mentioned, endurance training increased the ability of rat skeletal muscle to oxidize various lipid species (Mole & Holloszy 1970). Importantly, isolated mitochondria also oxidized these substrates, even when normalized to mitochondrial protein. These measurements reported for the first time that, in addition to the increases in mitochondrial content following training, alterations occurred within the mitochondria that enabled better utilization of substrates aerobically (Holloszy 1967). In addition, it appeared that the increase in mitochondrial volume was energetically relevant, as the P/O coupling ratios were ~2.5, which indicates the generation of ATP.

Carbohydrate oxidation

Similar to fatty acid metabolism, the substrate for carbohydrate metabolism can be derived from the plasma outside the cell, and from intracellular stores. Plasma glucose concentrations are highly regulated by insulin and glucagon, and following training the plasma glucose concentration prior to the start of exercise is not altered (Phillips et al. 1996a). As with fatty acid metabolism, there are also plasma membrane transporters that aid the movement of glucose into the cell. Basal glucose uptake is controlled by the so-called GLUT1 transporters, and insulin and exercise-related increases in glucose uptake are controlled by GLUT4 transporters (for a review see Furtado et al. 2002). There are three main similarities between GLUT4 and fatty acid transport proteins: (i) the amount of transporter on the membrane influences the transport rate; (ii) the transporter also exists in an intracellular location; and (iii) GLUT4 can be translocated to the plasma membrane under various metabolic perturbations (insulin and/or muscle contraction) (Wojtaszewski & Richter 1998; Czech & Corvera 1999; Bonen et al. 2002). The levels of GLUT4 are increased following training (Richter et al. 1998; Burgomaster et al. 2007), and therefore the capacity to transport glucose into the cell is increased. However, it appears that the translocation of GLUT4 to the plasma membrane following training is diminished (Phillips et al. 1996a; Richter et al. 1998) at a given absolute power output, and

that subsequently the transport of glucose is reduced (Richter et al. 1998). This occurs at the same time that fatty acid oxidation is increased. Physiologically, the increased capacity for glucose uptake plays a more important role during intense exercise at or around the new higher $\dot{V}O_{2peak}$ following training. Once inside the cell, glucose immediately undergoes phosphorylation by hexokinase, essentially trapping the glucose within the cell and maintaining a favorable concentration gradient across the membrane. Hexokinase has consistently been shown to increase following training, with the magnitude of increase typically greater than mitochondrial changes (50–200%; Baldwin et al. 1973; Phillips et al. 1995; Spina et al. 1996; MacDougall et al. 1998). Collectively, this suggests that the capacity for delivering glucose to the glycolytic pathway is enhanced following training. In addition, training has been shown to increase muscle glycogen stores substantially (~20–50%) following endurance training (Gollnick & King 1969; Green et al. 1995; Leblanc et al. 2004a; Gibala et al. 2006), sprint interval training (Burgomaster et al. 2005; Gibala et al. 2006), and high-intensity intermittent training (MacDougall et al. 1998). In addition, even a single bout of exercise has been shown to slightly elevate muscle glycogen stores following 24 h of recovery (Lamb et al. 1969). Therefore, it appears that the capacity to deliver glycolytic substrates is increased following training.

Prior to entering the mitochondria, glucose and glycogen go through a series of reactions ultimately generating pyruvate, which enters the mitochondria and is converted into acetyl-CoA and subsequently oxidized in the TCA cycle. Glycogen phopshorylase (PHOS) and phosphofructokinase (PFK) are regulated, non-equilibrium enzymes in the pathways that metabolize glycogen/glucose, and set the upper limit for maximal rates of carbohydrate use during exercise. Most of the remaining enzymes involved in glycolysis are near-equilibrium enzymes, and therefore are solely regulated by the enzyme content and the concentrations of substrates and products. It is generally agreed that "classic" endurance training does not normally alter enzyme levels in the glycolytic pathway; indeed, some endurance protocols have been found to decrease the maximal glycolytic capacity. Green and colleagues employed a cycling training protocol of 2 h·day^{-1} at 60% $\dot{V}o_{2peak}$ for seven consecutive days, and reported that maximum PFK activity decreased by about 20% (Green *et al.* 1992). While endurance training may decrease the maximum glycolytic capacity, it is important to consider the type of exercise, as more intense exercise has been shown to increase the functional ability of the glycolytic system (MacDougall *et al.* 1998). This controversy likely relates to the requirement for overloading in order for a response to be observed. The maximal capacity of the glycolytic system far exceeds the aerobic capacity as it is present for sprint type situations. Therefore, during "classic endurance training" the glycolytic system is not sufficiently stressed. However, with sprint interval training, and a greater stress on the glycolytic pathway to produce anaerobic energy, increases in glycolytic enzymes have been observed.

The maximum activity of PDH sets the upper limit for the aerobic use of carbohydrate in the mitochondria. Recent studies have shown that seven weeks of exercise training increased the maximum activity of PDH by about 30%, mainly as a result of increased expression of the E1a catalytic subunit (Leblanc *et al.* 2004a,b). It is important to remember that maximum activity assays only provide information on the capacity of an enzyme that would be relevant during exercise at ~100% $\dot{V}o_{2peak}$. Indeed, measurements of PDH in the active form (PDHa), which indicates actual flux through the enzyme, have revealed decreases at the same absolute intensity following training (Leblanc *et al.* 2004a), again an expected finding given the greater reliance on fatty acid oxidation. This can partially be explained through differences in allosteric regulators (as discussed below) and partially because of training-induced expression of PDH kinase 2 (PDK2). PDK2 phosphorylates and inactivates PDH, and has been shown to be upregulated by about 130% following training (LeBlanc *et al.* 2004b). This PDK isoform is more sensitive to the energy charge of the cell, and therefore "tightly" couples anaerobic with aerobic glycolysis following training – observed as a reduced muscle lactate production following training. This is an important consideration since acetyl-CoA, the product of both beta oxidation of fatty acids and PDH, has large influences on the interaction between fatty acid and carbohydrate oxidation.

Fatty acid-glucose substrate interactions

There are three main bioenergetic systems that provide the necessary ATP during exercise: the high-energy phosphate system (typically referred to as PCr), anaerobic ATP provision in the glycogenolysis/glycolysis pathway, and oxidative respiration (utilizing carbohydrate-derived pyruvate and fatty acids). Each bioenergetic system has unique properties, balancing the requirements of capacity (fuel storage) and maximal rates of ATP provision. Importantly, other than during very short, maximal sprint activities, the energy requirements of exercise are achieved through a balance of these systems. Each system contributes partially to the overall energy requirement, but different types and intensities of exercise require different strategies to maintain ATP homeostasis at any given point during the activity. This is illustrated graphically in Fig. 5.3, demonstrating that free fatty acids (either from intracellular or adipose TAG stores) provide the substrate for a larger proportion of ATP production at low intensity (55% $\dot{V}o_{2peak}$) vs. higher-intensity exercise (75% $\dot{V}o_{2peak}$). Following exercise training, the reliance on fatty acids for fuel is enhanced, such that at the same absolute intensity following training a greater proportion of energy is derived from fatty acid aerobic metabolism. The question that arises is therefore what mechanism is responsible for this adaptation. We have already discussed how exercise training increases the capacity and alters the control of the various bioenergetic systems. One way to approach this question is to examine the training-induced adaptations in mitochondrial ATP aerobic production and hence to study alterations that occur at various regulatory sites.

The hydrolysis of ATP is regulated by several ATPase enzymes, the end-products being ADP and P_i. The hydrolysis of ATP releases a large amount of energy, which is harnessed to pump ions against concentration gradients (Na$^+$-K$^+$-ATPase and Ca^{2+}-ATPase) and to create movement through actin myosin cross-bridge cycling. This reaction is also unidirectional and, for movement to be maintained, the regeneration of ATP must occur rapidly since muscle ATP concentrations are not large enough to maintain maximal sprint activities for more then a few seconds. The elegant design of the bioenergetic systems becomes apparent when considering the regulation of the enzymes involved in the generation of ATP. Once muscle contraction is initiated, the hydrolysis of ATP will subsequently increase the concentration of free ADP (ADP_f). An increase in ADP_f also increases the concentration of free AMP (AMP_f) through the adenylate kinase reaction. The increases in ADP_f and AMP_f concentrations have profound effects on the bioenergetic systems. Not only is ADP_f required for regenerating ATP in the mitochondria, but it also acts as feedback regulator to activate many enzymes responsible for the mobilization and metabolism of carbohydrate and fat, ultimately producing NADH for use in the ETC. While Ca^{2+} is seen as the feed-forward or early warning system to activate fuel uptake mechanisms and regulatory enzymes, ADP_f plays a role in activating PHOS, PFK, and PDH in the carbohydrate metabolizing pathways, by activating enzymes in the TCA cycle; AMP_f plays a feedback role in initiating glucose and fat transport into the cell, by activating PHOS and PDH. When oxygen and fuel or NADH (fat and carbohydrate) supply is abundant, ADP_f regulates the rate of mitochondrial ATP production and activation of the processes that provide NADH to the ETC in the mitochondria. ATP production is low at rest but can be elevated by ~100-fold during maximal activities (Spriet & Howlett 1999). The rise in ADP_f concentrations with exercise play a large role in increasing mitochondrial ATP production as ADP_f levels in muscle increase as a function of the exercise intensity (Howlett et al. 1998). Ultimately the tight relationship between ADP_f concentration and mitochondrial respiration is responsible for the greater reliance on fatty acids following a training program.

Holloszy pioneered the idea (for a review see Holloszy & Coyle 1984), and Dudley et al. (1987) and many others (Cadefau et al. 1994; Phillips et al. 1996b) have generated data to support the notion that increases in the mitochondrial volume and decreases in ADP_f following training have profound effects on substrate selection during exercise. Ultimately

Table 5.1 Muscle metabolites ($mmol \cdot kg$ dry weight^{-1}). Values are expressed as the means ± SEM before (Pre) and after (Post) 31 days of classic endurance training, comprising 2 h·day^{-1} at 60% $\dot{V}o_{2peak}$. (Redrawn from Phillips et al. 1996.)

		Rest	Exercise
ATP	Pre	24.3 ± 0.6	24.2 ± 0.8
	Post	24.6 ± 0.3	24.8 ± 0.8
ADP_f	Pre	0.088 ± 0.01	0.200 ± 0.03
	Post	0.085 ± 0.01	0.130 ± 0.03*
PCr	Pre	80.7 ± 0.7	46.6 ± 2.9
	Post	80.4 ± 0.7	62.7 ± 2.9*
Pyruvate	Pre	0.210 ± 0.01	0.320 ± 0.03
	Post	0.166 ± 0.02	0.218 ± 0.04*
Lactate	Pre	6.5 ± 0.4	29.8 ± 3.6
	Post	6.2 ± 0.5	12.3 ± 2.4*

*Significantly different from Pre ($p < 0.05$).

the ADP_f concentration drives mitochondrial respiration, and with an increase in mitochondrial volume it has been shown that a smaller rise in ADP_f is required to achieve the required $\dot{V}o_2$ following aerobic training (Table 5.1). This relationship is depicted in Fig. 5.5, as the untrained individual in this example requires an ADP_f concentration of 100 µM to attain a $\dot{V}o_2$ of 1.0 L·min^{-1}. In this example, the individual mitochondrial respiration is 0.5 L·min^{-1} (since there are two mitochondria). In contrast, following training-induced mitochondrial proliferation a smaller cytosolic ADP_f concentration must be reached (50 µM) to achieve the same $\dot{V}o_2$ of 1.0 L·min^{-1}, as the individual mitochondrial respiration is now reduced to 0.25 L·min^{-1} (since there are four mitochondria). In essence, the work of each individual mitochondrion is decreased and shared among a greater number of mitochondria, achieving the end goal of a $\dot{V}o_2$ of 1.0 L·min^{-1}.

While most enzymes in the glycolytic pathway are near equilibrium, there are a few reactions that are considered "rate-limiting," and are regulated allosterically and/or covalently, as mentioned above. Following training the cytosolic ADP_f concentrations are lower at the same absolute exercise intensity, and this decreases the flux rate of glycogenolysis/glycolysis. Allosterically, PHOS, PFK, and PDH

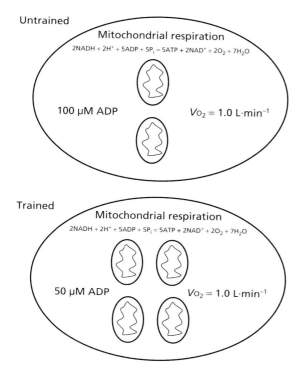

Untrained

Mitochondrial respiration

$2NADH + 2H^+ + 5ADP + 5P_i = 5ATP + 2NAD^+ + 2O_2 + 7H_2O$

100 μM ADP

$V_{O_2} = 1.0 \ L \cdot min^{-1}$

Trained

Mitochondrial respiration

$2NADH + 2H^+ + 5ADP + 5P_i = 5ATP + 2NAD^+ + 2O_2 + 7H_2O$

50 μM ADP

$V_{O_2} = 1.0 \ L \cdot min^{-1}$

Fig. 5.5 The effect of mitochondrial proliferation on the regulation of mitochondrial respiration rates. ADP, adenosine diphosphate; ATP, adenosine triphosphate; NADH, nicotinamide adenine dinucleotide (reduced); P_i, inorganic phosphate. (Reproduced with permission from Hood & Saleem 2007.)

are all "activated" with increasing levels of ADP_f. Therefore, following training smaller rises in ADP_f during exercise decrease the flux through the glycolytic pathway and the production of acetyl-CoA from pyruvate. With less reliance on carbohydrate for ATP production, fatty acid metabolism is increased.

As the mitochondrial volume increases following training so does the machinery for metabolizing fat and the capacity for ATP production from fat. Increased CPT-I activity, increased beta oxidation, and TCA enzyme capacities all contribute to this effect and to the greater reliance on fat at any given submaximal power output. Increases in the ability to transport fat into the muscle cell and in the ability to release FFA from intramuscular TAG may also provide more substrate to the mitochondria. In

addition, Garland and Randle (1964) proposed several mechanisms to explain the increased reliance on fat and decreased reliance on carbohydrate in skeletal muscle when FFA availability was high. They demonstrated that increased free fatty acid oxidation lead to enhanced NADH and acetyl-CoA levels in the mitochondria. This subsequently decreased the flux through PDH (both are allosteric inhibitors of PDH), and hence the aerobic metabolism of pyruvate (and ultimately glucose). The elevated acetyl-CoA levels increased mitochondrial and cytosolic citrate levels, which inhibited PFK. This increased glucose-6 phosphate levels, decreasing both the uptake of plasma glucose and the degradation of glycogen. The general premise was that there is an inverse relationship between fatty acid and carbohydrate metabolism. However, support for these specific mechanisms has been controversial over the years and more contemporary work suggests that the major effect of an increased availability of FFA to the muscle is a decrease in muscle ADP_f, resulting in the down-regulation of carbohydrate metabolism at the level of PHOS, PFK, and PDH (Dyck *et al.* 1993; Odland *et al.* 1998).

Summary

The regulatory changes observed following training are summarized in Fig. 5.6. The key change in skeletal muscle metabolism following training is the increase in mitochondrial volume and in the metabolic machinery contained within the mitochondria. A smaller rise in ADP_f is observed at the same absolute power output following training as the greater metabolic machinery is able to generate the required ATP with a lower ADP_f signal. This attenuated rise in ADP_f decreases the activation of PHOS, PFK, and PDH in the glycogenolytic/glycolytic pathways, resulting in less pyruvate and lactate production and less aerobic ATP production from carbohydrate. At the same time, the increased mitochondrial volume following training is accompanied by increases in CPT-I, beta oxidation, and TCA cycle enzyme levels, resulting in a greater capacity to oxidize fat. In addition, the capacity to transport FFA into the muscle cell and/or degrade FFA from intramuscular TAG is increased to provide more

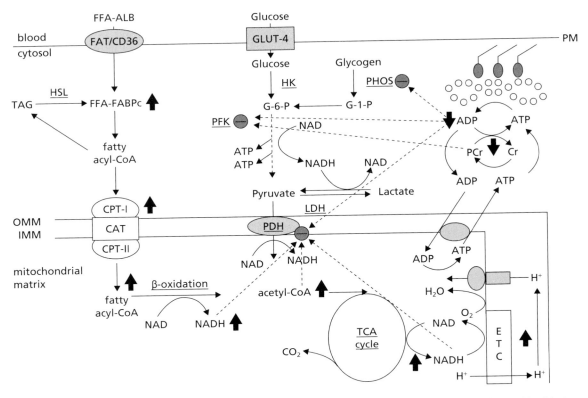

Fig. 5.6 Coordinated regulation of carbohydrate and fatty acid oxidation. Following aerobic training, fatty acid oxidation increases and carbohydrate oxidation decreases while exercising at a fixed intensity. One of the main reasons for these changes is the smaller rise in adenosine diphosphate (ADP) that occurs following training. ATP and ADP, adenosine tri and diphosphate; CAT, carnitine acylcarnitine translocase; CD36, fatty acid translocase CD36; CPTI & II, carnitine palmitoyltransferase I & II; Cr, creatine; ETC, electron transport chain; FABP, fatty acid binding protein; FFA, free fatty acid; G-1-P & G-6-P, glucose 1 and 6 phosphate; GLUT4, glucose transporter 4; HK, hexokinase; HSL, hormone sensitive lipase; LDH, lactate dehydrogenase; NAD & NADH, oxidized and reduced forms of nicotinamide adenine dinucleotide; OMM & IMM, outer and inner mitochondrial membranes; PCr, phosphocreatine; PDH, pyruvate dehydrogenase; PFK, phosphofructokinase; PHOS, glycogen phosphorylase; PM, plasma membrane; TCA tricarboxylic acid; TG, triacylglycerol. (Reproduced with permission from Spriet & Howlett 1999.)

FFA to the mitochondria. The net result of these changes is a greater reliance on fat as a fuel and less on carbohydrate for aerobic ATP production at submaximal power outputs. In addition, the muscle also has a greater overall capacity for aerobic ATP production from both carbohydrate (~100% $\dot{V}_{O_{2peak}}$) and fat (~65% $\dot{V}_{O_{2peak}}$) following training to match the increases in muscle and whole body $\dot{V}_{O_2}$.

References

Baldwin, K.M., Winder, W.W., Terjung, R.L. & Holloszy, J.O. (1973) Glycolytic enzymes in different types of skeletal muscle: adaptation to exercise. *American Journal of Physiology* **225**, 962–966.

Bonen, A., Luiken, J.J., Liu, S., Dyck, D.J., Kiens, B., Kristiansen, S., *et al.* (1998) Palmitate transport and fatty acid transporters in red and white muscles. *American Journal of Physiology* **275**, E471–E478.

Bonen, A., Luiken, J.J., Arumugam, Y., Glatz, J.F. & Tandon, N.N. (2000) Acute regulation of fatty acid uptake involves the cellular redistribution of fatty acid translocase. *Journal of Biological Chemistry* **275**, 14501–14508.

Bonen, A., Luiken, J.J. & Glatz, J.F. (2002) Regulation of fatty acid transport and membrane transporters in health and disease. *Molecular and Cellular Biochemistry* **239**, 181–192.

Bonen, A., Parolin, M.L., Steinberg, G.R., Calles-Escandon, J., Tandon, N.N., Glatz, J.F., *et al.* (2004) Triacylglycerol accumulation in human obesity and type 2 diabetes is associated with increased rates of skeletal muscle fatty acid transport and increased sarcolemmal FAT/CD36. *FASEB Journal* **18**, 1144–1146.

Bonen, A., Chabowski, A., Luiken, J.J. & Glatz, J.F. (2007) Is membrane transport of FFA mediated by lipid, protein, or both? Mechanisms and regulation of protein-mediated cellular fatty acid uptake: molecular, biochemical, and physiological evidence. *Physiology (Bethesda)* **22**, 15–29.

Bruce, C.R., Thrush, A.B., Mertz, V.A., Bezaire, V., Chabowski, A., Heigenhauser, G.J.F., *et al.* (2006) Endurance training in obese humans improves glucose tolerance and mitochondrial fatty acid oxidation and alters muscle lipid content. *American Journal of Physiology. Endocrinology Metabolism* **291**, E99–E107.

Burgomaster, K.A., Hughes, S.C., Heigenhauser, G.J.F, Bradwell, S.N. & Gibala, M.J. (2005) Six sessions of sprint interval training increases muscle oxidative potential and cycle endurance capacity in humans. *Journal of Applied Physiology* **98**, 1985–1990.

Burgomaster, K.A., Cermak, N.M., Phillips, S.M., Benton, C.R., Bonen, A. & Gibala, M.J. (2007) Divergent response of metabolite transport proteins in human skeletal muscle after sprint interval training and detraining. *American Journal of Physiology. Regulatory, Integrative and Comparative Physiology* **292**, R1970–R1976.

Cadefau, J., Green, H.J., Cusso, R., Ball-Burnett, M. & Jamieson, G. (1994) Coupling of muscle phosphorylation potential to glycolysis during work after short-term training. *Journal of Applied Physiology* **76**, 2586–2593.

Chabowski, A., Coort, S.L., Calles-Escandon, J., Tandon, N.N., Glatz, J.F., Luiken, J.J., *et al.* (2005) The subcellular compartmentation of fatty acid transporters is regulated differently by insulin and by AICAR. *FEBS Leters* **579**, 2428–2432.

Chesley, A., Heigenhauser, G.J.F. & Spriet, L.L. (1996) Regulation of muscle glycogen phosphorylase activity following short-term endurance training. *American Journal of Physiology* **270**, E328–E335.

Czech, M.P. & Corvera, S. (1999) Signaling mechanisms that regulate glucose transport. *Journal of Biological Chemistry* **274**, 1865–1868.

Dudley, G.A., Tullson, P.C. & Terjung, R.L. (1987) Influence of mitochondrial content on the sensitivity of respiratory control. *Journal of Biological Chemistry* **262**, 9109–9114.

Dyck, D.J., Putman, C.T., Heigenhauser, G.J.F., Hultman, E. & Spriet, L.L. (1993). Regulation of fat-carbohydrate interaction in skeletal muscle during intense aerobic cycling. *American Journal of Physiology* **265**, E852–E859.

Enevoldsen, L.H., Stallknecht, B., Langfort, J., Petersen, L.N., Holm, C., Ploug, T., *et al.* (2001) The effect of exercise training on hormone-sensitive lipase in rat intra-abdominal adipose tissue and muscle. *Journal of Physiology* **536**, 871–877.

Furtado, L.M., Somwar, R., Sweeney, G., Niu, W. & Klip, A. (2002) Activation of the glucose transporter GLUT4 by insulin. *Biochemistry and Cell Biology* **80**, 569–578.

Garland, P.B. & Randle, P.J. (1964) Control of pyruvate dehydrogenase in the perfused rat heart by the intracellular concentration of acetyl-coenzyme A. *Biochemistry Journal* **91**, 6C–7C.

Gibala, M.J., Little, J.P., van Essen, M., Wilkin, G.P., Burgomaster, K.A., Safdar, A., *et al.* (2006) Short-term sprint interval versus traditional endurance training: similar initial adaptations in human skeletal muscle and exercise performance. *Journal of Physiology* **575**, 901–911.

Glatz, J.F., Schaap, F.G., Binas, B., Bonen, A., van der Vusse, G.J. & Luiken, J.J. (2003) Cytoplasmic fatty acid-binding protein facilitates fatty acid utilization by skeletal muscle. *Acta Physiologica Scandinavica* **178**, 367–371.

Gollnick, P.D. & King, D.W. (1969) Effect of exercise and training on mitochondria of rat skeletal muscle. *American Journal of Physiology* **216**, 1502–1509.

Goodpaster, B.H., He, J., Watkins, S. & Kelley, D.E. (2001) Skeletal muscle lipid content and insulin resistance: evidence for a paradox in endurance-trained athletes. *Journal of Clinical Endocrinology and Metabolism* **86**, 5755–5761.

Gould, M.K. & Rawlinson, W.A. (1959) Biochemical adaptation as a response to exercise. Effect of swimming on the levels of lactic dehydrogenase, malic dehydrogenase and phosphorylase in muscles of 8-, 11- and 15-week-old rats. *Biochemistry Journal* **73**, 41–44.

Green, H.J., Helyar, R., Ball-Burnett, M., Kowalchuk, N., Symon, S. & Farrance, B. (1992) Metabolic adaptations to training precede changes in muscle mitochondrial capacity. *Journal of Applied Physiology* **72**, 484–491.

Green, H.J., Jones, S., Ball-Burnett, M., Farrance, B. & Ranney, D. (1995) Adaptations in muscle metabolism to prolonged voluntary exercise and training. *Journal of Applied Physiology* **78**, 138–145.

Han, X.-X., Chabowski, A., Tandon, N.N., Calles-Escandon, J., Glatz, J.F., Luiken, J.J., *et al.* (2007) Metabolic challenges reveal impaired fatty acid metabolism and translocation of FAT/CD36 but not FABPpm in obese zucker rat muscle. *American Journal of Physiology. Endocrinology and Metabolism* **293**, E566–E575.

Hearn, G.R. & Wainio, W.W. (1956) Succinic dehydrogenase activity of the heart and skeletal muscle of exercised rats. *American Journal of Physiology* **185**, 348–350.

Henriksson, J. & Reitman, J.S. (1977) Time course of changes in human skeletal muscle succinate dehydrogenase and cytochrome oxidase activities and maximal oxygen uptake with physical activity and inactivity. *Acta Physiologica Scandinavica* **99**, 91–97.

Henriksson, J., Chi, M.M., Hintz, C.S., Young, D.A., Kaiser, K.K., Salmons, S., *et al.* (1986) Chronic stimulation of mammalian muscle: changes in enzymes of six metabolic pathways. *American Journal of Physiology* **251**, C614–C632.

Holloszy, J.O. (1967) Biochemical adaptations in muscle. Effects of exercise on mitochondrial oxygen uptake and respiratory enzyme activity in skeletal muscle. *Journal of Biological Chemistry* **242**, 2278–2282.

Holloszy, J.O. & Coyle, E.F. (1984) Adaptations of skeletal muscle to endurance exercise and their metabolic consequences. *Journal of Applied Physiology* **56**, 831–838.

Holloszy, J.O. & Oscai, L.B. (1969) Effect of exercise on alpha-glycerophosphate dehydrogenase activity in skeletal muscle. *Archives of Biochemistry and Biophysics* **130**, 653–656.

Holloszy, J.O., Oscai, L.B., Don, I.J. & Mole, P.A. (1970) Mitochondrial citric acid cycle and related enzymes: adaptive response to exercise. *Biochemical and Biophysical Research Communications* **40**, 1368–1373.

Hood, D.A. & Saleem, A. (2007) Exercise-induced mitochondrial biogenesis in skeletal muscle. *Nutrition, Metabolism and Cardiovascular Diseases* **17**, 332–337.

Howlett, R.A., Parolin, M.L., Dyck, D.J., Hultman, E., Jones, N.L., Heigenhauser, G.J.F., *et al.* (1998) Regulation of skeletal muscle glycogen phosphorylase and pyruvate dehydrogenase at varying power outputs. *American Journal of Physiology* **275**, R418–R425.

Jocken, J.W., Langin, D., Smit, E., Saris, W.H., Valle, C., Hul, G.B., *et al.* (2007) Adipose triglyceride lipase and hormone-sensitive lipase protein expression is decreased in the obese insulin-resistant state. *Journal of Clinical Endocrinology and Metabolism* **92**, 2292–2299.

Koonen, D.P., Benton, C.R., Arumugam, Y., Tandon, N.N., Calles-Escandon, J., Glatz, J.F., *et al.* (2004) Different mechanisms can alter fatty acid transport when muscle contractile activity is chronically altered. *American Journal of Physiology. Endocrinology and Metabolism* **286**, E1042–E1049.

Koonen, D.P., Glatz, J.F., Bonen, A. & Luiken, J.J. (2005) Long-chain fatty acid uptake and FAT/CD36 translocation in heart and skeletal muscle. *Biochimica et Biophysica Acta* **1736**, 163–180.

Kushmerick, M.J. (1983). Energetics of muscle contraction. In: *Handbook of Physiology, Skeletal Muscle* (Peachey, L.D., Adrian, R.H. & Geiger, S.R., eds.) American Physiological Society, Bethesda: 315–353.

Lamb, D.R., Peter, J.B., Jeffress, R.N. & Wallace, H.A. (1969) Glycogen, hexokinase, and glycogen synthetase adaptations to exercise. *American Journal of Physiology* **217**, 1628–1632.

Leblanc, P.J., Howarth, K.R., Gibala, M.J. & Heigenhauser, G.J. (2004a) Effects of 7 wk of endurance training on human skeletal muscle metabolism during submaximal exercise. *Journal of Applied Physiology* **97**, 2148–2153.

Leblanc, P.J., Peters, S.J., Tunstall, R.J., Cameron-Smith, D. & Heigenhauser, G.J. (2004b) Effects of aerobic training on pyruvate dehydrogenase and pyruvate dehydrogenase kinase in human skeletal muscle. *Journal of Physiology* **557**, 559–570.

Lee, J.K., Lee, J.S., Park, H., Cha, Y.S., Yoon, C.S. & Kim, C.K. (2007) Effect of L-carnitine supplementation and aerobic training on FABPc content and beta-HAD activity in human skeletal muscle. *European Journal of Applied Physiology* **99**, 193–199.

Luiken, J.J., Koonen, D.P., Coumans, W.A., Pelsers, M.M., Binas, B., Bonen, A., *et al.* (2003) Long-chain fatty acid uptake by skeletal muscle is impaired in homozygous, but not heterozygous, heart-type-FABP null mice. *Lipids* **38**, 491–496.

MacDougall, J.D., Hicks, A.L., MacDonald, J.R., McKelvie, R.S., Green, H.J. & Smith, K.M. (1998) Muscle performance and enzymatic adaptations to sprint interval training. *Journal of Applied Physiology* **84**, 2138–2142.

Martin, W.H., 3rd, Dalsky, G.P., Hurley, B.F., Matthews, D.E., Bier, D.M., Hagberg, J.M., *et al.* (1993) Effect of endurance training on plasma free fatty acid turnover and oxidation during exercise. *American Journal of Physiology* **265**, E708–E714.

McGarry, J.D. & Brown, N.F. (1997) The mitochondrial carnitine palmitoyltransferase system. From concept to molecular analysis. *European Journal of Biochemistry* **244**, 1–14.

Mole, P.A. & Holloszy, J.O. (1970) Exercise-induced increase in the capacity of skeletal muscle to oxidize palmitate. *Proceedings of the Society for Experimental Biology and Medicine* **134**, 789–792.

Mole, P.A., Oscai, L.B. & Holloszy, J.O. (1971) Adaptation of muscle to exercise. Increase in levels of palmityl CoA synthetase, carnitine palmityltransferase, and palmityl CoA dehydrogenase, and in the capacity to oxidize fatty acids. *Journal of Clinical Investigation* **50**, 2323–2330.

Odland, L.M., Heigenhauser, G.J.F., Wong, D., Hollidge-Horvat, M.G. & Spriet, L.L. (1998). Effects of increased fat availability on fat-carbohydrate interaction during prolonged exercise in men. *American Journal of Physiology* **275**, R894–R902.

Oscai, L.B. & Holloszy, J.O. (1971) Biochemical adaptations in muscle. II. Response of mitochondrial adenosine triphosphatase, creatine phosphokinase, and adenylate kinase activities in skeletal muscle to exercise. *Journal of Biological Chemistry* **246**, 6968–6972.

Perry, C.G., Talanian, J.L., Heigenhauser, G.J.F. & Spriet, L.L. (2007) The effects of training in hyperoxia vs. normoxia on skeletal muscle enzyme activities and exercise performance. *Journal of Applied Physiology* **102**, 1022–1027.

Peters, S.J. (2003) Regulation of PDH activity and isoform expression: diet and exercise. *Biochemical Society Transactions* **31**, 1274–1280.

Phillips, S.M., Green, H.J., Tarnopolsky, M.A. & Grant, S.M. (1995) Decreased glucose turnover after short-term training is unaccompanied by changes in muscle oxidative potential. *American Journal of Physiology* **269**, E222–E230.

Phillips, S.M., Green, H.J., Tarnopolsky, M.A., Heigenhauser, G.J.F., Hill, R.E. & Grant, S.M. (1996a) Effects of training duration on substrate turnover and oxidation during exercise. *Journal of Applied Physiology* **81**, 2182–2191.

Phillips, S.M., Green, H.J., Tarnopolsky, M.A., Heigenhauser, G.J.F. & Grant, S.M. (1996b) Progressive effect of endurance training on metabolic adaptations in working skeletal muscle. *American Journal of Physiology* **270**, E265–E272.

Putman, C.T., Jones, N.L., Hultman, E., Hollidge-Horvat, M.G., Bonen, A., McConachie, D.R., *et al.* (1998) Effects of short-term submaximal training in humans on muscle metabolism in exercise. *American Journal of Physiology* **275**, E132–E139.

Randle, P.J. (1964) The interrelationships of hormones, fatty acid and glucose in the provision of energy. *Postgraduate Medicine Journal* **40**, 457–463.

Richter, E.A., Jensen, P., Kiens, B. & Kristiansen, S. (1998) Sarcolemmal glucose transport and GLUT-4 translocation during exercise are diminished by endurance training. *American Journal of Physiology* **274**, E89–E95.

Saltin, B. & Gollnick, P. (1983) Skeletal muscle adaptability: significance for metabolism and performance. In: *Handbook of Physiology, Skeletal Muscle* (Peachey, L.D., Adrian, R.H. & Geiger, S.R., eds.) American Physiological Society, Bethesda: 555–631.

Schantz, P.G., Sjoberg, B. & Svedenhag, J. (1986) Malate-aspartate and alpha-glycerophosphate shuttle enzyme levels in human skeletal muscle: methodological considerations and effect of endurance training. *Acta Physiologica Scandinavica* **128**, 397–407.

Spina, R.J., Chi, M.M., Hopkins, M.G., Nemeth, P.M., Lowry, O.H. & Holloszy, J.O. (1996) Mitochondrial enzymes increase in muscle in response to 7–10 days of cycle exercise. *Journal of Applied Physiology* **80**, 2250–2254.

Spriet, L.L. (2006) The metabolic systems: lipid metabolism. In: *ACSM's Graduate Textbook on Exercise Physiology* (Tipton, C.M., ed.) LWW, Philadelphia: 396–409.

Spriet, L.L. & Howlett, R.A. (1999) Metabolic control of energy production during physical activity. In: *The Metabolic Bases of Performance in Sport and Exercise* (Lamb, D.R. & Murray, R., eds.) Cooper Publishing Group, Indiana: 1–51.

Spriet, L.L. & Watt, M.J. (2003) Regulatory mechanisms in the interaction between carbohydrate and lipid oxidation during exercise. *Acta Physiologica Scandinavica* **178**, 443–452.

Starritt, E.C., Howlett, R.A., Heigenhauser, G.J.F. & Spriet, L.L. (2000) Sensitivity of CPT I to malonyl-CoA in trained and untrained human skeletal muscle. *American Journal of Physiology. Endocrinology and Metabolism* **278**, E462–E468.

Stellingwerff, T., Boon, H., Jonkers, R.A., Senden, J.M., Spriet, L.L., Koopman, R., *et al.* (2007) Significant intramyocellular lipid use during prolonged cycling in endurance-trained males as assessed by three different methodologies. *American*

Journal of Physiology. Endocrinology and Metabolism **292**, E1715–E1723.

Talanian, J.L., Galloway, S.D., Heigenhauser, G.J.F., Bonen, A. & Spriet, L.L. (2007) Two weeks of high-intensity aerobic interval training increases the capacity for fat oxidation during exercise in women. *Journal of Applied Physiology* **102**, 1439–1447.

Tansey, J.T., Sztalryd, C., HLavin, E.M., Kimmel, A.R. & Londos, C. (2004) The central role of perilipin a in lipid metabolism and adipocyte lipolysis. *IUBMB Life* **56**, 379–385.

Thamer, C., Machann, J., Bachmann, O., Haap, M., Dahl, D., Wietek, B., *et al.* (2003) Intramyocellular lipids: anthropometric determinants and relationships with maximal aerobic capacity and insulin sensitivity. *Journal of Clinical Endocrinology and Metabolism* **88**, 1785–1791.

Tunstall, R.J., Mehan, K.A., Wadley, G.D., Collier, G.R., Bonen, A., Hargreaves, M., *et al.* (2002) Exercise training increases lipid metabolism gene expression in human skeletal muscle. *American Journal of Physiology. Endocrinology and Metabolism* **283**, E66–E72.

Turcotte, L.P., Swenberger, J.R., Tucker, M.Z., Yee, A.J., Trump, G., Luiken, J.J., *et al.* (2000) Muscle palmitate uptake and binding are saturable and inhibited

by antibodies to FABP(PM). *Molecular and Cellular Biochemistry* **210**, 53–63.

van Loon, L.J.C. (2004) Use of intramuscular triacylglycerol as a substrate source during exercise in humans. *Journal of Applied Physiology* **97**, 1170–1187.

van Loon, L.J., Koopman, R., Manders, R., van der Weegen, W., van Kranenburg, G.P. & Keizer, H.A. (2004) Intramyocellular lipid content in type 2 diabetes patients compared with overweight sedentary men and highly trained endurance athletes. *American Journal of Physiology. Endocrinology and Metabolism* **287**, E558–E565.

Watt, M.J. & Spriet, L.L. (2004) Regulation and role of hormone-sensitive lipase activity in human skeletal muscle. *Proceedings of the Nutrition Society* **63**, 315–322.

Wojtaszewski, J.F. & Richter, E.A. (1998) Glucose utilization during exercise: influence of endurance training. *Acta Physiologica Scandinavica* **162**, 351–358.

Zimmermann, R., Strauss, J.G., Haemmerle, G., Schoiswohl, G., Birner-Gruenberger, R., Riederer, M., *et al.* (2004) Fat mobilization in adipose tissue is promoted by adipose triglyceride lipase. *Science* **306**, 1383–1386.

Part 2

Nutrition

Chapter 6

Nutrition Needs of Athletes

RONALD J. MAUGHAN

Many different factors contribute to success in sport, and the relative importance of these factors will depend on the sport involved. It is clear that the genetic endowment that confers talent on an individual is by far the most important of these factors in all sports. Not all of those who have the genetic inheritance that predisposes to success will choose to exploit it, but those who do are likely to excel. Achieving success requires consistent intensive training, and this in turn demands that the potential champion has the motivation to undertake such training, and can do so without succumbing to illness and injury. It is now also recognized that there are differences between individuals in their ability to respond to a training stimulus with an improved performance, although the mechanisms underpinning this are not well understood.

Nutrition is not one of the major factors that determine success in sport, and a good diet alone will not allow the mediocre athlete who lacks talent and the motivation to train hard to achieve success. Nonetheless, the talented athlete who has the motivation to do the necessary training will not achieve his or her potential without making good food choices. Each athlete needs to identify the nutritional goals that are necessary for training and competition and to devise an eating strategy that will meet those goals. The athlete's diet must supply energy to support the demands of training as well as the requirements of daily living activities, and must

also provide all of the necessary nutrients, including the energy-supplying macronutrients carbohydrate, protein and fat, a wide range of vitamins and minerals, and water. Alcohol is not an essential part of the human diet, but does form a part of the diet of many athletes. Choosing the foods that will supply all of these nutrients in appropriate amounts within the athlete's energy budget can present many challenges. Endurance athletes may expend several thousand calories in daily training, and may struggle to consume sufficient food to allow the training load to be sustained. Athletes in technical events, especially those where there is a premium on maintaining a low body mass and low body fat content, may train for prolonged periods each day, but the overall energy expenditure may be small and some may find it difficult to meet micronutrient needs.

Assessment of nutritional status

The first stage of assessing the nutrition needs of an athlete is to assess current status. Two approaches to the assessment of nutritional status are commonly applied to athletes, as indeed they are in the general population. One is to obtain an estimate of nutrient intake and to compare this with an estimate of requirement. This approach is limited by the inevitable errors inherent in the assessment of intake and requirement, but perhaps a more significant limitation is the absence of a standard by which any but the most gross inadequacies of intake can be identified. While it is undoubtedly true that the risk of deficiency falls with increasing intake, failure to meet a population-derived estimate of requirement

The Olympic Textbook of Science in Sport, 1st edition. Edited by R.J. Maughan. Published 2009 by Blackwell Publishing. ISBN: 978-1-4051-5638-7.

is not in itself an indication of inadequacy of intake (Gibson 1993). It should also be remembered that there are risks associated with the oversupply of most nutrients, and that these risks will also rise as intake increases.

The reference nutrient intake (RNI) is the amount of a nutrient deemed necessary to meet the needs of 98% of any given population, and this should not be mistaken for a recommended intake. Most of the members of any population will meet their requirements with an intake far below the RNI, and it is not necessary that all individuals should have an intake that matches the RNI. It is also important to recognize that the RNI applies to the general (sedentary) population, and there is an almost complete absence of athlete-specific data. It is tempting to believe that the requirement for essential nutrients is increased by the stresses of training, even though there is little evidence to support this in the case of most micronutrients. In the absence of definitive data, many athletes (and also many of those who advise them) subscribe to the "more is better" philosophy, failing to recognize that many nutrients may be harmful to health and to performance if taken in excessive amounts for prolonged periods.

A second, and usually preferable, approach to the assessment of nutritional status is to make measurements of relevant biomarkers in the individual. Most, but not all, nutritional parameters are amenable to measurement, and assessment of an athlete's nutritional status can be an important part of establishing whether current dietary habits are adequate or whether changes need to be made. In the case of some nutrients, routine clinical investigation will not be helpful because the markers themselves are disturbed by exercise, but there are some parameters that can usefully be measured.

One marker of nutritional status that is more easily measured is body mass and the related parameters of body composition. An individual's body mass and body composition represent a cumulative history of lifetime energy balance. For each athlete and each sport, there will be an optimum body mass and body composition. Too much body fat or too little and performance will be less than ideal. There will be no single value that is ideal, but rather a range of values within which the athlete should operate. An estimate of body fat content can therefore be an important tool in the identification of nutritional goals, but a single measure may present a false picture in a dynamic situation. Assessing the adequacy of intake of the essential macronutrients (protein, carbohydrate, and fat) is not so easy. Protein balance may be maintained with a wide range of protein intakes, and will depend not only on the protein intake but also on total energy intake and on physical activity levels (Millward 2004). Loucks (2004) has proposed that an inadequate energy intake, and more specifically an inadequate carbohydrate intake, can be identified by the appearance of ketone bodies in the blood or urine. While this is undoubtedly true when substantial deficiencies are imposed in an experimental setting, there has been no evidence that this method is useful in an applied setting.

Methods are available for the assessment of micronutrient status on the basis of measurements made on blood or other tissues. In some cases, the interpretation of these may be relatively straightforward, as in the diagnosis of iron deficiency based on serum ferritin and other related parameters (Bender & Bender 1997). In other cases interpretation of plasma concentrations is fraught with difficulty, as in the case of magnesium or zinc (Bender & Bender 1997). In the case of some nutrients, this is because of the effects of recent exercise on the distribution of nutrients between body compartments, while the plasma concentration of other nutrients may reflect recent intake rather than chronic nutrient status. Stress, injury, infection, pregnancy, and other factors may all result in values outside normal reference ranges. Where meaningful diagnostic tests are possible, these should be used as part of the needs assessment process when working with elite athletes. Once again, there is an almost total absence of evidence as to the optimum range for tissue biochemical parameters in athletes. Athletes and those who advise them should beware inappropriate interpretation of blood parameters and should be sceptical about the many companies promising assessment of status – usually antioxidants, minerals or vitamins – based on transcutaneous measurements or on analysis of hair or other tissue samples.

Identifying nutrition goals

The athlete's nutritional goal must be to ensure that all tissues are supplied with all the necessary nutrients in appropriate amounts at the correct time. Knowing the requirement for each of the macro- and micronutrients that are essential for health and performance is not easy, and the philosophy generally adopted by athletes is to err on the side of oversupply. This is not without risk, and excess is often more harmful that inadequacy. Translation of these nutritional goals into an eating strategy is the role of the dietitian, who must take account of the myriad of factors that influence individual food choices.

Athletes must also take account of the different needs at different stages of the competitive season. Nutrition may play its most important part by supporting consistent intensive training, but special nutrition strategies may be required before and during competition. In different sports, the balance between training and competition may be very different. Some athletes, including the professional boxer and the marathon runner, may spend many months preparing for a single competition, while others, such as the basketball player or the professional cyclist, may compete on most days of the week during the competitive season.

Nutrition needs for training

Training is not an end in itself, but rather the means of achieving the athlete's goal, which is an improved performance in competition. Nutrition has a key role in supporting the athlete during training. The diet must supply an appropriate amount of energy – neither too much nor too little – and must provide appropriate amounts of all of the macronutrients, water, and micronutrients.

Energy needs

The diet provides energy in the form of carbohydrate, fat, protein, and alcohol, and the proportions of these macronutrients is influenced by many factors. The energy requirements of training are largely met by oxidation of fat and carbohydrate. Protein typically constitutes about 12–15% of total energy intake, but oxidation of the carbon skeletons of protein makes only a small contribution to energy supply during prolonged exercise. This normally amounts to 5% or less of total energy demand, but may be more than this if the muscle glycogen stores are low (Lemon 1991). The higher the intensity of exercise, the greater the total energy demand, and the greater the reliance on carbohydrate as a fuel (Coyle 1991). At an exercise intensity corresponding to about 50% of maximum oxygen uptake ($\dot{V}o_{2max}$), approximately two-thirds of the total energy requirement is met by fat oxidation, with carbohydrate oxidation supplying about one-third. At about 75% of $\dot{V}o_{2max}$, which is closer to the typical training intensity in many endurance sports, the total energy expenditure is increased, and carbohydrate, especially muscle glycogen, is now the major fuel. The response is similar in men and women (Romijn et al. 2000). Alcohol is consumed by many athletes; in moderation this is not harmful, but excessive intakes will have both acute and chronic adverse effects on well-being and on performance (Maughan 2006).

Carbohydrate

The body stores of carbohydrate are small relative to the amount that can be used during exercise (Table 6.1). In prolonged hard exercise, carbohydrate can be oxidized at a rate of 3–4 g·min^{-1} by well-trained athletes; if this is sustained for 2 h or

Table 6.1 Normal body stores of fat and carbohydrate in a typical 70 kg male athlete and a typical 60 kg female athlete. The body fat content especially can vary greatly, from as little as perhaps 3% of body weight in very lean male individuals to 50% or more in the obese (including the sumo wrestler, one of the few sports where obesity is an advantage).

	Male	Female
Carbohydrate stores		
Liver glycogen	90 g	70 g
Muscle glycogen	400 g	300 g
Fat stores		
Intramuscular	500 g	500 g
Adipose tissue	7–10 kg	9–18 kg

more, a very large fraction of the total body carbohydrate content will be exhausted. In intense exercise, anaerobic metabolism provides most of the energy demand, and a large fraction of the muscle glycogen is rapidly converted to lactate by anaerobic glycolysis. In a single 6-s sprint, the muscle glycogen content may fall by as much as 16% of its initial value (Boobis 1987). Nevill *et al.* (1989) reported a 32% decrease in muscle glycogen content (from 317 to 215 mmol·kg^{-1}) after a single 30-s treadmill sprint. Many team games players will include multiple short sprints in their training program, but these individuals often do not consider that glycogen depletion is a significant factor in their training. Some of the lactate formed by anaerobic glycolysis will be used by the liver for conversion to glucose, but a large part will be oxidized by other tissues. Because the body cannot convert fat to carbohydrate (apart from the very small glycerol component of triglycerides), carbohydrate stores must be replenished from dietary carbohydrate.

During each strenuous training session, depletion of the glycogen stores in the exercising muscles takes place. In prolonged exercise, a substantial part of the liver glycogen reserve will also be mobilized: this has been demonstrated by both direct biopsy measurements (Hultman 1981) and by tracer methodologies (Romijn *et al.* 1993). If these carbohydrate stores are not replenished before the next exercise bout, training intensity must be reduced, leading to corresponding decrements in the training response. Any athlete training hard on a daily basis can readily observe this; if a low carbohydrate diet, consisting mostly of fat and protein, is consumed after a day's training, it will be difficult to repeat the same training load on the following day even though the total energy demand has been satisfied.

Recovery of the muscle and liver glycogen stores after exercise is a rather slow process, and complete recovery may not be achieved until 24–48 h after the end of unusually hard or prolonged exercise (Piehl 1974). The rate of glycogen resynthesis after exercise is determined largely by the amount of carbohydrate supplied by the diet (Ivy 2000), and the amount of carbohydrate consumed is of far greater importance for this process than the type of carbohydrate. The training diet therefore should be high in carbohydrate, and it is often recommended that 60% or more of total energy intake comes from carbohydrate. This suggestion conforms with the recommendations of various expert committees that carbohydrates provide more than 50% of dietary energy intake. However, it may not be helpful to athletes and those who advise them to express the carbohydrate requirements as a percentage of total energy intake; energy intake varies greatly between individuals, and a high carbohydrate intake may be achieved at very high energy intakes with a relatively low fraction of the total food intake consisting of carbohydrate. It may be better to think of an absolute requirement for carbohydrate, consisting of the amount used in training plus the amount used by body tissues during the remainder of the day, rather than relating the needs to total energy intake (Burke *et al.* 2004, 2006).

A daily dietary carbohydrate intake of 500–600 g may be necessary to ensure adequate glycogen resynthesis during periods of intensive training and, for some athletes, the amount of carbohydrate that must be consumed on a daily basis is even greater (Burke *et al.* 2004; Coyle 1991). Although the carbohydrate requirement is determined primarily by training volume and intensity, body size is also an important factor, so expressing the requirement in grams per kilogram body mass per day might be the best option. A daily requirement of about 8–10 g·kg^{-1} body mass is likely for endurance athletes in periods of hard training. It is important to recognize that not all athletes have a high carbohydrate requirement. The sprinter may train for several hours but a large part is flexibility and technical work which places little demand on carbohydrate metabolism.

Professional athletes can organize their days around training, resting, and eating, but the athlete who also has to work or study faces practical difficulties in meeting the demand for energy and carbohydrate, especially when training two or three times per day. Most athletes find it difficult to train hard for at least 3 h after food intake, and the appetite is also suppressed for a time after hard exercise. For athletes who train twice per day, it is particularly important to focus on ensuring a rapid recovery of the glycogen stores between training sessions. This is best achieved when carbohydrate is consumed as soon as possible after training, as the rate of glycogen synthesis if most rapid at this time. It is normally recommended that at least $1-2$ g·kg^{-1} body mass (a total of $50-100$ g carbohydrate) should be consumed in the first hour, and a high carbohydrate intake continued thereafter (Coyle 1991; Ivy *et al.* 1988). There is clearly a maximum rate at which muscle glycogen resynthesis can occur, and there appears to be no benefit in increasing the carbohydrate intake to levels in excess of 100 g every 2 h. The type of carbohydrate is less crucial than the amount consumed, but there may be some benefit from ingesting high glycemic index foods at this time to ensure a rapid elevation of the blood glucose level. Initial results suggesting that the addition of protein might be effective in stimulating faster rates of glycogen synthesis (Zawadzki *et al.* 1992) have not been supported by later studies where the energy content of meals has been more closely matched (van Hall *et al.* 2000a,b). Where there is a longer period of recovery between training sessions, there is less urgency to ensure that carbohydrate is eaten very soon after exercise, although the need for a high intake remains if the training intensity and duration are high.

High levels of carbohydrate intake may be difficult to achieve during periods of intensive training. In Chapter 7, Burke describes some of the strategies that athletes can adopt to ensure that they meet their carbohydrate needs.

Protein

It is clear that a prolonged period of training will cause substantial changes in the structural and functional characteristics of skeletal muscle and other tissues. Although major changes are not apparent in response to single exercise bouts, these changes must take place between training sessions. Numerous studies using isotopically labeled amino acids have shown that the rates of both protein synthesis and protein degradation are increased in the period after each training bout (Tipton & Wolfe 2004). If the exercise is carried out in the fasted state and no protein or amino acids consumed in the hours after exercise, breakdown is likely to exceed synthesis, leading to a net loss of muscle mass. However, if even a small amount (6 g) of essential amino acids is ingested after exercise, protein synthesis is stimulated, leading to net muscle protein synthesis (Tipton *et al.* 2001). This response may be linked to the need for free amino acids to be available within the muscle in adequate amounts to stimulate protein synthesis.

Not all training is intended to increase muscle mass: the training of the marathon runner, for example, is intended to change the functional characteristics of the muscle to improve aerobic energy supply and fatigue resistance without increasing muscle mass. This means that the response to training must be highly selective, with effects on specific proteins rather than on the muscle as a whole. There is good evidence that adaptive changes in muscle structure and function can take place in response to only a few exercise sessions (Green *et al.* 1991). These changes are different from those commonly observed to occur in untrained subjects after a single bout of intense exercise, when the observed responses are largely catabolic in nature and evidence themselves as muscle damage involving the efflux of cellular components into the extracellular space and are accompanied by a subjective sensation of soreness (Clarkson 1997). Nonetheless, there must be adaptive changes involving synthesis of new proteins in response to each training stimulus. It is likely that the methods currently available are simply inadequate to measure these changes with a sufficient degree of reliability. At the molecular level, adaptation is a consequence of changes in the tissue content of specific proteins, and training is the result of the accumulated effects of the changes in gene transcription that occur after each exercise bout, as evidenced by transient changes in mRNA levels for specific proteins (Fluck & Hoppeler 2003).

Athletes have been told for many years that muscle glycogen synthesis is a priority during the early stages of recovery, but synthesis of new proteins should perhaps be seen as being of equal or even greater importance. Because little attention has been paid to this area until recently, it is not at present apparent what factors may be manipulated to influence these processes. The supply of essential amino acids and the hormonal environment are two obvious factors that may be important. Nutritional status can influence the circulating concentration of a number of hormones that have anabolic properties, the most obvious and important example being insulin. The diet can also supply amino acids for incorporation into proteins. A fall in the intracellular amino acid concentration will restrict the rate of protein synthesis, and there is some evidence that the muscle amino acid concentration does fall after exercise (Tipton & Wolfe 2001). Ingestion of protein or amino acids immediately after exercise can prevent this fall and promote muscle protein synthesis (Biolo *et al.* 1997), but no long-term studies have yet been conducted to establish if these effects result in an improved adaptation of the muscle to the training stimulus (Tipton & Wolfe 2001).

In addition to these effects of nutrient intake, cell volume may be an important regulator of metabolic processes (Lang *et al.* 1998; Waldegger & Lang 1997), and there may be opportunities to manipulate the cell volume after exercise to promote synthesis of proteins and of glycogen. During and after exercise there may be large changes in cell volume, secondary to osmotic pressure changes caused by metabolic activity, hydrostatic pressure changes, or by loss of large volumes of hypotonic sweat. Alterations in cell volume induced by changes in osmolality are well known to alter the rate of glycogen synthesis in skeletal muscle (Low *et al.* 1997a). Amino acid transport into muscles is also affected by changes in cell volume induced by manipulation of the transmembrane osmotic gradient: skeletal muscle uptake of glutamine is stimulated by cell swelling and inhibited by cell shrinkage (Low *et al.* 1997b), and the intracellular glutamine concentration appears to have an important role in a number of processes, including protein and glycogen synthesis (Rennie *et al.* 1998).

The full significance of these recent findings for the post-exercise recovery process and the role that nutritional manipulation can have in adaptation to a training program remain to be established (Hawley *et al.* 2006). Manipulation of fluid and electrolyte balance and the ingestion of a variety of osmotically active substances or their precursors offers potential for optimizing the effectiveness of a training regimen. A number of commercial products consisting of combinations of carbohydrate with protein and/or amino acids are now available, but there is no evidence that these are likely to be more effective than normal foods. A sandwich made with ham, cheese, tuna, or even jam, or a chocolate milkshake, might be just as good at supplying both carbohydrate to replenish the muscle glycogen stores and amino acids to stimulate protein synthesis.

It must, of course, be recognized that many laboratory studies are conducted in highly unusual conditions. Subjects in most metabolic studies are fasted for some time – typically 6–12 h – before the experiment begins, and perhaps for much longer than this before the crucial measurements are made. Few athletes would abstain from food for more than a few hours before training, so the normal response to exercise may not be a fall in the muscle amino acid pool during the post-exercise period, and further increasing the availability of amino acids may have no effect on protein metabolism. It may be that the effects of food eaten in the pre-exercise period will make manipulation of intake after exercise irrelevant, but this is not at present known.

Fat

If carbohydrate is not available, or is available in only a limited amount, the contribution of fat to energy production will increase, with greater rates of oxidation of both plasma-derived free fatty acids and of intramuscular triglycerides. The maximum rate of oxidative energy supply from fat is only about half of that from carbohydrate, however, so the intensity of the exercise must be reduced to a level where the greater part of the energy requirement can be met by fat oxidation. One of the key adaptations to endurance training is to increase the capacity for oxidation of fat, and this is achieved by increasing muscle capillarity to enhance fatty acid delivery and increasing the muscle content of oxidative enzymes found in the mitochondria. Eating a high fat diet, without training, will result in some increase in the rate of oxidation of fat oxidation at rest and during exercise, and it has been suggested that there may be benefits for endurance athletes in training with reduced carbohydrate availability (Hawley *et al.* 2006).

Although it seems obvious that the ability to train at high intensities will be impaired if a high carbohydrate diet is not consumed, there is limited experimental evidence from studies on humans to support this (Williams 1998). Studies where subjects have trained on high fat diets have been more convincing, showing that a high carbohydrate diet during a period of training brings about greater improvements in performance, even when a high carbohydrate diet is fed for a few days to allow normalization of the muscle glycogen stores before exercise performance is measured (Burke *et al.* 2004). It must be recognized, however, that these short-term training studies usually involve relatively untrained individuals and may not reflect the situation of the highly trained elite endurance athlete where the capacity of the muscle for oxidation of fatty acids will be much higher (Henriksson & Hickner 1998). For the athlete with very high levels of energy expenditure in training, the exercise intensity will inevitably be reduced to a level where fatty acid oxidation will make a significant contribution to energy supply and fat will provide an important energy source in the diet. Once the requirements for protein and carbohydrate are met, the balance of energy intake can be in the form of fat.

Vitamins and minerals

For normal health to be maintained, a wide range of vitamins, minerals, and trace elements must be present in adequate amounts in the body tissues. There are ongoing losses from the body in urine, faeces, through shed skin cells and blood loss, so the dietary intake must be sufficient to maintain the tissue levels. The essentiality of the vitamins and minerals was recognized because of the deficiency states that exist when intake is inadequate: scurvy, rickets, goiter and cretinism, all of which are fortunately now rare. Many vitamins and minerals have key roles in energy metabolism, and the adverse effect of deficiencies of these components is well recognized and easily demonstrated. Marginal deficiency states may have little effect on the sedentary individual, but small impairments of exercise capacity may have profound consequences for the serious athlete. Regular intense exercise training may also increase micronutrient requirements, either by increasing degradation rates or by increasing losses

from the body. Consequently, there is a great interest shown by athletes in some of these dietary components because of their role in maintaining or enhancing physical performance. However, there is often a failure to appreciate that it is not inevitably, or indeed even generally, the case that increasing micronutrient intake to levels above those that are adequate for maintaining health will improve athletic performance.

Dietary micronutrient intake in athletes

With regular strenuous training, there must be an increased total food intake to balance the increased energy expenditure: without this, hard training cannot be sustained for long. Provided that a reasonably varied diet is consumed, this will supply more than adequate amounts of protein, minerals, vitamins, and other dietary requirements (van Erp-Baart *et al.* 1989). There are of course always exceptions – as with the general population, not all athletes eat a varied diet, and not all athletes have a high energy intake. Some athletes restrict energy intake to maintain low body mass and low levels of body fat. It must be remembered that the results of surveys that show intakes of vitamins and minerals below the recommended daily allowance (RDA) in some groups of athletes (most especially female athletes in sports where a low body fat content is considered essential, including ballet dancers, gymnasts, and long-distance runners) take no account of the very low body mass of most of these individuals. Indeed, the RDAs are so imprecise that there is generally no attempt to relate the requirement to body mass. However, it is likely that the increased energy intake of most athletes will ensure an adequate intake of most essential dietary components.

There is no good evidence to suggest that specific supplementation with any of these dietary components is necessary or that it will improve performance. Deficiencies can only be established by biochemical investigation or by the identification of specific symptoms as mentioned above. Where the presence of a specific deficiency is established, this should be treated wherever possible by directing the individual towards a more appropriate choice of foods to include those with a high content of the deficient component. In almost every case, it is possible to meet requirements from a normal varied diet, and only where clinical signs of an established deficiency are identified should vitamin or mineral supplementation be considered. The only exceptions to the generalization about the value of dietary supplements in meeting micronutrient needs may be iron and, in the case of very active women, calcium. There is also some experimental support for antioxidant supplementation in some situations.

Iron, hemoglobin, and oxygen transport

Iron has a number of essential functions in the human body, but the best-known one is its role – as a component of the protein hemoglobin – in the transport of oxygen from the lungs to the tissues where it is required. A fall in the circulating hemoglobin concentration is associated with a reduction in oxygen-carrying capacity and a decreased exercise performance (Maughan 1992). The body store of iron is small, and a regular intake is necessary to replace ongoing losses. Some iron is stored in the form of ferritin, and transport around the tissues is accomplished by another protein, transferrin. The first sign of iron deficiency is generally a fall in the circulating ferritin concentration. Anemia – a low blood hemoglobin concentration – may result from an inadequate iron intake in the diet, but may also be caused by inadequate absorption of dietary iron, or to a deficiency of vitamins B_{12} or folate, which are both involved in the formation of new red blood cells. The circulating transferrin level can rise sharply after exposure to any one of a number of stresses, so this cannot be used as an index of iron status.

An athlete's $\dot{V}o_{2max}$ can be increased by artificial elevation of the circulating hemoglobin concentration. This has been achieved in the laboratory by use of red cell reinfusion procedures (Ekblom *et al.* 1972, 1976), and it is well known that athletes have also used this procedure, either by removing their own blood some weeks before competition and replacing it in the last few days before competition, or by using someone else's blood. More recently, injections of recombinant erythropoietin (EPO) or related compounds have been used to stimulate increased red blood cell synthesis and thus enhance perform-

ance. Although the use of these procedures is, quite properly, banned under the World Anti-Doping Agency (WADA) code, the search for legitimate means of achieving the same end goes on. This explains in part the popularity of altitude training among athletes, as well as the widespread use of iron supplementation.

In view of the apparent importance of the oxygen-carrying capacity of the blood for oxygen transport, it seems odd that one commonly observed adaptation to endurance exercise is a decrease in the circulating hemoglobin concentration, commonly referred to as "sports anemia." This is not a true anemia and the decrease in hemoglobin concentration is a consequence of the disproportionate increase in plasma volume. The total circulating hemoglobin mass is usually increased or at least maintained in the trained state. This may be considered to be an adaptation to the trained state, but hard training may result in an increased iron requirement and exercise tolerance is certainly impaired in the presence of anemia. Low serum folate and serum ferritin levels are not associated with impaired performance, however, and correction of these deficiencies does not influence indices of fitness in trained athletes.

Stimulation of erythropoiesis – the formation of new red blood cells – is apparent within the first day or two of exercise training, and a similarly rapid response is observed on going to higher altitude. If the body's iron stores are inadequate at this time, there will certainly be some impairment of the process of adaptation. Special attention to dietary iron intake is therefore necessary for the sedentary individual who embarks on a strenuous training program or for the individual, whether sedentary or athletic, who plans to spend some time at an altitude of more than about 1500–2000 m.

Calcium

Osteoporosis is now widely recognized as a problem for both men and women, and an increased bone mineral content is one of the benefits of participation in an exercise program. Regular exercise results in increased mineralization of those bones subjected to stress and an increased peak bone mass may delay the onset of osteoporotic fractures; exercise may also delay the rate of bone loss (Bailey & McCulloch 1990). The specificity of this effect is demonstrated by the unilateral increase in forearm bone density observed in tennis players (Pirnay *et al.* 1987).

Because of the protective effect of weight-bearing exercise on bone density, it might be thought that athletes would have no need to be concerned about potential loss of bone mass. In athletes training hard on a regular basis, however, there is likely to be a decrease in circulating levels of sex steroids in both men and women. Estrogen has an important role in the maintenance of bone mass in women, and low estrogen levels are a major contributing factor to bone loss (Drinkwater *et al.* 1984). Many of these women also have low body fat and, because of their low body mass, also have low energy (and calcium) intakes in spite of their high activity levels. Dairy produce, the most important source of dietary calcium, is often excluded from the diet because of the perception that it is associated with a high fat intake. All of these factors are a threat to bone health, and when all are present together the risk is high. The loss of bone in these women may result in an increased predisposition to stress fractures and other skeletal injury and also raises concerns about bone health in later life (Martin & Bailey 1987). It should be emphasized that this condition appears to affect only relatively few athletes. Hard sustained training is a relatively new phenomenon, particularly among female athletes, and it remains to be seen whether there are clinically significant long-term effects on bone health.

It is important for everyone to ensure an adequate calcium intake, but calcium supplements themselves will not reverse bone loss in women while estrogen levels remain low. Although they are unlikely to result in harmful effects, calcium supplements should only be taken on the advice of a qualified practitioner after suitable investigative procedures have indicated an inadequate intake. The recommended dietary calcium intake varies between countries, but for men the recommended intake is normally about 800 mg·day^{-1}, and for women about 1200 mg·day^{-1}. Intakes of as much as 2000 mg·day^{-1} are sometimes recommended. Even

then, alternatives to supplementation, specifically alterations in the selection of foods to achieve a higher intake must also be considered, and should be sufficient to meet needs. Low fat dairy produce can make a significant contribution of calcium intake, but many athletes in weight-sensitive sports avoid dairy produce because they associate these foods with a high fat intake.

Antioxidant nutrients

Athletes engaged in very hard physical training and sedentary individuals participating in unaccustomed exercise show signs of muscle damage in the post-exercise period, and there is evidence of free radical-induced damage to muscle membranes and subcellular structures (Powers *et al.* 2004). There is some evidence for an adaptive increase in the activity of antioxidant enzymes in muscle in response to regular exercise, and this may help protect tissues against further damage. Supplementation of the diet with antioxidant nutrients has been proposed as a possible way of further reducing the harmful effects of exercise. Some studies suggest that the severity of muscle damage – as assessed by circulating levels of muscle-specific proteins – can be reduced by supplementation with large doses of vitamins A, C, and E, but the evidence is not entirely convincing, and further information is required before any specific recommendations can be made. Recent evidence suggests that curcumin, a constituent of the Indian spice turmeric, can reduce inflammation and offset some of the performance deficits associated with eccentric exercise-induced muscle damage (Davis *et al.* 2007). Again, further evidence on this and on other phytochemicals is required.

Training harder

An athlete's ability to sustain the consistent, intensive training that will optimize performance may be limited by any one of a number of nutritional factors. Among the most obvious are the immediate effects of an inadequate intake of carbohydrate to meet the metabolic needs of the muscles, or of water to maintain fluid balance. Failure to meet energy needs may be tolerated in the short term, provided carbohydrate intake is adequate, but a chronic energy deficit will result in deterioration of both physical and mental performance (Burke *et al.* 2006). Hard training can only be sustained if the athlete remains healthy, and there is some evidence that athletes may be at increased risk of opportunistic infections during periods of intense training (Nieman & Bishop 2006). Periods of unusually severe training may also lead to overtraining syndromes, which are typically characterized by underperformance, chronic fatigue, and depressed mood states (Fry *et al.* 1991; Gleeson *et al.* 2004). In both of these situations, inappropriate diet may be a contributing factor. Rather than resorting to exotic supplements that are promoted as stimulants of the immune system, athletes are advised to ensure an adequate energy intake and an adequate carbohydrate intake. Training while in a carbohydrate-depleted state will increase circulating levels of stress hormones, including cortisol and catecholamines, which are harmful to the cells of the immune system; carbohydrate intake before or during prolonged hard exercise can prevent excessive increases in stress hormone levels and thus help preserve immune function (Gleeson *et al.* 2004).

Training smarter

It was formerly thought that the primary role of nutrition in training was to allow faster and more effective recovery between training sessions, thus allowing an increased training load. Nutrition strategies, however, can allow the athlete to achieve the same functional outcome with less training. It is increasingly recognized that high training loads carry a risk of illness, injury, and underperformance. Achieving the same outcome in terms of improved functional capacity with a lower training load has many attractions, especially where there is a need for time to be devoted to skills training as well as fitness training. An adequate intake of protein is essential to prevent loss of muscle mass and to maintain the synthesis of new proteins. It is this synthesis of new proteins in the muscles in response to the imposed training stimulus that results in the adaptive changes in functional capacity that result from training (Hawley *et al.* 2006).

Nutrition for competition

Many athletes adopt specific nutritional strategies in preparation for competition, and these will vary greatly depending on the sport. These strategies are targeted at the factors that are thought to limit performance, and in general athletes are not concerned with their overall nutrition needs at these times. In some sports, however, competition is frequent, and athletes must ensure that their competition eating strategies do not compromise their overall nutrition goals. The most obvious example of a specific competition strategy is the high carbohydrate diet of the endurance athlete in the last few days before competition. There is good evidence that endurance performance, at least in laboratory cycling studies, is closely related to the pre-exercise muscle glycogen content (Bergstrom *et al.* 1967). Dehydration will also impair performance, and athletes are encouraged to ensure that they are well hydrated when they begin competition, especially in endurance events taking place in warm climates (Sawka *et al.* 2007).

In weight category sports, it is common for substantial losses of body mass to be achieved within the last few days prior to competition to make the competition weight limit. This often involves increased aerobic exercise in combination with restriction of energy intake and a combination of increased sweat losses and restricted fluid intake. These athletes then aim to recover as far as possible in the time period allowed between the weigh-in and the start of competition.

In some events, there are opportunities for intake of food and fluids during the event itself, and Burke (Chapter 7) and Shirreffs (Chapter 8) describe some of the strategies adopted by athletes to achieve this.

Dietary supplements

The use of dietary supplements in sport is widespread, and attracts a disproportional amount of attention. Supplements used by athletes range from the daily multivitamin tablet which is seen as some sort of health insurance policy to the more exotic supplements to be found on the shelves of health food stores. There are many published surveys of supplement use in athletes, and the type of supplement and the prevalence of use vary between sports (Maughan *et al.* 2004). Many athletes take multiple supplements, although many have nutritional habits that may be described as "unsatisfactory," implying that attention to the normal diet might be a more beneficial approach for these athletes (Ronsen *et al.* 1999). A survey of US university coaches and trainers revealed that nutrition supplements were provided for 94% of the athletes for whom the respondents were responsible (Rockwell *et al.* 2001). Reviews of the published literature suggest that the use of supplements is more prevalent in athletes (46%) than in the general population (35–40%), while use is more prevalent still among elite athletes, with 59% reporting supplement use (Sobal & Marquart 1994). All these surveys find that the overall prevalence and the types of supplements used vary with the nature of the sport, the sex of the athletes, and the level of competition.

When athletes are training to the limit of their capacity, it is perhaps not surprising that they seek to take advantage of any opportunity to gain an advantage over their competitors. Nutritional ergogenic aids are aimed primarily at enhancing performance, either by affecting some aspect of energy metabolism or by an effect on the central nervous system, at increasing lean body mass or muscle mass by stimulation of protein synthesis, or at reducing body fat content. Although not strictly ergogenic (i.e., capable of enhancing work performance), supplements aimed at increasing resistance to infection and improving general health are seen by athletes as important in reducing the interruptions to training that minor illness and infection can cause.

Of the wide range of supplements used by athletes, only a few have been comprehensively evaluated for efficacy and safety, and in many cases the limited research would not stand close scrutiny. The use of an inappropriate experimental design, with small subject numbers and the absence of proper control groups, is common. A few supplements have been the subject of closer scrutiny, and there is evidence to support the use of creatine, caffeine, alkalinizing agents, and perhaps also a small number of other compounds. These supplements form part of

the dietary strategy adopted by many athletes and are discussed in Chapter 7.

Problems with supplements

Unlike drugs, the regulations governing the purity of dietary supplements and of the claims that can be made as to their purity and efficacy are somewhat lax. The passing of the Dietary Supplements Health and Education Act (1994) by the US Congress resulted in a considerable liberalization of the regulations regarding the manufacture and sale of nutritional supplements. The lack of quality control in the manufacture of dietary supplements has caused the Food and Drugs Administration (FDA 2003) to require manufacturers to recall a number of products. Product recalls because of inadequate content include a folic acid product with 34% of the stated dose. The FDA has also recently recalled products containing excessive doses of vitamins A, D, B_6, and selenium because of potentially toxic levels of these components. Some products have been shown to contain potentially harmful impurities (e.g., lead, broken glass, animal faeces) because of poor manufacturing practice.

At present, dietary supplements are not evaluated by regulatory agencies and inaccurate labeling of ingredients is known to be a problem. Internet selling has also effectively removed most of the national controls that are in place to protect the consumer. Most dietary supplements will not cause problems for the athlete, and most of the companies that manufacture and supply these supplements are anxious to ensure the welfare of their customers. Nonetheless, there is now compelling evidence that dietary supplements may be responsible for at least some of the positive doping results recorded by athletes. This is reflected in the decisions by the governing bodies of some sports to apply reduced sanctions in the cases of some athletes who have tested positive, and by a recent decision in the game of tennis to absolve from guilt players who had tested positive for 19-nortestosterone (nandrolone).

The potential for a positive doping test from inadvertent ingestion of a prohibited compound has long been recognized in the case of some mild stimulants, including especially caffeine and ephedrine, that are present in over-the-counter herbal tonics. Many published studies have now shown contamination of supplements with prohibited compounds, including a range of anabolic androgenic steroids and stimulants (Ayotte *et al.* 2001; Catlin *et al.* 2000; Geyer *et al.* 2000; Kamber *et al.* 2000; Pipe & Ayotte 2002). Some investigations have shown that some products do not contain any measurable amount of the substances identified on the label while others may contain amounts greatly in excess of the stated dose (Gurley *et al.* 2000; Parasrampuria *et al.* 1998). Where relatively expensive ingredients are involved, it seems that some products contain little or no active ingredient (Green *et al.* 2001). According to data presented on the Internet, these are not isolated cases, and it is reported that, for some specific supplements, the majority of the available products fail to meet the expected standards.

Conclusions

Diet significantly influences athletic performance. Athletes can perform to their genetic potential only if they train consistently and intensively. This requires nutritional support during training to ensure that fatigue, injury, and illness do not interfere with training and also to maximize the molecular and cellular adaptations that take place in response to training. Specific nutritional needs apply during competition, but these vary greatly depending on the demands of the sport. Each athlete must identify their nutritional needs, but these then have to be translated into an eating strategy that will identify the types and amounts of foods that should be eaten and the timing of these meals, snacks, and drinks in relation to both training and competition.

It is important to recognize that most of what we know about the nutrition needs of athletes is derived from measurements made on healthy young males, of varying standards of athletic ability. It is assumed that the same general principles apply to the elite athlete, and it is also generally assumed that similar principles apply to the female athlete, the adolescent athlete, and the athlete who has a physical disability. This is not always the case and these athletes must be aware that their needs may be different.

References

Ayotte, C., Levesque, J.F., Cleroux, M., Lajeunesse, A., Goudreault, D. & Fakiran, A. (2001) Sport Nutritional supplements: quality and doping controls. *Canadian Journal of Applied Physiology* **26**, S120–S129.

Bailey, D.A. & McCulloch, R.G. (1990) Bone tissue and physical activity. *Canadian Journal of Sport Sciences* **15**, 229–239.

Bender, D.A. & Bender, A.E. (1997) *Nutrition: A Reference Handbook.* Oxford University Press, Oxford.

Bergstrom, J., Hermansen, L., Hultman, E. & Saltin, B. (1967) Diet, muscle glycogen and physical performance. *Acta Physiologica Scandinavica* **71**, 140–150.

Biolo, G., Tipton, K.D., Klein, S. & Wolfe, R.R. (1997) An abundant supply of amino acids enhances the metabolic effect of exercise on muscle protein. *American Journal of Physiology* **273**, E122–E129.

Boobis, L.H. (1987) Metabolic aspects of fatigue during sprinting. In: *Exercise Benefits, Limits and Adaptations* (Macleod, D. *et al.*, eds.) Spon, London: 116–143.

Burke, L.B., Kiens, B. & Ivy, J.L. (2004) Carbohydrates and fat for training and recovery. *Journal of Sports Sciences* **22**, 15–30.

Burke, L.M., Loucks, A.B. & Broad, N. (2006) Energy and carbohydrate for training and recovery. *Journal of Sports Sciences* **24**, 675–685.

Catlin, D.H., Leder, B.Z., Ahrens, B., Starcevic, B., Hatton, C.K., Green, G.A., *et al.* (2000) Trace contamination of over-the-counter androstenedione and positive urine test results for a nandrolone metabolite. *Journal of the American Medical Association* **284**, 2610.

Clarkson PM (1997) Eccentric exercise and muscle damage. *International Journal of Sports Medicine* **18**, S314–S317.

Coyle, E.F. (1991) Timing and method of increased carbohydrate intake to cope with heavy training, competition and recovery. *Journal of Sports Sciences* **9** (Special Issue), 29–52.

Davis, J.M., Murphy, E.A., Carmichael, M.D., Zielinski, M.R., Groschwitz, C.M., Brown, A.S. *et al.* (2007) Curcumin effects on inflammation and performance recovery following eccentric exercise-induced muscle damage. *American Journal of Physiology* **292**, R2168–R2173.

Drinkwater, B.L., Nilson, K., Chesnut, C.H., Bremner, W.J., Shainholtz, S. & Southworth, M.B. (1984) Bone mineral content of amenorrheic and eumenorrheic athletes. *New England Journal of Medicine* **311**, 277–281.

Ekblom, B., Goldberg, A.N. & Gullbring, B. (1972) Response to exercise after blood loss and reinfusion. *Journal of Applied Physiology* **33**, 175–180.

Ekblom, B., Wilson, G. & Astrand, P.O. (1976) Central circulation during exercise after venesection and reinfusion of red blood cells. *Journal of Applied Physiology* **40**, 379–383.

FDA (2003) Current good manufacturing practice in manufacturing, packing, or holding dietary ingredients and dietary supplements. *Federal Register* **68**(49), 12 157–12 263.

Fluck, M. & Hoppeler, H. (2003). Molecular basis of skeletal muscle plasticity: from gene to form and function. *Reviews in Physiology Biochemistry and Pharmacology* **146**, 159–216.

Fry, R.W., Morton, A.R. & Keast, D. (1991) Overtraining in athletes: an update. *Sports Medicine* **12**, 32–65.

Geyer, H., Mareck-Engelke, U., Reinhart, U., Thevis, M. & Schänzer, W. (2000) Positive doping cases with norandrosterone after application of contaminated nutritional supplements. *Deutsche Zeitschrift fur Sportmedizin* **51**, 378.

Gibson, R. (1993) *Nutritional Assessment.* OUP, New York.

Gleeson, M., Nieman, D.C. & Pedersen, B.K. (2004) Exercise, nutrition and immune function. *Journal of Sports Sciences* **22**, 115–125.

Green, H.J., Jones, S., Ball-Burnett, M.E., Smith, D., Livesey, J. & Farrance, B.W. (1991) Early muscular and metabolic adaptations to prolonged exercise training in man. *Journal of Applied Physiology* **70**, 2032–2038.

Gurley, B.J., Gardner, S.F. & Hubbard, M.A. (2000) Content versus label claims in ephedra-containing dietary supplements. *American Journal of Health Systems and Pharmacy* **57**, 963.

Hawley, J.A., Tipton, K.D. & Millard-Stafford, M.L. (2006) Promoting training adaptations through nutritional interventions. *Journal of Sports Sciences* **24**, 709–721.

Henriksson, J. & Hickner, R.C. (1998) Adaptations in skeletal muscle in response to endurance training. In: Harries, M., Williams, C., Stanish, W.D. & Micheli, L.J. (eds) *Oxford Textbook of Sports Medicine*, 2nd edn. Oxford University Press, Oxford: 45–69.

Hultman, E. (1981) Liver glycogen in man: effect of different diets and muscular exercise. In: Pernod, B. & Saltin, B. (eds) *Muscle metabolism during exercise.* Plenum, New York: 143–152.

Ivy, J.L. (2000) Optimization of glycogen stores. In: Maughan, R.J. (ed.) *Nutrition in Sport.* Blackwell Science, Oxford: 97–111.

Ivy, J.L., Katz, A.L., Cutler, C.L. & Coyle, E.F. (1988) Muscle glycogen synthesis after exercise: effects of time of carbohydrate ingestion. *Journal of Applied Physiology* **64**, 1480–1485.

Kamber, M., Baume, N., Saugy, M. & Rivier, L. (2000) Nutritional supplements as a source for positive doping cases? *International Journal of Sport Nutrition and Exercise Biochemistry* **11**, 258–262.

Lang, F., Busch, G.L. & Volkl, K. (1998) The diversity of volume regulatory mechanisms. *Cell Physiology and Biochemistry* **8**, 1–45.

Lemon, P.W.R. (1991) Effect of exercise on protein requirements. *Journal of Sports Sciences* **9** (Special Issue), 53–70.

Loucks, A.B. (2004) Energy balance and body composition in sports and exercise. *Journal of Sports Sciences* **22**, 1–14.

Low, S.Y., Rennie, M.J. & Taylor, P.M. (1997a) Signalling elements involved in amino acid transport responses to altered muscle cell volume. *FASEB Journal* **11**, 1111–1117.

Low, S.Y., Rennie, M.J. & Taylor, P.M. (1997b) Modulation of glycogen synthesis in rate skeletal muscle by changes in cell volume. *Journal of Physiology* **495**, 299–303.

Martin, A.D. & Bailey, D.A. (1987) Skeletal integrity in amenorrheic athletes. *Australian Journal of Science and Medicine in Sport* **19**, 3–7.

Maughan, R.J. (1992) Aerobic function. *Sports Science Reviews* **1**, 28–42.

Maughan, R.J. (2006) Alcohol and football. *Journal of Sports Sciences* **24**, 741–748.

Maughan, R.J., Depiesse, F., Geyer, H. (2007) The use of dietary supplements by athletes. *Journal of Sports Sciences* **25**, S103–S113.

Millward, D.J. (2004) Protein and amino acid requirements of athletes. *Journal of Sports Sciences* **22**, 143–144.

Nevill, M.E., Boobis, L.H., Brooks, S. & Williams, C. (1989) Effect of training on muscle metabolism during treadmill sprinting. *Journal of Applied Physiology* **67**, 2376–2382.

Nieman, D.C. & Bishop, N.C. (2006) Nutritional strategies to counter stress to the immune system in athletes, with special reference to football. *Journal of Sports Sciences* **24**, 763–772.

Parasrampuria, M., Schwartz, K. & Petesch, R. (1998) Quality control of dehydroepiandrosterone dietary supplement products. *Journal of the American Medical Association* **280**, 1565.

Piehl, K. (1974) Time-course for refilling of glycogen stores in human muscle fibers following exercise-induced glycogen depletion. *Acta Physiologica Scandinavica* **90**, 297–302.

Pipe, A. & Ayotte, C. (2002) Nutritional supplements and doping. *Clinical Journal of Sports Medicine* **12**, 245–249.

Pirnay, F., Bodeux, M., Crielaard, J.M. & Franchimont, P. (1987) Bone mineral content and physical activity. *International Journal of Sports Medicine* **8**, 331–335.

Powers, S.K., deRuisseau, K.C., Quindry, J. & Hamilton, K.L. (2004) Dietary antioxidants and exercise. *Journal of Sports Sciences* **22**, 81–94.

Rennie, M.J., Low, S.Y., Taylor, P.M., Khogali, S.E., Yao, P.C. & Ahmed, A. (1998) Amino acid transport during muscle contraction and its relevance to exercise. *Advances in Experimental Medicine and Biology* **441**, 299–305.

Rockwell, M.S., Nickols-Richardson, S.M. & Thye, F.W. (2001) Nutrition knowledge, opinions and practices of coaches and athletic trainers at a division 1 university. *International Journal of Sports Nutrition and Exercise Metabolism* **11**, 174–185.

Romijn, J.A., Coyle, E.F., Sidossis, L.S., Gastaldelli, A., Horowitz, J.F., Endert, E., *et al.* (1993) Regulation of endogenous fat and carbohydrate metabolism in relation to exercise intensity and duration. *American Journal of Physiology* **265**, E380–E391.

Romijn, J.A., Coyle, E.F., Sidossis, L.S., Rosenblatt, J. & Wolfe, R.R. (2000) Substrate metabolism during different exercise intensities in endurance-trained women. *Journal of Applied Physiology* **88**, 1707–1171.

Ronsen, O., Sundgot-Borgen, J. & Maehlum, S. (1999) Supplement use and nutritional habits in Norwegian elite athletes. *Scandinavian Journal of Medicine and Science in Sports* **9**, 28–35.

Sawka, M.N., Burke, L.M., Eichner, E.R., Maughan, R.J., Montain, S.J. & Stachenfeld, N.S. (2007) Exercise and fluid replacement. *Medicine and Science in Sports and Exercise* **39**, 377–390.

Sobal, J. & Marquart, L.F. (1994) Vitamin/mineral supplement use among athletes: a review of the literature. *International Journal of Sport Nutrition* **4**, 320–324.

Tipton, K.D. & Wolfe, R.R. (2004) Protein and amino acids for athletes. *Journal of Sports Sciences* **22**, 65–79.

Tipton, K.D., Rasmussen, B.B., Miller, S.L., Wolf, S.E., Owens-Stovall, S.K., Petrini, B.E., *et al.* (2001). Timing of amino acid-carbohydrate ingestion alters anabolic response of muscle to resistance exercise. *American Journal of Physiology* **281**, E197–E206.

van Erp-Baart, A.J.M., Saris, W.H.M., Binkhorst, R.A., Vos, J.A. & Elvers, J.W.H. (1989) Nationwide survey on nutritional habits in elite athletes. *International Journal of Sport Nutrition* **10**, S11–S16.

van Hall, G., Saris, W.H.M., van de Schoor, P.A.I. & Wagenmakers, A.J.M. (2000a) The effect of free glutamine and peptide ingestion on the rate of muscle glycogen resynthesis in man. *International Journal of Sports Medicine* **21**, 25–30.

van Hall, G., Shirreffs, S.M. & Calbet, J.A. (2000b) Muscle glycogen resynthesis during recovery from cycle exercise: no effect of additional protein ingestion. *Journal of Applied Physiology* **88**, 1631–1636.

Waldegger, S. & Lang, F. (1997) Cell volume and gene expression. *Journal of Membrane Biology* **162**, 95–100.

Williams, C. (1998) Diet and sports performance. In: Harries, M., Williams, C., Stanish, W.D. & Micheli, L.J. (eds.) *Oxford Textbook of Sports Medicine*, 2nd edn. Oxford University Press, Oxford: 77–97.

Zawadzki, K.M., Yaspelkis, B.B. & Ivy, J.L. (1992) Carbohydrate–protein complex increases the rate of muscle glycogen storage after exercise. *Journal of Applied Physiology* **72**, 1854–1859.

Chapter 7

Dietary Goals and Eating Strategies

LOUISE M. BURKE

The importance of a sound diet in optimizing sports performance is exemplified by the number of position stands on nutrition for athletes issued by international governing federations of sport (Federation International de Football Association 2006; International Association of Athletics Federations 2007; International Olympic Committee 2004) and expert bodies in sports medicine (American College of Sports Medicine *et al.* 2000). The relationship between exercise and diet, and the principles of sports nutrition, are summarized in these positions stands as well as in Chapters 6 and 8. Despite the sophistication of the knowledge available to guide athletes towards good eating practices, the results of studies of dietary practices of sports people and the observations of sports nutritionists suggest that many athletes make dietary choices that are not conducive to optimal performance.

A number of factors may explain poor eating practices by athletes. These include a reliance on myths and misconceptions rather than expert advice, and the pervasive influence of the marketers of supplements and specialized sports foods. Many athletes are hampered by their lack of practical nutrition knowledge and lifestyle skills (e.g., knowledge of food composition and the ability to undertake food purchasing, preparation, and cooking). Many athletes face an overcommitted lifestyle, with inadequate time and opportunities to obtain or consume appropriate foods because of the heavy workload of

The Olympic Textbook of Science in Sport, 1st edition. Edited by R.J. Maughan. Published 2009 by Blackwell Publishing. ISBN: 978-1-4051-5638-7.

sport, work, school, and family. This is compounded by the disruption of frequent travel. There are also the challenges of inadequate finances for emerging athletes (Burke *et al.* 2001).

The aim of this chapter is to explore the dietary risk factors and poor food choices that explain the common nutrition problems seen in athletes. Each section explores the eating patterns or manipulations of common dietary practices that will better help the athlete address a certain issue or challenge in sports nutrition. Although these issues are covered individually, it is important that the athlete is able to integrate several goals in achieving their overall dietary plan. It is impossible to cover the myriad food uses, cultural eating patterns or individual food likes and dislikes of all athletes, or their individual nutritional needs. These specific needs are best addressed by consulting a sports dietitian or nutrition expert for individual advice. Nevertheless, there are a number of ideas that may be useful for all athletes.

Achieving fuel needs for training, competition preparation, and recovery

The replenishment of body carbohydrate stores to meet the fuel needs of training and competition is an important goal of athletes (see Chapter 6). Inadequate refueling can be a cause of premature fatigue and reduced performance in a single bout of prolonged exercise (for review see Coyle 2004; Hargreaves 2000), and may compromise the ability to undertake periods of intensive training (Achten *et al.* 2004; Simonsen *et al.* 1991). Newer guidelines for carbohydrate intake by athletes focus on the

Table 7.1 Updated guidelines from the IOC consensus on nutrition for athletes for the intake of carbohydrate (CHO) in the everyday or training diets of athletes (Burke *et al.* 2004).

Recommendations for carbohydrate intake
1 Athletes should aim to achieve CHO intakes to meet the fuel requirements of their training program and to optimize restoration of muscle glycogen stores between workouts. General recommendations can be provided, but should be fine-tuned with individual consideration of total energy needs, specific training needs, and feedback from training performance
   - Immediate recovery after exercise (0–4 h): 1–1.2 $g \cdot kg^{-1} \cdot h^{-1}$ consumed at frequent intervals
   - Daily recovery: moderate duration/low intensity training: 5–7 $g \cdot kg^{-1} \cdot day^{-1}$
   - Daily recovery: moderate–heavy endurance training: 7–12 $g \cdot kg^{-1} \cdot day^{-1}$
   - Daily recovery: extreme exercise program (4–6 h+ per day): 10–12 $g \cdot kg^{-1} \cdot day^{-1}$

2 It is valuable to choose nutrient-rich CHO foods and to add other foods to recovery meals and snacks to provide a good source of protein and other nutrients. These nutrients may assist in other recovery processes, and in the case of protein, may promote additional glycogen recovery when CHO intake is suboptimal or when frequent snacking is not possible
3 When the period between exercise sessions is < 8 h, the athlete should begin CHO intake as soon as practical after the first workout to maximize the effective recovery time between sessions. There may be some advantages in meeting CHO intake targets as a series of snacks during the early recovery phase
4 During longer recovery periods (24 h), the athlete should organize the pattern and timing of CHO-rich meals and snacks according to what is practical and comfortable for their individual situation. There is no difference in glycogen synthesis when liquid or solid forms of CHO are consumed
5 CHO-rich foods with a moderate to high glycemic index provide a readily available source of CHO for muscle glycogen synthesis, and should be the major CHO choices in recovery meals
6 Adequate energy intake is also important for optimal glycogen recovery; the restrained eating practices of some athletes, particularly females, make it difficult to meet CHO intake targets and to optimise glycogen storage from this intake

Recommendations against carbohydrate intake
1 Guidelines for CHO (or other macronutrients) should not be provided in terms of percentage contributions to total dietary energy intake. Such recommendations are neither user-friendly nor strongly related to the muscle's absolute needs for fuel
2 The athlete should not consume excessive amounts of alcohol during the recovery period because it is likely to interfere with their ability or interest to follow guidelines for post-exercise eating. The athlete should follow sensible drinking practices at all times, but particularly in the period after exercise

individuality of the fuel requirements of exercise and recovery (Table 7.1; Burke *et al.* 2004). Surveys of the dietary practices of serious athletes find that many individuals, especially females, report intakes that appear to fall short of these guidelines (Burke *et al.* 2001). Risk factors that may lead to inadequate intakes of carbohydrate include:

1 High training volume, or sudden increase in training volume or intensity, unaccompanied by adequate dietary changes.
2 Inadequate energy intake. This reduces the "budget" available for intake of carbohydrate-rich foods. In addition, it impairs post-exercise refueling by reducing the dietary substrates available for storage.
3 Inadequate intake of carbohydrate-rich foods:

- food cultures or food environments where carbohydrate-rich foods are not plentiful;
- diets promoting avoidance or reduced intake of carbohydrate (e.g. Zone diet, Atkins diet);
- diets promoting avoidance or reduced intake of key carbohydrate-rich foods (e.g. diets for athletes with celiac disease or other diets restricting intake of wheat or gluten-containing foods);
- reliance on bulky high-fiber foods which limit total dietary intake; and
- poor nutrition knowledge.

4 Poor achievement of strategic timing of intake of carbohydrate-rich foods (before, during, or after training):

- poor knowledge of fueling practices for prolonged exercise;

Table 7.2 Specific eating strategies to allow increase carbohydrate intake to meet high carbohydrate requirements.

1 The athlete should be aware that the typical eating patterns in most countries or regions are not likely to achieve a high carbohydrate diet. When carbohydrate needs are high, the athlete may need to try new foods or to change the ratio of foods at meals to promote carbohydrate-rich sources while reducing the intake of other foods

2 Meals and snacks should be based around nutrient-dense carbohydrate-rich foods, with ideas for low fat eating helping to promote fuel intake rather than a high fat intake. The quantities of these foods should be scaled up or down according to the athlete's fuel goals:
  • wholegrain breads and breakfast cereals
  • rice, pasta, noodles, and other grain foods
  • fresh fruit, juices, dried fruit, stewed or canned fruit
  • starchy vegetables (e.g., potatoes, corn, kumera)
  • legumes (lentils, beans, soy-based products)
  • sweetened dairy products (e.g., fruit-flavored yoghurt, milkshakes, fruit smoothies)

3 Sugar and sugary foods (e.g., jam, honey, confectionery, syrups) are a compact carbohydrate source. These may be particularly useful in a high energy diet, or when carbohydrate is needed before, during, and after exercise

4 Carbohydrate-rich drinks (e.g., fruit juices, soft drinks, fruit/milk smoothies) also provide a compact fuel source for special situations or very high carbohydrate diets. This category includes many of the supplements specially made for athletes (e.g., sports drinks, sports gels, and liquid meal supplements)

5 When energy and carbohydrate needs are high, the athlete should increase the number of meals and snacks they eat, rather than the size of meals. This will mean being organized to have snacks on hand in a busy day

6 Lower fiber choices of carbohydrate-rich foods are useful when energy needs are high, or for pre-event meals

7 Carbohydrate consumed before, during, and after workouts and competition adds to the day's fuel intake, as well as addressing the acute needs of the exercise session. Table 7.4 provides ideas for pre-event and post-event eating

8 Information for planning or assessing carbohydrate intake can be found in ready-reckoners of carbohydrate-rich foods or from nutrient information on food labels. This information can help the athlete keep track when carbohydrate needs are very high

---

  • gastrointestinal discomfort associated with consuming food close to intensive exercise; and
  • poor access to food over the day or in relation to training sessions.

Of course, ideal fuel intakes can only be assessed in view of total energy and nutritional needs, and with feedback from training and competition performance. Practical suggestions to increase total intake of carbohydrate in the day are provided in Table 7.2. These should be undertaken in conjunction with strategies to address the acute need for carbohydrate in preparation for competition, during periods of prolonged exercise, or recovery after workouts.

Preparation for competition should involve the combination of an appropriate exercise taper and adequate intake of carbohydrate to achieve fuel stores that are adequate for the duration and intensity of exercise. Carbohydrate loading is a specialized technique to super-compensate muscle glycogen stores in anticipation of an endurance or ultra-endurance event that would otherwise be limited by the depletion of this critical muscle fuel. Pioneering

studies in sports nutrition, undertaken on healthy but untrained men, produced the classic 7-day model of carbohydrate loading; a 3–4 day depletion phase of hard training and low carbohydrate intake followed by a 3–4 day loading phase of high carbohydrate intake and exercise taper (Ahlborg et al. 1967). The super-compensation of glycogen achieved by such a practice can allow athletes to continue at an optimal race pace for longer, thus enhancing their performance (Karlsson & Saltin 1971). A modified version of carbohydrate loading was developed when well-trained athletes were shown to super-compensate their glycogen stores without the necessity of a severe depletion or glycogen stripping phase (Sherman et al. 1981). The modified protocol, consisting simply of 3 days of high carbohydrate intake and taper, was offered as a more practical competition preparation that avoided the fatigue and complexity of the extreme diet and training requirements of the previous depletion phase. More recently, it has been seen that well-trained athletes may be able to carbohydrate load with as little as 24–48 h of high carbohydrate eating in combination

Table 7.3 Carbohydrate loading menu providing carbohydrate intakes of 10 $g \cdot kg^{-1} \cdot day^{-1}$ before an endurance event (day 4) (Burke 2007).

Day	65 kg male athlete (~650 $g \cdot day^{-1}$ carbohydrate)	50 kg female athlete (~500 $g \cdot day^{-1}$ carbohydrate)
Day 1 The menu focuses on the carbohydrate-rich foods; other foods can be added to balance the meal. An exercise taper should accompany this menu to optimize muscle glycogen storage. It is possible that glycogen supercompensation can be achieved by 2 days of such a diet, at least in well-trained athletes who can arrange a suitable exercise taper	Breakfast: 2 cups flake cereal + milk + banana 250 mL sweetened fruit juice Snack: 500 mL bottle soft drink 2 slices thick toast + jam Lunch: 2 large bread rolls with fillings 200 g flavored yoghurt Snack: coffee scroll or muffin 250 mL sweetened fruit juice Dinner: 3 cups cooked pasta + $^3/_4$ cup sauce 2 cups jelly: 2 crumpets and honey 250 mL sweetened fruit juice	Breakfast: 2 cups flake cereal + milk + banana 250 mL sweetened juice Snack: 500 mL bottle soft drink Lunch: 1 large bread roll with fillings 200 g flavored yoghurt Snack: 2 slices toast + jam 250 mL sweetened fruit juice Dinner: 2 cups cooked pasta + $^1/_2$ cup sauce 2 cups jelly Snack: 250 mL sweetened fruit juice 2 crumpets and honey
Day 2	Breakfast: 2 cups flake cereal + milk + cup sweetened canned fruit 250 mL sweetened fruit juice Snack: 500 mL fruit smoothie Lunch: 3 stack pancake + syrup + 2 scoops ice cream 500 mL soft drink Snack: 100 g dried fruit 250 mL sweetened fruit juice Dinner: 3 cups rice dish (e.g., fried rice, risotto) Snack: 2 cups fruit salad + 2 scoops ice cream	Breakfast: 2 cups flake cereal + milk + cup sweetened canned fruit 250 mL sweetened fruit juice Snack: 500 mL fruit smoothie Lunch: 2 stack pancake + syrup + 2 scoops ice cream 500 mL soft drink Snack 50 g dried fruit 250 mL sweetened fruit juice Dinner: 2 cups rice dish (e.g., fried rice, risotto) Snack: 1 cup fruit salad + scoop ice cream
Day 3 Many athletes like to increase the focus on low-fiber and low-residue eating on day before race, allowing them to reach the start line feeling "light" rather than with gastrointestinal fullness	Breakfast: 2 cups cereal (low fiber) + milk + banana 250 mL sweetened fruit juice Lunch: 4 white crumpets + jam Dinner: 2 cups white pasta + $^1/_2$ cup sauce Over day 1 L liquid meal drink or 1 L sport drink + 3 sport gels 200 g jelly confectionery	Breakfast: 2 cups cereal (low fiber) + milk + banana 250 mL sweetened fruit juice Lunch: 2 white crumpets + jam Dinner: 1.5 cups white pasta + $^1/_2$ cup sauce Over day 1 L liquid meal drink or 1 L sport drink + 3 sport gels 200 g jelly confectionery

Athletes of differing sizes should scale this intake up or down according to their body mass.

with taper or rest (Bussau *et al.* 2002). However, this requires the athlete to have specific knowledge to consume carbohydrate intakes of approximately 8–10 g·kg^{-1}·day^{-1} from eating patterns that will not cause gastrointestinal discomfort during their event. A sample menu that might achieve these goals is provided in Table 7.3.

The goals of the pre-event meal are to continue to fine-tune fuel and hydration levels prior to competition while allowing the athlete to avoid gastrointestinal discomfort during the session. Typically, meals or snacks based on carbohydrate-rich foods are the preferred choice of most athletes. The timing, amount, and type of foods should be chosen according to the personal preferences of each athlete and fine-tuned with experience to meet the practical and physiological needs of their event. Some athletes who are at risk of gastrointestinal distress during high-intensity exercise may find it helpful to reduce the fat, protein, or fiber content of the pre-event meal, as well as experiment with liquid meal choices or altered timing of intake. Some of the common choices for pre-event meals are summarized in Table 7.4.

Achieving fluid and fuel needs during training and competition

In many sports events and exercise activities, athletes experience premature fatigue or suboptimal performance as a result of inadequate hydration or fuel status (see Chapter 8). Typically, in exercise activities lasting an hour or more there is opportunity for, and potential benefits from, consuming fluid and/or a source of carbohydrate during the session. The athlete should develop a personalized drinking plan to match rates of sweat loss as well as practical so that the total fluid deficit incurred during the event is kept below about 2% of body mass (Sawka *et al.* 2007). However, fluid intakes in excess of sweat rates are not warranted and can lead to the potentially fatal problem of hyponatremia (low blood sodium levels; Almond *et al.* 2005). Carbohydrate requirements during exercise are also specific to the event and individual. However, the athlete should experiment with a plan that provides 30–60 g·h^{-1} carbohydrate (Coyle 2004) to fine-tune a strategy

that meets their practical and performance goals. Competition strategies should be practiced during key training sessions so that the athlete is familiarized with successful strategies and the workout can benefit from nutritional support.

There are a range of challenges to achieving a suitable intake of fluid and food during events and key training sessions:
- Carry-over of glycogen depletion and fluid deficit from previous event or training session, or from strategies undertaken to "make weight" for a weight division sport;
- Lack of awareness of likely sweat losses and fluid deficit during exercise sessions;
- Lack of awareness of fuel requirements or benefits of refueling during exercise sessions;
- Restricted opportunities to consume fluids or foods during exercise activity (e.g., lack of breaks in activity, rules prohibiting intake during games);
- Poor access to fluids or appropriate refueling sources during activity (need for trainers or aid stations to provide supplies);
- Difficulties in maintaining the palatability of fluids and foods available during exercise activities;
- Gastrointestinal distress resulting from the type or amount of fluid or food consumed during exercise; or
- Reluctance to eat or drink to avoid need for toilet stops during exercise.

There are a variety of strategies that can address these challenges (Table 7.5).

Recovery after competition and workouts

Recovery is a major challenge for the athlete who undertakes two or even three workouts each day during certain phases of the training cycle, with 4–24 h between each session. Many athletes also compete in sports in which the final outcome of competition requires several heats or games. Recovery involves a complex range of processes of restoration and adaptation to physiological stress of exercise, including restoration of muscle and liver glycogen stores, replacement of fluid and electrolytes lost in sweat and synthesis of new protein following the catabolic state and damage induced by the exercise.

Table 7.4 Carbohydrate-rich choices suitable for special issues in sport (Burke 2007).

Carbohydrate-rich choices for pre-event meals
Breakfast cereal + low-fat milk + fresh/canned fruit
Muffins or crumpets + jam/honey
Pancakes + syrup
Toast + baked beans (note this is a high-fiber choice)
Creamed rice (made with low-fat milk)
Rolls or sandwiches
Fruit salad + low-fat fruit yoghurt
Spaghetti with tomato or low-fat sauce
Baked potatoes with low-fat filling
Fruit smoothie (low-fat milk + fruit + yoghurt/ice cream)
Liquid meal supplement

Carbohydrate-rich foods suitable for intake during exercise (50 g carbohydrate portions)
600–800 mL sports drink
2 × sachets sports gel
1–1.5 sports bars
2 cereal bars or granola bars
Large bread roll filled with jam/honey/cheese
2 bananas/3 medium pieces of other fruit
60 g jelly confectionery
450 mL cola drinks
80 g chocolate bar
100 g fruit bread or cake
80 dried fruit or 120 g trail mix

Recovery snacks – to be eaten post-exercise, or pre-exercise in the case of resistance training to promote refueling and protein responses
(Each serve provides 50 g carbohydrate and at least 10 g protein)
250–350 mL liquid meal supplement or milkshake/fruit smoothie
500 mL flavored low-fat milk
Sports bar + 200 mL sports drink
60 g (1.5–2 cups) breakfast cereal with $^{1}/_{2}$ cup milk
1 round sandwiches with cheese/meat/chicken filling, and 1 large piece of fruit or 300 mL sports drink
1 cup fruit salad with 200 g carton fruit-flavored yoghurt or custard
200 g carton fruit-flavored yoghurt or 300 mL flavored milk and 30–35 g cereal bar
2 crumpets or English muffins with thick spread of peanut butter
250 g tin baked beans on 2 slices of toast
250 g (large) baked potato with cottage cheese or grated cheese filling
150 g thick crust pizza

Portable carbohydrate-rich foods suitable for the traveling athlete
Breakfast cereal (and skim milk powder)
Cereal bars, granola bars
Dried fruit, trail mixes
Rice crackers, dry biscuits plus spreads – jam, honey, etc.
Quick-cook noodles and rice
Baked beans
Sports bars
Liquid meal supplements – powder and ready-to-drink tetra packs
Sports drink

Table 7.5 Guidelines for hydrating and refueling during and after exercise.

- The athlete should begin all exercise sessions well-hydrated, with particular focus on strategies to recover fluid losses from previous training sessions or weight-marking activities, and to drink adequate amounts of fluid when living in hot environments
- Hyperhydration techniques (acute fluid overloading) may be useful for specific situations of high sweat rates and reduced opportunities to drink during the session, but these tactics should be well practiced in advance and are best undertaken under the supervision of appropriate medical/scientific support staff
- During exercise, the athlete should develop a fluid intake plan to keep pace with sweat losses as much as it is practicable and tolerated. Ideally, the fluid deficit incurred during exercise should be kept below 2% of body mass, especially when exercise is undertaken in hot conditions. It is difficult to gauge sweat losses during an exercise session, but, monitoring changes in body mass before and after similar sessions can provide a guide to typical sweat losses and the athlete's typical success in replacing these losses. A loss of 1 kg is approximately equal to 1 L sweat loss. The athlete should undertake such fluid balance checks from time to time to obtain an estimate of expected sweat losses in different events and conditions
- The athlete should not consume excessive amounts of fluid during exercise so that they exceed their rate of sweat loss and gain weight over the session, unless they have begun exercise in a dehydrated state and this is a specific aim. This may be the case in the second training session of the day when sweat losses in the first session have not been fully replaced. Over-drinking may cause gastrointestinal discomfort and can lead to the potentially fatal condition of hyponatremia (low blood sodium)
- The athlete should examine their sport to identify opportunities to drink fluids during the session. Sometimes this can occur during formal breaks in play (time-outs, player substitutions, half-time) while in other sports the athlete must learn to drink "on the move." A successful fluid intake plan will also mean ensuring supplies of suitable drinks are available (e.g., at aid stations, carried by the athlete, or provided by trainers)
- The provision of cool, palatable drinks will encourage fluid intake. Sports drinks are ideal for providing fluids during events, as well as contributing to fuel needs. The replacement of electrolytes via sports drinks is probably valuable in very long events and contributes to the taste appeal of drinks. In prolonged events, it is useful to vary the flavours of drinks to continue to stimulate voluntary intake. Using insulated containers to keep drinks cool can also help
- Carbohydrate intake can be achieved during longer exercise sessions using sports drinks, special sports products (e.g., gels, bars), and other everyday foods. A carbohydrate intake of $30-60$ g$\cdot$h^{-1} is generally associated with successful refueling during events of $60-90$ min or longer and common fuel choices are presented in Table 7.4. Each athlete should experiment to find a plan that works for their event and their comfort
- Training sessions should also be targeted for fluid and fuel intake plans. Good hydration/fueling practices during training will mean better performance during that session, and a chance to practice the strategies intended for competition. There is considerable difference in individual (gastrointestinal) tolerance to drinking large volumes of fluid; however, there is some evidence that practice can increase the tolerance of even the most reluctant drinkers
- After each training session or event, the athlete should enhance recovery by undertaking active rehydration and refueling strategies. Rehydration requires an intake of greater volumes of fluid than the post-exercise fluid deficit. In general, the athlete will need to drink 150% of the post-race fluid deficit to ensure fluid balance is achieved (e.g., if the post-race fluid deficit is 2 kg (2 L), the athlete should drink 3 L fluid over the next hours to rehydrate)
- The replacement of sodium is important in restoring fluid balance, and can be achieved via the selection of sodium-containing fluids (sports drinks and oral rehydration solutions), snacks (pretzels, bread, breakfast cereal) or by adding a little extra salt to meals

Responses of the immune system are also important (see Chapter 10).

The various sections of this chapter provide guidelines to assist the athlete to consume carbohydrate, protein, fluid, electrolytes, and perhaps other nutrients that will be important in enhancing these recovery processes. However, there are often challenges to achieving these guidelines in the hours after competition or key workouts:

- Fatigue – interfering with ability or interest to obtain or eat food;
- Loss of appetite following high-intensity exercise;
- Limited access to (suitable) foods at exercise venue;
- Restricted energy intake during to real or perceived need to reduce body weight and body fat levels;
- Other post-exercise commitments and priorities (e.g., coaches' meetings, drug tests, equipment maintenance, warm-down activities); and

Table 7.6 Guidelines for manipulating energy intake for loss of weight and body fat in athletes.

- Targets for ideal body mass (BM) and body fat should be set on an individual basis. It is often useful to consider an ideal range of BM and body fat that the athlete may achieve at various times of the training and competitive season. Where fat loss is required, this should be achieved gradually and in conjunction with an appropriate exercise program
- Fat loss should be achieved via a moderate energy deficit (e.g., 2–4 MJ·day^{-1} or 500–1000 kcal·day^{-1}) achieved by manipulating diet and/or exercise. Excessive restriction of energy intake should be avoided such that energy availability (total intake minus the energy cost of training) is below 30 kcal (189 kJ) per kilogram body mass (see Table 7.7)
- Although reduced energy intake may reduce total intake of protein and carbohydrate, the athlete should consume these nutrients at strategic times, such as immediately after key training sessions. This may be achieved by altering the timetable of meals in relation to training
- There is no evidence to support the long-term success of currently fashionable weight loss diets such as low-carbohydrate, high-protein programs, or the Zone (40:30:30) diet. These diets are nutritionally unbalanced, and inconsistent with guidelines that are scientifically supported to optimize athletic performance
- The athlete should consume a wide variety of nutrient-dense foods, to meet protein and micronutrient requirements from a reduced energy intake. Micronutrient supplementation should be considered where restricted energy intake is a long-term issue
- Meals/snacks should be planned to avoid long periods without food intake and to promote post-exercise recovery
- A high volume of food intake can be achieved by making use of high-fiber, low energy-density foods such as fruits and vegetables. Carbohydrate-rich foods with a low glycemic index, and protein–carbohydrate food matches also help to promote satiety of meals and snacks
- Energy-rich fluids and energy-dense foods should not be consumed in excessive amounts
- A food diary may help to identify the athlete's *actual* intake rather than perceived intake, and note the occasions or situations in which the athlete is unable to adhere to their plan
- Behavior modification can overcome inappropriate eating practices such as eating for comfort or to relieve stress and boredom
- Athletes should seek professional advice from a sports dietitian, especially where nutritional goals are complex, or where previous dieting behaviors have already caused food-related stress

- Traditional post-competition activities (e.g., excessive alcohol intake).

Each athlete should be organized to have access to a range of palatable foods and drinks that allow them to meet their nutritional goals after exercise. In the case of a reduced energy intake, the athlete should schedule their timetable so that meals are eaten at strategic times in relation to key training sessions (Table 7.6).

Achieving a suitable physique – weight fat loss

Physique characteristics have a direct role in the performance of many sports. In fact, weight loss is the most popular reason for an athlete to consult a sports nutritionist, with common situations including:

- Athletes competing in a weight-controlled sport (e.g., boxing, judo, weightlifting, or lightweight rowing) who wish to compete at a weight division that is below their current weight.

- Athletes competing in an endurance sport or power sport, where a low body fat level, and an increased power to weight ratio, is a physical advantage to performance (e.g., distance running, cycling, triathlons, or gymnastics).
- Athletes competing in a sport where leanness and low body fat levels are of aesthetic advantage (e.g., gymnastics, diving, figure skating).
- Athletes competing in a skill-based sport where training hours are lengthy, but essentially low energy expenditure (and therefore do not contribute to a high energy turnover). These athletes may desire to lose weight for health or aesthetic reasons (e.g., golf, archery).
- Athletes who have been required by their sport to move away from a stable home environment. These athletes may have poor cooking and/or food preparation skills, lead an irregular and/or disorganized lifestyle, and be reliant on takeaway and restaurant meals (e.g., football codes and other team sports, tennis and other sports requiring extensive travel commitments).

• Athletes returning from injury or from a break from their sport where inactivity and a failure to adjust energy intake has led to body fat gain.

As displayed in these examples, low body mass and low levels of body fat are of value to the performance of a number of sports. A high level of muscularity is favorable for activities based on strength and power, as well as the aesthetics of some sports. Some high level athletes "naturally" display the physique characteristics that are required for their sport – as a result of the genetic traits that have caused them to gravitate to this activity as well as the conditioning effects of serious training. By contrast, other athletes have to undertake specific programs to manipulate their body mass, muscle mass, and body fat levels.

Many athletes pursue rigid criteria for the "ideal physique" for their sport, based on the characteristics of successful competitors or, in the case of sports favoring leanness, the attainment of minimum levels of body fat. However, there are several dangers and disadvantages to the establishment of rigid prescriptions for the body weight or body fat levels of individual athletes. First, it fails to acknowledge that there is considerable variability in the physical characteristics of successful athletes, even between individuals in the same sport. It also fails to take into account that it can take many years of training and maturation for an athlete to achieve their ideal shape and body composition. Finally, there are problems when changes in body mass or crude measures of body composition are assumed to be markers of fatness and muscle mass; unfortunately, many athletes and coaches rely on such crude markers.

There are a number of reliable and valid techniques for the assessment of body fat levels or lean body mass. These range from techniques that are best suited to the laboratory (e.g., hydro densitometry and dual-energy X-ray absorptiometry [DEXA] scans) to protocols that can be undertaken in the field (e.g., anthropometric data such as measurements of skinfold fat, body girths and circumferences; Kerr & Ackland 2006). Sports scientists who undertake these assessments on athletes should be appropriately trained to minimize their measurement error and to understand the limitations of their assessments. These techniques can then be used to set a range of acceptable values for body fat and body weight within each sport, and to monitor the health and performance of individual athletes within this range. Longitudinal profiling of an athlete can be used to monitor the development of physical characteristics that are associated with good performance for that individual, as well as to identify the changes in physique that can be expected over a season or period of specialized training.

In many "weight sensitive" sports, athletes strive to reduce their body mass and body fat below levels that seem "healthy" or to achieve these losses in a rapid manner. In the short term, a sudden improvement in the body's power to weight ratio may produce an improvement in performance. However, long-term disadvantages arise from the effects of excessive training, chronically low intakes of energy and nutrients, and psychological distress. These are likely to include illness, injury, reduced well-being, and impaired performance. Additional problems have been noted in "weight making" sports in which athletes undertake rapid weight loss in the days before competition in order to make their event "weight target." According to surveys of athletes in weight category sports (Moore et al. 2002; Oppliger et al. 2003; Steen & Brownell 1990), strategies used to achieve this weight loss include fasting, techniques causing dehydration (diuretics, saunas, or exercising in a hot environment), and purging (vomiting, laxatives). Various efforts by sports physicians and sports scientists to educate athletes and change the conditions under which they compete appear to have attenuated but not eliminated such unsafe weight loss practices (Oppliger et al. 1998). In extreme cases, athletes have died as a result of their "weight making" pursuits; in particular, undertaking prolonged and intense training sessions while dehydrated and following severe energy restriction (Centers for Disease Control and Prevention 1998).

Loss of body fat should be achieved through a program of eating and exercise that achieves a sustained and moderate energy deficit, but still allows the athlete to meet their nutritional needs and to enjoy some of the pleasure and social opportunities that food normally provides in our lives. Guidelines for such a plan are summarized in Table 7.6. It is important that successful weight control for an individual athlete considers measures of long-term health and performance. Some individuals are naturally light and have low levels of body fat, or can achieve these without paying a substantial penalty. Furthermore, some athletes vary their body fat levels over a season so that very low levels are achieved only for a specific and short time. In general, athletes should not undertake strategies to minimize body fat levels unless they can be sure there are no side effects or disadvantages.

Although it is difficult to obtain reliable figures on the prevalence of eating disorders or disordered eating behaviour and body image among athletes, there appears to be a higher risk of problems among female athletes, and among athletes in sports in which success is associated with specific weight targets or low body fat levels (Beals & Manore 1994; Sundgot-Borgen 2000). Even where clinical eating disorders do not exist, many athletes appear to restrict their energy intake – reporting energy intakes that are considerably less than expected energy requirements, and considerable stress related to food intake (Beals & Manore 1994). There is considerable evidence that a low level of "energy availability," defined as total energy intake minus the energy cost of the athlete's exercise program, has serious consequences on the hormonal, immunologic, and health status of the athlete (Loucks 2004).

The "female athlete triad," the coexistence of disordered or restricted eating, menstrual dysfunction, and impaired bone health has received considerable publicity (ACSM 2007). Incremental changes in "energy availability" lead to a dose-dependent relationship between energy restriction and metabolic and hormonal function. The threshold for maintenance of normal menstrual function in females is an energy availability of above 30 kcal (125 kJ) per kilogram fat-free mass (Table 7.7). Low energy availability is a potential outcome of the excessive pursuit of thinness by female athletes, but it is likely that male athletes also experience consequences that are not as yet well described. Expert advice from sports medicine professionals, including dietitians, psychologists, and physicians, is important in the early detection and management of problems related to body composition and nutrition. The reader is referred to the excellent textbook by Beals (2004) for

Table 7.7 Examples of energy availability.

Example of adequate energy availability
50 kg female with 20% body fat = 40 kg FFM
Daily energy intake 2500 kcal (10 500 kJ)
Cost of daily exercise (1.5 h·day^{-1}) = 1000 kcal (4200 kJ)
Energy availability = 2500 − 1000 = 1500 kcal (6300 kJ)
Energy availability = 1500/40 or 37.5 kcal (157 kJ) per kilogram FFM

Example of low energy availability
50 kg female with 20% body fat = 40 kg FFM
Daily energy intake 1500 kcal (6300 kJ)
Cost of daily exercise (1 h·day)$^{-1}$ = 500 kcal (2200 kJ)
Energy availability = 1500 − 500 = 1000 kcal (4200 kJ)
Energy availability = 1000/40 or 25 kcal (105 kJ) per kilogram FFM

FFM, fat-free mass.

more information on the treatment of disordered eating in athletes.

Achieving a suitable physique – increasing muscle size and strength

An increase in muscle mass is desired by many athletes whose performance is linked with size, strength, or power. In addition to the increase in muscle mass and strength that occurs during adolescence, particularly in males, many athletes pursue specific muscle hypertrophy through a program of progressive muscle overload. An important nutritional requirement to support such a program is adequate energy. This is required for the manufacture of new muscle tissue, as well as to provide fuel for the training program that supplied the stimulus for this muscle growth. Many athletes do not achieve a sufficiently positive energy balance to optimize muscle gains during a strength training program. Specialized nutrition advice can help the athlete improve this situation by making energy-dense foods and drinks accessible and easy to consume (Table 7.6). Despite the interest in gaining muscle size and strength, there is little rigorous scientific study of the amount of energy required, the optimal ratio of macronutrients supplying this energy, and the requirements for micronutrients to enhance this process.

Table 7.8 Guidelines for dietary strategies to support a gain in muscle mass or to achieve a high energy intake.

- The athlete should aim for a pattern of small frequent meals each day to achieve an adequate energy intake and promote recovery/adaptation to resistance training and other key training sessions
- A snack providing carbohydrate and protein will enhance recovery after key training sessions as well as contribute to total daily energy intake. Such a snack should also be consumed prior to resistance training sessions. Examples of foods combining these nutrients are provided in Table 7.4
- Carbohydrate should be consumed during prolonged exercise to provide additional fuel as well as contribute to total daily energy intake
- A food diary may help to identify the athlete's *actual* intake rather than perceived intake, and note the occasions or situations in which the athlete is unable to adhere to their plan of frequent meals and snacks
- The athlete is often faced with a chaotic and overcommitted lifestyle. Good skills in time management should see the athlete using quieter periods to undertake food shopping and meal preparation activities so that food is available during hectic periods
- The traveling athlete should take a supply of portable and non-perishable snacks which can be easily prepared and eaten (e.g., breakfast cereal and powdered milk, cereal bars, sports bars, liquid meal supplements, dried fruit/nuts and creamed rice)
- Specialized products such as sports drinks, sports gels, and sports bars provide a practical form of carbohydrate during exercise, while sports bars and liquid meal supplements provide an accessible form of carbohydrate and protein for post-exercise recovery
- Energy-containing drinks such as liquid meal supplements, flavored milk, fruit smoothies, sports drinks, soft drinks and juices provide a low-bulk way to consume energy and other important nutrients while meeting fluid needs
- Although fiber intake is important in a healthy diet, excessive intake of high-fiber foods may limit total energy intake or lead to gastrointestinal discomfort. It may be necessary to moderate intake of wholegrain or fiber-enriched versions of foods

It is tempting to hypothesize that an increase in dietary protein will stimulate muscle gain. Indeed, many strength trained athletes consume very large amounts of protein, in excess of 2–3 g per kilogram body mass per day in the belief that this will enhance the gains from resistance training programs. This is 2–3 times the recommended intake recognized in most countries. However, the value of very high protein intakes in optimizing muscle gains remains unsupported by the scientific literature (Tipton & Wolfe 2004).

There is emerging evidence that the strategic *timing* of intake of protein in relation to training may be the most important dietary factor in enhancing gains in muscle size and strength. Specifically, consuming protein after or even before a resistance training session has been shown to substantially increase net protein balance compared with a control condition (Rasmussen *et al.* 2000; Tipton *et al.* 2001). It is too early to provide specific details of amount and type of protein to achieve the optimal response in net protein balance. However, it appears that consuming a relatively modest amount of protein (a source providing approximately 3–6 essential amino acids or approximately 20 g of a high biologic value protein) either before or after a resistance workout causes a substantial increase in net protein synthesis (Borsheim *et al.* 2002; Miller *et al.* 2003; Tipton *et al.* 2001). This enhancement is still apparent in the 24-h picture of protein balance (Tipton *et al.* 2003). There may also be some benefits to net protein balance in combining carbohydrate with these protein "recovery" snacks (Borsheim *et al.* 2004a,b). These ideas are incorporated into the guidelines in Table 7.8, as well as the suggestions for carbohydrate-rich recovery snacks in Table 7.4.

Achieving requirements for vitamins and minerals

An adequate intake of the micronutrients and phytochemicals found in food is important for health and the optimization of training and performance. However, there is an inadequate body of research to make clear recommendations about increased intakes of vitamins and minerals resulting from a commitment to a substantial daily exercise program. Instead it is assumed that athletes who consume a moderate to high intake of energy from a range of nutrient-rich foods will meet all their requirements for dietary micronutrients and phytochemicals. There are several challenges to achieving these goals, resulting in the risk that some athletes will develop problems related to suboptimal micronutrient status. Nutrients that are well-known to be at risk of poor intake or to be a problem for athletes include iron and calcium. Suboptimal iron status is known to impair adaptations to training and the ability to undertake a single bout of exercise (Deakin 2006). Inadequate calcium intake is a risk factor in poor bone health and is recognized as a problem faced especially by female athletes (ACSM 2007).

Factors that can lead to inadequate intake of micronutrients are summarized below.

RISKS FOR POOR INTAKE OF ALL MICRONUTRIENTS

1 Chronic low energy intake (<2000 kcal·day^{-1} or 8 MJ·day^{-1}). Athletes at most risk are those who restrict energy intake to achieve their weight or body fat goals, especially female athletes and athletes in "weight division" sports.
2 Restriction of the range of foods included in eating patterns:
  • concentration on carbohydrate-rich meals to the exclusion of other foods;
  • poor finances or poor cooking skills leading to a limited food range;
  • travel to an environment or living in dormitory style accommodation with a restricted variety of foods on offer;
  • vegetarian eating on a whim;
  • fad diets; compulsive following of a rigid intake of "allowable" low fat foods;
  • overconsumption of micronutrient-poor convenience foods and sports foods (e.g., high carbohydrate powders, gels); and
  • disordered eating.

ADDITIONAL RISK FACTORS FOR IRON DEFICIENCY IN ATHLETES

1 Increased iron requirements:
  • recent growth spurt in adolescents;
  • pregnancy (current or within the past year).

2 Factors increasing iron loss or malabsorption:
  • sudden increase in heavy training load, particularly running on hard surfaces, causing an increase in intravascular hemolysis;
  • gastrointestinal bleeding (e.g., some anti-inflammatory drugs, ulcers);
  • gastrointestinal malabsorption problems (e.g., celiac disease, irritable bowel);
  • heavy menstrual blood losses;
  • excessive blood losses such as frequent nose bleeds, recent surgery, substantial contact injury;
  • frequent blood donation.
3 Additional factors leading to inadequate intake of bioavailable iron:
  • vegetarian eating – especially poorly constructed diets in which alternative food sources of iron are ignored (e.g., legumes, nuts, and seeds) and which contain large amounts of inhibitory factors for iron absorption (e.g., phytates);
  • failure to promote matching of iron-containing foods with dietary factors that promote iron absorption such as ascorbic and other food acids, meat factor;
  • natural food diets: failure to consume iron-fortified cereal foods such as commercial breakfast cereals and bread.

ADDITIONAL RISK FACTORS FOR POOR CALCIUM INTAKES IN ATHLETES

1 Lactose intolerance leading to avoidance of dairy foods.
2 Veganism with reliance on unfortified soy sources of milk and "dairy."
3 Other intolerances or fad diets excluding dairy foods.

Strategies to achieve better intakes of micronutrients are summarized in Table 7.9.

Meeting nutrition goals on the road

Most elite athletes are well-seasoned travelers, undertaking trips to training camps or specialized environments (e.g., altitude), and to compete. Athletes must be able to achieve their peak performance at important competitions such as Olympic Games or World Championships in an environment that is

Table 7.9 Strategies to promote adequate intake of vitamins and minerals.

- The athlete should be prepared to try new foods and new recipes to keep expanding their dietary range. Including a variety of foods in the day-to-day menu greatly reduces the risk of an inadequate intake of any individual micronutrient or dietary constituent
- The athlete should enjoy plenty of color at meals and snacks with the goodness of fruits and vegetables. Eat a rainbow of colors every day with representation from blue/purple, white, green, yellow/orange and red varieties
- It is a good idea to take advantage of foods that are in season to introduce new variety into menus
- The athlete should avoid popular diets that advise against "food combining," because these are unsound. Meals are usually improved nutritionally, and enhanced in flavor and color, when a number of ingredients or foods are integrated into the menu. This can be done by adding individual food items together on the plate, or by cooking recipes that already involve a mixture (e.g., stir fries, casseroles, main meal salads)
- Most foods provide some nutrient value, even if some features are not in line with other dietary principles. Banishing a food or food group from the diet can lead to the loss of important nutrients and to dietary boredom. There are often ways to reduce or modify the intake of particular food items rather than discarding the food totally. A sports dietitian can help an athlete to explore and maximize food variety – especially when there are sound reasons for restricting food choices (e.g., food allergies or intolerances, moral or religious sanctions)
- Because the haem form of iron found in many animal foods (e.g., red meats, shellfish, liver) is well-absorbed, it should be included regularly in meals – at least 3–5 times per week. These foods can be added as a partner to high-carbohydrate meal (e.g., meat sauce on a pasta dish; liver pate in a sandwich)
- The absorption of non-haem iron (found in wholegrains, cereal foods, eggs, leafy green vegetables etc.) is increased by including a vitamin C food at the same meal (e.g., a glass of orange juice consumed with breakfast cereal). The absorption is also enhanced by combining with a "meat" food (e.g., legumes and meat in a chilli con carne)
- Athletes who are at high-risk of iron deficiency should be aware that some food factors (e.g., excess bran, strongly brewed tea) interfere with iron absorption from non-haem iron foods. These items should be avoided or separated from meals
- Iron supplements should be taken only on the advice of a sports dietitian or doctor. They may be useful in the supervised treatment and prevention of iron deficiency, but do not replace a holistic assessment and treatment, including integrated dietary advice
- Calcium requirements are easy to meet if the athlete's eating patterns include at least three serves of dairy foods or a calcium-fortified soy equivalent each day (one serve is equal to a glass of milk or a carton of yoghurt). Low-fat and reduced-fat dairy products are available, as well as an increasing range of soy products
- Calcium requirements are increased in young athletes undergoing a growth spurt, or in females who are pregnant or breastfeeding. These athletes should increase their dairy intake to 4–5 serves a day. Female athletes who have irregular menstrual periods also require extra calcium and should seek expert advice from a sports doctor
- Fish eaten with its bones (e.g., tinned salmon, sardines) is a useful calcium source
- In some countries, everyday foods such as orange juice can be fortified with calcium to provide a substantial and regular source of calcium
- Athletes who are vegetarian, or unable to eat dairy products and red meat in the recommended amounts, should seek the advice of a sports dietitian. Creative ways can be found to include other foods or food uses to meet iron and calcium needs or to use mineral supplements correctly

often both far away and different from their home base. In some sports, national or regional competitions require athletes to travel weekly or bi-weekly to compete against the other members of their league. Frequent travel can pose a number of challenges:

- Disruptions to the normal training routine and lifestyle while the athlete is en route;
- Changes in climate and environment that create different nutritional needs;
- Jet lag;
- Changes to food availability including absence of important and familiar foods;
- Reliance on hotels, restaurants, and takeaways instead of home cooking;
- Exposure to new foods and eating cultures;
- Temptations of an "all you can eat" dining hall in an athlete village;
- Risk of gastrointestinal illnesses resulting from exposure to food and water with poor hygiene standards;

Table 7.10 Strategies to cope with the nutritional challenges of travel.

- The athlete should investigate food issues on travel routes (e.g., airlines) and at the destination before leaving home. Caterers and food organizers should be contacted well ahead of the trip to let them know meal timing and menu needs
- A supply of portable and non-perishable foods should be taken or sent to the destination to replace important items that are missing
- The athlete should be aware that many catering plans cover only meals. Because the athlete's nutrition goals are likely to include well-timed and well-chosen snacks, supplies should be taken to supplement meals en route and at the destination
- Many athletes will turn to "boredom eating" when confined. Instead, they should eat according to their real needs, taking into account the forced rest while traveling
- When moving to a new time zone, the athlete should adopt eating patterns that suit their destination as soon as the trip starts. This will help the body clock to adapt
- Unseen fluid losses in air-conditioned vehicles and pressurized plane cabins should be recognized and a drinking plan should be organized to keep the athlete well hydrated
- It is important to find out whether the local water supply is safe to drink. Otherwise the athlete should stick to drinks from sealed bottles, or hot drinks made from well-boiled water. Ice added to drinks is often made from tap water and may be a problem
- In high-risk environments, the athlete should eat only at good hotels or well-known restaurants. Food from local stalls and markets should be avoided, however tempting it is to have an "authentic cultural experience"
- Food that has been well-cooked is the safest; it is best to avoid salads or unpeeled fruit that has been in contact with local water or soil
- The athlete should choose the best of the local cuisine to meet their nutritional needs, supplementing with their own supplies where needed
- The athlete should be assertive in asking for what they need at catering outlets (e.g., low-fat cooking styles or an extra carbohydrate choice)
- The challenges of "all you can eat" dining should be recognized. The athlete should resist the temptation to eat "what is there" or "what everyone else is eating" in favor of their own meal plan

- Excitement and distraction of a new environment leading to inappropriate choice or quantity of food intake.

Table 7.10 provides a summary of strategies to cope with these challenges and achieve nutrition goals.

Conclusions

The specific nutritional needs of athletes vary according to their sport, the period of their training and competition program, and their individual issues and circumstances. There are some predictable challenges to achieving nutrition goals and some common strategies to address these issues. While athletes can often achieve a successful eating plan by following these ideas, they are also encouraged to seek professional advice from a sports nutrition expert when these challenges become substantial.

References

Achten, J., Halson, S.H., Moseley, L., Rayson, M.P., Casey, A. & Jeukendrup, A.E. (2004) Higher dietary carbohydrate content during intensified running training results in better maintenance of performance and mood state. *Journal of Applied Physiology* **96**, 1331–1340.

Ahlborg, B., Bergstrom, J., Brohult, J., Ekelund, L.G., Hultman, E. & Maschio, G. (1967) Human muscle glycogen content and capacity for prolonged exercise after different diets. *Forsvarsmedicin* **3**, 85–99.

Almond, C.S.D., Shin, A.Y., Fortescue, E.B., Mannix, R.C., Wypij, D., Binstadt, B.A., *et al.* (2005) Hyponatremia among runners in the Boston marathon. *New England Journal of Medicine* **352**, 1550–1556.

American College of Sports Medicine, American Dietetic Association, & Dietitians of Canada. (2000) Nutrition and athletic performance. *Medicine and Science in Sports and Exercise* **32**, 2130–2145.

American College of Sports Medicine (ACSM). (2007) Position Stand. The female athlete triad. *Medicine and Science in Sports and Exercise* **39**, 1867–1883.

Beals, K.A. (2004) *Disordered Eating Among Athletes: A Comprehensive Guide for Health Professionals.* Human Kinetics, Champaign, IL.

Beals, K.A. & Manore, M.M. (1994) The prevalence and consequences of subclinical eating disorders in female athletes. *International Journal of Sport Nutrition* **4**, 175–195.

Borsheim, E., Aarsland, A. & Wolfe, R.R. (2004a) Effect of an amino acid, protein, and carbohydrate mixture on net muscle protein balance after resistance exercise. *International Journal of Sport Nutrition and Exercise Metabolism* **14**, 255–271.

Borsheim, E., Cree, M.G., Tipton, K.D., Elliott, T.A., Aarsland, A. & Wolfe, R.R. (2004b) Effect of carbohydrate intake on net muscle protein synthesis during recovery from resistance exercise. *Journal of Applied Physiology* **96**, 674–678.

Borsheim, E., Tipton, K.D., Wolf, S.E. & Wolfe, R.R. (2002) Essential amino acids and muscle protein recovery from resistance exercise. *American Journal of Physiology. Endocrinology and Metabolism* **283**, E648–E657.

Burke, L. (2007) Training and competition nutrition. In *Practical Sports Nutrition* (Burke, L., ed.) Human Kinetics, Champaign, IL: 1–26.

Burke, L.M., Cox, G.R., Cummings, N.K. & Desbrow, B. (2001) Guidelines for daily CHO intake: do athletes achieve them? *Sports Medicine* **31**, 267–299.

Burke, L.M., Kiens, B. & Ivy, J.L. (2004) Carbohydrates and fat for training and recovery. *Journal of Sports Sciences* **22**, 15–30.

Bussau, V.A., Fairchild, T.J., Rao, A., Steele, P.D. & Fournier, P.A. (2002) Carbohydrate loading in human muscle: an improved 1 day protocol. *European Journal of Applied Physiology* **87**, 290–295.

Centers for Disease Control and Prevention. (1998) Hyperthermia and dehydration-related deaths associated with intentional rapid weight loss in three collegiate wrestlers – North Carolina, Wisconsin, and Michigan, November–December 1998. *JAMA* **279**, 824–825.

Coyle, E.F. (2004) Fluid and fuel intake during exercise. *Journal of Sports Sciences* **22**, 39–55.

Deakin, V. (2006) Iron depletion in athletes. In *Clinical Sports Nutrition* (3rd edn.) (Burke, L. & Deakin, V., eds.) McGraw-Hill, Sydney: 263–312.

Federation International de Football Association. (2006). Nutrition for football: the FIFA/F-MARC Consensus Conference. *Journal of Sports Sciences* **24**, 663–664.

Hargreaves, M. (2000) Carbohydrate replacement during exercise. In *Nutrition in Sport* (Maughan R.J., ed.) Blackwell Science, Oxford: 112–118.

International Association of Athletics Federations (2007) Nutrition for athletics: The 2007 IAAF consensus statement. Accessed at www.iaaf.org/mm/document/imported/38451.pdf

International Olympic Committee. (2004) IOC consensus statement on sports nutrition 2003. *Journal of Sports Sciences* **22**, x.

Karlsson, J. & Saltin, B. (1971) Diet, muscle glycogen, and endurance performance. *Journal of Applied Physiology* **31**, 203–206.

Kerr, D. & Ackland, T. (2006) Kinanthropometry: physique assessment of the athlete. In *Clinical Sports Nutrition* (3rd edn.) (Burke, L. & Deakin, V., eds.) McGraw-Hill, Sydney: 53–72.

Loucks, A.B. (2004) Energy balance and body composition in sports and exercise. *Journal of Sports Sciences* **22**, 1–14.

Miller, S.L., Tipton, K.D., Chinkes, D.L., Wolf, S.E. & Wolfe, R.R. (2003) Independent and combined effects of amino acids and glucose after resistance exercise. *Medicine and Science in Sports and Exercise* **35**, 449–455.

Moore, J.M., Timperio, A.F., Crawford, D.A., Burns, C.M. & Cameron-Smith, D. (2002) Weight management and weight loss strategies of professional jockeys. *International Journal of Sport Nutrition and Exercise Metabolism* **12**, 1–13.

Oppliger, R.A., Landry, G.L., Foster, S.W. & Lambrecht, A.C. (1998) Wisconsin minimum weight program reduces weight-cutting practices of high school wrestlers. *Clinical Journal of Sports Medicine* **8**, 26–31.

Oppliger, R.A., Steen, S.N. & Scott, J.R. (2003) Weight loss practices of college wrestlers. *International Journal of Sport Nutrition and Exercise Metabolism* **13**, 29–46.

Rasmussen, B.B., Tipton, K.D., Miller, S.L., Wolf, S.E. & Wolfe, R.R. (2000) An oral essential amino acid-carbohydrate supplement enhances muscle protein anabolism after resistance exercise. *Journal of Applied Physiology* **88**, 386–392.

Sawka, M.N., Burke, L.M., Eichner, E.R., Maughan, R.J., Montain, S.J. & Stachenfeld, N.S. for the American College of Sports Medicine. (2007) American College of Sports Medicine Position Stand. Exercise and fluid replacement. *Medicine and Science in Sports and Exercise* **39**, 377–390.

Sherman, W.M., Costill, D.L., Fink, W.J. & Miller, J.M. (1981). Effect of exercise-diet manipulation on muscle glycogen and its subsequent utilisation during performance. *International Journal of Sports Medicine* **2**, 114–118.

Simonsen, J.C., Sherman, W.M., Lamb, D.R., Dernbach, A.R., Doyle, J.A. & Strauss, R. (1991) Dietary carbohydrate, muscle glycogen, and power output during rowing training. *Journal of Applied Physiology* **70**, 1500–1505.

Steen, S.N. & Brownell, K.D. (1990) Patterns of weight loss and regain in wrestlers: has the tradition changed? *Medicine and Science in Sports and Exercise* **22**, 762–768.

Sundgot-Borgen, J. (2000) Eating disorders in athletes. In *Nutrition in Sport* (Maughan, R.J., ed.) Blackwell Science, Oxford: 510–522.

Tipton, K.D., Borsheim, E., Wolf, S.E., Sanford, A.P. & Wolfe, R.R. (2003) Acute response of net muscle protein balance reflects 24-h balance after exercise and amino acid ingestion. *American Journal of Physiology. Endocrinology and Metabolism* **284**, E76–E89.

Tipton, K.D., Rasmussen, B.B., Miller, S.L., Wolf, S.E., Owens-Stovall, S.K., Petrini, B.E., *et al.* (2001) Timing of amino acid-carbohydrate ingestion alters anabolic response of muscle to resistance exercise. *American Journal of Physiology. Endocrinology and Metabolism* **281**, E197–E206.

Tipton, K.D. & Wolfe, R.R. (2004) Protein and amino acids for athletes. *Journal of Sports Sciences* **22**, 65–79.

Chapter 8

Hydration

SUSAN M. SHIRREFFS

Many athletes are aware of the need to consider their hydration status on a regular basis, be that daily, around training sessions (before, during, and after), or when competing. This mirrors the increased interest and understanding in the general population of individual hydration status. This is not the situation that was apparent some years ago and the reasons for this change or apparent change of behavior are not the focus of this chapter. Rather, this chapter looks at the methods by which hydration status of athletes can be assessed, how it is altered, and the effects these alterations have on exercise.

Body water and its composition

Water is the largest component of the human body and the total body water content varies from approximately 45% to 70% of the total body mass (Sawka 1990), corresponding to about 33–53 L for a 75-kg man. Although body water content varies greatly between individuals, the water content of the various tissues is maintained relatively constant. For example, adipose tissue has a low water content (10%) and lean tissue such as muscle has a high water content (76%), so the total fraction of water in the body is determined largely by the total fat content. Therefore, a high body fat content is related to a lower total body water content as a percentage of body mass.

The body water can be divided into two components: the intracellular fluid (ICF) and the extra-

Table 8.1 The body water distribution between the different body fluid compartments in an adult male (Sawka 1990).

	Body mass (%)	Lean body mass (%)	Body water (%)
Total body water	60	72	100
Extracellular water	20	24	33
Plasma	5	6	8
Interstitium	15	18	25
Intracellular water	40	48	67

cellular fluid (ECF). ICF is the major component and comprises approximately two-thirds of total body water. ECF can be further divided into interstitial fluid (that between the cells) and plasma, with the plasma volume representing approximately one-quarter of the ECF volume. This is outlined in Table 8.1.

However, the water in the human body is not present as plain water. A wide range of electrolytes (compounds that dissociate into ions when in solution) and solutes are dissolved in varying concentrations in the body fluids. The major cations (positively charged electrolytes) in the body water are sodium, potassium, calcium, and magnesium; the major anions (negatively charged electrolytes) are chloride and bicarbonate. The osmolality of all the body water compartments is fairly similar, but the location of these electrolytes in the body water is not consistent throughout the body water compartments. Sodium is the major electrolyte present in ECF, while the potassium concentration in the extracellular space is much lower (Table 8.2). In ICF, the situation is

The Olympic Textbook of Science in Sport, 1st edition. Edited by R.J. Maughan. Published 2009 by Blackwell Publishing. ISBN: 978-1-4051-5638-7.

Table 8.2 The concentration (mmol·L^{-1}) of ions in the extracellular and intracellular body water compartments (Lentner 1981; Rose 1984). Plasma values are given to represent the extracellular compartment. The normal ranges of the plasma electrolyte concentrations are also shown.

Ion	Plasma: extracellular fluid	Intracellular fluid
Sodium	140 (135–145)	12
Potassium	4.0 (3.5–4.6)	150
Calcium	2.4 (2.1–2.7)	4.0
Magnesium	0.8 (0.6–1.0)	34
Chloride	104 (98–107)	4
Bicarbonate	29 (21–38)	12
Inorganic phosphate	1.0 (0.7–1.6)	40

reversed and the major electrolyte present is potassium, with sodium found in much lower concentrations. It is critical for the body to maintain this distribution of electrolytes because maintenance of the transmembrane electrical and chemical gradients is of paramount importance for assuring the integrity of cell function and allowing electrical communication throughout the body.

Control of body water and its composition

The composition of our body water and the distinctions in composition between the intracellular and extracellular compartments is a key homeostatic process in the body and central to the regulation of our hydration status.

Sodium and its associated chloride and bicarbonate anions form the major part of the osmotically active components of the plasma, with the plasma proteins making a smaller but important contribution. Cell membranes are freely permeable to water and exchange between body fluid compartments is rapid. The osmolality of the ECF and ICF compartments therefore remains very similar, in spite of the differences in the nature of the osmolytes present. Plasma osmolality is normally regulated in the range 280–290 mosmol·kg^{-1} by controlling water and solute loss by the kidneys and by regulating water intake by the thirst mechanism.

In humans, daily fluid intake in the form of food and drink (plus that formed from substrate oxidation) is usually in excess of the obligatory water loss (transcutaneous, pulmonary, and renal output), with renal excretion being the main mechanism regulating body water content (Fitzsimons 1990). However, conservation of water or electrolytes by the kidneys can only reduce the rate of loss; it cannot restore a deficit. The sensation of thirst, which underpins drinking behaviour, indicates the need to drink and hence is critical in the control of fluid intake and water balance. However, it is clear in many situations that the act of drinking may not be the direct result of a physiological need for water intake, but rather is initiated by habit, ritual, taste, or desire for nutrients, stimulants, or a warm or cooling effect. A number of the sensations associated with thirst are learned, with signals such as dryness of the mouth or throat inducing drinking, while distension of the stomach can stop ingestion before a fluid deficit has been restored. Nonetheless, the underlying regulation of thirst is controlled separately by the osmotic pressure and volume of the body fluids and as such is regulated by the same mechanisms that affect water and solute reabsorption in the kidneys and control central blood pressure. However, a full discussion of these processes is not within the scope of this chapter, and the interested reader is referred to the review by McKinley and Johnson (2004).

The volume of urine produced in a healthy individual is determined to a large extent by circulating hormone levels, and in particular by levels of vasopressin (also known as antidiuretic hormone). Vasopressin is released from the posterior pituitary after having been transported there along the axons of neurons whose cell bodies are located in the paraventricular and supraoptic nuclei of the hypothalamus, the site of synthesis (Sterns & Spital 1990). An increase in the circulating levels of vasopressin results in a reduction in urine production. Vasopressin acts on the renal distal tubules and collecting ducts in the kidney nephrons to cause an increased permeability to water and hence an increased reabsorption of water from the renal filtrate back into the circulation. This process also allows a hyperosmotic urine to be formed so that the excreted solute load can be accommodated in a small volume of water when necessary. A decrease in vasopressin secretion results in an increase in the volume of urine produced by causing a reduction in the permeability of the renal distal tubule and collecting ducts to water. This ensures less of the filtrate is reabsorbed back into the circulation. Vasopressin secretion is largely influenced by changes in plasma osmolality and an increase in plasma osmolality results in a increased vasopressin secretion and vice versa. Vasopressin is released rapidly in response to changes in plasma osmolality and begins to act within minutes. When secretion is inhibited in response to a decrease in plasma osmolality, the half-life of clearance from the circulation is approximately 10 min. Therefore, changes in body fluid tonicity are rapidly translated into changes in water excretion by this tightly regulated feedback system.

However, in addition to the influence of plasma osmolality on vasopressin secretion, other non-osmotic factors such as baroregulation, nausea, and pharyngeal stimuli also affect thirst and vasopressin levels. Aldosterone is a steroid hormone released into the circulation after synthesis by the zona glomerulosa cells of the adrenal cortex. Its primary role, in terms of renal function, is to increase renal tubular reabsorption of sodium. This results in an increased excretion of potassium and, in association with vasopressin, will increase water reabsorption in the distal segments of the nephron. The release of aldosterone is influenced by a number of factors, in particular the renin–angiotensin system. A fall in blood or extracellular fluid volume increases renin production by the kidneys and, via angiotensin II, results in an increase in aldosterone secretion.

Body water balance during exercise

Exercise elevates the metabolic rate, and only about 20–25% of the energy made available by the metabolic pathways is used to perform external work, with the remainder being dissipated as heat. When the energy demand is high, as occurs during periods of physical activity, high rates of heat production result. For example, the normal resting oxygen consumption is about 4 mL·kg body mass^{-1}·min^{-1} so for a 70-kg individual this gives a resting rate of heat production of about 60–70 W. Running a marathon in 2 h 30 min requires an oxygen consumption of about 4 L·min^{-1} to be sustained throughout the race for the average runner with a body mass of 70 kg (Maughan & Leiper 1983). The accompanying rate of heat production will now be about 1100 W so body temperature will begin to rise rapidly.

To limit the potentially harmful rise in core temperature, the rate of heat loss must be increased accordingly. Maintenance of a high skin temperature will facilitate heat loss by radiation and convection, but these mechanisms are effective only when the ambient temperature is low and the rate of air movement over the skin is high (Leithead & Lind 1964). A high skin temperature also requires a high skin blood flow and the cardiac capacity may not be permit this. At high ambient temperatures, skin temperature will be below ambient temperature, and the only mechanism by which heat can be lost from the body is evaporation. Evaporation of 1 L water from the skin will remove about 2.4 MJ (580 kcal) of heat from the body. For the 2 h 30 min marathon runner with a body mass of 70 kg to balance the rate of metabolic heat production by evaporative heat loss alone would therefore require sweat to be evaporated from the skin at a rate of about 1.6 L·h^{-1}. At such high sweat rates, an appreciable amount of sweat secreted onto the skin surface is likely to drip from the skin without evaporating and so a substantially higher sweat rate will to be necessary to achieve this rate of evaporative heat loss. This is possible, but a sweat rate of 2 L·h^{-1} in our marathon runner would result in the loss of about 5 L body water, corresponding to a loss of more than 7% of body mass. Some water will also be lost by evaporation from the respiratory tract. During hard exercise in a hot dry environment, this can amount to a significant water loss, although it is not generally considered to be a major heat loss mechanism in humans, unlike the dog, where panting is a major avenue of heat loss.

In most sporting activities, the energy demand varies continuously. Sweat losses for various sporting activities have been described in the published literature (Sawka et al. 2007; Shirreffs et al. 2006). What is clear from these data is that there is wide inter-individual variability even when the same activity is being undertaken at the same time in the same environmental conditions. It is also clear that even at low ambient temperatures, high sweat rates are sometimes observed when the energy demand is high or when insulative clothing is worn. Therefore, it cannot be concluded that dehydration is a problem only when the ambient temperature and humidity are high (Maughan 1985). However, sweat loss is closely related to the environmental conditions and substantial fluid deficits are much more common in warm weather months and in tropical climates.

When sweat loss occurs, the fluid losses are distributed in varying proportions among the plasma, extracellular water and intracellular water. The decrease in plasma volume that accompanies dehydration may be of particular importance in influencing work capacity. Blood flow to the muscles must be maintained at a high level to supply oxygen and substrates, but a high blood flow to the skin is also necessary to convect heat to the body surface where it can be dissipated (Nadel 1980). When the ambient temperature is high and blood volume has been decreased by sweat loss, there may be difficulty in meeting the requirement for a high blood flow to both of these tissues. In this situation, skin blood flow may be compromised, allowing central venous pressure and muscle blood flow to be maintained, thus maintaining exercise capacity and heat production but reducing heat loss and causing body temperature to rise (Rowell 1986).

A preferential loss of water from the extracellular space when sweat losses are high reflects the relatively high sodium and chloride concentration in sweat. Electrolyte losses in sweat are a function of both sweating rate and sweat composition and are highly influenced by the physiology of the individual. Sweat electrolyte losses can be assessed in the laboratory by using a whole body sweat collection methodology (Shirreffs & Maughan 1997) or an estimate can be obtained in the laboratory or field by using a sweat patch protocol (Shirreffs *et al.* 2006). However, despite the wide variation is sweat composition between individuals, sweat is invariably hypotonic with respect to plasma, and the major electrolytes are sodium and chloride, as in the extracellular space. Loss of 1 L sweat with a sodium

content of 50 mmol·L^{-1} represents a loss of approximately 2.9 g sodium chloride or salt. Therefore, an athlete who sweats 5 L sweat with this sodium concentration in a daily training session will lose almost 15 g salt. Even allowing for a reduced sweat sodium concentration and a decreased urinary output when sodium losses in sweat are large, this salt loss is large in comparison to normal intake, and it is clear that the salt balance of individuals exercising regularly in the heat may be precarious. The need for supplementary salt intake in these conditions is discussed below.

Hydration status and water turnover

Euhydration is the state or situation of being in water balance. However, although the dictionary definition is an easy one, establishing the physiological definition is not so simple. Hyperhydration is a state of being in positive water balance (a water excess) and hypohydration the state of being in negative water balance (a water deficit). Dehydration is the process of losing water from the body and rehydration the process of gaining body water. However, euhydration is not a steady state but rather is a dynamic state in that we continually lose water from the body – although the rate of loss varies – and there may be a time delay before replacing it or we may take in a slight excess and then lose this (Greenleaf 1992). When intake does occur, it is episodic, unlike the loss.

Many indices have been investigated to establish their potential as markers of hydration status. Body mass changes, blood indices, urine indices, and bioelectrical impedance analysis have been the most widely investigated to date. The current evidence and opinion tends to favor urine indices, and in particular urine osmolality, as the most promising marker available. A recent review by Armstrong (2005) provides a comparison of some of the more common methods used in exercise scenarios.

The body water content of an individual can be measured or estimated in a number of ways but the current consensus opinion is that tracer methodology gives the best measure of total body water. Deuterium oxide (D_2O or ^2H_2O) is the most commonly used tracer for this purpose and full details of the methods and protocols, assumptions, and limitations are well discussed elsewhere (Schoeller 1996). Briefly, the tracer is distributed relatively rapidly in the body (in the order of 3–4 h for an oral dose) and correction can be made for exchange with non-aqueous hydrogen. It is estimated that total body water can be measured with a precision and accuracy of 1–2%.

Hydration status has been assessed in a variety of situations, from clinical to exercise related, for a number of years. Measures such as serum osmolality and sodium concentration, blood urea nitrogen, hematocrit, urine osmolality, body mass, intake and output measurements, stool number and consistency, skin turgor, thirst, and mucous membrane moisture have all been investigated over the years.

In an exercise or sporting situation, hydration status is sometimes assessed in a laboratory, but assessment often takes place in the field with little or no scientific support. Clearly, this has implications for the markers that may be used for assessment.

Assessing hydration status and changes in hydration status in the laboratory and field

BODY MASS

Acute changes in body mass over a short time period are typically brought about by body water loss or gain; 1 mL water has a mass of 1 g (Lentner 1981). Therefore, changes in body mass can be used to quantify water gain or loss. However, there are confounding factors that need to be considered when using body mass changes to assess water loss (Maughan *et al.* 2007). These are loss of substrate mass used in the exercise, water of oxidation, and release of water stored with glycogen. These should be considered when using body mass changes to assess water loss or change in hydration status with exercise.

Nonetheless, throughout the exercise literature, changes in body mass over a period of exercise have been used as the main method of quantifying body water losses or gains brought about by sweating and drinking. Indeed, this method is frequently used as the method with which other methods are compared.

BLOOD INDICES

Collection of a blood sample for subsequent analysis has been both investigated and used as a hydration status marker.

Measurement of hemoglobin concentration and haematocrit have the potential to be used as a marker of hydration status or change in hydration status provided a reliable baseline can be established. In this regard, standardization of posture for a time prior to blood collection is necessary to distinguish between postural changes in blood volume, and therefore in hemoglobin concentration and hematocrit which occur (Harrison 1985), and changes resulting from water loss or gain.

Plasma or serum sodium concentration and osmolality will increase when the fluid loss inducing dehydration is hypotonic with respect to plasma. An increase in these concentrations would be expected therefore in the majority of cases of hypohydration including water loss by sweat secretion, urine production, or diarrhea. However, in subjects studied by Francesconi *et al.* (1987) who lost more than 3% of their body mass mainly through sweating, no change in hematocrit or serum osmolality was found although, as described below, certain urine parameters did show changes. Similar findings were reported by Armstrong *et al.* (1994, 1998). This perhaps suggests that plasma volume is defended in an attempt to maintain cardiovascular stability, and so plasma variables will not be affected by hypohydration until a certain degree of body water loss has occurred.

URINE INDICES

Collection of a urine sample for subsequent analysis has also been investigated and used as a hydration status marker. Urine osmolality has been extensively studied as a possible hydration status marker. In studies of fluid restriction, urine osmolality has increased to values greater than 900 mosmol·kg^{-1} for the first urine of the day passed in individuals dehydrated by 1.9% of their body mass as determined by body mass changes (Shirreffs & Maughan 1998a). Armstrong *et al.* (1994) have determined that measures of urine osmolality can be used interchangeably with urine specific gravity, opening this as another potential marker. Urine color is determined by the amount of urochrome present (Diem 1962). When large volumes of urine are excreted, the urine is dilute and the solutes are excreted in a large volume. This generally gives the urine a very pale color. When small volumes of urine are excreted, the urine is concentrated and the solutes are excreted in a small volume. This generally gives the urine a dark color. Armstrong *et al.* (1998) have investigated the relationship between urine color and specific gravity and conductivity. Using a scale of eight colors (Armstrong 2000), it was concluded that a linear relationship existed between urine color and both specific gravity and osmolality of the urine and that urine color could therefore be used in athletic or industrial settings to estimate hydration status when a high precision was not needed.

Urine indices of hydration status may be of limited use in identifying changes in hydration status during periods of rapid body fluid turnover, as in subjects studied who lost approximately 5% of their body mass with, on average, 62 min exercise in the heat before rehydrating by replacing this lost fluid (Popowski *et al.* 2001). In these subjects, in comparison to measures of plasma osmolality which increased and decreased in an almost linear fashion, urine osmolality and specific gravity were found to be less sensitive and demonstrated a delayed response, lagging behind the plasma osmolality changes. There now appears to be general agreement that measures of urine osmolality have the potential to be a marker of hydration status if there has been no large or rapid water intake in the hours prior to sample collection. For this reason, collection of an early morning urine sample, collected soon after waking, is a frequently reported parameter of hydration status in the literature.

Assessing water turnover

The non-invasive measurement of water turnover is typically made using deuterium as a tracer for body water. The body water pool is labeled with deuterium, and the water turnover is measured over a period of a few days from the rate of decrease in the concentration of the tracer in body water. The measurement can be made on blood, urine, saliva, or expired breath samples. An additional collection of 24-h urine output allows non-renal losses (consisting mainly of sweat and transcutaneous losses, respiratory water loss, and faecal loss) to be calculated by difference.

A higher rate of water turnover is typically seen in an exercising population in comparison to sedentary populations living in the same environmental conditions (Leiper *et al.* 1995, 1996). Studies of this nature also emphasize the variability in the normal pattern of fluid intake and loss in both sedentary and active individuals.

Pre-exercise hydration, drinking during exercise, and post-exercise rehydration

Pre-exercise hydration

For a person undertaking regular exercise, any fluid deficit that is incurred during one exercise session can potentially compromise the next exercise session if adequate fluid replacement does not occur. As such, fluid replacement after exercise can frequently be thought of as hydration prior to the next exercise bout. However, in addition to this, the issue of pre-exercise hyperhydration has been investigated in the last decade. In a healthy individual, the kidneys excrete any excess body water; therefore, ingesting excess fluid before exercise is generally ineffective at inducing pre-exercise hyperhydration. To overcome this, ingestion of either salt or glycerol solutions has been investigated as possible means of minimizing the diuresis that normally occurs when a euhydrated individual ingests a large volume of water. A small degree of temporary hyperhydration occurs when drinks with high concentrations (>100 mmol·L^{-1}) of sodium are ingested (Fortney *et al.* 1984), but palatability issues with high sodium drinks and nausea and vomiting with salt tablets bring some problems to this area. Glycerol has been shown to be an effective hyperhydrating agent. However, the subsequent effects on exercise capacity or performance and on thermoregulation have been inconsistent. A number of studies have suggested that ingesting 1–1.5 g glycerol per kilogram of body mass together with a large volume of water will significantly increase water retention and improve cycling time to fatigue (Hitchins *et al.* 1999; Lyons *et al.* 1990; Montner *et al.* 1996; Riedesel *et al.* 1987), but others (Latzka *et al.* 1997, 1998) have observed no differences in thermoregulatory or performance parameters. In addition, there have been a number of reports of side effects with glycerol ingestion that preclude this technique as a recommendation for pre-exercise hyperhydration. Latzka and Sawka (2000) came to the conclusion that "if euhydration is maintained during exercise-heat stress then [pre-exercise] hyperhydration appears to have no meaningful advantage."

However, the practice of drinking in the hours before exercise is effective in ensuring a situation of euhydration prior to exercise if there is any possibility that slight hypohydration is present. The current American College of Sports Medicine (ACSM) practical recommendation (Sawka *et al.* 2007) suggests that when optimizing hydration before exercise the individual should slowly drink a moderate amount (e.g., $5–7$ mL·kg body mass^{-1}) at least 4 h before exercise. If this does not result in urine production or the urine is dark or highly concentrated then more drink should be ingested slowly (e.g., $3–5$ mL·kg body mass^{-1}) about 2 h before exercise. This practice of drinking several hours before exercise gives sufficient time for urine output to return to normal. The guidelines also suggest that consuming beverages that contain some sodium and/or small amounts of salted snacks or sodium-containing foods at meals will help to stimulate thirst and retain the consumed fluids (Maughan *et al.* 1996; Ray *et al.* 1998; Shirreffs & Maughan 1998b).

Hydration during exercise

The diversity of sport and exercise training and competition including intensity, duration, frequency, and environmental conditions means that providing specific recommendations in terms of drink volumes and compositions and patterns of ingestions is not generally helpful. The current ACSM position stand (Sawka *et al.* 2007) on exercise and fluid replacement highlights the problems, and concludes that the goal of drinking during exercise should be to prevent excessive (>2%) body mass loss resulting

from a water deficit and to prevent excessive changes in electrolyte balance. By doing this, any compromise in performance should be minimized. They also concluded that, because there is considerable variability in sweating rates and sweat electrolyte content between individuals, as highlighted above, customized fluid replacement regimens are recommended to all. This is possible because individual sweat rates can be estimated as described above by measuring body mass before and after exercise.

Post-exercise rehydration

The primary factors influencing the post-exercise rehydration process are the volume and composition of the fluid consumed. The volume consumed will be influenced by many factors, including the palatability of the drink and its effects on the thirst mechanism, although with conscious effort some people can still drink large quantities of an unpalatable drink when they are not thirsty. The ingestion of solid food, and the composition of that food, may also be important factors, but there are many situations where solid food is avoided between exercise sessions or immediately after exercise.

BEVERAGE COMPOSITION

Sodium

Plain water is not the ideal post-exercise rehydration beverage when rapid and complete restoration of fluid balance is necessary and where all intake is in liquid form. This was established some time ago (Costill & Sparks 1973; Nielsen *et al.* 1986) when a high urine flow following ingestion of large volumes of electrolyte-free drinks did not allow subjects to remain in positive fluid balance for more than a very short time. These studies also established that the plasma volume was better maintained when electrolytes were present in the fluid ingested, and this effect was attributed to the presence of sodium in the drink.

The first studies to investigate the mechanisms of post-exercise rehydration showed that the ingestion of large volumes of plain water after exercise-induced dehydration resulted in a rapid fall in plasma osmolality and sodium concentration (Nose *et al.* 1988a), leading to a prompt and marked diuresis caused by a rapid return to control levels of plasma renin activity and aldosterone levels (Nose *et al.* 1988b). Therefore, the replacement of sweat losses with plain water will, if the volume ingested is sufficiently large, lead to hemodilution. The fall in plasma osmolality and sodium concentration that occurs in this situation reduces the drive to drink and stimulates urine output, as described above, and has potentially more serious consequences such as hyponatremia.

As sodium is the major ion lost in sweat, it is intuitive that sweat sodium losses should be replaced. It is not logical to think that the salty water that is lost as sweat would be best replaced in the body by plain water. This area has been systematically investigated and Shirreffs and Maughan (1998b) showed that, provided that an adequate volume is consumed, euhydration is achieved when the sodium intake is greater than the sweat sodium loss. The addition of sodium to a rehydration beverage is therefore justified on the basis that sodium is lost in sweat and must be replaced to achieve full fluid balance restoration. It has been demonstrated that the sodium concentration of the drink is more important than its osmotic content for increasing plasma volume after dehydration (Greenleaf *et al.* 1998). Sodium also stimulates glucose absorption in the small intestine via the active co-transport of glucose and sodium, which creates an osmotic gradient that acts to promote net water absorption. However, this sodium, to assist intestinal absorption, can either be consumed with the drink or can be secreted by the intestine. Sodium has been recognized as an important ingredient in rehydration beverages by an interassociation task force on exertional heat illnesses (American Physiological Society 2003) because sodium has a role in the etiology of exertional heat cramps, exertional heat exhaustion, and exertional hyponatremia (Armstrong & Casa 2003).

Potassium and magnesium

Potassium, as the major ion in the intracellular fluid, has been postulated to have a role in optimizing post-exercise rehydration by aiding the retention of water in the intracellular space. Potassium is lost in sweat in concentrations of about $5-10$ mmol·L^{-1}. Initial work using dehydrated rats supported this idea (Yawata 1990), indicating that the role of potassium in restoring intracellular volume is more modest that of sodium in restoring extracellular volume. However, subsequent work in humans has proved to be less conclusive (Maughan *et al.* 1994; Saat *et al.* 2002; Shirreffs *et al.* 2007). Potassium may therefore be important in enhancing rehydration by aiding intracellular rehydration, but further investigation is required to provide conclusive evidence. Importantly, no negative effect of including modest amounts of potassium in rehydration drinks has been demonstrated and indeed potassium, in small quantities, is an ingredient in most commercially available sports drinks that are promoted for post-exercise rehydration.

The importance of including magnesium in sports drinks has been the subject of much discussion. Magnesium is lost in sweat in small amounts (<0.2 mmol·L^{-1}) and many believe that this causes a reduction in plasma magnesium levels that are implicated in muscle cramp. Even though there can be a decline in plasma magnesium concentration during exercise, it is most likely to be caused by compartmental fluid redistribution rather than to sweat loss. There does not therefore seem to be any good reason for including magnesium in post-exercise rehydration and recovery sports drinks (Nielsen & Lukaski 2006).

DRINK VOLUME

Obligatory urine losses persist even in the dehydrated state, because of the need for elimination of metabolic waste products. The volume of fluid consumed after exercise-induced or thermal sweating must therefore be greater than the volume of sweat lost if effective rehydration is to be achieved. This contradicts earlier recommendations that after exercise athletes should match fluid intake exactly to the measured body mass loss.

Shirreffs *et al.* (1996) investigated the effect of drink volumes equivalent to 50%, 100%, 150%, and 200% of the sweat loss consumed after exercise-induced dehydration equivalent to approximately 2% of body mass. To investigate the possible interaction between beverage volume and its sodium content, a relatively low sodium drink (23 mmol·L^{-1}) and a moderately high sodium drink (61 mmol·L^{-1}) were compared. Subjects could not return to euhydration when they consumed a volume equivalent to, or less than, their sweat loss, irrespective of the drink composition. When a drink volume equal to 150% of the sweat loss was consumed, subjects were slightly hypohydrated 6 h after drinking when the test drink had a low sodium concentration, and they were in a similar condition when they drank the same beverage in a volume of twice their sweat loss. With the high sodium drink, enough fluid was retained to keep the subjects in a state of hyperhydration 6 h after drink ingestion when they consumed either 150% or 200% of their sweat loss. The excess would eventually be lost by urine production or by further sweat loss if the individual resumed exercise or moved to a warm environment.

While other studies have also shown the importance of drinking a larger volume of drink than the sweat volume lost (Mitchell *et al.* 1994), an interaction between sodium intake, volume intake, and whole body rehydration has not always been reported (Mitchell *et al.* 2000). However, it seems likely that in this study the length of subject observation after rehydration may not have been sufficient to observe the urine production response to the treatments. Additionally, evidence has recently emerged suggesting that the rate of drinking a large rehydration bolus can have important implications on the physiological handling of the drink (Archer & Shirreffs 2001; Kovacs *et al.* 2002). Drinking a large volume of fluid has the potential to induce a greater decline in plasma sodium concentration and osmolality which in turn may induce a greater diuresis by the mechanism described above.

FOOD AND FLUID CONSUMPTION

In many situations, there may be opportunities to consume solid food between exercise bouts, and this should be encouraged to meet other nutritional goals unless it is likely to result in gastrointestinal disturbances. Maughan *et al.* (1996) investigated the role of solid food intake in promoting rehydration from a 2.1% body mass sweat loss with consumption of either a solid meal plus flavored water or a commercially available sports drink. The urine volume produced following food and water ingestion was almost 300 mL less than that when the sports drink was consumed, resulting in a more favorable recovery and maintenance of hydration status. This was attributed to the higher electrolyte content of the meal relative to the sports drink. Subsequent studies have also highlighted a role for food products in post-exercise fluid balance restoration (Ray *et al.* 1998).

BEVERAGE PALATABILITY AND VOLUNTARY FLUID INTAKE

In the majority of scientific studies in the area, including those described above, a fixed volume of fluid was prescribed and consumed. However, in everyday situations that athletes find themselves in, intake is determined by the interaction of physiological and psychological factors. When the effect of palatability, together with the solute content of beverages in promoting rehydration after sweat loss, was studied (Wemple *et al.* 1997), subjects drank 123% of their sweat volume losses with flavored water and 163% and 133% when the solution had 25 and 50 mmol·L^{-1} sodium. Three hours after starting the rehydration process the subjects were in a better whole body hydration status after drinking the sodium-containing beverages than the flavored water. Similar results were reported by Maughan and Leiper (1993) and together these studies demonstrate the importance of palatability for promoting consumption, but also confirm earlier results showing that a moderately high electrolyte content is essential if the ingested fluid is to be retained in the body. The benefit of the higher intake with the more palatable drinks was lost because of the higher urine output. Other drink characteristics, including carbonation, influence drink palatability and therefore need to be considered when a beverage is being considered for effective post-exercise rehydration (Passe *et al.* 1997).

Conclusions

In healthy individuals, water is the largest single component of the body and although water balance is regulated around a range of volumes rather than a finite set point, its homeostasis is critical for virtually all physiological functions. To further assure proper regulation of physiological and metabolic functions, the composition of the individual body water compartments must also be regulated.

Humans continually lose water through the renal system, gastrointestinal system, skin, and respiratory tract, and this water must be replaced. Thirst is implicated in our water intake, although behavioral habits also have an important influence on drinking.

When exercise is undertaken or when an individual is exposed to a warm environment, a large part of the additional heat load is lost by sweating and this can greatly increase the individual's daily water loss and therefore the amount that must be consumed. Sweat rates in the order of $2-3$ L·h^{-1} can be reached and maintained by some individuals for a number of hours and it is not impossible for total losses to reach 10 L in a day. These losses must, of course, be replaced and when they are so extreme, the majority must be met from fluid consumption rather than food ingestion.

A variety of drink types and flavors are likely to be favored by individuals who have extreme losses to replace. Sports drinks have an important role in this recovery when no food is ingested, because their electrolyte content contributes to the replacement of sweat electrolyte losses, which is crucial for retention of the ingested water. The average sweat sodium concentration, typically about $40-50$ mmol·L^{-1}, is much higher than the sodium concentration of most sports drinks (typically about $20-25$ mmol·L^{-1}). Individuals whose sweat has a high sodium content may benefit from oral rehydration solutions or other drinks with high salt content.

For a person undertaking regular exercise, any fluid deficit that is incurred during one exercise session can potentially compromise the next exercise session if adequate fluid replacement does not occur. Fluid replacement after exercise can therefore frequently be thought of as hydration prior to the next exercise bout. However, additional specific issues in this area include ensuring euhydration before exercise and inducing a temporary hyperhydration with sodium salts or glycerol solutions.

Complete restoration of fluid balance after exercise is an important part of the recovery process, and becomes even more important in hot, humid conditions. If a second bout of exercise has to be performed after a relatively short interval, the rate of rehydration becomes of crucial importance. Rehydration after exercise requires not only replacement of volume losses, but also replacement of the sodium lost in the sweat. Daily sweat and sodium losses vary widely among individuals and depend on numerous factors including the environment, diet, physical fitness, and heat acclimatization status. However, where sweat losses are large, the total sodium loss will generally also be high. A moderate excess of salt intake would appear to be beneficial as far as hydration status is concerned without any detrimental effects on health, provided that fluid intake is in excess of sweat loss and that renal function is not impaired. Any excess sodium ingested will be excreted in the urine as the kidneys restore equilibrium. Drinks intended specifically for rehydration should therefore probably have higher electrolyte content than drinks formulated for consumption during exercise. Sodium is the most important electrolyte in terms of recovery after exercise and without its replacement, water retention is hampered. Potassium is also included in sports drinks in similar concentrations to that which it is lost in sweat. Unlike the strong evidence available for the inclusion of sodium, there is not the same evidence for the inclusion of potassium. There is no evidence for the inclusion of any other electrolytes.

Addition of an energy source seems unnecessary for rehydration, although a small amount of carbohydrate may improve the rate of intestinal uptake of sodium and water, and will improve palatability. Where sweat losses are high, rehydration with carbohydrate solutions has implications for energy balance (e.g., 10 L of soft drinks will provide approximately 1000 g carbohydrate, equivalent to about

17 000 kJ or 4000 calories). The volume of beverage consumed should be greater than the volume of sweat lost in order to make a provision for the ongo-ing obligatory urine losses, and palatability of the beverage is a major issue when large volumes of fluid have to be consumed.

References

American Physiological Society. (2003) Inter-association task force on exertional heat illnesses consensus statement. Accessed on 8/8/08 from http://www.the-aps.org/news/consensus.pdf/

Archer, D.T. & Shirreffs, S.M. (2001) Effect of fluid ingestion rate on post-exercise rehydration in man. *Proceedings of the Nutrition Society* **60**, 200A.

Armstrong, L.E. (2000) *Performing in Extreme Environments*. Human Kinetics, Champaign, IL.

Armstrong, L.E. (2005) Hydration assessment techniques. *Nutrition Reviews* **63**, S40–S54.

Armstrong, L.E. & Casa, D.J. (2003) Predisposing factors for exertional heat illnesses. In *Exertional Heat Illnesses* (Armstrong, L.E., ed.) Human Kinetics, Champaign, IL: 151–168.

Armstrong, L.E., Maresh, C.M., Castellani, J.W., Bergeron, M.F., Kenefick, R.W., LaGasse, K.E., *et al.* (1994) Urinary indices of hydration status. *International Journal of Sport Nutrition* **4**, 265–279.

Armstrong, L.E., Soto, J.A., Hacker, F.T. Jr, Casa, D.J., Kavouras, S.A. & Maresh, C.M. (1998) Urinary indices during dehydration, exercise, and rehydration. *International Journal of Sport Nutrition* **8**, 345–355.

Costill, D.L. & Sparks, K.E. (1973) Rapid fluid replacement following thermal dehydration. *Journal of Applied Physiology* **34**, 299–303.

Diem, K. (1962) *Documenta Geigy Scientific Tables*. Geigy Pharmaceutical Company Limited, Manchester: 538–539.

Fitzsimons, J.T. (1990) Evolution of physiological and behavioural mechanisms in vertebrate body fluid homeostasis. In *Thirst: Physiological and Psychological Aspects* (Ramsay, D.J., Booth, D.A., eds.) ILSI Human Nutrition Reviews, Springer-Verlag, London: 3–22.

Fortney, S.M., Wenger, C.B., Bove, J.R. & Nadel, E.R. (1984) Effect of hyperosmolality on control of blood flow and sweating. *Journal of Applied Physiology* **57**, 1688–1695.

Francesconi, R.P., Hubbard, R.W., Szlyk, P.C., Schnakenberg, D., Carlson, D., Leva, N. *et al.* (1987) Urinary and hematologic indexes of hypohydration. *Journal of Applied Physiology* **62**, 1271–1276.

Greenleaf, J.E. (1992) Problem: thirst, drinking behaviour, and involuntary dehydration. *Medicine and Science in Sports and Exercise* **24**, 645–656.

Greenleaf, J.E., Jackson, C.G.R., Geelen, G., Keil, L.C., Hinghofer-Szalkay, H. & Whittam, J.H. (1998) Plasma volume expansion with oral fluids in hypohydrated men at rest and during exercise. *Aviation Space and Environmental Medicine* **69**, 837–844.

Harrison, M.H. (1985) Effects of thermal stress and exercise on blood volume in humans. *Physiology Reviews* **65**, 149–209.

Hitchins, S., Martin, D.T., Burke, L. Yates, K., Fallon, K., Hahn, A., *et al.* (1999) Glycerol hyperhydration improves cycle time trial performance in hot humid conditions. *European Journal of Applied Physiology and Occupational Physiology* **80**, 494–501.

Kovacs, E.M., Schmahl, R.M., Denden, J.M. & Brouns, F. (2002) Effect of high and low rates of fluid intake on post-exeircse rehydration. *International Journal of Sport Nutrition and Exercise Metabolism* **12**, 14–23.

Latzka, W.A. & Sawka, M.N. (2000) Hyperhydration and glycerol: thermoregulatory effects during exercise in hot climates. *Canadian Journal of Applied Physiology* **25**, 536–545.

Latzka, W.A., Sawka, M.N., Montain, S.J., Skrinar, G.S., Fielding, R.A., Matott, R.P., *et al.* (1997) Hyperhydration: thermoregulatory effects during compensable exercise-heatstress. *Journal of Applied Physiology* **83**, 860–866.

Latzka, W.A., Sawka, M.N., Montain, S.J., Skrinar, G.S., Fielding, R.A., Matott, R.P., *et al.* (1998) Hyperhydration: tolerance and cardiovascular effects during uncompensable exercise-heat stress. *Journal of Applied Physiology* **84**, 1858–1864.

Leiper, J.B., Carnie, A. & Maughan, R.J. (1996) Water turnover rates in sedentary and exercising middle-aged men. *British Journal of Sports Medicine* **30**, 24–26.

Leiper, J.B., Pitsiladis, Y.P. & Maughan, R.J. (1995) Comparison of water turnover rates in men undertaking prolonged exercise and in sedentary men. *Journal of Physiology* **483**, 123P.

Leithead, C.S. & Lind, A.R. (1964) *Heat Stress and Heat Disorders*. Cassell, London.

Lentner, C. (1981) *Geigy Scientific Tables* (8th edn.) Ciba-Geigy Limited, Basle.

Lyons, T.P., Riedesel, M.L., Meuli, L.E. & Chick, T.W. (1990) Effects of glycerol-induced hyperhydration prior to exercise in the heat on sweating and core temperature. *Medicine and Science in Sports and Exercise* **22**, 477–483.

Maughan, R.J. (1985) Thermoregulation and fluid balance in marathon competition at low ambient temperature. *International Journal of Sports Medicine* **6**, 15–19.

Maughan, R.J. & Leiper, J.B. (1983) Aerobic capacity and fractional utilisation of aerobic capacity in elite and non-elite male and female marathon runners. *European Journal of Applied Physiology* **52**, 80–87.

Maughan, R.J. & Leiper, J.B. (1993) Post-exercise rehydration in man: effects of voluntary intake of four different beverages. *Medicine and Science in Sports and Exercise* **25** (Supplement): S2.

Maughan, R.J., Leiper, J.B. & Shirreffs, S.M. (1996). Restoration of fluid balance after exercise-induced dehydration: effects of food and fluid intake. *European Journal of Applied Physiology* **73**, 317–325.

Maughan, R.J., Owen, J.H., Shirreffs, S.M. & Leiper, J.B. (1994). Post-exercise rehydration in man: effects of electrolyte addition to ingested fluids. *European Journal of Applied Physiology* **69**, 209–215.

Maughan, R.J., Shirreffs, S.M. & Leiper, J.B. (2007) Errors in the estimation of hydration status from changes in body mass. *Journal of Sports Sciences* **25**, 797–804.

McKinley, M.J. & Johnson, A.K. (2004) The physiological regulation of thirst and fluid intake. *News in Physiological Sciences* **19**, 1–6.

Mitchell, J.B., Grandjean, P.W., Pizza, F.X., Starling, R.D. & Holtz, R.W. (1994) The effect of volume ingested on rehydration and gastric emptying following exercise-induced dehydration. *Medicine and*

Science in Sports and Exercise **26**, 1135–1143.

Mitchell, J.B., Phillips, M.D., Mercer, S.P., Baylies, H.L. & Pizza, F.X. (2000) Postexercise rehydration: effect of Na^+ and volume on restoration of fluid spaces and cardiovascular function. *Journal of Applied Physiology* **89**, 1302–1309.

Montner, P., Stark, D.M., Riedesel, M.L., Murata, G., Robergs, R., Timms, M., *et al.* (1996) Pre-exercise glycerol hydration improves cycling endurance time. *International Journal of Sports Medicine* **17**, 27–33.

Nadel, E.R. (1980) Circulatory and thermal regulations during exercise. *Federation Proceedings* **39**, 1491–1497.

Nielsen, B., Sjogaard, G., Ugelvig, J., Knudsen, B. & Dohlmann, B. (1986) Fluid balance in exercise dehydration and rehydration with different glucose-electrolyte drinks. *European Journal of Applied Physiology* **55**, 318–325.

Nielsen, F.H. & Lukaski, H.C. (2006) Update on the relationship between magnesium and exercise. *Magnesium Research* **19**, 180–189.

Nose, H., Mack, G.W., Shi, X. & Nadel, E.R. (1988a) Role of osmolality and plasma volume during rehydration in humans. *Journal of Applied Physiology* **65**, 325–331.

Nose, H., Mack, G.W., Shi, X.R. & Nadel, E.R. (1988b) Involvement of sodium retention hormones during rehydration in humans. *Journal of Applied Physiology* **65**, 332–336.

Passe, D.H., Horn, M. & Murray, R. (1997) The effects of beverage carbonation on sensory responses and voluntary fluid intake following exercise. *International Journal of Sports Nutrition* **7**, 286–297.

Popowski, L.A., Oppliger, R.A., Lambert, G.P., Johnson, R.F., Johnson, A.K. & Gisolfi, C.V. (2001) Blood and urinary measures of hydration status during progressive acute dehydration. *Medicine and Science in Sports and Exercise* **33**, 747–753.

Ray, M.L., Bryan, M.,W., Ruden, T.M., Baier, S.M., Sharp, R.L. & King, D.S. (1998) Effect of sodium in a rehydration beverage when consumed as a fluid or meal. *Journal of Applied Physiology* **85**, 1329–1336.

Riedesel, M.L., Allen, D.Y., Peake, G.T. & Al-Qattan, K. (1987) Hyperhydration with glycerol solutions. *Journal of Applied Physiology* **63**, 2262–2268.

Rose, B.D. (1984) *Clinical Physiology of Acid–Base and Electrolyte Disorders* (2nd edn.) McGraw-Hill, New York.

Rowell, L.B. (1986) *Human Circulation.* Oxford University Press, New York.

Saat, M., Singh, R., Sirisinghe, R.G. & Nawawi, M. (2002) Rehydration after exercise with fresh young coconut water, carbohydrate-electrolyte beverage and plain water. *Journal of Physiological Anthropology* **21**, 93–104.

Sawka, M.N. (1990) Body fluid responses and hypohydration during exercise-heat stress. In *Human Performance Physiology and Environmental Medicine at Terrestrial Extremes* (Pandolf, K.B., Sawka, M.N., Gonzalez, R.R., eds.) Cooper Publishing Group, Carmel: 227–266.

Sawka, M.N., Burke, L.M., Eichner, E.R., Maughan, R.J., Montain, S.J. & Stachenfeld, N.S. (2007) American College of Sports Medicine Position Stand. Exercise and fluid replacement. *Medicine and Science in Sports and Exercise* **39**, 377–390.

Schoeller, D.A. (1996) Hydrometry. In *Human Body Composition* (Roche, A.F., Heymsfield, S.B., Lohman, G., eds.) Human Kinetics, Champaign IL: 25–43.

Shirreffs, S.M., Aragon-Vargas, L.F., Keil, M., Love, T.D. & Phillips, S. (2007) Rehydration after exercise in the heat: a comparison of 4 commonly used drinks.

International Journal of Sport Nutrition and Exercise Metabolism **17**, 244–258.

Shirreffs, S.M. & Maughan, R.J. (1997) Whole body sweat collection in man: an improved method with preliminary data on electrolyte content. *Journal of Applied Physiology* **82**, 336–341.

Shirreffs, S.M. & Maughan, R.J. (1998a) Urine osmolality and conductivity as indices of hydration status in athletes in the heat. *Medicine and Science in Sports and Exercise* **30**, 1598–1902.

Shirreffs, S.M. & Maughan, R.J. (1998b) Volume repletion following exercise-induced volume depletion in man: replacement of water and sodium losses. *American Journal of Physiology* **274**, F868–F875.

Shirreffs, S.M., Sawka, M.N. & Stone, M. (2006) Water and electrolyte needs for football training and match-play. *Journal of Sports Sciences* **24**, 699–707.

Shirreffs, S.M., Taylor, A.J., Leiper, J.B. & Maughan, R.J. (1996) Post-exercise rehydration in man: effects of volume consumed and drink sodium content. *Medicine and Science in Sports and Exercise* **28**, 1260–1271.

Sterns, R.H. & Spital, A. (1990) Disorders of water balance. In *Fluids and Electrolytes* (2nd edn.) (Kokko, J.P. & Tannen, R.L., eds.) WB Saunders, Philadelphia: 139–194.

Wemple, R.D., Morocco, T.S. & Mack, G.W. (1997) Influence of sodium replacement on fluid ingestion following exercise-induced dehydration. *International Journal of Sport Nutrition* **7**, 104–116.

Yawata, T. (1990) Effect of potassium solution on rehydration in rats: comparison with sodium solution and water. *Japanese Journal of Physiology* **40**, 369–381.

Part 3

Anthropometry

Chapter 9

Body Composition and Sports Performance

TIMOTHY OLDS

Sport as a Darwinian system

Competitive sport constitutes an artificial Darwinian system. The essential elements of a Darwinian system are:

- A source population in which there is variability in certain characteristics;
- An environment where resources (rewards) are scarce;
- Competition for those scarce resources;
- Selection pressures resulting in the success of the best adapted; and
- Transmission of success characteristics to future members of the population.

Sport demonstrates all of these elements. Humans show variability in the kinds of characteristics, including body morphology, that predispose to sporting success. The sporting environment is a milieu where rewards (success and hence player salaries; kudos; financial returns to clubs, promoters, and media) are limited and subject to intense competition. There is a process of "artificial selection" whereby athletes with inferior success characteristics are culled, and only the "fittest" are retained. Successful characteristics are "transmitted" to new generations of players through training and nutritional regimens and genetic and cultural inheritance.

Like natural environments, the sporting environment is always changing, and teams and individuals who fail to adapt will not survive. The result

is a process of "optimization," whereby athletes develop optimal characteristics for success, in the same way as animals become ideally adapted to their environments. In the Darwinian world of sport, we would expect to see:

- Very large differences in success characteristics between the athletic and non-athletic populations;
- Superior success characteristics in higher level athletes than in lower level athletes;
- Secular increases in success characteristics; and
- Specialized adaptations to different sports and even different positions and roles within sports (i.e., to different "environmental niches").

The sporting environment

The sporting environment includes elements within the sport (such as rules, equipment, technology, training regimens) and elements outside the sport (such as financial support, the media, medical treatment options). This environment is constantly changing. For sport over the last 100 years, the most important change has been improvement in communication technologies. Consider a musical analogy. At the turn of the 20th century, the state of Iowa alone had 1300 opera houses, providing full if modest employment for over 1000 tenors (Frank 1999). A century later, we all listen to Iglesias and Pavarotti. The number of available places on the "opera team" has decreased, the standard of opera singing has increased, the reward structure has become much more skewed; as a result competition is much more intense. This intensification is the result of communications, first bringing us to Pavarotti by automobiles and

The Olympic Textbook of Science in Sport, 1st edition. Edited by R.J. Maughan. Published 2009 by Blackwell Publishing. ISBN: 978-1-4051-5638-7.

aeroplanes, and then bringing Pavarotti to us via television, CDs, and the Internet. The same has happened with sport. Local teams have atrophied, international competition attracts audiences in the billions, elite player salaries have increased exponentially and selection pressures have become much more intense. While the sport system supports fewer and fewer athletes, the pool of potential players has expanded with the increase in the world population, and the increased accessibility of populations in remote parts of the world and in formerly isolated ethnic and social ghettoes. The result is a very large pool of aspirants for a very small number of positions in a globalized "body market," greater variability within the population, and therefore the potential to select increasingly extreme sporting characteristics.

GLOBALIZATION

Globalization is the main driver of rapid changes in the anthropometrical, physiological, psychological, and skill characteristics of sports people. In 2004, the champion "English" soccer team Arsenal consisted of players from France, Germany, Sweden, Denmark, Iceland, Ireland, the Netherlands, Spain, Switzerland, Brazil, the Ivory Coast and the USA, plus a couple of Englishmen. The manager was French (Judt 2005). "National" teams are often heavily loaded with foreign-born players. In the 1999 Rugby World Cup, for example, there were enough New Zealanders playing for various countries to field two extra teams. Over 40% of the Scottish team were born outside of Scotland. An analysis of the players in the 2002 World Soccer Cup found that almost 50% of all World Cup players were playing in five wealthy European countries: England, Italy, Germany, Spain, and France. This indexes a kind of "body drain" from poor countries to wealthy countries. The globalization of sport is even more marked in "free" sports markets, such as the National Basketball Association (NBA). In 1999, 4.4% of NBA players were of foreign origin. The foreign-born players were taller (211.1 vs. 200.3 cm) and heavier (110.6 vs. 99.0 kg) than the American-born players. By 2002, the percentage had risen to 9%. Five of the 10 tallest and heaviest NBA players were foreign-born. The 2003 Women's National Basketball Association

(WNBA) had 96 American-born and 24 foreign-born players. The international players were significantly taller (188.4 vs. 181.6 cm) and heavier (78.3 vs. 73.5 kg) than the American-born players. Nine of the tallest 12 players were foreign-born.

As well as reaching into other countries, sports are also reaching into previously excluded ethnic groups. There were no black sprinters in any men's 100 m Olympic final until 1928; since 1984, almost all finalists have been black. There is a similar over-representation of Aboriginals in Australian football. Aboriginals constitute about 2% of the Australian population. In 1950, 1% of Australian Rules football players were Aboriginal; by 2005 this proportion had risen to 11%. The search for size and talent has had a positive influence on breaking down ethnic divisions.

PLAYER SALARIES

As the required sporting physiques become more extreme, and hence rarer, it has become necessary to pay much larger salaries to attract individuals with extreme physiques from other careers, and from other sports. Since 1975, player salaries in the four major US sports have increased from about five times the male median salary to 15–40 times the median male salary. Similar trends, although somewhat less extreme, have occurred in Rugby Union and Australian football. Size also means greater earnings in "winner-take-all" sports markets (i.e., markets where remuneration is very heavily skewed towards the top end; Frank 1999). In the NBA and National Football League (NFL), an extra 1 cm of stature may translate into an extra $35,000–70,000 in career earnings because of increased career longevity. One kilogram would equate to $15,000–30,000, and 1 body mass index (BMI) unit to $90,000–100,000. It is not surprising then that there is substantial investment in anthropometric talent identification and in artificial growth enhancement. It is also not surprising to see aggressive intersport poaching, such as the Australian Rugby Union's campaign to recruit players from Rugby League. The Australian Institute of Sport (AIS) recently launched a program (albeit unsuccessful) to win the Gold Medal in women's skeleton, an event being reintroduced into the Winter Olympics after a long absence. The AIS deliberately targeted beach sprinters from surf life-saving as having the right physical and physiological characteristics.

Transmission of anthropometric characteristics

The transmission of successful sporting adaptations, including body size and shape characteristics, which have been labeled "morphologic optimization" (Norton *et al.* 1996), has both cultural and genetic facets. There are many examples of sporting success within families: the Australian swimmers John and Ilsa Konrads, the three Italian Abbagnale brothers (rowing Gold Medallists 1988–2000), and the Russian throwers Tamara and Irina Press are examples of the aggregation of sporting talent within families. Sporting success is also transmissible across generations. The Austro-Hungarian Bogen-Gerevich family represents a three-generation dynasty, with Albert Bogen winning a silver medal in the sabre in 1912, and his daughter Erna picking up a bronze in the foil in 1932. Her husband, Aladár Gerevich won nine fencing medals between 1932 and 1960, while their son Pál medaled in the sabre in 1972. Germany's Keller family has three generations of Gold Medals in hockey. The Lunde family from Norway has three generations of yachting medals (Eugen in 1924; Peter in 1952; and his wife and brother; Peter junior in 1960). The transmission of successful characteristics doubtless has both genetic and cultural aspects. Elite sports people have greater opportunities for exposure to each other given the temporal and spatial constraints of tournaments, championships, and games villages, so that assortative mating has an important role. Some examples are Al Joyner and Florence Griffith-Joyner, Emil and Dana Zatopek, André Agassi and Steffi Graf. However, transmission is mainly cultural, in the form of training regimens, nutritional supplementation, and drugs.

Basic anthropometric measurements

In principle, an unlimited number of measurements can be taken on the human body. However, there is a small number of basic measurements that have been found to predict sporting success with some confidence. These include height (stature), weight (mass), and BMI (weight in kilograms divided by the square of height in meters). Body surface area is the total area of the skin, and is an important predictor of performance when the body moves through fluids such as air and water. Body surface area also relates to the body's potential to lose heat. Limb lengths and breadths, usually measured between bony landmarks, can determine the force and speed athletes can produce when jumping or striking. The percentage of fat in the body can be estimated from skinfolds, or measured by more complex methods such as underwater weighing using Archimedes' principle. One commonly used method of classification is somatotype, which describes body shape (independent of body size) in terms of three components: endomorphy, or fatness; mesomorphy, or muscularity; and ectomorphy, or relative linearity or "stretched-outness."

Which factors contribute to sporting success?

Clearly the characteristics contributing to sporting success are multifaceted, and include morphological, physiological, social, and psychological suitability. In some sports, morphology seems to be very important. Obvious examples are basketball, sumo, and bodybuilding. In others – yachting, shooting, golf – morphology is apparently largely irrelevant. We can quantify the importance of potential success characteristics by comparing the distribution of those characteristics in:
• The athlete group vs. the source population from which that group is drawn;
• Elite athlete groups vs. subelite groups; and
• The present athlete group vs. the past group.

ATHLETE GROUP VS. SOURCE POPULATION

Where the distribution of the potential success characteristic in the athlete group differs markedly from that of the source population, it is likely that the characteristic is important for sporting success. Norton and Olds (2000) have described methods – the Overlap Zone (OZ) and Bivariate Overlap Zone (BOZ) – for quantifying distributional differences. Both methods work by calculating the probability that a randomly chosen individual from the source population could be a member of the sports group. High OZ and BOZ values indicate substantial overlap

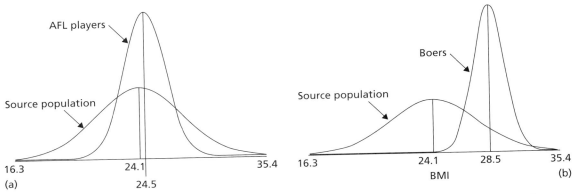

Fig. 9.1 Distribution of body mass index (BMI) values in: (a) Australian football (AFL) players; and (b) heavyweight boxers, compared with the source population of young Australian males. BMI values are plotted on a log scale.

between the source population and the athlete group, while small values indicate little overlap and therefore a low probability that the athlete could be randomly chosen from the source population. An example is shown in Fig. 9.1, which illustrates the distributions of BMI in Australian Football League (AFL) players, heavyweight boxers, and the source population. Note that while the mean values are relatively similar for AFL players and the source population, the variance is quite wide in the athlete group. The OZ value is 28.6%, indicating moderate overlap. Compare this with the situation for heavyweight boxers, where both the mean and the variance of the sports group differ greatly from those of the source population. The OZ value is 5.4%. The OZ and BOZ depend both on the difference in mean values and the relative size of the standard deviations (SD) of the two populations.

Table 9.1 shows the mean height and mass for athletes from 21 sports, using data gathered since 1980. The BOZ values are shown in the last column, quantifying the importance of these measures for sporting success. Clearly, height and mass are critical for heavyweight boxing, basketball, and rowing (BOZ <10%), but less important for swimming, soccer, and cycling (BOZ >28%).

COMPETITIVE LEVEL

Morphologic success characteristics should show gradients across competitive levels, with more extreme values occurring in elite athlete groups. Olds (2001) reviewed studies of male Rugby Union players. Elite players (Six Nations and Super 14 countries) were compared with national level (other rugby nations) and state level players. Table 9.2 shows the differences in muscularity or mesomorphy. There are clear gradients across competitive levels, with greater mesomorphy evident at the top levels. There are similar, but inverse, gradients in endomorphy.

In netball, Steele (1987) found that height increased from 165 cm at club level to 177 cm at national level, with a corresponding fall in the OZ from 54% (club) to 18% (national). Olds and Kang (2000) found similar gradients in Korean taekwondo players, with the most successful players being leaner, more ectomorphic, and less mesomorphic than their less successful counterparts (Table 9.3).

SECULAR TRENDS

Marked changes in an anthropometric dimension in the athlete group relative to the source population are strong evidence that this dimension is a success characteristic. Figure 9.2 shows the evolution of BMI in defensive tackles in the US National Football League between 1944 and 1999. BMI rose from about 30 in the 1940s to over 36 in the 1990s, with a marked upswing beginning in the late 1960s and early 1970s, perhaps associated with more widespread use of anabolic steroids. These trends strongly

Table 9.1 Data on 12,536 male athletes from 21 sports. The mean height and mass are shown, along with the overlap zone (OZ) values for height and mass separately, and bivariate overlap zone (BOZ) values for height and mass conjointly, relative to the population of young males.

Sport	n	Height Mean (cm)	Height OZ	Mass Mean (kg)	Mass OZ	BOZ
Source population		*178.6*		*78.7*		
Boxing (HW)	31	189.9	11.0	102.6	3.2	1.0
NBA	1480	200.3	7.0	97.0	18.7	5.4
Rowing (HW)	118	190.5	13.7	87.4	22.1	8.7
RU: forwards	636	187.6	30.7	103.6	7.5	9.5
NFL	7905	187.2	29.3	103.3	16.5	11.3
Hockey	31	179.2	34.9	74.1	21.4	15.2
Cycling: off-road	18	178.6	34.5	71.8	21.8	17.2
Waterpolo	190	186.3	28.1	86.0	28.9	17.6
Marathon	79	172.9	43.3	61.9	19.0	18.1
Running: sprint	33	179.6	32.3	76.1	36.2	22.8
Running: distance	43	174.5	40.5	63.2	30.4	23.8
Diving	43	169.9	36.5	67.1	40.4	25.7
AFL	315	184.9	39.8	82.8	36.2	25.9
Cycling: pursuit	24	178.9	36.7	73.1	36.4	26.8
Cycling: road	247	178.1	39.7	68.5	38.8	27.4
RU: backs	484	179.6	41.5	84.2	34.1	28.1
Soccer	283	174.3	43.7	66.9	32.8	28.1
Swimming	255	182.8	42.5	76.9	37.3	28.8

AFL, Australian Football League; HW, heavyweight; NBA, National Basketball Association; NFL, National Football League; RU, Rugby Union.

Table 9.2 Mesomorphy ratings for elite, national and state-level rugby players profiled since 1980, and the corresponding overlap zone (OZ) values.

Level	n	Mesomorphy [mean (SD)]	OZ
Source population		*4.5 (1.0)*	
Elite	36	7.4 (1.4)	24.0
National	105	6.5 (1.1)	34.9
State	142	5.1 (1.5)	54.3

SD, standard deviation.

suggest that BMI is an important success characteristic in American football.

There have been less spectacular changes in body shape. Figure 9.3 shows the evolution of somatotype in male athletes from 11 sports between the 1960s and the 1990s. Two general trends can be detected. In endurance sports, there is a tendency for athletes to become more ectomorphic and less mesomorphic. In power sports, there has been a tendency towards increased mesomorphy and decreased ectomorphy, with little change in endomorphy. This suggests that changes in relative mass are almost entirely

Table 9.3 Characteristics of taekwondo players of different competitive levels.

Level	n	Endomorphy	Mesomorphy	Ectomorphy	Body fat (%)
International	11	1.4	4.1	3.2	7.3
State	90	2.2	4.5	2.7	10.7
Club	45	2.5	4.9	2.5	11.9

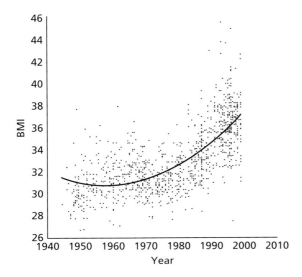

Fig. 9.2 Evolution of body mass index (BMI) in 1045 defensive tackles in the US National Football League since World War II.

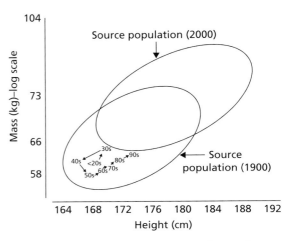

Fig. 9.4 Changes in the average stature and mass of male marathon runners in the 20th century. The ellipses are the 67% density ellipses for the source populations (Australian norms) in 1900 and 2000. The arrows represent shifts in the average stature and mass of 668 elite marathon runners between 1897 and 1999, through the decades of the 20th century.

a result of changes in muscularity. Changes in the running events are particularly interesting, with middle-distance, distance, and marathon runners decreasing in mesomorphy and increasing in ecto-morphy, and sprinters and 400 m runners decreasing in ectomoprhy and increasing or staying the same in mesomorphy. In terms of somatotype, the running disciplines are moving further apart.

Secular trends in athlete groups need to be quantified against the backdrop of secular changes in the source population. In the general population, height has been increasing by about 1 cm and mass

by >1 kg each decade for over 100 years (Meredith 1976). Given this background trend, even a lack of change in the athlete group can represent a relative shift. Figure 9.4 describes changes in the height and mass of elite marathon runners in the 20th century. In spite of increases of about 8 cm and 7 kg in the source population, there have been almost no changes in these characteristics in marathon runners. This suggests that there is an ideal absolute size for marathon runners (about 60 kg and 170 cm), possibly a result of complex physiological trade-offs involving power : weight ratio (important for relative aerobic power),

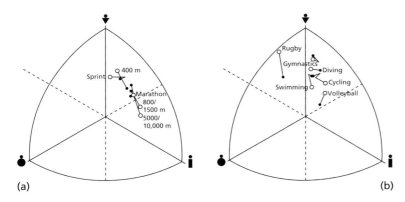

Fig. 9.3 Changes in the somatotype of athletes since the 1960s. The solid circles indicate the starting point and the open circles the endpoint. The starting point is in the 1960s and the endpoint in the 1990s, the exceptions being volleyball and rugby (1980s to 1990s), and gymnastics and swimming (1960s to 1980s). (a) Running events; (b) other sports.

body surface area : mass ratio (important for thermoregulation), increased reuse of elastic energy, and injury risk.

Norton and Olds (2001) distinguish three types of morphologic optimization:

1 *Open-ended optimization:* when the success characteristic in the athlete group becomes more and more extreme in absolute terms (e.g., when athletes get bigger and bigger, or, more rarely, smaller and smaller). Ackland *et al.* (1994), for example, reported that the mean height of female basketballers had increased by 3.1 cm in a decade, about three times the rate of increase in the source population.

2 *Relative optimization:* when the body size of the athlete group may differ from that of the source population, but changes over time in step with the source population. The changes in morphologic characteristics seen in the athlete group are of a similar magnitude to those in the source population. One example is rugby players. Between 1905 and 1999, the stature of top level rugby players increased at a rate of 0.9 cm·year^{-1}, which is not different from the rate of increase in the source population (about 1 cm·year^{-1}).

3 *Absolute optimization:* when the morphology of the athlete group does not change, despite secular changes in the body size of the source population. The stature of international level male divers, for example, did not change between 1950 and 1991, with a mean of 170.8 cm. Another example is the median mass of southern hemisphere jockeys, which stayed at 49–52 kg throughout the 20th century. Over the same period, the spread of jockeys' masses decreased dramatically. The difference between the 10th and 90th percentiles was 14 kg for jockeys who rode between 1900 and 1910, but only 2.7 kg in the 1990s. This probably reflects laws against the use of child jockeys, and the declining popularity of races such as highweights.

Specialization

A corollary of morphologic optimization is increasing specialization of morphologic characteristics, as each body type finds its niche in the sporting ecology. The tendency in most sports has been towards more similar physiques within sports, but towards very different physiques between sports – a "big bang" of sporting physiques. One consequence has been that very few athletes now excel in more than sport. In the history of the Olympics, 39 athletes have medaled in more than one sport, but only three have achieved that feat since 1936. Such improbable cross-sport successes as diving and water polo (American Frank Kehoe in 1904), boxing and bobsled (American Eagen Edward 1920–1932) or water polo and fencing (Belgian Boin Victor in 1908–1920) have become morphologically impossible.

The idea of extreme anthropometric specialization in sports is relatively new. To late 19th century physical educators, the athlete was seen as the embodiment of the perfect form of man – which was seen as the destiny of the race – meaning the white race. "There is a perfect form or type of man, and the tendency of the race is to attain this type" (*Statistics, Medical and Anthropological of the Provost-Marshal-General's Bureau* 1880, cited in Sargent 1887). The athlete's proportions remained ideal, and perfect form meant perfect function. For this reason, athletes were isomorphic but polyvalent, excelling in a wide range of sports. The functional was also the beautiful, and the "typical athlete" conformed to the ideal canons of body proportions from classical art. Clearly, many philosophic streams flow together in this notion, including neo-Platonism, social Darwinism, and nostalgic classicism. The concept of the "athletic type" influenced anthropometric and analytical methods. A physical educator from 1900 felt justified in lumping together the measurements of long, standing broad, high and triple jumpers, pole vaulters, shot putters, 800–1500 m runners and walkers to profile the "athletic type" (Bemies 1900). It also affected athletic practice, encouraging participation in a wide range of sports. The intercollegiate champions documented by Sargent (1887) demonstrated excellence across a range of sports which would be impossible today. One held all amateur running records from 100 to 400 m. Another held collegiate records in broad jump, high jump, and pole vault. Three were several who were college representatives in both rowing and football, another was a wrestler, broad jumper, and hammer thrower. Yet another was a champion weightlifter, baseball pitcher, and footballer.

By the 1920s, this view had changed. The anthropometric and medical survey of the Amsterdam

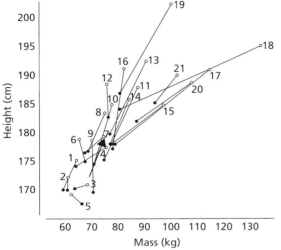

1 Running – distance
2 Running – marathon
3 Diving
4 Running – sprint
5 Gymnastics
6 Running – 800 –1500 m
7 Running – 400 m
8 Long jump
9 Cycling – road
10 Swimming
11 Waterpolo
12 High jump
13 Rowing
14 Australian football
15 Rugby Union
16 Volleyball
17 Throwing (other than shot)
18 Shot-put
19 Basketball – NBA
20 American football
23 Boxing – heavyweight

Fig. 9.5 Changes in the heights and masses of international level male athletes in 21 sports between 1925 (solid circles) and 2000 (open circles). The trend in the source population (here, young Australian males) is indicated by the black arrow.

Olympics conducted by Buytendijk in 1928 analyzed sports people by their athletic speciality, although subtypes within sports (e.g., road and track cyclists) were lumped together. On the basis of his studies of the Amsterdam athletes, Kohlrausch (1930) postulated three major athletic body types, classified into 15 subtypes: slender (runners, jumpers); medium (swimmers, ball players); and massive (throwers, weightlifters, wrestlers). Arnold (1931) also identified three major classes: gymnastic, wrestler, and pentathlon types. In each case, classification was formalized by specific anthropometric measurements. The polyvalent athletic type at the beginning of the 20th century has splintered into rapidly diverging specialist bodies, and specialization was the rule. "Today is the age of specialization in athletics," wrote Boardman in 1933, "Athletes run very much to types in the various events of sport." This fragmentation has continued since, with markedly different morphologies appearing for individual sports, and on a positional or speciality basis within sports.

Figure 9.5 shows trends in the mean heights and masses of international level male athletes in 21 sports between about 1925 and 2000. The athletes were Olympic, World Championship or national representatives. The striking aspect of this graph is the "expanding universe" of sporting bodies. In 1925, 15 of the sports fall in the region bounded by 170–180 cm in height and 60–80 kg in mass. By 2000,

the data points are spread over a very wide swathe of the height–mass graph, and only eight sports fall into that region. Individual sports have followed quite different trajectories. It is quite conceivable, from a morphologic viewpoint, that an elite volleyballer could also have been an elite thrower in 1925. Their mean height differed by <1 cm and their mean mass by <1 kg. In 2000, however, while the heights are almost identical, the volleyballer is more than 32 kg lighter. In 1925, the masses of high jumpers and shot putters differed by barely 4 kg. In 2000, the difference was almost 60 kg.

Mechanisms linking morphology and sporting performance

While statistical comparisons can give useful clues as to which morphologic characteristics are important, it is of interest to consider the mechanisms linking morphology and sporting success. Too often, anthropometric characteristics have been assumed to be success characteristics, based on statistical analyses, but prove to be sample-specific or epiphenomenal. Statistical associations should be supported by plausible and quantifiable mechanisms.

Theories about mechanistic links between body morphology and performance should take into account both demand- and supply-side variables. Demand-side variables refer to how body size and shape can affect the external demands of the sporting task (e.g., the power required to accelerate to a certain speed in a certain time is proportional to body mass). Supply-side variables refer to how body size and shape make it possible for the individual to meet those requirements (e.g., peak leg power is proportional to thigh muscle mass). In many cases, optimal morphology is a compromise between the effects of body size and shape on different demand-side variables, or between effects on demand and supply-side variables. For example, in rugby, greater mass is associated with greater momentum (and hence ability to withstand tackles), but also with poorer acceleration for any given power output. In cycling, a larger muscle mass is associated with a greater power output, but also with increased air resistance, rolling resistance, kinetic energy, and increased power requirements for riding up a grade. In most sports, these competing demands keep body size and shape within relatively restrained limits.

Height and limb length

Height is clearly an advantage in sports where projectiles are thrown for maximum distance, such as javelin and discus, because they can travel greater horizontal distances before striking the ground if released from a greater height. It is also an advantage when a ball is thrown or struck downwards over a barrier such as a net in sports such as tennis and volleyball. This is because the striker has more options for placing the ball in different parts of the opponent's court. In tennis, by simple trigonometry, a 1 cm increase in height will allow about an extra 4 cm of the opponent's court in which a ball can be placed in serves from the baseline.

Some sports, such as diving and gymnastics, require rapid twisting and turning of the body and body segments (i.e., high angular acceleration). Angular acceleration is described by the equation

$$\alpha = T/(Mk^2)$$

where α is angular acceleration in rad·s^{-2}, T is torque in Nm, M is mass in kg and k is the radius of gyration in m. The radius of gyration is the distance of the center of mass from the axis of rotation. It therefore generally increases with limb and body length.

A 1% increase in the radius of gyration will result in a reduction of about 2% in angular acceleration. It is not surprising, therefore, that divers (mean stature 169.9 cm for males and 161.2 cm for females), gymnasts (169.4 and 157.0 cm) and figure skaters (170.7 and 157.7 cm) are relatively short.

For any given angular velocity, long levers will achieve a higher linear speed at the end of the lever. This is advantageous in movements where speed is important, such as throwing and striking. In water polo players, the ratio of lower arm (radiale–stylion) length to height is 14.9 ± 0.4%, compared to source population norms of 14.5 ± 0.8%. Furthermore, there have been secular increases in the arm length of elite Croatian water polo players, from 80.3 cm in 1980 to 83.1 cm in 1998 – about five times the rate of increase in the source population (Leo Pavicic, personal communication, October 2004). In weightlifters, by contrast, the ratio is 13.4 ± 1.2%. Limb length is also important in events where reaching is important, such as swimming. Because a relatively high proportion of a sprint swim involves the start, turn, and stretch for the wall, sprint swimmers tend to be taller than distance swimmers. In the 1990 World Championships, 50–100 m male and female sprint swimmers were taller (186.4 ± 7.5 and 173.9 ± 8.6 cm, respectively) than distance swimmers (179.6 ± 8.6 and 162.6 ± 4.6 cm) (Mazza et al. 1994).

Body fat

Low body fat is generally desirable in sports, because body fat constitutes a metabolically non-productive load, resulting in a lower power : mass ratio. Olds et al. (1995) have calculated that on the flat, a 1 kg increase in fat mass would increase 40 min time-trial time by about 0.2% (about 7 s). On a 2% slope, the decrease would be 0.5%. The same increase in fat mass in a middle-distance runner would increase 1500 m time by 1.6%, or about 3–4 s. If a 70 kg athlete with an 80 cm vertical jump were to put on 1 kg of body fat, the jump would be reduced by 1.5 cm. These effects are relatively small, but likely to be critical at the elite level. Low body fat is also required in sports where success is at least partly depends on aesthetic considerations, such as figure skating, body building, and competitive aerobics.

Subcutaneous body fat reduces the rate of transfer of heat from the body core to the skin, and decreases the body surface area : mass ratio, both of which impair heat loss (Pyke 1981). This is likely to be significant in sports such as distance running, especially in events held in hot climates. Finally, levels of body fat limit muscle mass in sports where there are weight classes, such as karate and rowing.

However, there are some benefits to moderate levels of body fat. Certain minimal levels of body fat (about 4% body fat in males) appear to be necessary for normal physiological and immunological function (Friedl *et al.* 1993). Body fat may also provide some protection against injury in contact sports such as Rugby Union. In swimming, body fat increases buoyancy, thereby reducing hydrodynamic drag, and reduces heat loss in marathon swimmers. In some sports people, such as sumo wrestlers and defensive linemen in American football, absolute body mass is important as it increases the inertia of the athlete. On the other hand, a large body mass requires a great deal of power to accelerate rapidly to speed. Ignoring air resistance, a 100 kg quarterback will need to generate a power output of at least 1225 W for 2 s to accelerate to 7 m·s^{-1}. Because kinetic energy is proportional to mass, a 1 kg (1%) increase in body mass would increase the required acceleration time to 2.02 s, or alternatively reduce the final velocity to 6.965 m·s^{-1}. This equates to a loss of about 7 cm in distance – enough to make the difference between being tackled or avoiding a tackle. The opposing requirements of rapid acceleration and high inertia may explain why quarterbacks and other sportsmen, although very big, are not as big as linemen. In this aspect, as in most others, morphologic optimization is probably a matter of compromise.

Table 9.4 shows mean skinfold thicknesses in international level athletes in 12 sports, measured since 1980. Skinfold thicknesses are lower than the source population average in each case. Very low OZ values (high selection pressures) are associated with gymnastics and running events.

Body surface area : mass ratio

Smaller body size is usually associated with a larger body surface area (BSA) : mass ratio. The BSA : mass

Table 9.4 Mean (SD) triceps skinfolds in selected sports. The overlap zone (OZ) value relative to the reference population (Australian males aged 18–35 years) is also shown.

Sport	Triceps skinfold thickness (mm)		
	Mean	SD	OZ
Source population	*12.9*	*6.2*	
Gymnastics	5.6	1.2	6.3
Distance running	6.7	1.4	8.4
Running: 800–1500 m	6.5	1.5	9.3
Running: sprint	6.2	2.1	12.2
Taekwondo	7.8	3.3	13.9
Rugby Union: backs	7.5	2.3	15.0
Australian football	7.2	2.3	15.3
Field hockey	9.1	2.3	18.9
Rowing	7.8	2.0	22.2
Soccer	8.8	2.8	22.4
Volleyball	8.9	2.7	22.8
Rugby Union: forwards	10.9	3.0	27.6

ratio has implications for thermoregulatory ability, and may partially explain a lower tolerance to exercise in the heat in children. Heat production is theoretically proportional to mass (more specifically, metabolically active mass), and heat loss is proportional to body surface area, although subcutaneous fat also has an insulating role. We would therefore expect to see a high BSA : mass ratio in sports where heat loss is important, such as distance running. This indeed the case. The lowest ratios in men are in sumo (188 cm^2·kg^{-1}, compared to an average of 254 cm^2·kg^{-1} for young Australian males), shot put (205 cm^2·kg^{-1}), Rugby Union forwards (212 cm^2·kg^{-1}), and American football (214 cm^2·kg^{-1}). These values are 2 SD or more below the source population values. The highest values in men are for 800 m running (276 cm^2·kg^{-1}), marathon (267 cm^2·kg^{-1}), steeplechase (268 cm^2·kg^{-1}) and distance running (10,000 m to marathon) (271 cm^2·kg^{-1}) – all 0.5 SD or more above the values in the source population. In women, the lowest values are found in discus (173 cm^2·kg^{-1}, 1.75 SD below the average of 273 cm^2·kg^{-1} in the source population), and the highest values are found in marathon runners (315 cm^2·kg^{-1}, or almost 2 SD above the population average). These patterns may result from a selection pressure for smaller body size in sports where heat loss is important.

Fluid resistance

The resistance of a body moving through fluid is proportional to the body's projected frontal area. In theory, projected frontal area is proportional to body surface area, which is in turn a function of height and mass (Olds & Olive 1999). Larger athletes are therefore relatively disadvantaged, given equal power output and similar body shape and posture, in sports such as cycling, downhill skiing, and speed skating. The degree of disadvantage increases with speed, because the power required to overcome air resistance is proportional to the cube of speed. The degree of disadvantage will differ according to the competitive context. Different size relationships apply for flat vs. uphill cycling, where the main resistance is mass (successful Tour de France hill climbers are typically very light), and downhill riding (where greater mass is an advantage). Using mathematic models developed by Olds et al. (1995), comparisons can be made between riders of different sizes. A rider 180 cm tall and weighing 70 kg (close to the average for a Tour de France cyclist) will be 2.1% slower than a rider weighing 70 kg and 165 cm tall, but with the same power output over 40 km on the flat. On a 2.5% uphill grade, he or she will be 3.4% slower, and on a 2.5% downhill grade, 1.3% slower.

Methods of physique assessment

The assessment of physique in athletes has not always been rationally based. In general, *anatomic* body composition is more relevant to sports performance than *chemical* body composition. We should, for example, be more interested in quantifying muscle mass than protein mass. In spite of this, there has been an inordinate amount of effort devoted to the estimation of percentage body fat in athletes, driven more by the development of new technologies than by any useful information likely to be derived.

Too much attention has also been given to whole-body assessments (e.g., somatotype, fat-free mass) at the expense of segmental analysis, such as limb volumes. Nevill et al. (2004) found that skinfold-corrected thigh girth showed group-specific variation it its relation to body mass in a sample of 478 athletes, with exponents ranging from 0.96 for endurance athletes to 1.49 for speed athletes. Stewart (2006) discusses the use of dual-energy X-ray absorptiometry (DEXA) to calculate segmental lean and fat masses.

Finally, the emphasis has been too much on the accuracy of measurements rather than their precision. In monitoring athletes, the accurate estimation of an anthropometric characteristic at one point of time is generally less important than tracking changes with serial measurements of high precision. While estimates of percentage body fat based on skinfold thicknesses, for example, may vary wildly between themselves and therefore cannot all be accurate, they can reliably track changes in fatness in athletes.

Traditional anthropometry

Surface anthropometric measurements of skinfolds, girths, lengths, and breadths remain the standard fare of sports anthropometrists. Measurement sites and protocols have been standardized by the International Society for the Advancement of Kinanthropometry (ISAK; Marfell-Jones et al. 2006), and are widely used around the world. Skinfolds are a simple and sensitive measure of training status, and girths a reasonable estimate of changes in segmental muscle mass in athletes. Lengths and breadths are useful in anthropometric talent identification, but are largely unresponsive to training in adult athletes. Surface anthropometric measurements can be fed into algorithms to calculate somatotype (Carter 1996) and indices of corpulence and limb ratios; to estimate muscle mass (Lukaski 2005), body density, and hence percentage body fat (Norton 1996); and for fractionation of body mass (Drinkwater & Ross 1980). While these derived variables can discriminate between different types of athletes, and between competitive levels, they are generally insufficiently sensitive to monitor small changes in athletes' physiques. For example, a 30% decrease in triceps skinfold or a 10% increase in flexed arm girth would be necessary to shift endomorphy and mesomorphy ratings by a half-point in a male athlete. Using the formula for estimated muscle mass of Martin *et al.* (1990), a 3% increase in corrected girths would be required before one could be 95% confident that muscle mass had increased.

Much has been said about the use of raw skinfold thicknesses as opposed to converting to estimated percentage body fat. There are some 200 equations used to estimate percentage body fat based on surface anthropometric values. These equations yield very different values for the same inputs. For one male athlete, for example, seven common equations yielded estimated body fat percentages ranging from 5.6 to 12.7%. Furthermore, 10% increases in all skinfolds resulted in changes in estimated percentage body fat ranging from 7.8% to 16.1%. Converting to percentage body fat is therefore a suspect procedure from the point of view of accuracy. However, a single percentage body fat value is simpler to comprehend and sensitive to change across serial measurements.

New methods

In the last 20 years a number of new technologies have become available or more widely used for anthropometric research. Table 9.5 briefly summarizes the rationale behind some of these technologies. Most exploit the differential effects of various types of electromagnetic radiation on different types of body tissues. Some depend on the assumption that various body components have fixed proportions of certain substances (e.g., that fat-free mass contains 68.1 mmol·kg^{-1} potassium, or that it is 73% water). Because of the expense and expertise required for many of these technologies, they have not so far been widely used with athletic populations.

DEXA in particular shows great promise and has emerged as a rival gold standard to hydrodensitometry, which relies on the differential densities of fat and lean tissue. It has the ability to determine fat, fat-free, and bone masses both on a whole-body and

Table 9.5 Some of the more common new technologies used in anthropometric assessment.

Technology	Rationale	Reference
CT	Internal image reconstructed based on attenuation of X-rays	Ross & Jansen (2005)
MRI	A powerful magnet causes protons to realign. Protons in different tissues return to their original state at different rates	Ross & Jansen (2005)
DEXA	X-rays of different strengths are passed through the body and absorbed differentially by different tissues	Stewart (2006)
Ultrasound	High-frequency sound waves are deflected at tissue boundaries	Bellisari & Roche (2005)
3D laser scanning	A laser beam passes over the body and its reflection is recorded by cameras. The body surface is captured as 3D points	Honey & Olds (2006)
Hydrometry	Isotopic tracers spread throughout body water, and the amount of dilution is used to estimate total body water and hence FFM	Schoeller (2005)
Whole-body counting	Counters measure the rate of decay of radioactive potassium (K), which has a fixed concentration in FFM	Ellis (2005)
Neutron activation analysis	In a neutron field, atoms (e.g., of Ca, C, N) undergo nuclear reactions which can be measured by counters	Ellis (2005)
BIA	A weak electric current is passed through the body. Impedance is proportional to the body's water content, and hence to FFM	Forbes *et al.* (1992)
Air displacement plethysmography (Bod-Pod)	Uses pressure–volume relationships to estimate body volume and hence density	Nunez *et al.* (1999)

BIA, Bioelectrical impedance analysis; CT, Computerized tomography; FFM, fat-free mass; DEXA, dual-energy X-ray absorptiometry; MRI, magnetic resonance imaging.

segmental basis. Recently, three-dimensional whole-body laser scanning has enriched surface anthropometry, facilitating the measurement of volumes, cross-sectional and surface areas, and surface contours. This technique has been shown to be valid and reliable (Honey & Olds 2006). It offers scope for serial monitoring of changes in limb volumes and cross-sectional areas with training, characteristics closely linked to strength and power performance. Three-dimensional shape analysis (morphometrics) may also prove to be a useful tool in describing morphologies.

Both DEXA and three-dimensional laser scanning require cumbersome and expensive equipment and substantial operator expertise. Other technologies are more portable and practical in field settings. Bioelectrical impedance analysis (BIA) measures the impedance of an electric current passed through the body. Because the current is conducted by water, impedance is proportional to the concentration of water in the body, and hence to fat-free mass. BIA units are cheap and portable, and yield quite accurate estimates of body composition at the group level, but can be inaccurate at the individual level, and unreliable in tracking changes over time (Forbes *et al.* 1992). The fact that BIA readings change with changes in posture, which clearly do not alter total body water content, suggests that the method may be sensitive to the distribution of the body water between the intracellular and extracellular compartments (Shirreffs & Maughan 1994).

Measurement error

The accuracy (validity) and precision (reliability) of any measurement should be determined using equipment, anthropometrists, and subjects similar to the target population. A wide variety of statistics have been used to quantify validity and reliability (Atkinson & Nevill 1998), not always appropriately. Some anthropometrists speak of measurements as being "valid" or "not valid," "reliable" or "not reliable," often citing arbitrary cut-offs for coefficients such as the intraclass correlation coefficient (ICC). Validity and reliability are not characteristics that measurement methods either possess or do not possess – they are a matter of degree. Any quantifica-

tion of validity or reliability should express validity and reliability in a way that makes it possible to calculate the confidence limits of a measurement, the number of subjects needed to discriminate between groups, or the confidence we can have in saying that an anthropometric characteristic has changed over time. Correlation coefficients such as Pearson, Spearman, and the ICC do not allow us to do this. In general, whether statistically significant differences exist between the test and retest measurements, or between the trial method and the criterion method, is not of interest. The analysis of choice for both accuracy and precision is Bland–Altman analysis (Bland & Altman 1986). ISAK recommends the technical error of measurement (TEM; Pederson & Gore 1996), which is useful as a global measure but does not distinguish between systematic error (bias) and random error (Olds 2002).

The quantification of measurement error makes it possible to determine how much an anthropometric characteristic measured on a single subject needs to change before we can say with 95% confidence that a real change has occurred. Highly trained ISAK anthropometrists can consistently achieve intratester TEMs of 5% for skinfold measurements. Even with this level of precision, a change of $2 \times \sqrt{2} \times 5\% = 14\%$ would be required between two measurements for the anthropometrist to say with 95% confidence that a real change has occurred. These confidence limits can be reduced by taking multiple measurements or by improving technique.

Conclusions

Anthropometric success characteristics are not fixed within the athlete group; they are constantly evolving as a response to changes in the sporting and external environment. The most dramatic changes have been the increasing degree of specialization and the search for "extreme physiques." Sports anthropmetrists should keep in mind the following guidelines:

• Reference data should be up-to-date, and event- and position-specific.
• The precision and accuracy of anthropometric data should always be assessed and reported.
• Data should, as much as possible, be compatible

with existing databases. This requires a high degree of standardization in measurement. The ISAK guidelines are recommended.

- When choosing which dimensions to measure, consider plausible mechanistic associations between anthropometric characteristics and sporting success.

References

Ackland, T., Schreiner, A. & Kerr, D. (1994) Anthropometric profiles of world championship female basketball players. *International Conference of Science and Medicine in Sport, Brisbane, September, 1994.* Sports Medicine Australia.

Arnold, A. (1931) *Körperentwicklung und Leibesübungen für Schul und Sportärzte.* Johann Barth, Leipzig.

Atkinson, G. & Nevill, A.M. (1998) Statistical methods for assessing measurement error (reliability) in variables relevant to sports medicine. *Sports Medicine* **26**, 217–238.

Bellisari, A. & Roche, A.F. (2005) Anthropometry and ultrasound. In: *Human Body Composition*, 2nd edn. (Heymsfield, S.B., Lohman, T.G., Wang, Z. & Going, S.B., eds.) Human Kinetics, Champaign, IL: 89–108.

Bemies, C.O. (1900) Physical characteristics of the runner and jumper. *American Physical Education Review* **5**, 235–245.

Bland, J.M. & Altman, D.G. (1986) Statistical methods for assessing agreement between two methods of clincial measurement. *Lancet* **1**, 307–310.

Boardman, R. (1933) World's champions run to types. *Journal of Health and Physical Education* **4**, 32–33.

Buytendijk, F.J.J. (1929) *Ergebnisse der sportärztlichen Untersuchungen bei den IX. Olympischen Spielen in Amsterdam 1928.* Verlag von Lulius Springer, Berlin.

Carter, J.E.L. (1996) Somatotyping. In: *Anthropometrica* (Norton, K.I. & Olds, T.S., eds.) UNSW Press, Sydney: 147–170.

Drinkwater, D. & Ross, W. (1980) Anthropometric fractionation of body mass. In: *Kinanthropometry II* (Ostyn, W., Beunen, G. & Simons, J., eds.) University Park Press, Baltimore: 177–188.

Ellis, K.J. (2005) Whole-body counting and neutron activation analysis. In: *Human Body Composition*, 2nd edn. (Heymsfield, S.B., Lohman, T.G., Wang, Z. & Going, S.B., eds.) Human Kinetics, Champaign, IL: 51–62.

Forbes, G., Simon, W. & Amatruda, J. (1992) Is bioimpedance a good predictor of body composition changes? *American Journal of Clinical Nutrition* **56**, 4–6.

Frank, R.H. (1999) *Luxury Fever*. Princeton University Press, Princeton.

Friedl, K.E., Moore, R.J., Martinez-Lopez, L.E., *et al.* (1993) Lower limit of body fat in healthy active men. *Journal of Applied Physiology* **77**, 933–940.

Honey, F. & Olds, T. (2006) The use of whole-body 3D scanners in anthropometry. In: *Kinanthropometry IX* (Marfell-Jones, M., Stewart, A. & Olds, T., eds.) Routledge, London: 1–13.

Judt, T. (2005) *Postwar: A History of Europe Since 1945.* William Heinemann, London.

Kohlrausch, W. (1930) Zusammenhänge von Körperform und Leistung. Ergebnisse der anthropometrischen Messungen an den Athleten der Amsterdamer Olympiade. *Arbeitsphysiologie* **2**, 187–204.

Lukaski, H.C. (2005) Assessing muscle mass. In: *Human Body Composition*, 2nd edn. (Heymsfield, S.B., Lohman, T.G., Wang, Z. & Going, S.B., eds.) Human Kinetics, Champaign, IL: 203–218.

Marfell-Jones, M., Olds, T., Stewart, A. & Carter, J.E.L. (2006) *International Standards for Anthropometric Assessment.* North-West University, Potchefstroom, South Africa.

Martin, A.D., Spenst, L.F., Drinkwater, D.T. & Clarys, J.P. (1990) Anthropometric estimation of muscle mass. *Medicine and Science in Sports and Exercise* **22**, 729–733.

Mazza, J.C., Ackland, T.R., Bach, T.M. & Cosolito, P. (1994) Absolute body size. In: *Kinanthropometry in Aquatic Sports* (Carter, J.E.L. & Ackland, T.R., eds.) Human Kinetics, Champaign, IL: 15–54.

Meredith, H.V. (1976) Findings from Asia, Australia, Europe and North America on secular change in mean height of children, youths and young adults. *American Journal of Physical Anthropology* **44**, 315–326.

Nevill, A., Stewart, A., Olds, T. & Holder, R. (2004) Are adult physiques geometrically similar? The dangers of allometric scaling using body mass power laws. *American Journal of Physical Anthropology* **124**(2), 177–182.

Norton, K.I. (1996) Anthropometric estimation of body fat. In: *Anthropometrica* (Norton, K.I. & Olds, T.S., eds.) UNSW Press, Sydney: 171–198.

Norton, K.I. & Olds, T.S. (2000) The evolution of the size and shape of athletes: causes and consequences. In: *Kinanthropometry VI* (Norton, K. & Olds, T., eds.) ISAK, Adelaide: 3–36.

Norton, K.I. & Olds, T.S. (2001) Morphological evolution of athletes over the 20th century: causes and consequences. *Sports Medicine* **31**, 763–783.

Norton, K.I., Olds, T.S., Olive, S.C. & Craig, N.P. (1996) Anthropometry and sports performance. In: *Anthropometrica* (Norton, K.I. & Olds, T.S., eds.) UNSW Press, Sydney: 287–364.

Nunez, C., Kovera, A.J., Pietrobelli, A., *et al.* (1999) Body composition in children and adults by air displacement plethysmography. *European Journal of Clinical Nutrition* **53**, 382–387.

Olds, T.S. (2001) The evolution of physique in male Rugby Union players in the twentieth century. *Journal of Sports Sciences* **19**, 253–262.

Olds, T.S. (2002) Five errors about error. *Journal of Science and Medicine in Sport* **5**, 336–340.

Olds, T.S. & Kang, S. (2000) Anthropometric characteristics of adult male Korean taekwondo players. In: *Taekwondo and the New Millennium. Proceedings of the First Olympic Taekwondo Scientific Congress, Seoul, May, 2000.* OTSC, Seoul: 69–75.

Olds, T.S. & Olive, S.C. (1999) Methodological considerations in the determination of projected frontal area in cyclists. *Journal of Sports Sciences* **17**, 335–345.

Olds, T.S., Norton, K.I., Lowe, E.L.A., Reay F., Olive, S.C. & Ly S.V. (1995) Modeling road cycling performance. *Journal of Applied Physiology* **78**, 1596–1611.

Pederson, D. & Gore, C. (1996) Anthropometry measurement error. In: *Anthropometrica* (Norton, K.I. & Olds, T.S., eds.) UNSW Press, Sydney: 77–96.

Pyke, F. (1981) Physiological considerations during exercise in hot climates. *Transactions of the Menzies Foundation* **2**, 213–220.

Ross, R. & Janssen, I. (2005) Computed tomography and magnetic resonance imaging. In: *Human Body Composition*, 2nd edn. (Heymsfield, S.B., Lohman, T.G., Wang, Z. & Going, S.B., eds.) Human Kinetics, Champaign, IL: 89–108.

Sargent, D.A. (1887) The physical characteristics of the athlete. *Scribner's Magazine* **2**, 541–561.

Schoeller, D. (2005) Hydrometry. In: *Human Body Composition*, 2nd edn. (Heymsfield, S.B., Lohman, T.G., Wang, Z. & Going, S.B., eds.) Human Kinetics, Champaign, IL: 35–49.

Shirreffs, S.M. & Maughan, R.J. (1994) The effect of posture change on blood volume, serum potassium and whole body electrical impedance. *European Journal of Applied Physiology* **69**, 461–463.

Steele, J.R. (1987) *The relationship of selected anthropometric and lower extremity characteristics to the mechanics of landing in netball.* Technical Report I, Part B. Australian Sports Commission, Canberra.

Stewart, A. (2006) Athletic morphology: approaches and limitations using dual X-ray absorptiometry and anthropometry. In: *Kinanthropometry IX* (Marfell-Jones, M., Stewart, A. & Olds, T., eds.) Routledge, London: 53–64.

Part 4

Immunology

Chapter 10

Exercise Immunology

MICHAEL GLEESON

This chapter examines the effects of exercise and training on immune function and discusses the methodologic problems that limit the interpretation of many exercise immunology studies. Acute bouts of exercise cause a temporary depression of various aspects of immune function, such as neutrophil oxidative burst, lymphocyte proliferation, monocyte antigen presentation, and natural killer cell cytotoxic activity, which will usually last for approximately 3–24 h after exercise, depending on the intensity and duration of the exercise bout. Several studies indicate that the incidence of symptoms of upper respiratory tract illness (URTI) is increased in the days following prolonged strenuous endurance events and it has been generally assumed that this is a result of the temporary depression of immune function induced by prolonged exercise. More recently, it has been proposed that at least some of these symptoms are attributable to inflammation of the upper respiratory tract rather than to infectious episodes. Post-exercise immune function depression is most pronounced when the exercise is continuous, prolonged (>1.5 h), of moderate to high intensity (55–75% $\dot{V}o_{2max}$), and performed without food intake. Periods of intensified training that result in overreaching have been shown to chronically depress immune function; in other words, immune cell functions measured at rest are still depressed 24 h after the last exercise bout. Although elite athletes are not clinically immunodeficient, it is possible that

the combined effects of small changes in several immune parameters may compromise resistance to common minor illnesses such as upper respiratory tract infection. Protracted immune depression linked with prolonged intensive training may determine susceptibility to infection, particularly at times of major competitions.

Role of the immune system

The immune system protects against, recognizes, attacks, and destroys elements that are foreign to the body, and the major function of the immune system is to protect the body against infectious diseases. A comprehensive description of the human immune system can be found in many textbooks (e.g., Gleeson 2005) and only a very brief summary is provided here. The immune system operates at the systemic as well as at the local level, which includes the mucosal tissue such as in the upper airways and the gut. The immune system can be divided into two broad functions: innate (natural and non-specific) and acquired immunity (adaptive and specific), which work together synergistically. The attempt of an infectious agent to enter the body immediately activates the innate system. This so-called "first line of defense" comprises three general mechanisms with the common goal of restricting micro-organism entry into the body:

1 *Physical/structural barriers:* skin, epithelial linings, mucosal secretions;

2 *Chemical barriers:* pH of bodily fluids and soluble factors such as lysozymes and complement proteins; and

The Olympic Textbook of Science in Sport, 1st edition. Edited by R.J. Maughan. Published 2009 by Blackwell Publishing. ISBN: 978-1-4051-5638-7.

3 *Phagocytic cells* (e.g., neutrophils and monocytes/macrophages) *and cytotoxic cells* (natural killer cells).

Failure of the innate system and the resulting infection activates the acquired system, which aids recovery from infection. Monocytes or macrophages ingest, process, and present foreign material (antigens) to lymphocytes. This is followed by clonal proliferation of T and B lymphocytes that possess receptors that recognize the antigen, engendering specificity and "memory" that enable the immune system to mount an augmented cell-mediated and humoral (antibody) response when the host is reinfected by the same pathogen. Critical to the activation and regulation of immune function is the production of cytokines, including interferons, interleukins, and colony-stimulating factors. A fundamental characteristic of the immune system is that it involves multiple functionally different cell types which permits a large variety of defense mechanisms. Resistance to infection is strongly influenced by the effectiveness of the immune system in protecting the host against pathogenic micro-organisms. Immune function is influenced by genetic as well as environmental factors and thus there is some degree of variability in resistance to infection within the normal healthy adult population. Resistance to specific infections is also affected by previous exposure to the disease-causing pathogen or inoculation with vaccines used for immunization. Vaccines contain dead or attenuated pathogens that trigger immune responses including the development of specific memory without eliciting symptoms of disease which are associated with inoculation by wild-type pathogens.

Exercise and susceptibility to infection

Athletes engaged in heavy training programs, particularly those involved in endurance events, appear to be more susceptible to infection. According to some surveys, sore throats and flu-like symptoms are more common in athletes than in the general population and, once athletes are infected, colds may last longer (Peters & Bateman 1983; Nieman *et al.* 1990; Heath *et al.* 1991). There is some evidence that this increased susceptibility to infection arises because of a depression of immune system function

and there are several detailed reviews on the subject (Shephard 1997; Gleeson & Bishop 1999; Mackinnon 1999; Gleeson 2005).

The circulating numbers and functional capacities of leukocytes (white blood cells) may be decreased by repeated bouts of intense prolonged exercise. The reason for this is probably related to increased levels of stress hormones during exercise and entry into the circulation of less mature leukocytes, particularly neutrophils, from the bone marrow. Falls in the blood concentration of glutamine have also been suggested as a possible cause of the immunodepression associated with heavy training, although the evidence for this is less compelling. During exercise there is an increased production of reactive oxygen species and some immune cell functions can be impaired by an excess of free radicals (Niess *et al.* 1999). Exposure to airborne pathogens is increased as a result of the higher rate and depth of breathing. An increase in gut permeability may also allow increased entry of gut bacterial endotoxins into the circulation, particularly during prolonged exercise in the heat. The cause of the increased incidence of infection in athletes is therefore likely to be multifactorial: a variety of stressors, physical, psychological, environmental, or nutritional, can suppress immune function. These effects, together with increased exposure to pathogens, can make the athlete more susceptible to infection (Fig. 10.1).

The relationship between exercise and susceptibility to infection has been modeled in the form of a

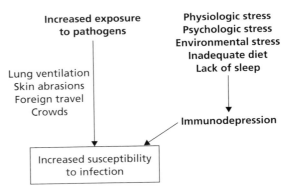

Fig. 10.1 Factors affecting susceptibility to infection in athletes. From Gleeson (2005) with permission from Elsevier Ltd.

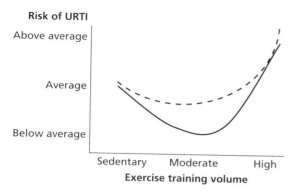

Fig. 10.2 The J-shaped model of the relationship between risk of upper respiratory tract infection (URTI) and exercise volume. The dashed line may give a more realistic interpretation of the relationship. From Gleeson (2005) with permission from Elsevier Ltd.

J-shaped curve as illustrated in Fig. 10.2 (Nieman 1994). This model suggests that while engaging in moderate activity may enhance immune function above sedentary levels, excessive amounts of prolonged high intensity exercise induce detrimental effects on immune function. Although the literature provides strong evidence in support of the latter point (Peters & Bateman 1983; Nieman *et al.* 1990; Heath *et al.* 1991; Nieman 1994; Pedersen & Bruunsgaard 1995; Shephard 1997), relatively little evidence is available to suggest that there is any clinically significant difference in immune function between sedentary and moderately active persons. Thus, it may be more realistic to flatten out the portion of the curve representing this part of the relationship, as indicated by the dashed line in Fig. 10.2. Recently, an epidemiologic study on infection incidence and habitual physical activity reported that the regular performance of about 2 h of moderate exercise per day was associated with a 29% reduction in risk of picking up a URTI as compared the risk of infection associated with a sedentary lifestyle (Matthews *et al.* 2002). In contrast, it has been reported that there is a 100–500% increase in risk of picking up an infection in the weeks following a competitive ultra-endurance running event (Nieman *et al.* 1990; Peters *et al.* 1993, 1996).

Effects of exercise on immune function

Acute effects of exercise on immune function

A single, acute bout of prolonged strenuous exercise has a temporary depressive effect on immune function and has been associated with an increased incidence of infection, or at least an increased incidence of symptoms of upper airway illness. For example, several studies have described a substantially higher (two- to sixfold increase) frequency of self-reported symptoms of URTI in athletes who completed long-distance foot races compared to control runners who did not compete in the events (Peters & Bateman 1983; Nieman *et al.* 1990; Peters *et al.* 1993, 1996). However, as infections were not clinically confirmed, it cannot be ruled out that some of the reported symptoms (e.g., sore throat) were caused by non-infectious airway inflammation brought about by drying of the mucosal surfaces and/or the inhalation of dry air or pollutants.

An acute bout of physical activity is accompanied by physiological responses that are remarkably similar in many respects to those induced by infection, sepsis, or trauma (Northoff *et al.* 1998; Gleeson & Bishop 1999): there is a substantial increase in the number of circulating leukocytes (mainly lymphocytes and neutrophils), the magnitude of which is related to both the intensity and duration of exercise. There are also increases in the plasma concentrations of various substances that are known to influence leukocyte functions, including inflammatory and anti-inflammatory cytokines such as tumour necrosis factor-α, interleukin 1β (IL-1β), IL-6, IL-10, macrophage inflammatory protein-1, granulocyte colony-stimulating factor (GCSF) and IL-1 receptor antagonist (IL-1ra), acute phase proteins such as C-reactive protein and activated complement fragments. The large increases in plasma IL-6 concentration observed during exercise can be entirely accounted for by release of this cytokine from contracting muscle fibers (Steensberg *et al.* 2000). However, IL-6 production by monocytes (Starkie *et al.* 2001) and IL-2 and γ-interferon (IFN-γ), but not IL-4, production by T lymphocytes are inhibited during and for several hours after prolonged exercise (Northoff *et al.* 1998; Lancaster *et al.* 2004). These

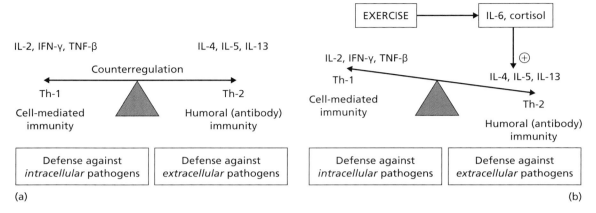

Fig. 10.3 T helper 1 (Th1) and Th2 cytokines and the influence of exercise on their production by T-helper (CD4⁺) lymphocytes. (a) Whether humoral or cell-mediated immunity will dominate depends largely on the type of cytokines that are released by the activated T-helper cells. Cell-mediated immunity depends on a so-called Th1 profile of cytokines, including particularly γ-interferon (IFN-γ). Th1 cytokines activate macrophages and induce killer mechanisms, including T-cytotoxic cells. A Th2 profile includes mainly interleukin-4 (IL-4), IL-5, and IL-13, which are necessary for promotion of humoral immunity, IgE-mediated allergic reactions and activation of eosinophils. IL-4 and IL-13 primarily drive B-cell differentiation to antibody production, while IL-5 stimulates and primes eosinophils. (b) Exercise results in elevated levels of IL-6 and cortisol which promote Th2 and inhibit Th1 cytokine production.

cytokine changes suggest a shift in the T-helper cell type 1–type 2 (Th1–Th2) balance towards a Th2 response which would be expected to decrease defense against intracellular pathogens (Fig. 10.3) as explained in more detail below.

Hormonal changes also occur in response to exercise, including rises in the plasma concentration of several hormones, such as epinephrine, cortisol, growth hormone, and prolactin, that are known to have immunomodulatory effects. Muscle-derived IL-6 appears to be at least partly responsible for the elevated secretion of cortisol during prolonged exercise. Infusion of recombinant human IL-6 (rhIL-6) into resting humans to mimic the exercise-induced plasma levels of IL-6 increases plasma cortisol in a similar manner (Steensberg *et al.* 2003). In contrast, the same rhIL-6 infusion does not change plasma epinephrine, norepinephrine or insulin levels in resting healthy young subjects. Therefore, muscle-derived IL-6 may be partly responsible for the cortisol response to exercise, whereas other hormonal changes cannot be ascribed to IL-6. Stimulation of cortisol secretion by IL-6 may be caused by an effect of IL-6 on the hypothalamus, stimulating the release of adrenocorticotrophic hormone from the anterior

pituitary gland or by a direct effect of IL-6 on cortisol release from the adrenal glands; evidence for both mechanisms exists. In addition, it was recently demonstrated that relatively small increases in plasma levels of IL-6 induce the two anti-inflammatory cytokines IL-1ra and IL-10 together with C-reactive protein (Steensberg *et al.* 2003). During exercise the increase in IL-6 precedes the increase in these two cytokines, arguing circumstantially for muscle-derived IL-6 to be the initiator of this response. IL-6 and IL-4 stimulate monocytes and macrophages to produce IL-1ra, which inhibits the effect of pro-inflammatory IL-1. Type 2 T lymphocytes, monocytes, and B cells are the main producers of IL-10 which, together with IL-4, can inhibit type 1 T-cell cytokine production. In accordance with this, strenuous exercise decreases the percentage of type 1 T cells in the circulation, whereas the percentage of type 2 T cells does not change. Both cortisol and epinephrine suppress the type 1 T-cell cytokine production, whereas IL-6 directly stimulates type 2 T-cell cytokine production. Type 1 T cells drive the immune system towards protection against intracellular pathogens such as viruses; therefore exercise, possibly working through muscle-derived IL-6, may decrease virus protection in the host and thus may account for why athletes appear to be more prone to acquire URTI. However, it is very important to stress that the shift toward type 2 T-cell dominance might be beneficial, because it also suppresses the ability of the immune system to induce tissue damage and inflammation.

Phagocytic neutrophils appear to be activated by an acute bout of exercise, but show a diminished responsiveness to stimulation by bacteria, including both reduced oxidative burst and diminished degranulation responses, which can last for many hours after exercise (Pyne 1994; Robson et al. 1999b). Prolonged continuous exercise at moderate intensity (55–70% $\dot{V}o_{2max}$) appears to have a greater and longer lasting effect on neutrophil responsiveness than shorter more intensive bouts of exercise.

Acute exercise temporarily increases the number of circulating natural killer (NK) cells, but following exercise NK cell counts drop to less than half of normal levels for a couple of hours; normal resting values are usually restored within 24 h (Shephard & Shek 1999). NK cell cytolytic activity (per cell) may increase, remain unchanged, or fall after exercise. If the exercise session is both prolonged and vigorous, the decrease in NK cell counts and cytolytic activity may begin during the exercise session (Shephard & Shek 1999). During recovery from exercise, lymphokine-activated NK cell numbers and activity also fall below pre-exercise levels. Acute exercise has been shown to diminish the proliferative response of lymphocytes to mitogens (Mackinnon 1999) and decrease the expression of an early activation marker (CD69) in response to stimulation with mitogen (Ronsen et al. 2001). When the exercise bout is strenuous and very prolonged (>1.5 h), the number of circulating lymphocytes may be decreased below pre-exercise levels for several hours after exercise and the T-lymphocyte $CD4^+ : CD8^+$ (helper : suppressor) ratio is decreased (Berk et al. 1986; Pedersen & Bruunsgaard 1995). It may be worth mentioning here that the abbreviation CD refers to clusters of differentiation or cluster designators that are specific proteins expressed on the cell surface which can be identified through the use of fluorescent-labeled monoclonal antibodies. These CD markers can be used to identify and enumerate particular cell types

using fluorescence-activated flow cytometry. For example, T lymphocytes all express the protein CD3 on the cell surface. B lymphocytes do not express CD3, but express CD19, CD20, and CD22. A particular subset of T lymphocytes called helper T cells specifically express the CD4 protein, whereas the cytotoxic/suppressor T cells express CD8.

Antigen-presenting cell function is also affected by exercise: exercise-induced reductions in macrophage major histocompatibility complex (MHC) class II expression and antigen-presenting capacity have been documented (Woods et al. 2000). Both T memory ($CD45RO^+$) and T naive ($CD45RA^+$) cells increase temporarily during exercise, but the CD45RO : CD45RA ratio tends to increase because of the relatively greater mobilization of the $CD45RO^+$ subset (Gannon et al. 2002; Lancaster et al. 2003b). Following prolonged strenuous exercise, the production of immunoglobulins by B lymphocytes is inhibited and delayed-type hypersensitivity responses (an in vivo measure of cell-mediated immunity as measured by skin swelling 48 h following antigen injection) are diminished (Bruunsgaard et al. 1997). These changes during early recovery from exercise would appear to weaken the potential immune response to pathogens and have been suggested to provide an "open window" for infection, representing the most vulnerable time period for athletes in terms of their susceptibility to contracting an infection (Pedersen & Bruunsgaard 1995).

A new and potentially important finding is that following a prolonged bout of strenuous exercise the expression of some toll-like receptors on monocytes is decreased (Lancaster et al. 2005a). Toll-like receptors enable antigen-presenting cells to recognize pathogens and control the activation of the adaptive immune response (Schnare et al. 2001). Prolonged exercise also results in a decreased induction of co-stimulatory molecules and cytokines following stimulation with known toll-like receptor ligands/activators (Lancaster et al. 2005a). These effects may represent a mechanism through which exercise stress impairs immune function and increases susceptibility to infection. However, this may not be entirely detrimental to the host and may, by reducing immune activation and subsequent inflammation, be one of the mechanisms through which regular exercise benefits long-term health. Blood markers of inflammation are strongly associated with cardio-vascular and metabolic disease in the middle-aged and elderly population (Dandona *et al.* 2004).

Can exercise-induced immunodepression be prevented?

Studies from Bente Pedersen's group in Copenhagen indicate that the release of IL-6 from contracting muscle can be attenuated by long-term antioxidant supplementation. In a recent single-blind placebo-controlled study it was reported that 4 weeks of oral supplementation with a combination of vitamin C (500 mg·day^{-1}) and vitamin E (400 IU·day^{-1}) mar-kedly attenuated the release of IL-6 from active muscle and the plasma IL-6 and cortisol response to 3 h of dynamic two-legged knee-extensor exercise at 50% of maximal power output compared with placebo (Fischer *et al.* 2004). High levels of circulat-ing IL-6 stimulate cortisol release and this study provides some strong evidence that the mechanism of action of the antioxidant supplementation was via a reduction in IL-6 release from the muscle of the exercising legs. Attenuating the IL-6 and cortisol response would be expected to limit the exercise-induced depression of immune function and this may be the mechanism for the reported lower incid-ence of URTI symptoms following an ultramarathon race in runners supplemented for several weeks be-fore the race with vitamin C compared with placebo (Peters *et al.* 1993, 1996).

Consumption of carbohydrate (CHO) during exercise also attenuates rises in plasma IL-6, cate-cholamines, adrenocorticotropic hormone, and cor-tisol (Nehlsen-Cannarella *et al.* 1997; Nieman 1998). CHO intake during exercise also attenuates the trafficking of most leukocyte and lymphocyte sub-sets, including the rise in the neutrophil : lymphocyte ratio, prevents the exercise-induced fall in neutrophil function, and reduces the extent of the diminution of mitogen-stimulated T-lymphocyte proliferation following prolonged exercise (Gleeson *et al.* 2004a). Very recently, it was shown that consuming 30–60 g·h^{-1} CHO during 2.5 h of strenuous cycling prevented both the decrease in the number and percentage of IFN-γ positive T lymphocytes and the suppression of IFN-γ production from stimulated T lymphocytes observed on the placebo controlled trial (Lancaster *et al.* 2005b). IFN-γ production is crit-ical to antiviral defense and it has been suggested that the suppression of IFN-γ production may be an important mechanism leading to an increased risk of infection after prolonged exercise bouts (Northoff *et al.* 1998).

However, Pedersen's group has argued that the reduction in the IL-6 response to exercise may be a two-edged sword, as IL-6 has several metabolic effects and shared mechanisms exist regarding immune impairment and training adaptation (Starkie *et al.* 2003). Attenuating the IL-6 response to exercise will also inhibit lipolysis (Starkie *et al.* 2003), reduce the anti-inflammatory effects of exercise, and attenuate the expression of a number of metabolic genes in the exercised muscle (Pilegaard *et al.* 2002). The concern for athletes is that although these nutritional inter-ventions may reduce their risk of infection, another effect may be to limit their hard-earned adaptation to training. However, it can also be argued that CHO intake during training allows the athlete to work harder and longer and as yet there is no evid-ence that physiological and performance adapta-tions are impaired by CHO intake during training sessions.

Further research is needed to determine how nutrient intake might affect the transcriptional regu-lation of metabolic genes in skeletal muscle and what, if any, consequences this has for training adap-tation. In the case of adaptation to resistance train-ing, it is worth noting that consumption of CHO or a combination of CHO and essential amino acids appears to attenuate cortisol responses to the exer-cise and actually improves physiological (muscle protein synthesis and fiber cross-sectional area) and functional (strength gain) adaptations (Andersen *et al.* 2005; Koopman *et al.* 2005; Bird *et al.* 2006).

Chronic effects of exercise training on immune function

The effects of exercise training on immune function have been investigated using:
1 Cross-sectional studies that have compared im-mune function in athletes and non-athletes;

2 Longitudinal studies that have reported the effect of a training program – typically 4–12 weeks' duration – in previously sedentary people;

3 Short-term longitudinal studies that have reported the effect of a period – typically 1–3 weeks' duration – of intensified training on immune function in already well-trained athletes;

4 Longitudinal studies that have monitored immune function in athletes over the course of a competitive season lasting typically 4–10 months; and

5 Cross-sectional studies that have compared immune function in athletes diagnosed as "overtrained" with healthy athletes.

Following an acute bout of exercise, changes in circulating leukocyte numbers and functions normally return to pre-exercise values within 3–24 h. Cross-sectional studies that have compared leukocyte numbers and functions in blood samples taken from athletes more than 24 h after their last training session with those of sedentary individuals have generally reported very few differences. Thus, in the true resting state, immune function appears to be broadly similar in athletes and non-athletes, and clinically normal levels are observed in most athletes (Nieman 2000). However, circulating numbers of leukocytes are generally lower in endurance athletes at rest than in sedentary people. A low blood leukocyte count may arise from the hemodilution (expansion of the plasma volume) associated with training, or may represent increased apoptosis (programmed cell death) or altered leukocyte kinetics including a diminished release from the bone marrow. Indeed, the large increase in circulating neutrophil numbers that accompanies a bout of prolonged exercise could, over periods of months or years of heavy training, deplete the bone marrow reserve of these important cells. Certainly, the blood population of these cells seems to be less mature than those found in sedentary individuals (Pyne 1994; Keen *et al.* 1995) and the phagocytic and oxidative burst activity of stimulated neutrophils has been reported to be lower in well-trained cyclists than in age- and weight-matched sedentary controls (Blannin *et al.* 1996).

Some studies have indicated that well-trained individuals have a lower serum complement concentration than in sedentary controls (Mackinnon 1999), but this may reflect only a training-induced hemodilution. There is a weak suggestion of a slightly elevated NK cell count and cytolytic action in trained individuals (Shephard & Shek 1999), but these effects are small and unlikely to be of any clinical significance. Levels of secretory immunoglobulins such as salivary IgA (s-IgA) vary widely between individuals and, although some early studies indicated that s-IgA concentrations are lower in endurance athletes than in sedentary individuals (Tomasi *et al.* 1982), the majority of studies indicate that s-IgA levels are generally not lower in athletes than in non-athletes except when athletes are engaged in very heavy training (Gleeson 2000).

Longitudinal studies in which previously sedentary people are subjected to weeks or months of exercise training have shown that marked changes in immune function do not occur provided that blood samples are taken at least 24 h after the last exercise bout. Furthermore, moderate exercise training in healthy young adults does not appear to have an effect on the initiation of a specific antibody response to vaccination or cell-mediated (delayed-type hypersensitivity) responses as measured by the swelling that arises 48 h after injecting antigens into the skin (Bruunsgaard *et al.* 1997). These *in vivo* measures of immune function are probably more meaningful than *in vitro* individual cell-type functional measures as they represent the whole system response to challenge.

Athletes commonly intensify their training for a few days or weeks at certain stages of the season. This may induce a state of overreaching in which performance is temporarily reduced but, following a period of taper with only light training, results in supercompensation and an increase in performance. Several studies in recent years have investigated the effects of short periods of intensified training on resting immune function and on immunoendocrine responses to endurance exercise. These studies indicate that several indices of neutrophil function appear to be sensitive to the training load. A 2-week period of intensified training in already well-trained triathletes was associated with a 20% fall in the bacterially stimulated neutrophil degranulation response (Robson *et al.* 1999a). Other leukocyte functions including T-lymphocyte $CD4^+ : CD8^+$ ratios, mitogen-stimulated lymphocyte proliferation and antibody synthesis and NK cell cytotoxic activity have been shown to be sensitive to increases in the training load in already well-trained athletes (Verde *et al.* 1992). Levels of secretory immunoglobulins such as s-IgA are lower in athletes engaged in heavy training (Gleeson 2000). However, exercise training in healthy young adults does not appear to have an effect on the initiation of a specific antibody response to vaccination or delayed-type hypersensitivity responses (Bruunsgaard *et al.* 1997). Thus, with chronic periods of very heavy training, several aspects of both innate and adaptive immunity are depressed, but athletes are not clinically immunodeficient. In other words, exercise-induced immunodepression does not put athletes in danger of serious illness, but it could be sufficient to increase the risk of picking up common infections.

Several studies have examined changes in immune function during periods of intensive military training (Shephard 1997; Carins & Booth 2002). Several studies have documented a fall in s-IgA concentration and some (Carins and Booth 2002), although not all (Gomez-Merino *et al.* 2005; Tiolier *et al.* 2005), have observed a negative relationship between s-IgA concentration and occurrence of URTI. In one recent study, an increased URTI incidence during 4 weeks of intense military training was significantly correlated with decreased numbers of circulating NK cells (Gomez-Merino *et al.* 2005). S-IgA was evaluated as a marker of the severity of stress during a 19-day Royal Australian Air Force survival course, during which the 29 participants experienced hunger, thirst, boredom, loneliness, and extreme heat and cold combined with demanding physical effort (Carins & Booth 2002). Reduced food energy intake, consumption of alcohol, body mass loss, occurrence of URTI, and negative emotions were negatively associated with s-IgA concentration or the ratio of s-IgA : albumin and the authors concluded that this ratio is a useful marker of the severity of stresses encountered during stressful training. However, in these situations the training often involves not only strenuous physical activity, but also negative energy balance, sleep deprivation, and psychological challenges. These multiple stressors are likely to induce a pattern of immunoendocrine responses that amplify the exercise-induced alterations.

Few studies have investigated the effects of intensified training on multiple markers of immune function. However, in one such study (Lancaster *et al.* 2003a, 2004), seven healthy endurance-trained men completed three trials consisting of cycling exercise until volitional fatigue at a work rate equivalent to 74% $\dot{V}o_{2max}$. The trials took place in the morning, before and after a 6-day period of intensified training (IT), and after 2 weeks of light recovery training (RT). Normal training (NT) consisted of approximately 10 h of cycling per week; during the IT period, training volume was increased on average by 73%. During RT, exercise was limited to no more than 4 hours per week for 2 weeks. Training intensity and duration were confirmed by the use of heart rate monitors. The percentage and number of T cells producing IFN-γ were lower at rest following the IT period than after normal training. *Ex vivo* stimulated neutrophil oxidative burst activity and lymphocyte proliferation fell after acute exercise and were markedly depressed at rest after the IT period compared with normal training (Fig. 10.4). *Ex vivo* stimulated monocyte oxidative burst activity was unchanged after acute exercise, but was lower at rest following the IT period compared with normal training. Following all acute exercise trials the circulating number of IFN-γ^+ T cells and the amount of IFN-γ produced per cell was decreased. The 6 days of IT did not affect resting s-IgA concentration, but the latter was significantly lower at the end of RT. S-IgA values were 74.2 ± 13.1, 64.6 ± 12.5, and 49.0 ± 10.4 mg·L^{-1} during NT, IT, and RT, respectively. Except for s-IgA, all measured immune parameters were back to normal after 2 weeks of RT. These results indicate that:

1 Acute exhausting exercise causes a temporary fall in several aspects of immune cell function and a decrease in IFN-γ production by T cells;

2 Resting immune function is decreased after only 6 days of IT and these effects are reversible with 2 weeks of relative rest; and

3 In general, the immune response to an acute bout of exhausting exercise is not affected by the weekly training load (or at least not by short-term changes in the weekly training load).

Several longitudinal studies have monitored immune function in high-level athletes over the course of a competitive season. In a recent study of Amer-

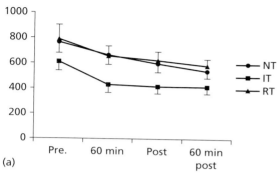 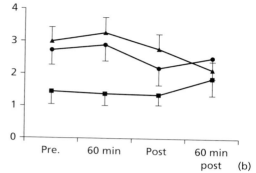

Fig. 10.4 Effect of an exhaustive exercise bout performed during normal training (NT), intensified training (IT), and recovery training (RT) periods on: (a) neutrophil oxidative burst activity (mean fluorescence intensity, MFI); ANOVA revealed significant main effects of time and treatment. (b) Mitogen-stimulated lymphocyte proliferation (stimulation index, SI); ANOVA revealed significant main effects of time and treatment (Lancaster *et al.* 2004). From Gleeson (2005) with permission from Elsevier Ltd.

ican football players, the incidence of URTI was increased during intense training and it was reported that the secretion rate of s-IgA (which represents the amount of s-IgA available on the mucosal surfaces for protection against pathogens) was significantly and inversely related to URTI incidence (Fahlmann & Engels 2005).

In an earlier, much cited study, the impact of long-term training on systemic and mucosal immunity was assessed prospectively in a cohort of elite Australian swimmers over a 7-month training season in preparation for national championships (Gleeson *et al.* 1995, 2004b). The results indicated significant suppression of resting serum IgA, IgG and IgM, and s-IgA concentration in athletes, associated with long-term training at an intensive level. Furthermore, resting s-IgA concentrations at the start of the training period showed significant correlation with infection rates, and the number of infections observed in the swimmers was predicted by the pre-season and mean pre-training s-IgA levels (Fig. 10.5). These studies on mucosal immunity in elite athletes are representative of a very small number of studies that have established a relationship between some measure of immune function and infection incidence in athletes. Among the markers of systemic immunity that were also measured in the study on swimmers (Gleeson *et al.* 1995) there were no significant changes in numbers or percentages of B or T cell subsets, but there was a significant fall in both

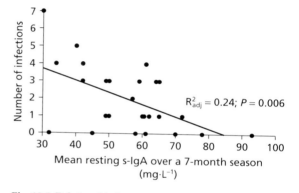

Fig. 10.5 Relationship between numbers of upper respiratory tract infection (URTI) episodes and resting salivary IgA (s-IgA) concentration during a 7-month training season in elite Australian swimmers (Gleeson *et al.* 1995). From Gleeson (2005) with permission from Elsevier Ltd.

NK cell numbers and percentages over the training season.

In a study on competitive cyclists, the total number of leukocytes, T-lymphocyte subsets, mitogen-induced lymphocyte proliferation, and IL-2 production, adherence capacity, and oxidative burst activity of neutrophils were measured at rest at the beginning of a training season, and after 6 months of intensive training and a racing season, during which the athletes were cycling approximately 500 km·week^{-1} (Baj *et al.* 1994). Baseline values of the tested immune parameters were within the range observed in non-trained healthy controls. Significant decreases in absolute numbers of CD3+ and CD4+ cells, diminished IL-2 production, and reduced oxidative burst activity of neutrophils were noted at the end of the season.

A few studies have examined immunologic changes in professional soccer players before, during, and after a full season. In 15 Belgian professional soccer players, a competitive season did not produce any change in the total number of leukocytes but increased neutrophil counts and decreased CD4+ T-lymphocyte counts (Bury *et al*. 1998). There was also a slight decrease in T-cell proliferation and a significant decrease in neutrophil function. On the other hand, training and competitions did not induce significant changes in the number of NK cells or NK cytotoxic activity (Bury *et al*. 1998). In 13 Portuguese players, total leukocyte, and neutrophil numbers and CD8+ cells were increased at the end of the season compared to pre-season values, and the CD4 : CD8 ratio was decreased (Rebelo *et al*. 1998). In an unpublished study of an English premier league squad that was monitored during the 2001–2002 season, we found that the mean total leukocyte, neutrophil, monocyte and lymphocyte counts, and the CD4 : CD8 ratio did not change. During the season, however, the concentrations of some lymphocyte subpopulations were changed: CD45RO+ (memory) T cells showed significant decreases, falling to very low levels by the end of the season whereas the numbers of CD45RA+ (naïve) T cells increased. CD45RO expression on T cells also fell after 22 and 33 weeks and a significant fall in NK cells was evident at the end of the season. During the competitive period, s-IgA concentration and MHC class II expression on monocytes were lowest at 11 weeks when form (wins : losses ratio and league position) was lowest. Plasma cortisol levels were unchanged at the end of the season but testosterone levels were approximately 20% lower than pre-season. Cells positive for CD45RO are actually a mixture of memory cells, important in long-term recognition of antigens and in generating the acquired immune response to recall antigens, and short-term activated T cells. The loss of these cell types and the fewer number of circulating NK cells could be viewed as disadvantageous to the body's defense against viral infection.

There are several possible causes of the diminution of immune function associated with heavy training. One mechanism may simply be the cumulative effects of repeated bouts of intense exercise with the consequent elevation of stress hormones, particularly glucocorticoids such as cortisol, causing temporary immunosuppression. It is known that both acute glucocorticosteroid administration (Moynihan *et al*. 1998) and exercise (Northoff *et al*. 1998; Lancaster *et al*. 2004) cause a temporary inhibition of IFN-γ production by T lymphocytes and it has been suggested that this may be an important mechanism in exercise-induced depression of immune cell functions (Northoff *et al*. 1998). When exercise is repeated frequently there may not be sufficient time for the immune system to recover fully. Furthermore, plasma glutamine levels can change substantially after exercise and may become chronically depressed after repeated bouts of prolonged strenuous training. Glutamine is an important fuel for lymphocytes and is also a precursor for the synthesis of nucleotide bases needed for the replication of DNA during lymphocyte proliferation. However, the evidence for a role of decreased plasma glutamine availability in exercise-induced immune depression is weak (Walsh *et al*. 2000; Hiscock & Pedersen 2002; Gleeson *et al*. 2004a).

Methodologic problems in exercise immunology studies

The response of various components of the immune system to exercise is transient and quite variable, depending upon the type of exercise, the immunologic methodology used, the intensity of effort relative to the fitness of the individual, and the timing of the observations. Effects disappear usually within 24 h post-exercise. Many findings are method-dependent; blood analyses are time-consuming, and so some investigators collect few blood samples. Delaying sample-taking by 30 min after exercise may lead to quite different results, and all blood measures will be affected by hemoconcentration. Responses may also be influenced by natural circadian variations in circulating lymphocyte numbers and plasma hormone (e.g., cortisol) concentrations, yet many studies do not include non-exercising time-controls in their protocols. Overall and differential white blood cell counts can also be modified by changes in blood volume, margination and demargination of cells, modification of leukocyte–endothelial interactions, sympathetic and parasympathetic neural activity, and cell redistribution with the release of granulocytes from bone marrow. Thus, changes in populations of cells may be responsible for some apparent changes in leukocyte functions.

Numerous studies report effects of exercise on functions of isolated leukocytes when these cells are stimulated *in vitro* by added antigens or mitogens. However, it is difficult to extrapolate from the *ex vivo* stimulated response of isolated cells how these same cells would respond in the far more complex *in vivo* environment. In addition to the presence of antigens, leukocyte function is also influenced by endogenous chemicals including hormones, neurotransmitters and cytokines, and the plasma concentration of these may change during exercise. The pH and temperature of the blood also change during exercise, but these factors are often ignored in experiments on isolated cell types. Thus, separating cells from their *in vivo* environment is somewhat artificial and to a large degree excludes the effects of exercise-induced chemical changes in the blood that will undoubtedly modify leukocyte function. The closest one can get to the *in vivo* condition is by performing measurements on whole blood, in which the proximity between the leukocytes and the extracellular milieu is retained. Another limitation in the interpretation of such studies, even where multiple parameters are assessed, is that no instruments are presently available to predict the cumulative effects of several small changes in immune system parameters on host resistance (Keil *et al.* 2001). Furthermore, it should be borne in mind that only 0.2% of the total leukocyte mass is circulating at any moment; the remainder is in lymphoid tissue, the bone marrow, and other tissues. It may thus be more important to assess the status of leukocytes in the skin, mucosa, and lymph nodes rather than in the blood.

Self-reporting of symptoms of URTI using questionnaires has been used in a number of studies designed to evaluate the effects of acute prolonged exercise (e.g., running a marathon) or periods of intensified training on infection incidence. This approach leaves such studies open to the criticism that the reporting of symptoms, such as sore throat, runny nose, congestion, or fever is subjective and that factors other than infection, such as allergies, inhalation of air pollutants, and airway inflammation, could also cause some of these symptoms. Of course, infection risk not only depends on immune system status, but also on the degree of exposure to pathogens and the experience of previous exposure. The average incidence of URTI in adults in developed countries is 1–2 episodes per individual per year (Matthews *et al.* 2002) and URTI incidence is highest in the winter months (Heath *et al.* 1991; Matthews *et al.* 2002). Thus, epidemiologic or exercise intervention studies require large numbers of subjects who are followed over a time period that is sufficiently long to detect potential differences in infection incidence resulting from differences in exercise participation. Questionnaires may also be used to evaluate duration and severity of episodes of symptomatic illness, and similar limitations apply to these.

Furthermore, in studies using postal questionnaires, if the reported incidence of respiratory symptoms is compared with anticipated infection rates for the general population, there may be a response bias. For example, in a study on infection incidence following a marathon race (Nieman *et al.* 1990), only 47% of questionnaires were returned, and the respondents may have been mainly those who developed symptoms. Thus, it is preferable that infections are clinically confirmed rather than self-reported. The presence of an infection verified by the isolation of a virus or bacterium from body fluid samples or an increase in the pathogen-specific antibody titre would be the gold standard in this regard.

Recently, a surveillance study was conducted over a 5-month summer/autumn competition season to identify the pathogenic aetiology and symptomatology of upper respiratory illness (URI) in highly trained elite athletes ($n = 32$), recreationally competitive athletes ($n = 31$), and untrained sedentary controls ($n = 20$) (Spence *et al.* 2005). Nasopharyngeal and throat swabs were collected on subjects presenting with two or more defined upper respiratory symptoms. Swabs were analyzed using microscopy/

culture/sensitivity and polymerase chain reaction (PCR) testing for bacterial, viral, chlamydial, and mycoplasmal respiratory pathogens. The Wisconsin Upper Respiratory Symptom Survey (WURSS-44) questionnaire was administered to assess the daily symptomatology and functional impairment. A total of 37 URI episodes in 28 subjects were reported (9 controls, 7 recreationally competitive exercisers, and 21 elite athletes). The overall distribution mimicked the J-shaped curve with rate ratios for illness higher in both the control (1.93; 95% CI, 0.72–5.18) and elite (4.50; 95% CI, 1.91–10.59) cohorts than the referent recreationally competitive athlete cohort. However, of these 37 episodes, infectious agents were identified in only 11 (30%) (two control, three recreationally competitive exercisers, and six elite athletes). No pathogens were identified in 26 episodes of URI. Specific global symptom, total symptom, and functional impairment severity scores were higher in subjects with an infectious URI episode, particularly on illness days 3–5. These findings strongly suggest that URI in elite athletes is seldom infectious and the symptomatology is distinct between infectious and non-infectious episodes. Non-infectious causes of URI should be considered and investigated to identify alternative mechanisms and mediators.

Conclusions

Despite the aforementioned limitations, there are sufficient reliable data to establish the immunologic response to acute exercise and periods of intensified training. In summary, acute bouts of prolonged strenuous exercise cause a temporary depression of various aspects of immune function, such as neutrophil oxidative burst, lymphocyte proliferation, monocyte MHC class II expression, and NK cell cytotoxic activity that lasts approximately 3–24 h after exercise, depending on the intensity and duration of the exercise bout. Post-exercise immune function depression is most pronounced when the exercise is continuous, prolonged (>1.5 h), of moderate to high intensity (55–75% $\dot{V}o_{2max}$), and performed without food intake. Periods of intensified training that result in overreaching are associated with chronically depressed immune function. Although elite athletes are not clinically immunodeficient, it is possible that the combined effects of small changes in several immune parameters may compromise resistance to common minor illnesses such as URTI. Protracted immune depression linked with prolonged training may determine susceptibility to infection, particularly at times of major competitions. Hundreds of studies have now been conducted that confirm both acute and chronic effects of exercise on the immune system, yet there are still very few studies that have been able to show a link between exercise-induced immune depression and increased incidence of illness in athletes. This is an important issue that needs to be addressed in future studies, although it must be recognized that this will be a difficult task. Even amongst the general population, we do not know the impact of small changes in specific immune parameters on risk of infection. Most clinical studies have been concerned only with the risk of life-threatening illness in immunodeficient patients, and not with the risk of picking up common infections such as colds and flu.

References

Andersen, L.L., Tufekovic, G., Zebis, M.K., et al. (2005) The effect of resistance training combined with timed ingestion of protein on muscle fiber size and muscle strength. *Metabolism* **54**, 151–156.

Baj, Z., Kantorski, J., Majewska, E., et al. (1994) Immunological status of competitive cyclists before and after the training season. *International Journal of Sports Medicine* **15**, 319–324.

Berk, L.S., Ton, S.A., Nieman, D.C. & Eby, E.C. (1986) The suppressive effect of stress from acute exhaustive exercise on T-lymphocyte helper/suppressor ratio in athletes and non-athletes. *Medicine and Science in Sports and Exercise* **18**, 706–710.

Bird, S.P., Tarpenning, K.M. & Marino, F.E. (2006) Independent and combined effects of liquid carbohydrate/essential amino acid ingestion on hormonal adaptations and muscle fibre size following resistance training. *European Journal of Applied Physiology* **97**, 225–238.

Blannin, A.K., Chatwin, L.J., Cave, R. & Gleeson, M. (1996) Effects of submaximal cycling and long-term endurance training on neutrophil phagocytic activity in middle-aged men. *British Journal of Sports Medicine* **30**, 125–129.

Bruunsgaard, H., Hartkopp, A., Mohr, T., et al. (1997) In vivo cell-mediated immunity and vaccination response following prolonged, intense exercise. *Medicine and Science in Sports and Exercise* **29**, 1176–1181.

Bury, T., Marechal, R., Mahieu, P. & Pirnay, F. (1998) Immunological status of competitive football players during the training season. *International Journal of Sports Medicine* **19**, 364–368.

Carins, J. & Booth, C. (2002) Salivary immunoglobulin-A as a marker of stress during strenuous physical training. *Aviation Space and Environmental Medicine* **73**, 1203–1207.

Dandona, P., Aljada, A. & Bandyopadhyay, A. (2004) Inflammation: the link between insulin resistance, obesity and diabetes. *Trends in Immunology* **25**, 4–7.

Fahlman, M.M. & Engels, H.J. (2005) Mucosal IgA and URTI in American college football players: A year longitudinal study. *Medicine and Science in Sports and Exercise* **37**, 374–380.

Fischer, C.P., Hiscock, N.J., Penkowa, M., *et al.* (2004) Vitamin C and E supplementation inhibits the release of interleukin-6 from contracting human skeletal muscle. *Journal of Physiology* **558**, 633–645.

Gannon, G.A., Rhind, S., Shek, P.N. & Shephard, R.J. (2002) Naïve and memory T cell subsets are differentially mobilized during physical stress. *International Journal of Sports Medicine* **23**, 223–229.

Gleeson, M. (2000) Mucosal immune responses and risk of respiratory illness in elite athletes. *Exercise Immunology Review* **6**, 5–42.

Gleeson, M., ed. (2005) *Immune Function in Sport and Exercise. Advances in Sport and Exercise Science Series*. Elsevier, Edinburgh.

Gleeson. M. & Bishop, N.C. (1999) Immunology. In: *Basic and Applied Sciences for Sports Medicine* (Maughan, R.J., ed.) Butterworth Heinemann, Oxford: 199–236.

Gleeson, M., McDonald, W.A., Cripps, A.W., Pyne, D.B., Clancy, R.L. & Fricker, P.A. (1995) The effect on immunity of long-term intensive training in elite swimmers. *Clinical and Experimental Immunology* **102**, 210–211.

Gleeson, M., Nieman, D.C. & Pedersen, B.K. (2004a) Exercise, nutrition and immune function. *Journal of Sports Sciences* **22**, 115–125.

Gleeson, M., Pyne, D.B. & Callister, R. (2004b) The missing links in exercise effects on mucosal immunity. *Exercise Immunology Review* **10**, 107–128.

Gomez-Merino, D., Drogou, C., Chennaoui, M., Tiollier, E., Mathieu, J. & Guezennec, C.Y. (2005) Effects of combined stress during intense training on cellular immunity, hormones and respiratory infections. *Neuroimmunomodulation* **12**, 164–172.

Heath, G.W., Ford, E.S., Craven, T.E., Macera, C.A., Jackson, K.L. & Pate, R.R. (1991) Exercise and the incidence of upper respiratory tract infections. *Medicine and Science in Sports and Exercise* **23**, 152–157.

Hiscock, N. & Pedersen, B.K. (2002) Exercise-induced immunodepression: plasma glutamine is not the link. *Journal of Applied Physiology* **93**, 813–822.

Keen, P., McCarthy, D.A., Passfield, L., Shaker, H.A.A. & Wade, A.J. (1995) Leukocyte and erythrocyte counts during a multi-stage cycling race ("The Milk Race"). *British Journal of Sports Medicine* **29**, 61–65.

Keil, D., Luebke, R.W. & Pruett, S.B. (2001) Quantifying the relationship between multiple immunological parameters and host resistance: probing the limits of reductionism. *Journal of Immunology* **167**, 4543–4552.

Koopman, R., Wagenmakers, A.J., Manders, R.J., *et al.* (2005) Combined ingestion of protein and free leucine with carbohydrate increases postexercise muscle protein synthesis *in vivo* in male subjects. *American Journal of Physiology* **288**, E645–E653.

Lancaster, G.L., Halson, S.L., Khan, Q., *et al.* (2003a) Effect of acute exhaustive exercise and a 6-day period of intensified training on immune function in cyclists. *Journal of Physiology* **548P**, O96.

Lancaster, G.L., Halson, S.L., Khan, Q., *et al.* (2003b) Effect of exhaustive exercise and intensified training on human T-lymphocyte CD45RO expression. *Journal of Physiology* **548P**, O97.

Lancaster, G.L., Halson, S.L., Khan, Q., *et al.* (2004) The effects of acute exhaustive exercise and intensified training on type 1/type 2 T cell distribution and cytokine production. *Exercise Immunology Review* **10**, 91–106.

Lancaster, G.L., Halson, S.L., Khan, Q., *et al.* (2005a) The physiological regulation of toll-like receptor expression and function in humans. *Journal of Physiology* **563**, 945–955.

Lancaster, G.I., Khan, Q., Drysdale, P.T., *et al.* (2005b) Effect of prolonged strenuous exercise and carbohydrate ingestion on type 1 and type 2 T lymphocyte distribution and intracellular cytokine production in humans. *Journal of Applied Physiology* **98**, 565–571.

Mackinnon, L.T. (1999) *Advances in Exercise and Immunology*. Human Kinetics, Champaign, IL.

Matthews, C.E., Ockene, I.S., Freedson, P.S., Rosal, M.C., Merriam, P.A. & Hebert, J.R. (2002) Moderate to vigorous physical activity and the risk of upper-respiratory tract infection. *Medicine and Science in Sports and Exercise* **34**, 1242–1248.

Moynihan, J.A., Callahan, T.A., Kelley, S.P. & Campbell, L.M. (1998) Adrenal hormone modulation of type 1 and type 2 cytokine production by spleen cells: dexamethasone and dehydroepiandrosterone suppress interleukin-2, interleukin-4, and interferon-gamma production *in vitro*. *Cell Immunology* **184**, 58–64.

Nehlsen-Cannarella, S.L., Fagoaga, O.R., Nieman, D.C., *et al.* (1997) Carbohydrate and the cytokine response to 2.5 h of running. *Journal of Applied Physiology* **82**, 1662–1667.

Nieman, D.C. (1994) Exercise, infection and immunity. *International Journal of Sports Medicine* **15**, S131–S141.

Nieman, D.C. (1998) Influence of carbohydrate on the immune responses to intensive, prolonged exercise. *Exercise Immunology Review* **4**, 64–76.

Nieman, D.C. (2000) Is infection risk linked to exercise workload? *Medicine and Science in Sports and Exercise* **32**, S406–S411.

Nieman, D.C., Johansen, L.M., Lee, J.W. & Arabatzis, K. (1990) Infectious episodes in runners before and after the Los Angeles Marathon. *Journal of Sports Medicine and Physical Fitness* **30**, 316–328.

Niess, A.M., Dickhuth, H.H., Northoff, H. & Fehrenbach, E. (1999) Free radicals and oxidative stress in exercise: immunological aspects. *Exercise Immunology Review* **5**, 22–56.

Northoff, H., Berg, A. & Weinstock, C. (1998) Similarities and differences of the immune response to exercise and trauma: the IFN-γ concept. *Canadian Journal of Physiology and Pharmacology* **76**, 497–504.

Pedersen, B.K. & Bruunsgaard, H. (1995) How physical exercise influences the establishment of infections. *Sports Medicine* **19**, 393–400.

Peters, E.M. & Bateman, E.D. (1983) Ultramarathon running and URTI: an epidemiological survey. *South African Medical Journal* **64**, 582–584.

Peters, E.M., Goetzsche, J.M., Grobbelaar, B. & Noakes, T.D. (1993) Vitamin C supplementation reduces the incidence of post-race symptoms of upper respiratory tract infection in ultramarathon runners. *American Journal of Clinical Nutrition* **57**, 170–174.

Peters, E.M., Goetzsche, J.M., Joseph, L.E. & Noakes, T.D. (1996) Vitamin C as effective as combinations of anti-oxidant nutrients in reducing symptoms of upper respiratory tract infections in ultramarathon runners. *South African Journal of Sports Medicine* **11**, 23–27.

Pilegaard, H., Keller, C., Steensberg, A., *et al.* (2002) Influence of pre-exercise muscle glycogen content on exercise-induced transcriptional regulation of metabolic genes. *Journal of Physiology* **541**, 261–271.

Pyne, D.B. (1994) Regulation of neutrophil function during exercise. *Sports Medicine* **17**, 245–258.

Rebelo, A.N., Candeias, J.R., Fraga, M.M., *et al.* (1998) The impact of soccer training on the immune system. *Journal of Sports Medicine and Physical Fitness* **38**, 258–261.

Robson, P.J., Blannin, A.K., Walsh, N.P., Bishop, N.C. & Gleeson, M. (1999a) The effect of an acute period of intense interval training on human neutrophil function and plasma glutamine in endurance-trained male runners. *Journal of Physiology* **515**, 84–85.

Robson, P.J., Blannin, A.K., Walsh, N.P., Castell, L.M. & Gleeson, M. (1999b) Effects of exercise intensity, duration and recovery on *in vitro* neutrophil function in male athletes. *International Journal of Sports Medicine* **20**, 128–135.

Ronsen, O., Pedersen, B.K., Oritsland, T.R., Bahr, R. & Kjeldsen-Kragh, J. (2001) Leukocyte counts and lymphocyte responsiveness associated with repeated bouts of strenuous endurance exercise. *Journal of Applied Physiology* **91**, 425–434.

Schnare, M., Barton, G.M., Holt, A.C., Takeda, K., Akira, S. & Medzhitov, R. (2001) Toll-like receptors control activation of adaptive immune responses. *Nature Immunology* **2**, 947–950.

Shephard, R.J. (1997) *Physical Activity, Training and the Immune Response.* Cooper, Carmel, CA.

Shephard, R.J. & Shek, P.N. (1999) Effects of exercise and training on natural killer cell counts and cytolytic activity: a meta-analysis. *Sports Medicine* **28**, 177–195.

Spence, L., Nissen, M.D., Sloots, T.P., *et al.* (2005) Upper respiratory illness aetiology and symptomatology in elite and recreationally competitive athletes. *Brain, Behavior and Immunity* **19**, 469–470.

Starkie, R.L., Ostrowski, S.R., Jauffred, S., Febbraio, M. & Pedersen, B.K. (2003) Exercise and IL-6 infusion inhibit endotoxin-induced TNF-alpha production in humans. *FASEB Journal* **17**, 884–886.

Starkie, R.L., Rolland, J., Angus, D.J., Anderson, M.J. & Febbraio, M. (2001) Circulating monocytes are not the source of elevations in plasma IL-6 and TNF-alpha levels after prolonged running. *American Journal of Physiology* **280**, C769–C774.

Steensberg, A., Fischer, C.P., Keller, C., Moller, K. & Pedersen, B.K. (2003) IL-6 enhances plasma IL-1ra, IL-10, and cortisol in humans. *American Journal of Physiology* **285**, E433–E437.

Steensberg, A., van Hall, G., Osada, T., Sacchetti, M., Saltin, B. & Pedersen, B.K. (2000) Production of interleukin-6 in contracting human skeletal muscles can account for the exercise-induced increase in plasma interleukin-6. *Journal of Physiology* **529**, 237–242.

Tiollier, E., Gomez-Merino, D., Burnat, P., *et al.* (2005) Intense training: mucosal immunity and incidence of respiratory infections. *European Journal of Applied Physiology* **93**, 421–428.

Tomasi, T.B., Trudeau, F.B. & Czerwinski, D. (1982) Immune parameters in athletes before and after strenuous exercise. *Journal of Clinical Immunology* **2**, 173–178.

Verde, T.J., Thomas, S.G., Moore, R.W., Shek, P. & Shephard, R.J. (1992) Immune responses and increased training of the elite athlete. *Journal of Applied Physiology* **73**, 1494–1499.

Walsh, N.P., Blannin, A.K., Bishop, N.C., Robson, P.J. & Gleeson, M. (2000) Effect of oral glutamine supplementation on human neutrophil lipopolysaccharide-stimulated degranulation following prolonged exercise. *International Journal of Sport Nutrition and Exercise Metabolism* **10**, 39–50.

Woods, J., Lu, Q., Ceddia, M.A. & Lowder, T. (2000) Special feature for the Olympics: effects of exercise on the immune system: exercise-induced modulation of macrophage function. *Immunology and Cell Biology* **78**, 545–553.

Chapter 11

Exercise, Inflammation, and Metabolism

BENTE K. PEDERSEN

During the past few years, skeletal muscle has been identified as an endocrine organ, which produces and releases cytokines, also named myokines. This discovery suggests a new scientific paradigm: skeletal muscle is an endocrine organ which by contraction stimulates the production and release of cytokines, which can influence metabolism and modify cytokine production in other tissues and organs (Fig. 11.1). The discovery of adipose tissue as a secretory organ in the mid 1990s has been a dominating research area in the past decade, giving rise to the identification of new regulatory peptides (e.g., leptin and adiponectin) and their receptors. Visceral and subcutaneous adipose tissues have been regarded as the major sources of cytokines (adipokines); however, the finding that muscles produce and release cytokines (myokines) suggests that working skeletal muscle may be an alternative major source of secreted molecules. Muscle-derived myokines are likely to be important "messengers" conveying the beneficial health effects of exercise. In particular, they may play a role in combating chronic diseases associated with low-grade inflammation. This chapter describes the link between exercise, inflammation, and metabolism and discusses to what extent anti-inflammatory activity induced by regular exercise may exert its beneficial health effects.

Chronic diseases linked with low-grade systemic inflammation

Cardiovascular disease and type 2 diabetes are not only primary causes of morbidity and mortality in developed countries, but are also becoming the dominating health problem worldwide (Murray & Lopez 1997). Regular exercise offers protection against all-cause mortality, primarily by protecting against atherosclerosis and type 2 diabetes (Blair et al. 2001). In addition, physical training is effective in the treatment of patients with ischemic heart disease and type 2 diabetes (Pedersen & Saltin2006).

Over the past decade there has been an increasing focus on the role of inflammation in the pathogenesis of atherosclerosis (Libby 2002). Furthermore, inflammation has been suggested to be a key factor in insulin resistance (Dandona et al. 2004). Low-grade chronic inflammation is reflected by an increase in the systemic levels of some cytokines (Ross 1999) as well as in C-reactive protein (CRP). Several reports investigating various markers of inflammation have confirmed an association between low-grade systemic inflammation on one hand and atherosclerosis and type 2 diabetes on the other (Festa et al. 2002).

Evidence for prescribing exercise as therapy in chronic diseases

Considerable knowledge has accumulated in recent decades concerning the significance of physical activity in the treatment of a number of diseases, including those that do not primarily manifest as

The Olympic Textbook of Science in Sport, 1st edition. Edited by R.J. Maughan. Published 2009 by Blackwell Publishing. ISBN: 978-1-4051-5638-7.

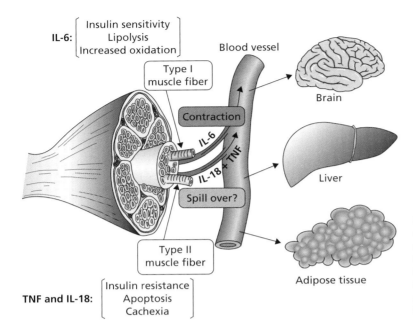

Fig. 11.1 Skeletal muscle is an endocrine organ, which expresses and releases cytokines (myokines) into the circulation and potentially influences the metabolism and inflammatory status in other tissues and organs. IL, interleukin; TNF, tumor necrosis factor.

disorders of the locomotive apparatus (Pedersen & Saltin 2006).

Insulin resistance

Few studies have examined the isolated effect of training on the prevention of diabetes in patients with impaired glucose tolerance, but there is good evidence for a beneficial effect of combined physical training and dietary modification. Two randomized controlled trials including people with impaired glucose tolerance have found that lifestyle modification protects against the development of type 2 diabetes (Tuomilehto *et al.* 2001; Knowler *et al.* 2002). A Finnish trial randomized 522 overweight, middle-aged people with impaired glucose tolerance to physical training combined with diet, or to a control group, and followed them for 3.2 years (Tuomilehto *et al.* 2001). The results showed that the risk of type 2 diabetes was reduced by 58% in the intervention group, with the greatest effect seen with the patients who made the biggest lifestyle modification. An American trial randomized 3234 people with impaired glucose tolerance to either treatment with metformin, lifestyle modification entailing dietary

change and at least 150 min of physical exercise weekly, or to a placebo group, and followed them for 2.8 years (Knowler *et al.* 2002). In support of the results of the Finnish study (Tuomilehto *et al.* 2001) it was found that modifying lifestyle reduced the risk of type 2 diabetes by 58%, whereas treatment with metformin only reduced the risk by 31%. Although it is not possible to determine the isolated effect of increased physical activity in these trials, results strongly suggest that exercise protects against the development of type 2 diabetes in patients with insulin resistance.

Type 2 diabetes

The beneficial effect of training in patients with type 2 diabetes is well-documented, and there is international consensus that physical training comprises one of the three cornerstones of the treatment of diabetes, together with diet and medicine. A meta-analysis published in 2001, including 14 controlled clinical trials encompassing a total of 504 patients, examined the effect of a minimum of eight weeks of physical training on glycemic control (Boule *et al.* 2001). Twelve of the trials examined the effect of aerobic training [mean (SD): 3.4 (0.9) times·wk^{-1} for 18 (15) wk], while two examined the effect of strength conditioning [mean (SD): 10 (0.7) exercises, 2.5 (0.7) sets, 13 (0.7) repetitions, 2.5 (0.4) times·wk^{-1} for 15 (10) wk]. No differences could be identified between the effect of aerobic training and strength conditioning. Neither could any dose-response effect be demonstrated relative to either the intensity or the duration of training. Post-intervention glycosylated hemoglobin (HbA1c) was lower in the exercise groups than in the control groups (7.65 vs. 8.31%; weighted mean difference, 0.66%; $P < 0.001$). In comparison, intensive glycemic control with metformin reduced HbA1c by 0.6%, whereas it reduced the risk of diabetes-related complications by 32%, and the risk of diabetes-related mortality by 42% [UK Prospective Diabetes Study (UKPDS) Group 1998]. A meta-analysis encompassing 95 783 non-diabetic individuals showed that cardiovascular morbidity is strongly correlated to fasting blood glucose levels (Coutinho et al. 1999). The effect of physical training on HbA1c is thus clinically relevant and there is evidence to support exercise recommendations in patients with type 2 diabetes.

Coronary heart disease

The evidence for a beneficial effect of physical training in patients with coronary heart disease is strong. Physical training improves survival and is believed to have direct effects on the pathogenesis of the disease (Pedersen & Saltin 2006). A meta-analysis was published in 2004 (Taylor et al. 2004) based on 48 randomized, controlled trials and 8940 patients. The patients were typically randomized at the time of acute myocardial infarction or up to six weeks thereafter. Exercise was predominantly aerobic training, but varied considerably with regard to frequency, intensity, and duration. Exercise-based cardiac rehabilitation reduced all-cause mortality by 20% [odds ratio (OR): 0.80; 95% confidence interval (CI) 0.68–0.93]. Exercise-based cardiac rehabilitation reduced cardiac mortality by 26% (OR 0.74; 95% CI 0.61–0.96), although there was no effect on non-fatal myocardial infarction. Total cholesterol and triglyceride levels and systolic blood pressure were also found to be reduced in the exercise-based group,

and more of these patients ceased smoking (OR 0.64; 95% CI 0.50–0.83). In summary, exercise has pronounced health outcome effects in patients with cardiac disease.

The players in chronic low-grade inflammation and its link with chronic disease

The local inflammatory response is accompanied by a systemic response, known as the acute-phase response (Petersen & Pedersen 2005). This response includes the production of a large number of hepatocyte-derived acute phase proteins, such as CRP, and can be mimicked by the injection of the cytokines tumor necrosis factor-alpha (TNF-α), interleukin-1beta (IL-1β), and interleukin-6 (IL-6) into laboratory animals or humans. The initial cytokines in the cytokine cascade are (named in order): TNF-α, IL-1β, IL-6, interleukin-1 receptor antagonist (IL-1ra), and soluble TNF receptors (sTNF-R). IL-1ra inhibits IL-1 signal transduction, and sTNF-R represents the naturally occurring inhibitors of TNF-α. In response to an acute infection or trauma, cytokine and cytokine inhibitor levels may increase three- to four-fold, and then decrease again after recovery. Chronic low-grade systemic inflammation has been introduced as a term for conditions in which a two- to three-fold increase in the systemic concentrations of TNF-α, IL-1, IL-6, IL-1ra, sTNF-R, and CRP is seen. The stimuli for cytokine production during low-grade inflammation are not known, but the likely origin of TNF in chronic low-grade systemic inflammation is mainly the adipose tissue.

The systemic cytokine response to exercise

In sepsis and experimental models of sepsis, the cytokine cascade consists of (in named order): TNF-α, IL-1β, IL-6, IL-1ra, sTNF-R, and IL-10 (Akira et al. 1993). The first two cytokines in the cytokine cascade, TNF-α and IL-1β, which are produced locally. These are usually referred to as pro-inflammatory cytokines, and can stimulate the production of IL-6, which has been classified as both a pro- and an anti-inflammatory cytokine. The cytokine response to

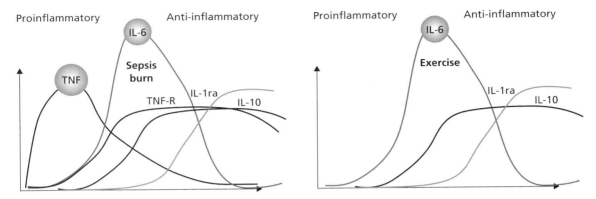

Fig. 11.2 In sepsis, the cytokine cascade within the first few hours consists of tumor necrosis factor-alpha (TNF-α), interleukin-6 (IL-6), interleukin-1 receptor antagonist (IL-1ra), tumor necrosis factor receptor (TNF-R), and interleukin-10 (IL-10). The cytokine response to exercise does not include TNF-α but does show a marked increase in IL-6, which is followed by IL-1ra, TNF-R, and IL-10. Increased C-reactive protein (CRP) levels do not appear until 8–12 h later.

exercise differs from that elicited by severe infections (Fig. 11.2). Typically, IL-6 is the first cytokine released into the circulation; the levels of circulating IL-6 increase in an exponential fashion (up to 100-fold) in response to exercise, and decline in the post-exercise period (Pedersen & Hoffman-Goetz 2000; Pedersen *et al.* 2001; Febbraio & Pedersen 2002; Suzuki *et al.* 2002).

The fact that the classic pro-inflammatory cytokines, TNF-α and IL-1β, in general do not increase with exercise indicates that the cytokine cascade induced by exercise markedly differs from the cytokine cascade induced by infections. In the post-exercise period the circulating levels of well-known anti-inflammatory cytokines – cytokine inhibitors such as IL-1ra and sTNF-R – rise and the levels of chemokines such as IL-8 may or may not increase. Taken together, exercise provokes an increase in the systemic concentrations of cytokines, primarily in IL-6, followed by an increase in IL-1ra and IL-10 (Pedersen & Febbraio 2008).

Searching for the exercise factor

The question is whether a cytokine should be classified as an exercise factor. For most of the last century researchers have searched for a muscle contraction-induced factor that mediates some of the exercise effects in other tissues such as the liver and adipose tissue.

Erling Asmussen discussed this factor in his introductory talk in a symposium held in Dallas in January 1966. He stated that: "For every state of physical exercise, there is a carefully controlled level of pulmonary function, ventilation of cardiac output, and of deep body temperature. These levels are maintained at least as precisely as the resting level, and the controlling feedback systems are the same in exercise as during rest; only the set-point has been changed. For years the search for the stimulus that initiates and maintains this change of excitability or sensibility of the regulating centers in exercise has been going on. For lack of more precise knowledge, it has been called the 'work stimulus' or 'the work factor.'" It has recently been suggested that the term "exercise factor" should be used to cover the effects of muscle contractions as such. It has become clear that the signaling pathways from contracting muscles to other organs are not associated with the nervous system, as electrical stimulation of paralyzed muscles in patients with spinal cord injuries induces, in essence, the same physiological changes as those in intact subjects (Pedersen *et al.* 2003).

Presently, two cytokines are candidates for the term "exercise factor:" Muscle-derived IL-6 represents a link between skeletal muscle and peripheral organs such as adipose tissue and the liver, whereas IL-8 may be released from skeletal muscle to exert its actions mainly locally within the muscle itself.

The biologic role of muscle-derived IL-8 has not yet been defined, but it is likely that it is involved in mediating exercise-induced angiogenesis. It has been suggested that muscle-derived cytokines that fulfill the criteria of "exercise factors" are termed "myokines." Only IL-6 will be discussed in the present review as IL-8 does not seem to play a major role in metabolism (Akerstrom *et al.* 2005).

IL-6 and its receptor

IL-6 is a pleiotropic cytokine that is produced by many cell types (e.g., macrophages, monocytes, and endothelial cells). Until recently, IL-6 was regarded a cytokine with mainly immunomodulatory effects, and immune cells were believed to be the major source of production. However, the findings that high amounts are produced and released from skeletal muscle in response to muscle contractions, suggest that IL-6 may be an important mediator of the beneficial effects of exercise and that muscle-derived IL-6 works in a hormone-like manner and exerts its effects on glucose and lipid metabolism.

IL-6 belongs to the IL-6 family of cytokines, including IL-11, oncostatin M, leukemia inhibitory factor, ciliary neurotrophic factor, cardiotrophin-1, and cardiotrophin-like cytokine. These cytokines are characterized by their common use of the gp130 (also known as IL-6Rβ or CD130) receptor as a signaling subunit. The two IL-6 receptors, gp130 and IL-6Rα (also known as gp80 or CD126), belong to the type I cytokine receptor family, which, in addition to the above cytokines, comprises leptin, growth hormone, prolactin, erythropoietin, thrombopoietin, and granulocyte- and granulocyte/macrophage-colony stimulating factors (Kamimura *et al.* 2003; Kristiansen & Mandrup-Poulsen 2005).

The human IL-6 gene (IL6, Online Mendelian Inheritance in Man #147620) maps to chromosome 7p21. *Escherichia coli*-derived non-glycosylated recombinant human or mouse IL-6 exhibits the same potency as the glycosylated natural IL-6, suggesting that the carbohydrate moieties are not important for *in vitro* biological activity. In comparison with mouse IL-6, human IL-6 exhibits only approximately 65 and 42% sequence identity at the nucleotide and amino acid levels, respectively (Kamimura *et al.* 2003).

There are several polymorphisms in and close to IL-6. Studies investigating the genetic association between IL-6 polymorphisms and disease have mainly focused on the three common single nucleotide polymorphisms (SNP) in the IL-6 promoter: IL-6-174G > C, IL-6-572A > G, and IL-6-597A > G. IL-6-174G > C, which has been suggested to functionally affect IL-6 promoter activity, is a suitable haplotype marker for the common IL-6 promoter polymorphisms.

The human IL-6 protein comprises 212 amino acids with a signal peptide of 27 amino acids and two potential amino (NH_2)-linked glycosylation sites. The molecular weight ranges from 21 to 28 kDa. Human IL-6Rα comprises 449 amino acids in its mature form but has only 82 amino acids in its cytoplasmic domain. IL-6Rα occurs as a membrane-bound form and at least two soluble forms generated by proteolytic cleavage of the membrane-bound form or by alternative splicing are also produced.

Exercise and IL-6

Compared to other cytokines, the appearance of IL-6 in the circulation is by far the most marked and its appearance precedes that of the other cytokines (Pedersen & Hoffman-Goetz 2000; Pedersen *et al.* 2001, 2003; Febbraio & Pedersen 2002). A marked increase in circulating levels of IL-6 after exercise in the absence of muscle damage has been a remarkably consistent finding. Plasma-IL-6 increases in an exponential fashion with exercise and is related to exercise intensity, duration, the mass of muscle recruited, and to endurance capacity. A two-fold increase in plasma IL-6 is seen after only 6 min of maximal rowing exercise. In contrast, during prolonged endurance activity, IL-6 does not appear until later during exercise (Pedersen & Fischer 2007). Data from the Copenhagen Marathon race (n = 56) suggested a correlation between intensity of exercise and the increase in plasma IL-6 (Pedersen & Fischer 2007). Although these studies suggest that exercise intensity plays a role in the IL-6 response, these results may be related to the mode of exercise in that the mass of skeletal muscle recruitment may play a role. In support of the notion that the mass of muscle recruited is important in the appearance of

IL-6 in the plasma, studies have observed higher systemic concentrations of IL-6 during running compared with cycling exercise. The fact that the IL-6 response was higher during running, which involves the recruitment of more muscle groups than cycling, provides sound evidence that the mass of muscle recruited has a major effect on the systemic concentration of IL-6. Indeed, during studies using either the one- or two-legged concentric knee extensor exercise model, which recruits only muscles from the upper legs, the appearance of IL-6 in the plasma is observed later and is less pronounced compared with exercise that results in the recruitment of more motor units.

The type of muscle contraction also appears to have a large effect on the time-course of the systemic appearance of IL-6 (Pedersen & Bruunsgaard 2003). During prolonged eccentric, one-legged knee extensor exercise or two-legged eccentric knee extensor exercise the IL-6 level does not peak until well after the cessation of exercise. In contrast, during running, cycling, or concentric knee-extensor exercise the IL-6 level peaks at the cessation of exercise before progressively declining into recovery. It is clear, therefore, that the kinetics of IL-6 differs depending on whether the stimulus for release was concentric muscle contraction or eccentric exercise associated with muscle damage. In fact, using an eccentric exercise model, peak IL-6 was associated not with exercise intensity or duration but with creatine kinase (CK), a traditional marker of muscle damage. Due to these observations, it was commonly thought that the IL-6 response to exercise represented a reaction to exercise-induced muscle injury, in that the exercise-induced increase in IL-6 was a consequence of an immune response due to local damage in the working muscles. Although an earlier study provided some evidence that the increase in plasma IL-6 was a consequence of an immune response due to local damage in the working muscles, recent studies fail to show an association between peak IL-6 and peak CK levels. It can be thus be concluded that the large increase in plasma levels of IL-6 in exercise models where the CK level does not change or is enhanced only a few fold, is related to mechanisms other than muscle damage. It is most likely that the marked and immediate increase in plasma

IL-6 in response to long-duration exercise is independent of muscle damage, whereas muscle damage *per se* is followed by repair mechanisms including invasion of macrophages into the muscle leading to IL-6 production. The IL-6 production in relation to muscle damage occurs later and is of lower magnitude compared with the IL-6 production related to muscle contraction (Pedersen & Febbraio 2008).

IL-6 is derived from working muscle during concentric exercise

Steensberg *et al.* (2002) published the first article demonstrating that most of the IL-6 seen in the circulation was likely to be derived from the contracting limb. Using a single-legged kicking model and measuring arteriovenous difference and blood flow across the contracting and non-contracting limb, it was clear that net release from the contracting limb was marked. This study has been followed by many others that confirmed that the net limb release of IL-6 is marked and that mRNA levels in biopsy samples taken from the contracting limb rapidly increase above baseline levels. However, it was only recently confirmed that the myocytes *per se* produce IL-6. A qualitative elevation in IL-6 protein expression was recorded in muscle cells within human muscle biopsy sections by immunohistochemistry (Penkowa *et al.* 2003). A follow-up study provided definitive evidence that myocytes *are* a major source of contraction-induced IL-6 release (Hiscock *et al.* 2004). In addition to immunohistochemistry techniques, *in situ* hybridization assays have been performed on muscle cross-sections before and after exercise (Hiscock *et al.* 2004). Consistent with the immunohistochemistry data, IL-6 mRNA was almost absent prior to exercise, but prominent after contraction (Pedersen & Hoffman-Goetz 2000; Pedersen *et al.* 2001; Febbraio & Pedersen 2002; Suzuki *et al.* 2002). In summary, evidence exists that contracting muscle fibers produce IL-6.

Intracellular signaling

The nuclear transcriptional rate of the IL-6 gene is remarkably rapid after the onset of exercise, with a 10- to 20-fold increase when comparing 30 min of exercise with rest. It was therefore hypothesized that this rapid increase in nuclear transcriptional rate was related to a glycogen-independent mechanism, possibly the cytosolic Ca^{2+} levels, since mechanical load is a potent stimulus for liberating Ca^{2+} from the lateral sacs of the sarcoplasmic reticulum. To test this hypothesis, muscle cells isolated from human biopsies were harvested and grown in a culture medium until they fused into myotubes. The cell cultures were then stimulated with the Ca^{2+} ionophore, ionomycin, and IL-6 mRNA was measured by real-time polymerase chain reaction (PCR) over the next 48 h. IL-6 mRNA increased progressively compared with pre-incubation levels. It is clear from an examination of the literature that there is a signaling cascade in other cell types, which indeed implicates intracellular Ca^{2+} ion concentrations ($[Ca^{2+}]_i$) as a potent signaling factor for IL-6 transcription. It is well known that $[Ca^{2+}]_i$ controls a diverse range of cellular functions, including gene expression and proliferation. In B lymphocytes, the amplitude and duration of $[Ca^{2+}]_i$ controls the differential activation of the pro-inflammatory transcriptional regulators nuclear factor- kappa B (NF-κB), c-Jun amino-terminal kinase (JNK), and nuclear factor of activated T cells (NFAT). NF-κB and JNK were selectively activated by a large $[Ca^{2+}]_i$ rise, whereas activation of NFAT was induced by a low, sustained increase in $[Ca^{2+}]_i$. It is therefore possible that during prolonged contractile activity that results in an increase in IL-6 mRNA in skeletal muscle, initial IL-6 transcription occurs via a $Ca^{2+}/$ NFAT-dependent pathway. Several factors would fit with such a hypothesis. First, NFAT is activated in many cells, including skeletal myocytes, via the upstream activation of calcineurin. Calcineurin, also called protein phosphatase 2B, is a serine-threonine protein phosphatase located in the cytosol. Although it was first shown to be activated by Ca^{2+} in T cells, it is present in ~10-fold higher concentrations in neuronal and muscle cells than in other cell types. Second, when activated, calcineurin binds to and dephosphorylates NFAT, allowing it to translocate to the nucleus where it associates with other transcription factors. Although NFAT in itself can lead to cytokine gene transcription, it can bind to the transcription factor activator protein-1 (AP-1), which

can lead to cytokine gene transcription. Although this pathway is likely to lead to IL-6 gene transcription during sustained muscular contractions, it is possible that large Ca^{2+} transients as seen with maximal contraction can activate IL-6 via NF-kappaB and JNK. It is known that skeletal muscle expresses JNK and muscle contraction markedly increases JNK activation. In summary, the degree to which IL-6 is activated in skeletal muscle by these signaling pathways is not known, it is possible that during more intense muscular activity serial activation of these various pathways gives rise to a more pronounced IL-6 response (Febbraio & Pedersen 2002).

Role of carbohydrate and glycogen

Studies have reported that carbohydrate ingestion attenuates elevations in plasma IL-6 during both running and cycling (Nieman *et al.* 1998), and that glucose ingestion during exercise attenuates leg IL-6 release without decreasing intramuscular expression of IL-6 mRNA. The data suggest that IL-6 release by the contracting muscles during exercise is regulated by substrate availability (Febbraio *et al.* 2003; Fig. 11.3), whereas low muscle glycogen concentrations further enhances IL-6 mRNA and transcription rates.

It is well known that exercise of this duration results in glycogen depletion and possibly hypoglycemia. This led us to the hypothesis that IL-6 gene transcription and ultimately protein translation and release was linked to glycogen depletion. To test this hypothesis we conducted a study where subjects completed 1 h of single-legged bicycle exercise, followed by 1 h of double-arm cranking 16 h before performing 4–5 h of exhaustive two-legged knee extensor exercise at 40% of their maximal knee extensor power output. In the intervening 16 h, subjects consumed a low-carbohydrate diet. This protocol was designed to deplete glycogen content in one leg and it allowed us to test the hypothesis that pre-exercise glycogen availability affected IL-6 production. The experimental model had the advantage that delivery of substrates and hormones to each limb was the same. Subjects commenced exercise with a 40% lower glycogen content in the low- vs. high-glycogen leg (Steensberg *et al.* 2001). We found that in the post-exercise samples, those with

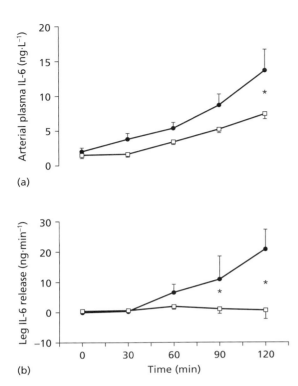

(a)

(b)

Fig. 11.3 Arterial plasma (a) and leg (b) interleukin-6 (IL-6) release before (0 min) and during 120 min of semi-recumbent cycling at 62 ± 2 % of maximal oxygen uptake with (□) or without (●) the ingestion of glucose throughout exercise.* Significant difference ($P < 0.05$) between trials. Data expressed as means ± SEM ($n = 7$). (Adapted with permission from Febbraio *et al*. 2003.)

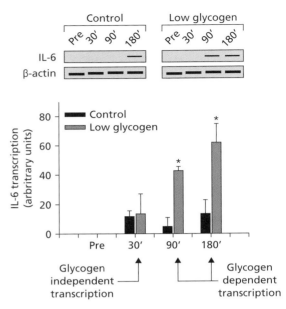

Fig. 11.4 IL-6 mRNA content before (Pre) and after 30, 90, and 180 minutes of a two-legged knee extensor exercise with normal or low pre-exercise levels of muscle glucogen. Total RNA was isolated from biopsy samples of the vastus lateralis muscle at the indicated time points and subjected to RT-PCR. The top panels show representative negative images of PCR products (stained with ethidium bromide) for the IL-6 and β-actin genes, and the graph at the bottom shows the data (mean ± SE) for IL-6 mRNA (relative to β-actin) during exercise with normal (control, dark bars) or low (gray bars) pre-exercise levels of muscle glycogen. *Significantly ($P < 0.05$) different from control. (Adapted with permission from Keller *et al*. 2001.)

the lowest glycogen content expressed the highest levels of IL-6 mRNA. The release of IL-6 from the low-glycogen exercising leg occurred after only 60 min of exercise, whereas it occurred after 120 min in the other limb Thus, we concluded that muscle glycogen content is a determining factor for production of IL-6 across contracting limbs. One potential concern from the previous study was that one leg performed exercise the day before and the other did not. Since a mechanical load can activate the calcineurin/NFAT signaling cascade, we could not rule out the possibility that the exercise the day before was the stimulus for the IL-6 transcription, even though resting IL-6 on the day of the experiment was similar when comparing legs. To rule out this possibility, we had subjects perform exercise on

two different occasions, once with a normal and once with a low pre-exercise muscle glycogen content (Keller *et al*. 2001). We demonstrated that prolonged exercise activated transcription of the IL-6 gene in skeletal muscle of humans, a response that was dramatically enhanced under conditions in which muscle glycogen concentrations were low (Fig. 11.4). Therefore, pre-exercise intramuscular glycogen content appears to be an important determinant of IL-6 gene transcription and ultimate release.

The signaling cascade that would result in IL-6 gene transcription due to altered glycogen availability is not well understood, but it has been suggested that this process may involve the activation of p38 mitogen-activated protein (MAP) kinase. In summary, pre-exercise intramuscular glycogen content appears to be an important stimulus for IL-6 gene transcription, whereas carbohydrate inhibits the release of muscle-derived IL-6 (Pedersen & Hoffman-Goetz 2000; Pedersen *et al.* 2001; Febbraio & Pedersen 2002; Suzuki *et al.* 2002).

Role of epinephrine and lactate

Apart from exercise, intensity duration, and mode, it has been suggested that the exercise-induced increase in plasma IL-6 is related to the sympatho-adrenal response. A study performed in animals suggested that the increase in epinephrine during stress was responsible for the increase in IL-6. However, when epinephrine was infused into volunteers to closely mimic the increase in plasma epinephrine during 2.5 h of running exercise, plasma IL-6 increased only four-fold during the infusion but 30-fold during the exercise. It therefore seems that epinephrine plays only a minor role in the exercise-induced increase in plasma IL-6 (Febbraio & Pedersen 2002). It was previously demonstrated that peak plasma IL-6 during exercise correlated with plasma lactate. However, a study examined patients with mitochondrial myopathy, characterized by high plasma lactate levels. These patients were treated with dichloroacetate (DCA) for 15 days, an agent that increases the activity of the pyruvate-dehydrogenase complex. The same exercise test was repeated on days with and without treatment. DCA lowered the plasma lactate levels and increased plasma IL-6 at rest; IL-6 increased in response to exercise only during DCA treatment. In summary, IL-6 production during exercise is not a direct result of high lactate levels and epinephrine has only a minor role in the exercise-induced increase in circulating IL-6 levels (Febbraio & Pedersen 2002).

IL-6 production from trained and untrained muscle

Most studies of muscle-derived IL-6 have been performed in healthy young volunteers that exercised at high intensities. However, the clinical relevance of muscle-derived IL-6 is supported by the findings that even moderate exercise has a major effect on muscle-derived IL-6. Young healthy individuals performed 3 h of dynamic two-legged knee-extensor exercise at 50% of their individual maximal power output. This exercise induced an only moderate increase in heart rate (113 to 122 beats·min^{-1}), but resulted in a 16-fold increase in IL-6 mRNA expression, a 20-fold increase in plasma IL-6, and a marked IL-6 release from working muscle. When the same model was applied in elderly, healthy, untrained subjects, even higher amounts of IL-6 were released from working muscle during exercise at the same relative intensity. In accordance, the magnitude of the exercise-induced IL-6 mRNA response in contracting skeletal muscle was markedly reduced by 10 weeks of training, possibly related to the training-induced increase in basal muscle glycogen content (Fischer *et al.* 2004). In summary, the IL-6 production in response to an acute bout of exercise is more pronounced in untrained vs. trained muscle when comparing exercise at the same relative intensities.

Sources of contraction-induced production of IL-6

Skeletal muscle is the main source of IL-6 during exercise. Studies have demonstrated that monocytes are not major contributors to the IL-6 response during exercise. However, small amounts of IL-6 are also produced and released from adipose tissue, and studies indicate that the brain and peri-tendon tissue may release IL-6 in response to exercise. Accumulating data supports the hypothesis that the role of IL-6 released from contracting muscle during exercise is to act in a hormone-like manner to mobilize extracellular substrates and/or augment substrate delivery during exercise.

Exercise and IL-6 receptors

IL-6 exerts its actions via the IL-6 receptor (IL-6R) in conjunction with the ubiquitously expressed gp130 receptor. IL-6 is regulated in an autocrine fashion (Keller *et al.* 2003). In accordance, acute exercise induces IL-6 receptor expression after exercise, suggesting a post-exercise-sensitizing mechanism. Furthermore, after a 10-week training period, IL-6 receptor mRNA production was increased in skeletal muscle, suggesting a sensitization of skeletal muscle to IL-6 at rest.

Inflammation, insulin resistance, and atherosclerosis

Role of TNF

Mounting evidence suggests that TNF-α plays a direct role in the metabolic syndrome (Plomgaard *et al.* 2005a). Patients with diabetes demonstrate high TNF and protein expression in skeletal muscle and high TNF levels in plasma (Plomgaard *et al.* 2007). In addition, it is likely that adipose tissue, which produces TNF-α, is the main source of this cytokine in diabetic patients. Mounting evidence points to an effect of TNF-α on insulin signaling. For example, TNF-α impairs insulin-stimulated glucose storage in cultured human muscle cells (Halse *et al.* 2001) and insulin-mediated glucose uptake in rats (Youd, Rattigan & Clark 2000). Furthermore, obese mice with a knock-out (KO) of the TNF-α gene are protected from insulin resistance, and inhibition of TNF-α using a specific antibody has been shown to enhance insulin sensitivity in a rat model of insulin-resistance (Uysal *et al.* 1997).

In vitro studies have demonstrated that TNF-α has direct inhibitory effects on insulin signaling, and it has been shown to directly impair glucose uptake and metabolism by altering signal transduction pathways. Recently, it was demonstrated that TNF-α infusion in healthy humans induces insulin resistance in skeletal muscle, whilst having no effect on endogenous glucose production. These data provide a direct molecular link between low-grade systemic inflammation and insulin resistance (Plomgaard *et al.* 2005a). It has also been proposed that TNF-α indirectly causes insulin resistance *in vivo* by increasing the release of free fatty acids (FFA) from adipose tissue. The cytokine has been shown to increase lipolysis in human, rat, and 3T3-L1 adipocytes. Recently, it was found that TNF-α had no effect on muscle fatty acid oxidation, but increased fatty acid incorporation into diacylglycerol, which may be involved in the development of TNF-α-induced insulin resistance in skeletal muscle.

Recent evidence suggests that TNF-α plays a key role in linking insulin resistance to vascular disease. Several downstream mediators and signaling pathways seem to provide the crosstalk between inflammatory and metabolic signaling. These include JNK and I kappa beta kinase (IκK), which act as critical regulators of insulin action activated by TNF-α (Hotamisligil 2003). In human TNF-α infusion studies, TNF-α increases phosphorylation of p70 S6 kinase, extracellular signal-regulated kinase-1/2, and c-Jun NH(2)-terminal kinase, concomitant with increased serine and reduced tyrosine phosphorylation of insulin receptor substrate-1. These signaling effects are associated with impaired phosphorylation of Akt substrate 160, the most proximal step identified in the insulin signaling cascade regulating GLUT4 translocation and glucose uptake (Plomgaard *et al.* 2005b).

Role of IL-6

While IL-6 appeared to play a role in endogenous glucose production during muscular activity in humans, its action on the liver was totally dependent on a yet unidentified muscle contraction-induced factor (Febbraio *et al.* 2004). During resting conditions, acute IL-6 administration at physiological concentrations did not impair whole-body glucose disposal, net leg glucose uptake, or increased endogenous glucose production in resting healthy young humans (Lyngso *et al.* 2002; Steensberg *et al.* 2003; Petersen *et al.* 2004). In patients with type 2 diabetes, plasma insulin levels decreased in response to IL-6 infusion, suggesting an insulin sensitizing effect of IL-6 (Petersen *et al.* 2004; Fig. 11.5). Recently, it was demonstrated that IL-6 increased glucose infusion rate (Carey *et al.* 2006) and glucose oxidation without affecting the suppression of endogenous glucose production during a hyperinsulinemic euglycemic clamp in healthy humans. These data are in contrast with observations reported in mice (Kim *et al.* 2004). Therefore, the generally negative effects of IL-6 on hepatic insulin sensitivity observed in murine models *in vivo* must be interpreted with caution. The finding of an insulin-sensitizing effect of IL-6 during conditions where endogenous glucose production was completely suppressed underlines

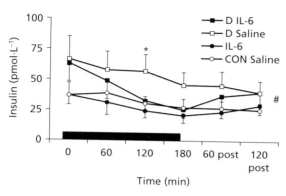

Fig. 11.5 Plasma insulin before (0 min), during, and after IL-6 or saline infusion in patients with type 2 diabetes (D) or healthy controls (CON). # = Main group effect (D > CON, $P < 0.05$); * = difference between IL-6 and Saline (treatment × time interaction). (Adapted with permission from Petersen *et al.* 2004.)

the fact that, in humans, the main effects of IL-6 with regard to glucose metabolism are likely to be in peripheral tissues (muscle, adipose), with no effect on glucose output from the liver.

Infusion of recombinant human IL-6 (rhIL-6) into healthy subjects (Lyngso *et al.* 2002; van Hall *et al.* 2003; Petersen *et al.* 2004) and patients with type 2 diabetes (Petersen *et al.* 2004) to achieve physiological concentrations was found to increase lipolysis in the absence of hypertriacylglyceridemia or changes in catecholamines, glucagon, insulin; no adverse effects were recorded (Fig. 11.6). These findings, together with cell culture experiments demonstrating that IL-6 alone markedly increased both lipolysis and fat oxidation, identify IL-6 as a novel lipolytic factor.

Blocking IL-6 in clinical trials rheumatoid arthritis patients leads to enhanced cholesterol and plasma glucose levels, indicating that a functional lack of IL-6 may lead to insulin resistance and an atherogenic lipid profile rather than the opposite (Choy *et al.* 2002; Adis R&D Profile 2003; Nishimoto *et al.* 2004). In accordance, IL-6KO mice develop late-onset obesity and impaired glucose tolerance. In addition, when treated with IL-6 there was a significant decrease in body fat mass in the IL-6 knock-out, but not in the wild-type mice (Wallenius *et al.* 2002).

In isolated hepatocytes and in *in vivo* studies in mice, IL-6 has a negative effect on hepatic insulin sensitivity. However, these findings have no clin-

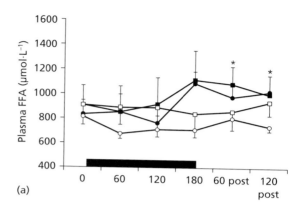

(a)

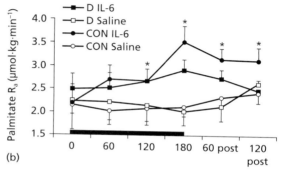

(b)

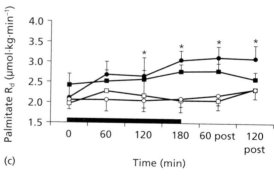

(c)

Fig. 11.6 (a) Plasma free fatty acids (FFA), (b) palmitate R_a, and (c) palmitate R_d before (0 min), during, and after interleukin-6 (IL-6) or Saline infusion in D or CON. Filled bar, infusion. *Difference between IL-6 and saline (treatment × time interaction). (Adapted with permission from Petersen *et al.* 2004.)

ical relevance as *in vivo* studies in humans clearly demonstrate that neither splanchnic glucose output, determined by the arteriovenous balance across the hepatosplanchnic tissue, nor endogenous glucose production, measured using an isotopic tracer, is increased following acute infusion of rhIL-6 (Lyngso *et al.* 2002; Steensberg *et al.* 2003; Petersen *et al.* 2004). *In vitro*, IL-6 either enhances (Stouthard *et al.* 1996; Carey *et al.* 2006) or has no effect (Lagathu *et al.* 2003; Rotter *et al.* 2003) on glucose transport in adipocytes. The fact that IL-6 infusion increases subcutaneous adipose tissue glucose uptake in humans (Lyngso *et al.* 2002) argues against IL-6 as an insulin resistance-inducing agent in adipocytes. In addition, several studies have reported that IL-6 increases intramyocellular (Bruce & Dyck 2004; Petersen *et al.* 2004) or whole body (van Hall *et al.* 2003; Petersen *et al.* 2004) fatty acid oxidation, which is likely to decrease intramyocellular fatty acid accumulation, which can in turn impair insulin signaling (Shulman 2004). With regard to myocytes, IL-6 enhances insulin-stimulated glucose transport (Carey *et al.* 2006) and glycogen synthesis (Weigert *et al.* 2004, 2005). *In vivo* experiments demonstrated that IL-6 increases basal and insulin-stimulated glucose uptake via an increase in the translocation of GLUT4 from intracellular pools to the plasma membrane (Carey *et al.* 2006).

Studies have shown that IL-6 can enhance lipid oxidation *in vitro* (Petersen *et al.* 2004), *ex vivo* (Bruce & Dyck 2004), and *in vivo* (van Hall *et al.* 2003; Petersen *et al.* 2004). A link between IL-6 and AMP-activated protein kinase (AMPK) has been established. AMPK plays a central role in the regulation of fuel metabolism in skeletal muscle because its activation stimulates fatty acid oxidation and increases glucose uptake via mechanisms thought to involve enhanced insulin signal transduction (Kahn *et al.* 2005). IL-6 was shown to enhance AMPK in both skeletal muscle and adipose tissue (Kelly *et al.* 2004). Furthermore, the effects of IL-6 on glucose metabolism were abolished in L6 myotubes infected with a dominant-negative AMPK α-subunit (Carey *et al.* 2006), indicating that the effects of IL-6 *in vitro* are mediated by this protein. In this respect, the biological profiles of TNF and IL-6 are very different: TNF has direct inhibitory effects on insulin signaling, whereas IL-6 enhances glucose uptake in skeletal muscle via activation of AMPK.

The anti-inflammatory effects of IL-6

IL-6 may exert inhibitory effects on TNF-α (Petersen & Pedersen 2005). IL-6 inhibits lipopolysaccharide (LPS)-induced TNF-α production both in cultured human monocytes and in the human monocytic cell line U937. Furthermore, levels of TNF-α are markedly elevated in anti-IL-6-treated mice and in IL-6KO mice, indicating that circulating IL-6 is involved in the regulation of TNF-α. In addition, rhIL-6 infusion inhibits the endotoxin-induced increase in circulating levels of TNF-α in healthy humans. Lastly, IL-6 stimulates the release of soluble TNF-α receptors, but not IL-1β or TNF-α, and appears to be the primary inducer of the hepatocyte-derived acute-phase proteins, many of which have anti-inflammatory properties.

The anti-inflammatory effects of IL-6 are also demonstrated by the fact that IL-6 stimulates the production of IL-1ra and IL-10. The appearance of these cytokines in the circulation following exercise appears to contribute to the anti-inflammatory effects observed post-exercise. IL-10 inhibits the production of IL-1α, IL-1β, and TNF-α, as well as the production of chemokines, including IL-8 and macrophage inflammatory protein (MIP)-α, from LPS-activated human monocytes. These cytokines and chemokines play a critical role in the activation of granulocytes, monocytes/macrophages, and lymphocytes and in their recruitment to sites of inflammation. Whereas IL-10 influences multiple cytokines, the biological role of IL-1ra is to inhibit signaling transduction through the IL-1 receptor complex.

IL-6 also influences leukocyte subpopulations. Infusion of rhIL-6 into humans increases plasma cortisol, which increases the circulating pool of neutrophils by inhibiting their ability to bind to the endothelial membrane and hence to infiltrate into the tissue. The increased neutrophil count observed is therefore a result of the anti-inflammatory effect of cortisol. Exercise increases circulating neutrophils numbers in a similar manner, and to approximately equivalent levels (Pedersen & Hoffman-Goetz 2000). It is therefore likely that muscle-derived IL-6 mediates this effect. A small decrease in the circulating pool of lymphocytes towards the end of the rhIL-6 infusion supports the observation that the late lymphopenia seen during the recovery from exercise may also in part be caused by IL-6. Exercise-induced loss of type 1 cytokine-producing cells from the circulation may be related to elevated levels of IL-10, and the increases in both IL-10 and plasma IL-1ra seen during exercise are likely to be mediated by IL-6.

Increased levels of both TNF-α and IL-6 are observed in obese individuals, in smokers, and in patients with type 2 diabetes mellitus (Bruunsgaard *et al.* 1999; Bruunsgaard 2005), and plasma concentrations of IL-6 have been shown to predict all-cause mortality as well as cardiovascular mortality. Based on observational studies, it cannot be concluded if a causal relationship exists. The G-174-C genotype, where the C allele shows lower IL-6 expression than the G allele (Terry *et al.* 2000), is a disease "risk genotype" (Petersen & Pedersen 2005), although its association with type 2 diabetes has been somewhat contradictory (Kristiansen & Mandrup-Poulsen 2005). Compared with the G-308G genotype, the –308A allele of the TNF-α gene has been shown to increase transcription two-fold (Petersen & Pedersen 2005). Subjects with risk genotypes for both TNF-α and IL-6 have the highest incidence of diabetes (Kubaszek *et al.* 2003), favoring the theory that high levels of TNF-α and low production of IL-6 are determining factors in the metabolic syndrome.

Given the different biological profiles of TNF-α and IL-6, and given that TNF-α can trigger IL-6 release, one theory that holds is that it is adipose tissue-derived TNF-α that is the "driver" behind the metabolic syndrome, and that increased systemic levels of IL-6 reflects locally produced TNF-α (Petersen & Pedersen 2005). Furthermore, as it is described in the following paragraph, evidence exists that IL-6 suppresses TNF-α production in humans (Starkie *et al.* 2003) and it is likely that that the anti-inflammatory effects of exercise, which is mediated by muscle-derived IL-6, may offer protection against TNF-induced insulin resistance.

The anti-inflammatory effects of acute exercise

An association between physical inactivity and low-grade systemic inflammation has been demonstrated in cross-sectional studies involving healthy younger individuals, elderly people, as well as in patients with intermittent claudication (Tisi *et al.* 1997). These data, however, do not provide any information with regard to a possible causal relationship. Longitudinal studies show that regular training

induces a reduction in CRP levels and suggest that physical activity *per se* may suppress systemic low-grade inflammation. To study whether acute exercise induces a true anti-inflammatory response, a model of "low-grade inflammation" was established in which a low dose of *E. coli* endotoxin was injected to healthy volunteers that had been randomized to either rest or exercise prior to endotoxin administration. In resting subjects, endotoxin induced a two- to three-fold increase in circulating levels of TNF-α. In contrast, when the subjects performed 3 h of ergometer cycling and received the endotoxin bolus at 2.5 h, the TNF-α response was totally blunted.

Post-exercise, the high circulating levels of IL-6 are followed by an increase in IL-1ra and IL-10, and the latter two anti-inflammatory cytokines can be induced by IL-6. Therefore, IL-6 induces an anti-inflammatory environment by inducing the production of IL-1ra and IL-10, but *in vitro* and animal studies suggest that it also inhibits TNF-α production. In addition, rhIL-6 infusion inhibited endotoxin-induced increase in plasma-TNF-α in humans. The possibility exists that with regular exercise, the anti-inflammatory effects of an acute bout of exercise will protect against chronic, systemic low-grade inflammation, but such a link between the acute effects of exercise and the long-term benefits has not yet been proven. Given that the atherosclerotic process is characterized by inflammation, one alternative explanation would be that regular exercise, which offers protection against atherosclerosis, indirectly offers protection against vascular inflammation and hence systemic low-grade inflammation.

Conclusion

Muscle contraction-induced factors, so-called myokines, may be involved in mediating the health beneficial effects of exercise and play important roles in the protection against diseases associated with low-grade inflammation, such as cardiovascular disease and type 2 diabetes.

Acknowledgements

The Centre of Inflammation and Metabolism is supported by a grant from the Danish National Research Foundation (# 02-512-55).

References

Adis R&D Profile (2003) Atlizumab: anti-IL-6 receptor antibody-Chugai, anti-interleukin-6 receptor antibody-Chugai, MRA-Chugai. BioDrugs **17**(5), 369–372.

Akerstrom, T., Steensberg, A., Keller, P., Keller, C., Penkowa, M. & Pedersen, B.K. (2005) Exercise induces interleukin-8 expression in human skeletal muscle. *Journal of Physiology* **563**, 507–516.

Akira, S., Taga, T. & Kishimoto T. (1993) Interleukin-6 in biology and medicine. *Advances in Immunology* **54**, 1–78.

Blair, S.N., Cheng, Y. & Holder, J.S. (2001) Is physical activity or physical fitness more important in defining health benefits? *Medicine and Science in Sports and Exercise* **33**(6 Suppl), S379–S399.

Boule, N.G., Haddad, E., Kenny, G.P., Wells, G.A. & Sigal, R.J. (2001) Effects of exercise on glycemic control and body mass in type 2 diabetes mellitus: a meta-analysis of controlled clinical trials. *JAMA* **286**(10), 1218–1227.

Bruce, C.R. & Dyck, D.J. (2004) Cytokine regulation of skeletal muscle fatty acid metabolism: effect of interleukin-6 and tumor necrosis factor-alpha. *American Journal of Physiology. Endocrinology and Metabolism* **287**(4), E616–E621.

Bruunsgaard, H. (2005) Physical activity and modulation of systemic low-level inflammation. *Journal of Leukocyte Biology* **78**(4), 819–835.

Bruunsgaard, H., Andersen-Ranberg, K., Jeune, B., Pedersen, A.N., Skinhoj, P. & Pedersen, B.K. (1999) A high plasma concentration of TNF-alpha is associated with dementia in centenarians. *Journals of Gerontology. Series A, Biological Sciences and Medical Sciences* **54**(7), M357–M364.

Carey, A.L., Steinberg, G.R., Macaulay, S.L., Thomas, W.G., Holmes, A.G., Ramm, G., *et al.* (2006) IL-6 increases insulin stimulated glucose disposal in humans and glucose uptake and fatty acid oxidation *in vitro* via AMPK. *Diabetes* **55**, 2688–2697.

Choy, E.H., Isenberg, D.A., Garrood, T., Farrow, S., Ioannou, Y., Bird, H., *et al.* (2002) Therapeutic benefit of blocking interleukin-6 activity with an anti-interleukin-6 receptor monoclonal antibody in rheumatoid arthritis: a randomized, double-blind, placebo-controlled, dose-escalation trial. *Arthritis and Rheumatism* **46**(12), 3143–3150.

Coutinho, M., Gerstein, H.C., Wang, Y. & Yusuf, S. (1999) The relationship between glucose and incident cardiovascular events. A metaregression analysis of published data from 20 studies of 95 783 individuals followed for 12.4 years. *Diabetes Care* **22**(2), 233–240.

Dandona, P., Aljada, A. & Bandyopadhyay, A. (2004) Inflammation: the link between insulin resistance, obesity and diabetes. *Trends in Immunology* **25**(1), 4–7.

Febbraio, M.A. & Pedersen, B.K. (2002) Muscle-derived interleukin-6: mechanisms for activation and possible biological roles. *FASEB Journal* **16**(11), 1335–1347.

Febbraio, M.A., Steensberg, A., Keller, C., Starkie, R.L., Krustrup, P., Ott, P., *et al.* (2003) Glucose ingestion attenuates interleukin-6 release from contracting skeletal muscle in humans. *Journal of Physiology* **549**, 607–612.

Febbraio, M.A., Hiscock, N., Sacchetti, M., Fischer, C.P. & Pedersen, B.K. (2004) Interleukin-6 is a novel factor mediating glucose homeostasis during skeletal muscle contraction. *Diabetes* **53**(7), 1643–1648.

Festa, A., D'Agostino, R., Jr., Tracy, R.P. & Haffner, S.M. (2002) Elevated levels of acute-phase proteins and plasminogen activator inhibitor-1 predict the development of type 2 diabetes: the insulin resistance atherosclerosis study. *Diabetes* **51**(4), 1131–1137.

Fischer, C.P., Plomgaard, P., Hansen, A.K., Pilegaard, H., Saltin, B. & Pedersen, B.K. (2004) Endurance training reduces the contraction-induced interleukin-6 mRNA expression in human skeletal muscle. *American Journal of Physiology. Endocrinology and Metabolism* **287**(6), E1189–E1194.

Halse, R., Pearson, S.L., McCormack, J.G., Yeaman, S.J. & Taylor, R. (2001) Effects of tumor necrosis factor-α on insulin action in cultured human muscle cells. *Diabetes* **50**, 1102–1109.

Hiscock, N., Chan, M.H., Bisucci, T., Darby, I.A. & Febbraio, M.A. (2004) Skeletal myocytes are a source of interleukin-6 mRNA expression and protein release during contraction: evidence of fiber type specificity. *The FASEB Journal* **18**(9), 992–994.

Hotamisligil, G.S. (2003) Inflammatory pathways and insulin action. *International Journal of Obesity and Related Metabolic Disorders* **27**(Suppl 3), S53–S55.

Kahn, B.B., Alquier, T., Carling, D. & Hardie, D.G. (2005) AMP-activated protein kinase: ancient energy gauge provides clues to modern understanding of metabolism. *Cell Metabolism* **1**(1), 15–25.

Kamimura, D., Ishihara, K. & Hirano, T. (2003) IL-6 signal transduction and its physiological roles: the signal orchestration model. *Reviews of Physiology, Biochemistry and Pharmacology* **149**, 1–38.

Keller, C., Steensberg, A., Pilegaard, H., Osada, T., Saltin, B., Pedersen, B.K., *et al.* (2001) Transcriptional activation of the IL-6 gene in human contracting skeletal muscle: influence of muscle glycogen content. *FASEB Journal* **15**(14), 2748–2750.

Keller, P., Keller, C., Carey, A.L., Jauffred, S., Fischer, C.P., Steensberg, A., *et al.* (2003) Interleukin-6 production by contracting human skeletal muscle: Autocrine regulation by IL-6. *Biochemical and Biophysical Research Communications* **319**(2), 550–554.

Kelly, M., Keller, C., Avilucea, P.R., Keller, P., Luo, Z., Xiang, X., *et al.* (2004) AMPK activity is diminished in tissues of the IL-6 knockout mice: the effect of exercise. *Biochemical and Biophysical Research Communications* **320**(2), 449–454.

Kim, H.J., Higashimori, T., Park, S.Y., Choi, H., Dong, J., Kim, Y.J., *et al.* (2004) Differential effects of interleukin-6 and -10 on skeletal muscle and liver insulin action *in vivo*. *Diabetes* **53**(4), 1060–1067.

Knowler, W.C., Barrett-Connor, E., Fowler, S.E., Hamman, R.F., Lachin, J.M., Walker, E.A., *et al.* (2002) Reduction in the incidence of type 2 diabetes with lifestyle intervention or metformin. *New England Journal of Medicine* **346**(6), 393–403.

Kristiansen, O.P. & Mandrup-Poulsen, T. (2005) Interleukin-6 and diabetes: the good, the bad, or the indifferent? *Diabetes* **254**(Suppl 2), S114–S124.

Kubaszek, A., Pihlajamaki, J., Komarovski, V., Lindi, V., Lindstrom, J., Eriksson, J., *et al.* (2003) Promoter polymorphisms of the TNF-alpha (G-308A) and IL-6 (C-174G) genes predict the conversion from impaired glucose tolerance to type 2 diabetes: the Finnish Diabetes Prevention Study. *Diabetes* **52**(7), 1872–1876.

Lagathu, C., Bastard, J.P., Auclair, M., Maachi, M., Capeau, J. & Caron, M. (2003) Chronic interleukin-6 (IL-6) treatment increased IL-6 secretion and induced insulin resistance in adipocyte: prevention by rosiglitazone. *Biochemical and Biophysical Research Communications* **311**(2), 372–379.

Libby, P. (2002) Inflammation in atherosclerosis. *Nature* **420**(6917), 868–874.

Lyngso, D., Simonsen, L. & Bulow, J. (2002) Interleukin-6 production in human subcutaneous abdominal adipose tissue: the effect of exercise. *Journal of Physiology* **543**(1), 373–378.

Murray, C.J. & Lopez, A.D. (1997) Global mortality, disability, and the contribution of risk factors: Global Burden of Disease Study. *Lancet* **349**(9063), 1436–1442.

Nieman, D.C., Nehlsen-Canarella, S.L., Fagoaga, O.R., Henson, D.A., Utter, A., Davis, J.M., *et al.* (1998) Influence of mode and carbohydrate on the cytokine response to heavy exertion. *Medicine and Science in Sports and Exercise* **30**(5), 671–678.

Nishimoto, N., Yoshizaki, K., Miyasaka, N., Yamamoto, K., Kawai, S., Takeuchi, T., *et al.* (2004) Treatment of rheumatoid arthritis with humanized anti-interleukin-6 receptor antibody: a multicenter, double-blind, placebo-controlled trial. *Arthritis and Rheumatism* **50**(6), 1761–1769.

Pedersen, B.K. & Bruunsgaard, H. (2003) Possible beneficial role of exercise in modulating low-grade inflammation in the elderly. *Scandinavian Journal of Medicine and Science in Sports* **13**(1), 56–62.

Pedersen, B.K. & Febbraio, M.A. (2008) Muscle as an endocrine organ – focus on muscle-derived IL-6. *Physiological Reviews* in press.

Pedersen, B.K. & Fischer, C.P. (2007) Beneficial health effects of exercise – the role of IL-6 as a myokine. *Trends in Pharmacological Sciences* **28**, 149–196.

Pedersen, B.K. & Hoffman-Goetz, L. (2000) Exercise and the immune system: regulation, integration and adaption. *Physiology Reviews* **80**, 1055–1081.

Pedersen, B.K. & Saltin, B. (2006) Evidence for prescribing exercise as therapy in chronic disease. *Scandinavian Journal of Medicine and Science in Sports* **16**(Suppl 1), 3–63.

Pedersen, B.K., Steensberg, A. & Schjerling, P. (2001) Muscle-derived interleukin-6: possible biological effects. *Journal of Physiology* **536**(2), 329–337.

Pedersen, B.K., Steensberg, A., Fischer, C., Keller, C., Keller, P., Plomgaard, P., *et al.* (2003) Searching for the exercise factor – is IL-6 a candidate. *Journal of Muscle Research and Cell Motility* **24**(2–3), 113–119.

Penkowa, M., Keller, C., Keller, P., Jauffred, S. & Pedersen, B.K. (2003) Immunohistochemical detection of interleukin-6 in human skeletal muscle fibres following exercise. *The FASEB Journal* **17**(14), 2166–2168.

Petersen, A.M. & Pedersen, B.K. (2005) The anti-inflammatory effect of exercise. *Journal of Applied Physiology* **98**(4), 1154–1162.

Petersen, E.W., Carey, A.L., Sacchetti, M., Steinberg, G.R., Macaulay, S.L., Febbraio, M.A., *et al.* (2004) Acute IL-6 treatment increases fatty acid turnover in elderly humans *in vivo* and in tissue culture *in vitro*: evidence that IL-6 acts independently of lipolytic hormones. *American Journal of Physiology* **288**(1), E155–E162.

Plomgaard, P., Bouzakri, K., Krogh-Madsen, R., Mittendorfer, B., Zierath, J.R. & Pedersen, B.K. (2005a) Tumor necrosis factor-alpha induces skeletal muscle insulin resistance in healthy human subjects via inhibition of Akt substrate 160 phosphorylation. *Diabetes* **54**(10), 2939–2945.

Plomgaard, P., Keller, P., Keller, C. & Pedersen, B.K. (2005b) TNF-alpha, but not IL-6, stimulates plasminogen activator inhibitor-1 expression in human subcutaneous adipose tissue. *Journal of Applied Physiology* **98**(6), 2019–2023.

Plomgaard, P., Nielsen, A.R., Fischer, C.P., Mortensen, O.H., Broholm, C., Penkowa, M. *et al.* (2007) Associations between insulin resistance and TNF-α in plasma, skeletal muscle and adipose tissue in humans with and without type 2 diabetes. *Diabetologia* **50**(12), 2562–2571.

Ross, R. (1999) Atherosclerosis – an inflammatory disease. *New England Journal of Medicine* **340**(2), 115–126.

Rotter, V., Nagaev, I. & Smith, U. (2003) Interleukin-6 (IL-6) induces insulin resistance in 3T3-L1 adipocytes and is, like IL-8 and tumor necrosis factor-alpha, overexpressed in human fat cells from insulin-resistant subjects. *Journal of Biological Chemistry* **278**(46), 45777–45784.

Shulman, G.I. (2004) Unraveling the cellular mechanism of insulin resistance in humans: new insights from magnetic resonance spectroscopy. *Physiology* **19**,183–190.

Starkie, R., Ostrowski, S.R., Jauffred, S., Febbraio, M. & Pedersen, B.K. (2003) Exercise and IL-6 infusion inhibit endotoxin-induced TNF-alpha production in humans. *FASEB Journal* **17**(8), 884–886.

Steensberg, A., Febbraio, M.A., Osada, T., Schjerling, P., van Hall, G., Saltin, B., *et al.* (2001) Interleukin-6 production in contracting human skeletal muscle is influenced by pre-exercise muscle glycogen content. *Journal of Physiology* **537**(2), 633–639.

Steensberg, A., Keller, C., Starkie, R.L., Osada, T., Febbraio, M.A. & Pedersen, B.K. (2002) IL-6 and TNF-alpha expression in, and release from, contracting human skeletal muscle. *American Journal of Physiology. Endocrinology and Metabolism* **283**(6), E1272–E1278.

Steensberg, A., Fischer, C.P., Sacchetti, M., Keller, C., Osada, T., Schjerling, P., *et al.* (2003) Acute interleukin-6 administration does not impair muscle glucose uptake or whole body glucose disposal in healthy humans. *Journal of Physiology* **548**(2), 631–638.

Stouthard, J.M., Oude Elferink, R.P. & Sauerwein, H.P. (1996) Interleukin-6 enhances glucose transport in 3T3-L1 adipocytes. *Biochemical and Biophysical Research Communications* **220**(2), 241–245.

Suzuki, K., Nakaji, S., Yamada, M., Totsuka, M., Sato, K. & Sugawara, K. (2002) Systemic inflammatory response to exhaustive exercise. Cytokine kinetics. *Exercise and Immunology Reviews* **8**, 6–48.

Taylor, R.S., Brown, A., Ebrahim, S., Jolliffe, J., Noorani, H., Rees, K., *et al.* (2004) Exercise-based rehabilitation for patients with coronary heart disease: systematic review and meta-analysis of randomized controlled trials. *American Journal of Medicine* **116**(10), 682–692.

Terry, C.F., Loukaci, V. & Green, F.R. (2000) Cooperative influence of genetic polymorphisms on interleukin 6 transcriptional regulation. *Journal of Biological Chemistry* **275**(24), 18138–18144.

Tisi, P.V., Hulse, M., Chulakadabba, A., Gosling, P. & Shearman, C.P. (1997) Exercise training for intermittent claudication: does it adversely affect biochemical markers of the exercise-induced inflammatory response? *European Journal of Vascular and Endovascular Surgery* **14**(5), 344–350.

Tuomilehto, J., Lindstrom, J., Eriksson, J.G., Valle, T.T., Hamalainen, H.,

Ilanne-Parikka, P., *et al.* (2001) Prevention of type 2 diabetes mellitus by changes in lifestyle among subjects with impaired glucose tolerance. *New England Journal of Medicine* **344**(18), 1343–1350.

UK Prospective Diabetes Study (UKPDS) Group. (1998) Effect of intensive blood-glucose control with metformin on complications in overweight patients with type 2 diabetes (UKPDS 34). *Lancet* **352**(9131), 854–865.

Uysal, K.T., Wiesbrock, S.M., Marino, M.W. & Hotamisligil, G.S. (1997) Protection from obesity-induced insulin resistance in mice lacking TNF-α function. *Nature* **389**(6651), 610–614.

van Hall, G., Steensberg, A., Sacchetti, M., Fischer, C., Keller, C., Schjerling, P., *et al.* (2003) Interleukin-6 stimulates lipolysis and fat oxidation in humans. *Journal of Clinical Endocrinology and Metabolism* **88**(7), 3005–3010.

Wallenius, V., Wallenius, K., Ahren, B., Rudling, M., Carlsten, H., Dickson, S.L., *et al.* (2002) Interleukin-6-deficient mice develop mature-onset obesity. *Nature Medicine* **8**(1), 75–79.

Weigert, C., Brodbeck, K., Staiger, H., Kausch, C., Machicao, F., Haring, H.U., *et al.* (2004) Palmitate, but not unsaturated fatty acids, induces the expression of interleukin-6 in human myotubes through proteasome-dependent activation of nuclear factor kappa B. *Journal of Biological Chemistry* **279**(23), 23942–23952.

Weigert, C., Hennige, A.M., Brodbeck, K., Haring, H.U. & Schleicher, E.D. (2005) Interleukin-6 (IL-6) acts as insulin sensitizer on glycogen synthesis in human skeletal muscle cells by phosphorylation of Ser-473 of Akt. *American Journal of Physiology. Endocrinology and Metabolism* **289**, E251–E257.

Youd, J.M., Rattigan, S. & Clark, M.G. (2000) Acute impairment of insulin-mediated capillary recruitment and glucose uptake in rat skeletal muscle *in vivo* by TNF-α. *Diabetes* **49**, 1904–1909.

Part 5

Cell Biology

Chapter 12

Genetic Determinants of Physical Performance

CLAUDE BOUCHARD AND TUOMO RANKINEN

Physical performance of any type is always complex and multifactorial in nature. All physical performance traits pose extraordinary challenges to the geneticist trying to understand the specific contribution of DNA sequence variation, not only to the range of inter-individual differences, but also to the probability that one may join the ranks of the world elite. A thorough review of this field would require that we consider a number of performance domains, including those in which being very tall and muscular or very short and light or very fast or very strong and powerful or very skilled or very tolerant to fatigue or having great endurance is an absolute necessity to succeed. Such a review would be beyond the limit set for the present publication. The emphasis of this chapter is therefore on endurance performance determinants, recognizing that there are many areas and studies that will not be covered as a result of this choice.

Endurance performance depends on a large number of factors, including physique, biomechanical, physiological, metabolic, behavioral, and psychological as well as social and economic characteristics and circumstances. Some of these determinants and concomitants of endurance performance are probably little influenced by our genes, but most of them are affected to a significant extent. Because little is known about the genetics of biomechanical, behavioral, psychological, and social determinants of endurance performance, the focus of the chapter is on physiological and metabolic factors. Three classes of

The Olympic Textbook of Science in Sport, 1st edition. Edited by R.J. Maughan. Published 2009 by Blackwell Publishing. ISBN: 978-1-4051-5638-7.

determinants are considered: maximal oxygen uptake ($\dot{V}o_{2max}$), stroke volume (SV) and cardiac output ($\dot{Q}$), and skeletal muscle characteristics. All of them have been shown to be strongly correlated with indicators of endurance performance, not only in the laboratory, but also with success in endurance sports. For instance, maximal $\dot{Q}$ can be twice as high in well-trained endurance athletes as in untrained subjects, and the difference is mainly explained by a larger SV (Saltin & Strange 1992; Mitchell & Raven 1994). The skeletal muscle capillary bed and mitochondrial content are substantially larger in endurance-trained individuals, and they favorably alter the exchange of gases, substrates, and metabolites that is taking place between the systemic capillaries and the core of the muscle cell. The activities of the aerobic-oxidative and lipid metabolizing enzyme in human skeletal muscle are significantly increased with exercise training (Simoneau 1995). In addition, an increased utilization of muscle triglycerides and a greater fatty acid mobilization are observed during exercise in the trained compared with the untrained state. These factors are thought to be involved in the ability to sustain high intensity exercise over long periods of time.

The fundamental questions are whether there is evidence that genetic factors contribute to the commonly observed variations in endurance performance, which genes are involved, and what are the specific mutations of interest? The evidence for a role of genetic factors is reviewed, based on the genetic epidemiology literature, with an emphasis on key determinants in the sedentary state and on responsiveness to exercise training. Then, results from candidate gene studies and other molecular markers are summarized. It is important at the outset to recognize that few genetic investigations have been undertaken to date on performance in endurance sports or endurance athletes per se.

Human variation among sedentary people

In this section, we deal with the following questions:
• Is there a familial concentration for indicators of endurance performance?
• What is the relative contribution of the estimated genetic effect (heritability) to the total population variation in these traits?
• Do we have evidence for a stronger maternal or paternal influence in the transmission pattern?

We review first the evidence for $\dot{V}o_{2max}$, then for selected cardiovascular and skeletal muscle determinants of $\dot{V}o_{2max}$. One approach to assessing the importance of familial resemblance in relevant phenotypes is to compare the variance between families or sibships to that observed within nuclear families or sibships after adjustment for relevant concomitant variables such as age, gender, and body mass.

Endurance performance phenotypes

At the outset, it is useful to recognize that studies on animal models strongly support the hypothesis that there is a significant genetic component to variation in endurance performance in the untrained state. For instance, six rats of each sex from 11 different inbred strains were tested for maximal running capacity on a treadmill (Barbato *et al.* 1998). The COP rats were the lowest performers while the DA were the best runners based on duration of the run, distance run, and vertical work performed. There was a 2.5-fold difference between the COP and DA rats. These observations are depicted in Fig. 12.1 for males' and females' performance scores combined. The heritability of aerobic endurance performance was estimated at 50% in these untrained rodents. Selective breeding for three successive generations using the lowest performing pairs vs. the highest performing pairs resulted in divergent lines for endurance performance: the high performance line averaging 659 m (standard deviation [SD] 36 m) in a run test to exhaustion, the low performance line averaging 388 m (SD 28 m) (Koch *et al.* 1998). It was observed that 39% of the variation in running performance between the high and low lines was determined by genetic differences.

Maximal oxygen uptake ($\dot{V}o_{2max}$)

The maximal heritability of a trait can be estimated using data from family and twin studies. The heritability estimates are based on comparisons of phenotypic similarities between pairs of relatives with different level of biologic relatedness. For example, biologic siblings, who share about 50% of their genes identical by descent (IBD), should be phenotypically more similar than their parents (biologically unrelated individuals) if genetic factors contribute to the trait of interest. Likewise, a greater

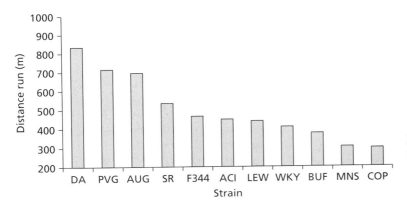

Fig. 12.1 Comparison of distances run among 11 inbred strains of rats. From Barbato *et al.* (1998). Reproduced with permission from the *Journal of Applied Physiology*.

Table 12.1 Intraclass correlations from twin studies of maximal oxygen intake. From Bouchard *et al.* (2000b). Reproduced with permission from Blackwell Science Ltd.

| Source | n Pairs | | Cohort | Test | MZ | DZ |
	MZ	DZ				
Klissouras (1971)	15	10	Males	$\dot{V}o_{2max} \cdot kg^{-1}$	0.91	0.44
Klissouras *et al.* (1973)	23	16	Males and females	$\dot{V}o_{2max} \cdot kg^{-1}$	0.95	0.36
Bouchard *et al.* (1986a)	53	33	Males and females	$\dot{V}o_{2max} \cdot kg^{-1}$	0.71	0.51
Fagard *et al.* (1991)	29	19	Males	$\dot{V}o_{2max} \cdot kg^{-1}$	0.77	0.04
Maes *et al.* (1993)	41	50	Males and females	$\dot{V}o_{2max} \cdot kg^{-1}$	0.85	0.56
Sundet *et al.* (1994)	436	622	Males	$\dot{V}o_{2max} \cdot kg^{-1}$ Predicted*	0.62	0.29
Maes *et al.* (1996)	43	61	10-year-old boys and girls	$\dot{V}o_{2max} \cdot kg^{-1}$†	0.75	0.32

DZ, dizygotic, MZ, monozygotic.

*Maximal aerobic power was predicted from a nomogram and the predicted $\dot{V}o_{2max}$ was subsequently transformed to a categorical score from 1 to 9. The intraclass correlations are based upon the categorical scores.

†$\dot{V}o_{2max}$ not adjusted for body mass.

phenotypic resemblance between monozygotic twins (MZ; 100% of genes IBD) than between dizygotic twins (DZ; 50% of genes IBD) strongly suggest a genetic effect on the phenotype.

The heritability of $\dot{V}o_{2max}$ has been estimated from a few family and twin studies. Table 12.1 summarizes intraclass correlations in pairs of DZ and MZ twins from seven studies. The data vary in test protocol (measured or predicted aerobic power, maximal or submaximal tests), the number of twin pairs, uncontrolled age or sex effects, and differences in means or variances between twin types. The intraclass correlations for MZ twins ranged from about 0.6 to 0.9, whereas correlations for DZ twins with one exception ranged from 0.3 to 0.5. The largest of the twin studies (Sundet *et al.* 1994) was derived from a population-based twin panel of conscripts. The data were based on predicted $\dot{V}o_{2max}$ values, which were subsequently transformed to categorical scores, from low to high maximal aerobic power, but intraclass correlations for the categorical scores were similar to those found in other twin studies (Sundet *et al.* 1994). These twin studies have yielded heritability estimates in the range 25–65%.

$\dot{V}o_{2max}$ in the sedentary state is characterized by a significant familial resemblance as demonstrated by four studies (Montoye & Gayle 1978; Lortie *et al.*

1982; Lesage *et al.* 1985; Bouchard *et al.* 1998). The most comprehensive of these is the HERITAGE Family Study in which two cycle ergometer $\dot{V}o_{2max}$ tests were performed on separate days in members of sedentary families of Caucasian descent (Bouchard *et al.* 1998). In the latter, an F ratio of 2.72 was found when comparing the between-family variance to the within-family variance for $\dot{V}o_{2max}$ in the sedentary state adjusted for age, sex, body mass, and body composition (Fig. 12.2). The concept of family lines with low and high $\dot{V}o_{2max}$ phenotypes in the sedentary state is clearly demonstrated by the data shown in the figure. Parents and offspring of Caucasian descent of both sexes were included and the age range was 17–65 years. The intraclass coefficient for the familial resemblance was 0.41 (Bouchard *et al.* 1998). Maximum likelihood estimation of familial correlations (spouse, four parent–offspring, and three sibling correlations) revealed a maximal heritability of 51% for $\dot{V}o_{2max}$ adjusted for age, sex, body mass, fat-free mass, and fat mass. However, the significant spouse correlation indicated that the genetic heritability was likely less than 50% (Bouchard *et al.* 1998).

Cardiac performance phenotypes

The ability to deliver oxygen to the active tissues is a major determinant of endurance performance. This

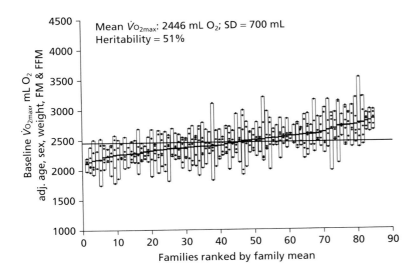

Fig. 12.2 Family lines with low and high $\dot{V}o_{2max}$ phenotypes in the sedentary state based on data from the HERITAGE Family Study. From Bouchard *et al.* (1998). Reproduced with permission from Lippincott Williams & Wilkins.

has been repeatedly shown in human and animal model studies. For instance, in the study comparing 11 inbred strains of rats of both sexes, the highest performing DA line had also the highest cardiac output ($\dot{Q}$) while the COP rats that ran for the shortest distance had the lowest $\dot{Q}$. The correlation between average distance run and $\dot{Q}$ among the 11 strains reached 0.868, corresponding to a common variance of about 75% (Barbato *et al.* 1998). Even though selection for high or low endurance performance was primarily associated with a greater oxygen uptake and utilization by skeletal muscle in the high endurance line in the early generations (Henderson *et al.* 2002), which correlated with skeletal muscle capillarity and enzyme activities at markers of oxidative metabolism (Howlett *et al.* 2003), the capacity to deliver O_2 to the exercising muscle became progressively more important. Thus, at generation 15, the high endurance performance line exhibited a $\dot{V}o_{2max}$ normalized for body weight 50% higher than the low performance line (Gonzalez *et al.* 2006). This higher $\dot{V}o_{2max}$ in the high performer line was accompanied by a 41% higher $\dot{Q}$ and a 48% higher SV under normoxic conditions.

A larger SV is commonly associated with a larger heart volume and left ventricular mass. The inheritance of left ventricular structure adjusted for body mass has been considered in a number of studies. In one experiment, 32 MZ and 21 DZ pairs of healthy

male twins were studied for cardiac dimensions (Bielen *et al.* 1991a). A path analysis model allowed the phenotypic variance to be partitioned into genetic, shared environmental, and non-shared environmental components. The data were adjusted for the effects of age and body mass. All heart structures, except left ventricular internal diameter, were significantly influenced by genetic factors, with heritability estimates ranging from 29% to 68%. The strong relationship between body size and cardiac dimensions raises the question of how much of the covariation between these two variables is explained by common genetic factors. This question was addressed in a bivariate genetic analysis of left ventricular mass and body mass in 147 MZ and 107 DZ pubertal twin pairs of both sexes (Verhaaren *et al.* 1991). Heritabilities of adjusted left ventricular mass reached 39% in males and 59% in females. Bivariate genetic analyses showed that the correlation between left ventricular mass and body mass was almost entirely of genetic origin, 90% being attributed to common genes (Verhaaren *et al.* 1991). These studies suggest that genetic factors are important in determining cardiac dimensions under resting conditions. One study of 21 MZ and 12 DZ twin pairs considered the inheritance of cardiac changes during submaximal supine cycle exercise at a heart rate of 110 beats·min^{-1} (Bielen *et al.* 1991b). The increases in left ventricular internal diameter and fractional shortening in response to exercise showed genetic effects of 24% and 47%, respectively.

In the HERITAGE Family Study, subjects completed two submaximal exercise tests at 50 W and at 60% of the initial $\dot{V}o_{2max}$, both prior to and after completing a 20-week endurance training protocol. Steady state heart rate (HR), SV, and $\dot{Q}$ were measured twice during each test. Submaximal exercise SV and $\dot{Q}$ were characterized by a significant familial aggregation in the sedentary state. Maximal heritabilities reached 40% and 42% for stroke volume and cardiac output at 50 W, and were 46% for both phenotypes at 60% $\dot{V}o_{2max}$ (An *et al.* 2000).

Skeletal muscle phenotypes

Skeletal muscle fiber type distribution is thought to be a significant determinant of endurance performance. Human variation in the proportion of a given fiber type is strikingly large, as illustrated by the data in Fig. 12.3. Sampling variation and laboratory error variance must be taken into account when attempting to quantify the importance of genetic differences based on human muscle biopsies. For instance, repeated measurements within the adult vastus lateralis muscle indicate that sampling variability and technical error together account for about 15% of the variance in the proportion of type 1 muscle fibers (Simoneau *et al.* 1986b; Simoneau & Bouchard 1995). The variability in the percentage of type 1 fibers within pairs of MZ twins provides useful information on the role of non-genetic factors. The mean difference in percentage of type 1 fibers

between a member of a MZ pair and his or her co-twin reached $9.5 \pm 6.9\%$ in 40 pairs of MZ twins that we were able to study (Simoneau & Bouchard 1995). The difference was less than 6% in 16 pairs but ranged from 18% to 23% in eight pairs. Research thus far has not been able to account for the fact that about 25% of sedentary adult Caucasians exhibit quite low ($\leq 35\%$) or quite high ($\geq 65\%$) proportion of skeletal muscle type 1 fibers in the vastus lateralis, which is the most studied skeletal muscle in humans. Genetic variation has undoubtedly something to do with this human heterogeneity but it is likely not the only cause.

These results combined with those on pairs of DZ twins and regular brothers (Bouchard *et al.* 1986a; Simoneau *et al.* 1986b) have led to the conclusion that a genetic component accounts for about 45% of variance in the proportion of type 1 muscle fibers in humans (Simoneau & Bouchard 1995). A summary of genetic, environmental, and methodologic sources of variation in the proportion of type 1 fibers in human skeletal muscle is illustrated in Fig. 12.4. Fiber type distributions were also examined in 78 sedentary subjects from 19 families of the HERITAGE Family Study (Rico-Sanz *et al.* 2003). There was no evidence for a genetic contribution to the proportion of the various fiber types, although a trend was observed for the proportion of type 1 fibers. However, significant familial aggregation was found in the same study for the number of capillaries around fiber types 1 and 2A.

There is considerable interindividual variation in the enzymatic activity profile of skeletal muscle.

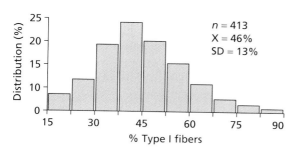

Fig. 12.3 Human variation in vastus lateralis percentage type 1 fibers among sedentary adults. After Simoneau and Bouchard (1989).

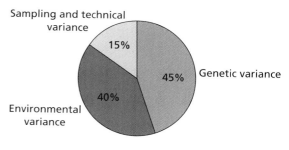

Fig. 12.4 Proportion of type 1 fibers in human skeletal muscle among sedentary people. From Simoneau and Bouchard (1995). Reproduced with permission from *FASEB Journal*.

One can distinguish individuals with high or low activity levels of enzyme markers for the catabolism of different substrates in the skeletal muscle among healthy sedentary and moderately active individuals of both sexes (Simoneau & Bouchard 1989). Many factors probably contribute to these interindividual differences, and it is likely that the genotype has a role in determining the amount of protein for several important enzymes in skeletal muscle.

Studies of MZ ($n = 35$) and DZ ($n = 26$) twin pairs of both sexes and pairs of biologic brothers ($n = 32$) indicate significant inheritance of variation in several key enzymes of skeletal muscle (Bouchard *et al.* 1986b). There was significant within pair resemblance in MZ twins for all skeletal muscle enzyme activities ($r = 0.30-0.68$), but the within pair correlations for DZ twins and brothers suggested that variation in several enzyme activities was also related to non-genetic factors and environmental conditions. After adjusting for variation in enzyme activities associated with age and sex, genetic factors were responsible for about 25–50% of the total phenotypic variation in the activities of the regulatory enzymes of the glycolytic (phosphofructokinase, PFK) and citric acid cycle (oxoglutarate dehydrogenase, OGDH) pathways, and in the ratio of glycolytic : oxidative activities (PFK : OGDH ratio) (Bouchard *et al.* 1986b). Results from the HERITAGE Family Study based on biopsies of the vastus lateralis muscle in 78 sedentary subjects from 19 families of Caucasian descent confirmed that there was significant familial aggregation for activities of enzymes of the glycolytic and oxidative pathways (Rico-Sanz *et al.* 2003; Rankinen *et al.* 2005).

Responsiveness to training

The concept of heterogeneity in responsiveness to standardized exercise programs was first introduced in the early 1980s (Bouchard 1983). In a series of carefully controlled and standardized exercise training studies conducted with young and healthy adult volunteers, it was shown that the individual differences in training-induced changes in several physical performance and health-related fitness phenotypes were large, with the range between low and high responders reaching several folds (Bouchard

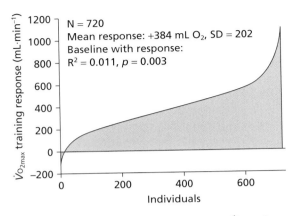

Fig. 12.5 Distribution of training responses in $\dot{V}O_{2max}$ in individuals of the HERITAGE Family Study. Black and white people are combined. From Bouchard & Rankinen (2001). Reproduced with permission from Lippincott Williams & Wilkins.

1983, 1995; Lortie *et al.* 1984; Simoneau *et al.* 1986a; Bouchard *et al.* 1992).

However, the most extensive data on the individual differences in trainability come from the HERITAGE Family Study, where healthy but sedentary subjects followed a highly standardized, well-controlled, laboratory-based, endurance-training program for 20 weeks. The average increase in $\dot{V}O_{2max}$ was 384 mL O_2 (SD 202 mL). The training responses varied from no change to increases of more than 1000 mL $O_2 \cdot min^{-1}$ (Bouchard *et al.* 1999; Bouchard & Rankinen 2001). The response distribution for $\dot{V}O_{2max}$ is depicted in Fig. 12.5. This high degree of heterogeneity in responsiveness to a fully standardized exercise program in the HERITAGE Family Study was not accounted for by baseline level, age, gender, or ethnic differences. These data underline the notion that the effects of endurance training on cardiovascular and other relevant traits should be evaluated not only in terms of mean changes but also in terms of response heterogeneity.

A similar picture emerged for training-induced changes in SV, $\dot{Q}$, and skeletal muscle traits. For instance, in the HERITAGE Family Study, at the same absolute power output (50 W), HR and $\dot{Q}$ decreased significantly (9.5% and 5%, respectively), whereas SV increased by 4% after 20 weeks of endurance

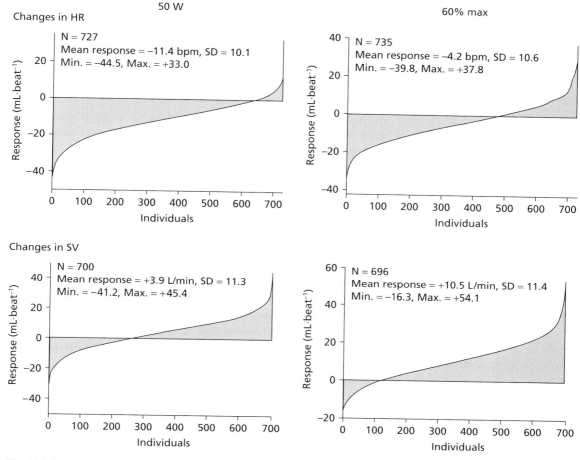

Fig. 12.6 Changes in heart rate and stroke volume in the HERITAGE Family Study at two levels of submaximal exercise. From Rankinen and Bouchard, unpublished data.

training. At 60% $\dot{V}_{O_{2max}}$, HR decreased 3.1%, while $\dot{Q}$ and SV increased 7.3% and 10.8%, respectively (Wilmore *et al.* 2001a,b). There were marked inter-individual differences in all these training-induced changes as revealed by the magnitude of the standard deviations for the training-induced changes and as illustrated in Fig. 12.6.

A similar pattern of variation in training responses was observed for other phenotypes, including insulin and plasma lipid levels, submaximal exercise HR, and blood pressure (Leon *et al.* 2000; Wilmore *et al.* 2001b; Boule *et al.* 2005). For example, systolic and diastolic blood pressure (SBP, DBP) measured during steady state submaximal (50 W) exercise decreased,

on average, by 7 and 3.5 mmHg, respectively, in response to exercise training (Wilmore *et al.* 2001b). However, the responses varied from marked decreases (SBP >25 mmHg and DBP >12 mmHg) to no changes or, in some cases, even to slight increases (Bouchard & Rankinen 2001; Wilmore *et al.* 2001b). Similar heterogeneity in responsiveness to exercise training has been reported also in other populations (Kohrt *et al.* 1991; Hautala *et al.* 2003).

Two questions come to mind as a result of the observations such as those depicted in Figs 12.5 and 12.6. Are the high and low responses to regular exercise characterized by significant familial aggregation (i.e., are there families with mainly low responders

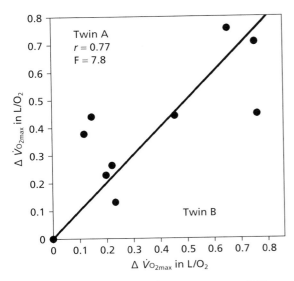

Fig. 12.7 Training changes in $\dot{V}O_{2max}$ in 10 pairs of MZ twins subjected to a standardized 20-week training program. From Bouchard *et al.* (1992). Reproduced with permission from Lippincott Williams & Wilkins.

ardized training programs showed 6–9 times more variance between genotypes (between pairs of twins) than within genotypes (within pairs of twins) based on the findings of three independent studies (Prud'homme *et al.* 1984; Hamel *et al.* 1986; Bouchard *et al.* 1992). Thus, gains in absolute $\dot{V}O_{2max}$ were much more heterogeneous between pairs of twins than within pairs of twins. The results of one such study are summarized in Fig. 12.7. The MZ twins exercised for 20 weeks using a standardized and demanding endurance-training program (Bouchard *et al.* 1992).

These observations were corroborated by the results of the HERITAGE Family Study. The increase in $\dot{V}O_{2max}$ in 481 individuals from 99 two-generation families of Caucasian descent showed 2.6 times more variance between families than within families, and the model-fitting analytical procedure yielded a maximal heritability estimate of 47% (Bouchard *et al.* 1999). Thus, the extraordinary heterogeneity observed for the gains in $\dot{V}O_{2max}$ among adults is not random and is characterized by a strong familial aggregation (Fig. 12.8). These observations support the notion that individual variability is a normal biologic phenomenon, which may largely reflect genetic diversity (Bouchard 1995; Bouchard & Rankinen 2001).

In addition to $\dot{V}O_{2max}$, the heritability of training-induced changes in several other phenotypes, such as submaximal aerobic performance, resting and

and others in which all family members show significant improvements)? Is individual variability a normal biologic phenomenon reflecting genetic diversity?

Of relevance to the first question are the early studies that we undertook with identical twins. In pairs of MZ twins, the $\dot{V}O_{2max}$ response to stand-

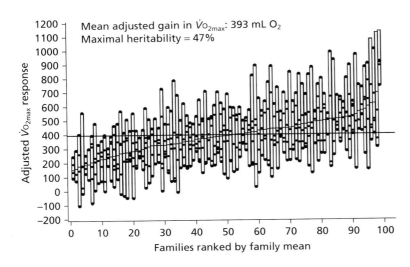

Fig. 12.8 Familial aggregation of $\dot{V}O_{2max}$ changes in response to exercise training in the HERITAGE Family Study (Bouchard *et al.* 1999). Reproduced with permission from the *Journal of Applied Physiology.*

submaximal exercise blood pressure, HR, SV and $\dot{Q}$, as well as skeletal muscle characteristics have all been investigated in the HERITAGE Family Study. Submaximal exercise SV and $\dot{Q}$ were characterized by a significant familial aggregation both in the sedentary state and in response to endurance training. The between-family variation in age, sex, body surface area, and baseline phenotype level-adjusted SV and $\dot{Q}$ training responses at 50 W were 1.5–2.2 times greater than the within-family variation. The maximal heritability estimates were 29% and 38% for SV and $\dot{Q}$ training responses at 50 W, and 24% and 30% for the training-induced changes in SV and $\dot{Q}$ at 60% of $\dot{V}o_{2max}$ (An et al. 2000).

Investigation of the role of the genotype in the response of skeletal muscle tissue to standardized training programs has only just begun. Two experimental studies of the responses of young adult MZ twins to relevant training programs provide some insights into potential genotypic contributions to the skeletal muscle training response. The studies included male and female MZ twins, and there were no sex differences in training-related gains. The effects of high-intensity intermittent training are summarized in Table 12.2. The training program involved 15 weeks of both continuous and interval cycle ergometer work in 12 pairs of MZ twins of both sexes. Program-related changes in fiber-type proportions showed no significant within-pair resemblance. However, about 50–60% of the response of hexokinase (HK), lactate dehydrogenase (LDH), malate dehydrogenase (MDH), OGDH, and the PFK : OGDH ratio to the intermittent training program was genotype-associated, while about 80% of the creatine kinase (CK) training response appeared to be determined by the genotype (Simoneau et al. 1986a).

The second study followed six pairs of young adult MZ twins (three males and three females) through 15 weeks of endurance training on a cycle ergometer (Hamel et al. 1986). Genotype–training interactions were evaluated for the proportion of muscle fibers and several enzymes after 7 and 15 weeks of training. There were no significant changes in the proportions of type 1 and type 2A and 2B fibers. Changes in skeletal muscle enzyme activities during the first half of training were only weakly related to genotype. However, changes in the activities of PFK, MDH, HADH, and OGDH across the whole 15 weeks were characterized by significant within-pair resemblance. This suggests that early in the program, adaptation to endurance training may be under less stringent genetic control; however, as training continues and perhaps nears maximal trainability, the response becomes more genotype dependent. Taken together, these two studies provide

Table 12.2 Effects of training and genotype-training interactions in the response to high intensity intermittent training for muscle fiber types and enzyme activities. From Simoneau et al. (1986a). Reproduced with permission from Georg Thieme Verlag KG.

Enzyme	Before training mean ± SD	After training mean ± SD	Genotype–training interaction F ratio	Intrapair resemblance in response
CK	237.0 ± 48	278.0 ± 98	9.8**	0.82
HK	1.3 ± 0.4	1.41 ± 0.36	3.8*	0.59
PFK	152.0 ± 27	155.0 ± 52	2.2	0.38
LDH	239.0 ± 122	201.0 ± 93	4.6**	0.64
MDH	220.0 ± 56	246.0 ± 44*	3.0*	0.50
HADH	3.7 ± 1.2	5.03 ± 1.55**	1.3	0.15
OGDH	0.7 ± 0.2	1.04 ± 0.23**	3.0*	0.50
PFK : OGDH ratio	558.0 ± 173	231.0 ± 109	4.5**	0.64

All enzymes were expressed in μmol of NADH or NADPH per gram of wet weight per minute. $N = 12$ pairs of MZ twins. CK, creatine kinase; HADH, 3-hydroxyacyl CoA dehydrogenase; HK, hexokinase; LDH, lactate dehydrogenase; MDH, malate dehydrogenase; OGDH, oxoglutarate dehydrogenase; PFK, phosphofructokinase.
*$P < 0.05$ **$P < 0.01$.

Phenotype	Pre-training			Training response		
	n	F	P	n	F	P
PCr metabolism						
CK	78	6.25	<0.0001	76	3.97	<0.0001
Glycolysis						
PHOS	78	6.85	<0.0001	75	2.14	0.0169
HK	78	1.69	0.069	75	4.01	<0.0001
PFK	78	3.83	<0.0001	76	1.85	0.043
GAPDH	78	5.62	<0.0001	76	2.39	0.0072
Oxidative metabolism						
CPT	78	2.55	0.0039	75	2.47	0.0058
HADH	78	3.80	<0.0001	76	2.13	0.017
CS	78	1.66	0.076	76	2.73	0.0023
COX	78	3.03	0.0008	76	2.07	0.0213

Table 12.3 Familial aggregation of maximal enzyme activities in the vastus lateralis muscle in a subset of families of Caucasian descent of the HERITAGE Family Study. From Rankinen *et al.* (2005). Reproduced with permission from Lippincott Williams & Wilkins.

CK, creatine kinase; COX, cyclo-oxygenase; CPT, carnitine palmitoyltransferase; CS, citrate synthase; GAPDH, gluceraldehyde phosphate dehydrogenase; HADH, 3-hydroxyacyl CoA dehydrogenase; HK, hexokinase; PFK, phosphofructokinase; PHOS, phosphorylase.

strong support for the notion that genetic variation accounts for some of the heterogeneity in skeletal muscle metabolic responses to exercise training.

Training-induced changes in muscle enzyme activities were also investigated in the HERITAGE Family Study (Rico-Sanz *et al.* 2003; Rankinen *et al.* 2005). Results confirmed that there was consistent familial resemblance for the training responses in activities of marker enzymes of the glycolytic and oxidative pathways (Table 12.3). In contrast, no evidence for familial aggregation was found for the changes in capillary density, even though capillarity increased around all fiber types in response to 20 weeks of endurance training.

The human heterogeneity described in this section is an example of normal biologic diversity, is observed in most populations, is beyond measurement error and day-to-day fluctuation, and is potentially very informative in terms of the adaptive mechanisms involved.

Candidate gene studies

The evidence from genetic epidemiology studies suggests that there is a genetically determined component affecting physical performance phenotypes.

Moreover, the latter traits are complex and multifactorial in nature, and the search for genes and mutations responsible for the genetic effects must target both the sedentary state and the responsiveness to exercise training.

Lessons from exercise intolerance cases

Although exercise-related traits are mainly polygenic and multifactorial in nature, much can be learned from some monogenic disorders characterized by compromised exercise capacity or exercise intolerance. These disorders affect only a few individuals, but they provide examples of biologic defects that have profound consequences on the ability to perform physical activity, usually because of compromised energy metabolism. However, although these genetic defects compromise exercise capacity, there is no evidence that overexpression of these genes leads to improved physical performance. We believe that important lessons can be learned by a brief review of the genes harboring mutations resulting in diminished endurance performance.

Muscle glycogen phosphorylase deficiency (McArdle disease) was the first documented carbohydrate metabolism disorder associated with exercise intolerance (McArdle 1951). The condition is characterized by partial or total absence of glycogen phosphorylase in skeletal muscles, which results in impaired glycogenolysis. Identification of three mutations in the muscle glycogen phosphorylase (*PYGM*) gene in 1993 established the molecular genetic basis for McArdle disease. These mutations were found in almost 90% of the investigated patients (Tsujino *et al.* 1993a). Additional mutations have been reported in subsequent studies, and currently the Online Mendelian Inheritance in Man (OMIM, entry 232600) database lists 17 *PYGM* mutations related to McArdle disease. Phosphorylase kinase is a multimeric protein composed of four subunits, which regulates the activity of glycogen phosphorylase. The gene encoding the muscle-specific isoform of the α subunit of phosphorylase kinase (PHKA1) is located on chromosome Xq12–q13, and two mutations have been identified in patients with phosphorylase kinase deficiency: a nonsense mutation (G3334T) changing a glutamic acid residue to a stop codon (Wehner *et al.* 1994); and a guanine to cytosine splice-junction substitution at the 5′ end of an intron, which causes skipping of the preceding exon (Bruno *et al.* 1998).

Muscle phosphofructokinase deficiency is a hereditary disorder of glycolysis featuring exercise intolerance as a clinical symptom. Phosphofructokinase is a rate-limiting enzyme in the glycolytic energy production pathway, and several mutations in the gene encoding the muscle form have been reported in patients with muscle phosphofructokinase deficiency (Sherman *et al.* 1994; Tsujino *et al.* 1994a; Vorgerd *et al.* 1996). Phosphoglycerate kinase 1 and phosphoglycerate mutase are also involved in glycolysis. Deficiencies of both enzymes have been shown to cause myopathy and exercise intolerance. At least four mutations in the muscle phosphoglycerate mutase gene have been identified in the phosphoglycerate mutase deficient patients (Tsujino *et al.* 1993b; Toscano *et al.* 1996; Hadjigeorgiou *et al.* 1999). Several mutations have been identified in the phosphoglycerate kinase gene; however, only four of these have been found in the myopathic form of phosphoglycerate kinase (*PGK1*) deficiency (Tsujino *et al.* 1994c; Ookawara *et al.* 1996; Sugie *et al.* 1998; Hamano *et al.* 2000).

Comi *et al.* (2001) have reported two heterozygous missense mutations in the beta enolase gene in a patient with severe muscle enolase deficiency, exercise intolerance, and myalgias. Muscle lactate dehydrogenase deficiency is also characterized by exercise intolerance. Three mutations in the lactate dehydrogenase A (*LDHA*) gene have been identified, and they all induce a premature stop codon and result in a truncated gene product (Maekawa *et al.* 1990; Tsujino *et al.* 1994b).

Carnitine palmitoyltransferase II (CPT II) deficiency is the most common recessively inherited lipid metabolism disorder affecting skeletal muscle. Patients with CPT II deficiency have recurrent episodes of myoglobinuria triggered by exercise, fasting, or infection. Some patients also manifest muscle stiffness and soreness following exercise (Bonnefont *et al.* 1999). Another lipid metabolism-related gene pertaining to exercise intolerance is that encoding very-long-chain acyl-CoA dehydrogenase (ACADVL). A patient with a long history of exercise intolerance, myoglobinuria, low fasting ketogenesis, impaired palmitoylcarnitine oxidation by muscle mitochondria, and lack of palmitoyl-CoA dehydrogenase enzyme in muscle and fibroblasts was found to be homozygous for a 3 base pair (bp) deletion in exon 9 of the *ACADVL* gene. The mutation deleted a lysine residue at position 238 of the mature gene product (Scholte *et al.* 1999).

The fitness and performance gene map

The 2005 human gene map for physical performance and health-related phenotypes included 165 autosomal and five X chromosome gene entries and quantitative trait loci (QTLs) (Rankinen *et al.* 2006b). Moreover, there were 17 mitochondrial genes in which sequence variants have been shown to influence relevant fitness and performance phenotypes. A total of 29 autosomal genes and three genes encoded by mitochondrial DNA were reported in at least one study to be associated with physical performance-related phenotypes: 18 autosomal and three mitochondrial genes were associated with endurance phenotypes, whereas 14 genes (all autosomal) were associated with speed and muscle strength-related traits (Rankinen *et al.* 2006a).

Angiotensin-converting enzyme as a candidate gene

A clear favorite gene among exercise scientists has been the angiotensin-converting enzyme (*ACE*) gene, which was investigated in 42 reports. A 287 bp insertion (I)/deletion (D) polymorphism in intron 16 of the *ACE* gene was first reported to be strongly associated with plasma ACE activity in Caucasians in 1990 (Rigat *et al*. 1990). The ACE activity was lowest in subjects with two copies of the I allele (I/I homozygotes), highest in the D/D homozygotes, and intermediate in the I/D heterozygotes. In subsequent studies, the D allele was reported to be associated with increased risks of coronary heart disease and other chronic disorders, although the evidence to date is still inconsistent.

In exercise performance-related studies, the I allele has been reported to be more frequent in Australian elite rowers, Spanish endurance athletes, Italian Olympic aerobic endurance athletes, and fastest South African triathletes than in sedentary controls (Gayagay *et al*. 1998; Alvarez *et al*. 2000). Likewise, British long-distance runners tended to have a greater frequency of the I allele than sprinters (Myerson *et al*. 1999). In a group of postmenopausal women, who were selected on the basis of their physical activity levels, the I/I genotype was associated with greater $\dot{V}o_{2max}$ and maximal arterial–venous oxygen difference compared to the D/D homozygotes (Hagberg *et al*. 1998), while in Chinese males the D/D genotype was associated with the highest $\dot{V}o_{2max}$ level (Zhao *et al*. 2003). The I allele was also associated with greater increase in muscular endurance and efficiency after 10 weeks of physical training in British Army recruits (Montgomery *et al*. 1998; Williams *et al*. 2000; Woods *et al*. 2002).

In contrast, the frequency of the D allele was found to be higher in elite swimmers and short-distance athletes than in sedentary controls (Woods *et al*. 2001). The D allele was also more frequent in Spanish elite cyclists than in runners (Lucia *et al*. 2005). The D/D genotype was associated with better middle-distance running performance in non-elite Turkish athletes (Cam *et al*. 2005) and with higher $\dot{V}o_{2max}$ in Turkish wrestlers (Kasikcioglu *et al*. 2004). In almost 300 sedentary but healthy white offspring

of the HERITAGE Family Study, the D/D homozygotes showed the greatest improvements in $\dot{V}o_{2max}$ and maximal power output following a controlled and supervised 20-week endurance-training program, although similar trends were not seen in their parents or in black HERITAGE families (Rankinen *et al*. 2000).

Some cross-sectional studies suggest that the D allele is associated with greater muscle strength than the I allele (Hopkinson *et al*. 2004; Williams *et al*. 2005). Greater gains in muscle strength in response to isometric, but not to dynamic resistance training in D/D vs. I/I homozygotes have been reported (Folland *et al*. 2000). On the other hand, the largest strength training study conducted so far reported greater increases in maximal voluntary contraction of the elbow flexor muscles in the I/I rather than the D/D homozygotes (Pescatello *et al*. 2006). However, the fact that the genotype effect was greater for the untrained arm than the trained arm complicates the interpretation of the results. Along the same lines, a study in 1027 teenage Greeks reported greater hand grip strength and vertical jump height in females (*n* = 448) who were I/I homozygotes than the D allele carriers. The *ACE* genotype was not associated with any of the performance phenotypes in 535 boys (Moran *et al*. 2006).

The observations on the *ACE* gene need to be put in perspective. The statistical evidence for or against an association is not very strong in the published reports to date. In fact, of the 42 studies dealing with the *ACE* genotype and performance phenotypes, the primary hypothesis was statistically significant only in six reports. Another 22 studies reported at least one positive finding based on *post hoc* subgroup analyses, while the tests for the main hypotheses, and in many cases tests for several additional subgroup analyses, were negative. Furthermore, even among the positive studies the findings tend to be inconsistent. Only one study corrected the results or interpretations of the results for multiple testing. Finally, 14 studies found no support for an association between performance and the *ACE* I/D polymorphism. The most likely explanation for seemingly inconsistent results from association studies in different populations is typically the overinterpretation of marginal statistical evidence (Cardon & Palmer

2003). Thus, the available data are still too fragmented to evaluate fully the part played by the *ACE* gene in the variation of human physical performance level, if any. The same conclusion can be reached for all other genes studied to date.

Alpha-actinin 3 as a candidate

Another candidate gene that recently has been associated with performance phenotypes is alpha-actinin 3 (*ACTN3*). Alpha-actinin 3 is an actin-binding protein expressed in fast (type 2) muscle fibers, where it cross-links actin thin filaments. *ACTN3* deficiency caused by a premature stop codon mutation in position 577 (R577X mutation) is fairly common. Yang *et al.* (2003) reported that the frequency of the stop-codon mutation was significantly lower among Australian sprint and power athletes than in non-athlete controls (Table 12.4). In a small group of Finnish top sprinters (*n* = 23), none of the athletes were homozygotes for the stop codon. However, the genotype and allele frequencies did not differ from control subjects or endurance athletes (Niemi & Majamaa 2005). Likewise, the *ACTN3* genotype frequencies in Spanish cyclists and runners did not differ from controls (Lucia *et al.* 2006). Clarkson *et al.* (2005) reported a greater improvement in dynamic elbow flexor strength after a 12-week strength training program among women who were *ACTN* X577X homozygous compared to heterozygous and R577R-homozygous women. However, the *ACTN3* genotypes were not associated with muscle strength phenotypes in men (Clarkson *et al.* 2005). However, Moran *et al.* (2007) reported that the *ACTN3* 577R allele was associated with faster 40 m sprint times in adolescent boys from Greece, whereas no associations were found in girls. Furthermore, other performance phenotypes, such as hand grip test, basketball throw, vertical jump, agility run, and aerobic capacity, were not associated with the *ACTN3* genotypes in boys or girls. Thus, it seems that the *ACTN3* genotype association study results are beginning to reflect a level of heterogeneity comparable to the studies dealing with the *ACE* I/D polymorphism.

Gene expression studies and novel candidates

Acute or chronic adaptation to exercise is dependent on the expression level of multiple genes.

Table 12.4 Summary of the ACTN3 R577X genotype studies with performance phenotypes.

Study	Group (sample size)	577X allele frequency	X577X genotype frequency	Main findings
Yang *et al.* (2003)	Sprint (*n* = 73)	0.28	0.06	X allele frequency lower in sprinters vs. controls and endurance
	Endurance (*n* = 40)	0.46	0.24	
	Controls (*n* = 120)	0.44	0.18	
Niemi & Majamaa (2005)	Sprint (*n* = 73)	0.29	0.09	No difference in frequencies between athletes and controls
	Endurance (*n* = 40)	0.30	0.10	
	Control (*n* = 120)	0.32	0.09	
Lucia *et al.* (2006)	Cyclists (*n* = 50)	0.49	0.26	No difference in frequencies between athletes and controls
	Runners (*n* = 52)	0.46	0.17	
	Controls (*n* = 123)	0.45	0.18	
Clarkson *et al.* (2005)	Men (*n* = 182)	0.51	0.264	Greater training-induced increase in strength in the X/X vs. R/R homozygotes in women. No difference in men
	Women (*n* = 287)	0.49	0.268	
Moran *et al.* (2007)	Boys (*n* = 507)	0.42	0.183	R allele associated with faster 40 m sprint time in boys but not in girls
	Girls (*n* = 439)	0.41	0.17	

Advances in microarray technology have opened new opportunities to investigate the expression levels of thousands of genes simultaneously in a single experiment. This allows the exploration of the effects of a specific stimulus, such as exercise, on the expression patterns of several gene families, such as transcription factors or genes involved in specific metabolic or physiological pathways.

This technology has been applied to strength training with a focus on the vastus lateralis gene expression changes in sedentary young and older adults of both sexes (Roth *et al.* 2002). A total of 69 genes showed >1.7-fold difference in expression levels after the training period in the pooled data. Bronikowski *et al.* (2003) investigated cardiac expression levels of 11 904 genes in middle-aged and old male mice derived from sedentary and spontaneously physically active selective breeding lines. In the sedentary animals, 137 genes showed significant aging-related changes in expression levels. These genes were involved in inflammatory and stress responses, signal transduction, and energy metabolism. However, in the physically active animals, the number of genes showing expression changes with age was significantly lower ($n = 62$) than in the sedentary animals.

To find novel candidate genes for exercise-induced improvement in insulin sensitivity (S_I), total RNA was isolated from vastus lateralis before and after 20 weeks of exercise from individuals participating in the HERITAGE Family Study (Teran-Garcia *et al.* 2005). Sixteen subjects were selected: eight showing no changes in S_I (low responders; LS_IR) and eight displaying marked improvement in S_I (high responders; HS_IR) with endurance training. The S_I increase was about four times greater in HS_IR than LS_IR ($+3.6 \pm 0.5$ vs. -1.2 ± 0.5 $\mu U \cdot mL^{-1} \cdot min^{-1}$, mean $\pm$ SE), whereas age, body mass index (BMI), percentage body fat, and baseline S_I were similar between the groups. Almost twice as many genes showed greater than twofold differences between HS_IR and LS_IR after training compared with pre-training. The differentially expressed genes were involved in energy metabolism and signaling, novel structural genes, and transcripts of unknown functions. Genes of interest upregulated in HS_IR included V-Ski oncogene (*SKI*), four and half LIM domain 1 (*FHL1*), and titin (*TTN*).

These gene expression studies and others not reviewed here suggest that the genes most commonly responsive to acute or regular exercise pertain to energy metabolism, cell signaling, cytoskeleton, and inflammatory pathways. Understanding the profile of acute exercise- or training-related changes in gene expression and their time dependence can potentially provide us with new strong candidates for variation in performance or trainability. An example of this translational path comes from the development of a transgenic mouse in which the peroxisome proliferator-activated receptor delta (PPARD) was overexpressed in skeletal muscle (Wang *et al.* 2004). Targeted expression of an activated form of PPARD in skeletal muscles increased the formation of type 1 muscle fibers and improved running capacity in mice. These mice were able to run as much as twice the distance compared to wild-type littermates, and they were resistant to high-fat diet-induced obesity and glucose intolerance. In wild-type mice, treatment with PPARD agonist produced similar increase in type 1 fibers as PPARD activation in transgenic mice (Wang *et al.* 2004). It has also been reported that endurance training promotes accumulation of PPARD protein in skeletal muscle of mice (Luquet *et al.* 2003). Globally, these results suggest that PPARD is potentially a molecular regulator of muscle fiber type and a modifier of endurance training induced changes in muscular performance.

More recently, it has been proposed to combine the power of RNA microarray technologies with the advantages of classic mapping techniques by using gene expression levels as quantitative traits, to be mapped as quantitative trait loci (Secko 2005). Even though this has not been widely applied to humans yet, the approach has great potential. This should make it possible to define the nature of the sequence variation that contributes to complex phenotypes or disease traits from the point of view of systems or pathways that can be captured in the expression studies. The method could be applied to the study of the genetics of adipose tissue, skeletal muscle, or other organs in relevant experimental or observational study designs for performance phenotypes.

Genome-wide scans as a tool to identify new targets

An alternative strategy to identify genes affecting performance-related phenotypes relies on linkage analysis. The basic idea of genetic linkage is to test whether a genetic locus is transmitted from one generation to the next together with a trait (or another genetic locus) of interest. The process is fairly straightforward when the trait is influenced by only one (major) gene. In these cases, the underlying genetic architecture can be deducted by observing the transmission of the trait in affected families, which allows generation of powerful models for linkage testing with genetic markers. However, multifactorial and oligogenic traits such as performance phenotypes rarely follow a specific inheritance model. In this case, it is not possible to use traditional parametric or model-based linkage methods. Instead, the linkage test for oligogenic traits is based on the idea that a pair of relatives (usually siblings) who are genetically similar should also be alike in terms of phenotypic values. The genetic similarity of the pair is determined by estimating how many common alleles at a given locus the individuals have inherited from the same ancestors (allele sharing IBD).

The statistical testing of linkage is usually carried out by using either regression-based methods (Haseman & Elston 1972; Elston *et al*. 2000) or by a variance components modeling. Briefly, in the original Haseman–Elston regression method, the phenotypic resemblance of a sibling pair, modeled as a squared sib-pair trait difference, is regressed on the genotypic resemblance (alleles shared IBD). In the variance component linkage methods, the total phenotypic variance is decomposed into additive effects of a trait locus, a residual familial background, and a residual non-familial component, and the phenotypic covariance of the pair of relatives is modeled as a function of allele sharing IBD. The linkage testing is performed using likelihood ratio test contrasting a null hypothesis model of no linkage with an alternative hypothesis model in which the variance brought about by the trait locus is estimated (Rao & Province 2003).

Thus, linkage analysis can be used to identify chromosomal regions that harbor gene(s) affecting a phenotype, even if there is no *a priori* knowledge of the existence of such genes. By definition, linkage analysis always requires family data. Therefore, data collection is more challenging than in case–control and cohort studies with unrelated subjects. The usefulness of linkage analysis to study elite athletes is predictably quite limited. However, in studies on interindividual differences in responsiveness to acute exercise and exercise training, the family design can provide exploratory data that are not available in association studies with independent subjects.

The HERITAGE Family Study is the first and thus far the only study employing a family design in exercise-related questions (Bouchard *et al*. 1995). Several genome-wide linkage scans dealing with endurance training response and acute exercise response phenotypes have been published based on the HERITAGE Family Study data.

An example of a QTL for endurance training-induced changes in submaximal exercise stroke volume on chromosome 10 is given in Fig. 12.9. The

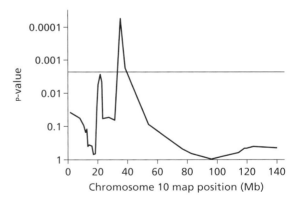

Fig. 12.9 A quantitative trait locus for submaximal exercise (50 W) stroke volume training response on chromosome 10 in the HERITAGE Family Study. *P* values from the regression-based multipoint linkage analysis are shown on the *y* axis, and chromosomal location derived from the Location Database is on the *x* axis. The reference line indicates the criteria for promising linkage (*P* < 0.0023). For further details, see Rankinen *et al*. (2002). Reproduced with permission from Human Kinetics.

QTL covers approximately 15 million bp in the short arm of chromosome 10 (10p11.2) and the maximum linkage (LOD = 1.96) was detected with the microsatellite marker D10S1666 (Rankinen *et al.* 2002). In the same study, promising linkages were also found on chromosome 8q24.3 and on 10q23–q24 for SBP measured during submaximal exercise or its response to training.

The first genome-wide linkage scan for $\dot{V}o_{2max}$ did not produce any strong QTLs, but several suggestive linkage signals were found, such as for the sedentary state $\dot{V}o_{2max}$ on chromosome 4q12 and for $\dot{V}o_{2max}$ training response on 4q26 and 6p21.33 (Bouchard *et al.* 2000a). The lack of particularly strong QTLs most likely reflects the polygenic nature of $\dot{V}o_{2max}$, which is influenced by several intermediate phenotypes (e.g., cardiac output, oxygen transport capacity, oxidative capacity of the working muscles), and multiple genes contribute to the variation in each of these subphenotypes. A denser panel of genetic markers (509) was used in a subsequent study with a focus on $\dot{V}o_{2max}$ and maximal power output as well as their responses to the standardized HERITAGE training program (Rico-Sanz *et al.* 2004). Again, no strong evidence for linkage was uncovered. However, stronger evidence of linkage was found on chromosome 11p15 and 10q23 for $\dot{V}o_{2max}$ and maximal power output in the sedentary state and on 1p31 and 5q23 for their responsiveness to training. More work remains to be done to clarify the true nature of these linkage signals.

It is important to remember that the identification of a QTL is only the first step in the gene discovery process. Because linkage analysis provides information about a genomic region, a typical QTL may span several million base pairs. Such a vast region may contain dozens or even hundreds of genes. How to proceed from a QTL to a gene and eventually to a causal DNA sequence variant is beyond the scope of this chapter.

Comments on major challenges for research

The study of the genetics of human physical performance and the genetics of the biologic basis of human variation in the ability to respond to exercise training is an extremely complex undertaking. However, progress made in genomics and transgenic technologies has opened new avenues for experimental investigations that could not be contemplated even in the recent past. For instance, the International HapMap Consortium published the first detailed haplotype map of the human genome (Altshuler *et al.* 2005). We are likely to see further refinement of the HapMap in the coming years. Already we have a tool that should improve our ability to identify the complex genotypes that contribute to complex traits such as physical performance or trainability.

Moreover, introduction of microarray-based SNP genotyping methods has drastically increased the throughput and reduced the cost of SNP genotyping. The ability to assay hundreds of thousands of DNA sequence variants in a single experiment has also made genome-wide association studies a reality, and the first such studies have been already published (Klein *et al.* 2005). It is clear that genome-wide association scans will be an important part of the performance-related genetic studies in the future. However, a genome-wide association study is a major intellectual and financial investment, and several questions remain to be addressed to optimize the benefits from such an investment. These include the optimum number of SNPs, the optimum sample size and study design (e.g., case–control vs. family studies), the optimum statistical methods for a given study design, and the control of multiple testing bias. All these questions are topics of lively discussion and detailed research in the genetic community around the world.

One important issue that has not received any attention thus far is that of the role of the fetal life on postnatal biologic and behavioral determinants of performance and perhaps even trainability. For instance, it has been hypothesized that a low birth weight, taken as a marker of maternal nutritional deficiencies, is associated with childhood and adulthood obesity (Barker 2004). However, nothing is known about the role of maternal nutritional deficiencies and the physiological fitness of the fetus and the newborn child. Most of us are certainly prepared to accept that maternal nutrition has consequences on the fetus, and some of these effects have been shown to translate into individual differences in the risk for diseases later in life. There is a need for a major research effort designed to address this issue for physiological fitness, physical performance, and trainability. Interestingly, a recent study has shown that Wistar rat offspring of mothers who were undernourished during pregnancy had a diminished locomotor activity level shortly after birth and subsequently later in life (14 months) compared to rats born from mothers who were fed *ad libitum* during pregnancy (Vickers *et al.* 2003).

Finally, a growing body of data strongly suggests that epigenetic events may be implicated in altering gene expression modulating a phenotype or creating a predisposition over and above that inscribed in the DNA sequence of genes. The nature of epigenetic modifications of DNA and histones as well as their potential relevance to human physical performance and trainability is beyond the scope of this chapter. However, epigenetic modifications provide a new research path that may help us understand some of the variance unaccounted for in more classic genetic studies. For instance, one should look beyond sequence variation to take full advantage of studies performed with identical twins. Indeed, recent data suggesting that epigenetic differences arising during the lifetime of an individual are of particular interest when it comes to accounting for differences to standardized protocols or for discordance in phenotypes between brothers or sisters identical by descent. In an experiment performed on 40 pairs of MZ twins, it was observed that the patterns of epigenetic modifications diverged in older twins compared to infant twin pairs (Fraga *et al.* 2005). Using a combination of whole genome and locus-specific methods, it was found that about one-third of MZ pairs harbored epigenetic differences in DNA methylation and histone modification that had an impact on gene expression. These epigenetic events were more pronounced in MZ pairs who were older, had different lifestyles, and had spent less of their lives together, thus emphasizing the key role of environmental factors in fostering a different phenotype on an identical genotype (Fraga *et al.* 2005). The full implications of these observations remain to be understood.

Conclusions

Human variation in physical performance, including determinants of endurance performance as reviewed here, is ubiquitous among sedentary people. Several studies have focused on the genetic component of this extensive human heterogeneity and have conclusively found that there is a significant genetic component to it. Thus, low to moderate heritability levels have been reported for such traits as maximal oxygen uptake, stroke volume and cardiac output, skeletal muscle fiber type distribution and muscle maximum enzyme activities. There is also considerable human heterogeneity in the response to regular exercise even when the exercise dose is fully standardized. Twin and family studies have revealed that there are family lines composed of high responders and other lineages in which family members are non-responders or exhibit low trainability when challenged by a standardized endurance training program. Again, the phenomenon is observed for the gains in maximal oxygen uptake, stroke volume and other hemodynamic traits, and skeletal muscle metabolism.

The search for the genes and DNA sequence variants associated with this human heterogeneity has yielded several candidates but the results are equivocal. For instance, two of the most studied candidates, *ACE* and *ACTN3*, are characterized by a range of contradictory findings. A common weakness in studies of candidate genes reported to date is that of a low and inadequate statistical power. Genome-wide screen with hundreds of markers have made it possible to identify a few chromosomal regions likely to harbor genes of relevance to endurance or its trainability. Expression studies have the potential to generate new gene targets to be explored for their contributions to performance and trainability. While genetic studies will eventually yield very important information on the biology of human performance and the response to exercise training, an in-depth understanding of the complex causal network of human variation in these attributes will also require that *in utero* and early postnatal influences, including the role of DNA methylation and histone modifications, on programming of physiological and metabolic pathways as well as on behavioral patterns be incorporated in our conceptual framework.

References

Altshuler, D., Brooks, L.D., Chakravarti, A., Collins, F.S., Daly, M.J. & Donnelly, P. (2005) A haplotype map of the human genome. *Nature* **437**, 1299–1320.

Alvarez, R., Terrados, N., Ortolano, R., *et al.* (2000) Genetic variation in the renin–angiotensin system and athletic performance. *European Journal of Applied Physiology* **82**, 117–120.

An, P., Rice, T., Gagnon, J., *et al.* (2000) Familial aggregation of stroke volume and cardiac output during submaximal exercise: the HERITAGE Family Study. *International Journal of Sports Medicine* **21**, 566–572.

Barbato, J.C., Koch, L.G., Darvish, A., Cicila, G.T., Metting, P.J. & Britton, S.L. (1998) Spectrum of aerobic endurance running performance in eleven inbred strains of rats. *Journal of Applied Physiology* **85**, 530–536.

Barker, D. (2004) Fetal origins of obesity. In: *Handbook of Obesity* (Bray, G.A. & Bouchard, C., eds.) Marcel Dekker, New York: 109–116.

Bielen, E., Fagard, R. & Amery, A. (1991a) The inheritance of left ventricular structure and function assessed by imaging and Doppler echocardiography. *American Heart Journal* **121**, 1743–1749.

Bielen, E.C., Fagard, R.H. & Amery, A.K. (1991b) Inheritance of acute cardiac changes during bicycle exercise: an echocardiographic study in twins. *Medicine and Science in Sports and Exercise* **23**, 1254–1259.

Bonnefont, J.P., Demaugre, F., Prip-Buus, C., *et al.* (1999) Carnitine palmitoyltransferase deficiencies. *Molecular Genetics and Metabolism* **68**, 424–440.

Bouchard, C. (1983) Human adaptability may have a genetic basis. In: *Health Risk Estimation, Risk Reduction and Health Promotion.* Proceedings of the 18th annual meeting of the Society of Prospective Medicine (Landry, F., ed.). Canadian Public Health Association, Ottowa: 463–476.

Bouchard, C. (1995) Individual differences in the response to regular exercise. *International Journal of Obesity and Related Metabolic Disorders* **19** (Supplement 4), S5–S8.

Bouchard, C., An, P., Rice, T., *et al.* (1999) Familial aggregation of $\dot{V}o_{2max}$ response to exercise training: results from the HERITAGE Family Study. *Journal of Applied Physiology* **87**, 1003–1008.

Bouchard, C., Daw, E.W., Rice, T., *et al.* (1998) Familial resemblance for $\dot{V}o_{2max}$ in the sedentary state: the HERITAGE family study. *Medicine and Science in Sports and Exercise* **30**, 252–258.

Bouchard, C., Dionne, F.T., Simoneau, J.A. & Boulay, M.R. (1992) Genetics of aerobic and anaerobic performances. *Exercise and Sport Sciences Reviews* **20**, 27–58.

Bouchard, C., Leon, A.S., Rao, D.C., Skinner, J.S., Wilmore, J.H. & Gagnon, J. (1995) The HERITAGE family study. Aims, design, and measurement protocol. *Medicine and Science in Sports and Exercise* **27**, 721–729.

Bouchard, C., Lesage, R., Lortie, G., *et al.* (1986a) Aerobic performance in brothers, dizygotic and monozygotic twins. *Medicine and Science in Sports and Exercise* **18**, 639–646.

Bouchard, C. & Rankinen, T. (2001) Individual differences in response to regular physical activity. *Medicine and Science in Sports and Exercise* **33**, S446–S451.

Bouchard, C., Rankinen, T., Chagnon, Y.C., *et al.* (2000a) Genomic scan for maximal oxygen uptake and its response to training in the HERITAGE Family Study. *Journal of Applied Physiology* **88**, 551–559.

Bouchard, C., Simoneau, J.A., Lortie, G., Boulay, M.R., Marcotte, M. & Thibault, M.C. (1986b) Genetic effects in human skeletal muscle fiber type distribution and enzyme activities. *Canadian Journal of Physiological Pharmacology* **64**, 1245–1251.

Bouchard, C., Wolfarth, B., Rivera, M.A., Gagnon, J. & Simoneau, J.A. (2000b) Genetic determinants of endurance performance. In: *Endurance in Sport* (Shephard, R.J. & Åstrand, P.O., eds.) Blackwell Science, Oxford: 223–242.

Boule, N.G., Weisnagel, S.J., Lakka, T.A., *et al.* (2005) Effects of exercise training on glucose homeostasis: the HERITAGE Family Study. *Diabetes Care* **28**, 108–114.

Bronikowski, A.M., Carter, P.A., Morgan, T.J., *et al.* (2003) Lifelong voluntary exercise in the mouse prevents age-related alterations in gene expression in the heart. *Physiological Genomics* **12**, 129–138.

Bruno, C., Manfredi, G., Andreu, A.L., *et al.* (1998) A splice junction mutation in the alpha(M) gene of phosphorylase kinase in a patient with myopathy. *Biochemical and Biophysical Research Communications* **249**, 648–651.

Cam, F.S., Colakoglu, M., Sekuri, C., Colakoglu, S., Sahan, C. & Berdeli, A. (2005) Association between the ACE I/D gene polymorphism and physical performance in a homogeneous non-elite cohort. *Canadian Journal of Applied Physiology* **30**, 74–86.

Cardon, L.R. & Palmer, L.J. (2003) Population stratification and spurious allelic association. *Lancet* **361**, 598–604.

Clarkson, P.M., Devaney, J.M., Gordish-Dressman, H., *et al.* (2005) ACTN3 genotype is associated with increases in muscle strength in response to resistance training in women. *Journal of Applied Physiology* **99**, 154–163.

Comi, G.P., Fortunato, F., Lucchiari, S., *et al.* (2001) Beta-enolase deficiency, a new metabolic myopathy of distal glycolysis. *Annals of Neurology* **50**, 202–207.

Elston, R.C., Buxbaum, S., Jacobs, K.B. & Olson, J.M. (2000) Haseman and Elston revisited. *Genetic Epidemiology* **19**, 1–17.

Fagard, R., Bielen, E. & Amery, A. (1991) Heritability of aerobic power and anaerobic energy generation during exercise. *Journal of Applied Physiology* **70**, 357–362.

Folland, J., Leach, B., Little, T., *et al.* (2000) Angiotensin-converting enzyme genotype affects the response of human skeletal muscle to functional overload. *Experimental Physiology* **85**, 575–579.

Fraga, M.F., Ballestar, E., Paz, M.F., *et al.* (2005) Epigenetic differences arise during the lifetime of monozygotic twins. *Proceedings of the National Academy of Science USA* **102**, 10604–10609.

Gayagay, G., Yu, B., Hambly, B., *et al.* (1998) Elite endurance athletes and the ACE I allele: the role of genes in athletic performance. *Human Genetics* **103**, 48–50.

Gonzalez, N.C., Kirkton, S.D., Howlett, R.A., *et al.* (2006) Continued divergence in $\dot{V}o_{2max}$ of rats selected for running endurance is mediated by greater convective blood O_2 delivery. *Journal of Applied Physiology* **101**, 1288–1296.

Hadjigeorgiou, G.M., Kawashima, N., Bruno, C., *et al.* (1999) Manifesting heterozygotes in a Japanese family with a novel mutation in the muscle-specific phosphoglycerate mutase (PGAM-M) gene. *Neuromuscular Disorders* **9**, 399–402.

Hagberg, J.M., Ferrell, R.E., McCole, S.D., Wilund, K.R. & Moore, G.E. (1998) $\dot{V}o_{2max}$ is associated with ACE genotype in postmenopausal women. *Journal of Applied Physiology* **85**, 1842–1846.

Hamano, T., Mutoh, T., Sugie, H., Koga, H. & Kuriyama, M. (2000) Phosphoglycerate kinase deficiency: an adult myopathic form with a novel mutation. *Neurology* **54**, 1188–1190.

Hamel, P., Simoneau, J.A., Lortie, G., Boulay, M.R. & Bouchard, C. (1986) Heredity and muscle adaptation to endurance training. *Medicine and Science in Sports and Exercise* **18**, 690–696.

Haseman, J.K. & Elston, R.C. (1972) The investigation of linkage between a quantitative trait and a marker locus. *Behavior Genetics* **2**, 3–19.

Hautala, A.J., Makikallio, T.H., Kiviniemi, A., *et al.* (2003) Cardiovascular autonomic function correlates with the response to aerobic training in healthy sedentary subjects. *American Journal of Physiology Heart and Circulatory Physiology* **285**, H1747–H1752.

Henderson, K.K., Wagner, H., Favret, F., *et al.* (2002) Determinants of maximal O₂ uptake in rats selectively bred for endurance running capacity. *Journal of Applied Physiology* **93**, 1265–1274.

Hopkinson, N.S., Nickol, A.H., Payne, J., *et al.* (2004) Angiotensin converting enzyme genotype and strength in chronic obstructive pulmonary disease. *American Journal of Respiratory Critical Care Medicine* **170**, 395–399.

Howlett, R.A., Gonzalez, N.C., Wagner, H.E., *et al.* (2003) Selected contribution: skeletal muscle capillary and enzyme activity in rats selectively bred for running endurance. *Journal of Applied Physiology* **94**, 1682–1688.

Kasikcioglu, E., Kayserilioglu, A., Ciloglu, F., *et al.* (2004) Angiotensin-converting enzyme gene polymorphism, left ventricular remodeling, and exercise capacity in strength-trained athletes. *Heart Vessels* **19**, 287–293.

Klein, R.J., Zeiss, C., Chew, E.Y., *et al.* (2005) Complement factor H polymorphism in age-related macular degeneration. *Science* **308**, 385–389.

Klissouras, V. (1971) Heritability of adaptive variation. *Journal of Applied Physiology* **31**, 338–344.

Klissouras, V., Pirnay, F. & Petit, J.M. (1973) Adaptation to maximal effort: genetics and age. *Journal of Applied Physiology* **35**, 288–293.

Koch, L.G., Meredith, T.A., Fraker, T.D., Metting, P.J. & Britton, S.L. (1998) Heritability of treadmill running endurance in rats. *American Journal of Physiology* **275**, R1455–R1460.

Kohrt, W.M., Malley, M.T., Coggan, A.R., *et al.* (1991) Effects of gender, age, and fitness level on response of $\dot{V}o_{2max}$ to training in 60–71 year olds. *Journal of Applied Physiology* **71**, 2004–2011.

Leon, A.S., Rice, T., Mandel, S., *et al.* (2000) Blood lipid response to 20 weeks of supervised exercise in a large biracial population: the HERITAGE Family Study. *Metabolism: Clinical and Experimental* **49**, 513–520.

Lesage, R., Simoneau, J.A., Jobin, J., Leblanc, J. & Bouchard, C. (1985) Familial resemblance in maximal heart rate, blood lactate and aerobic power. *Human Heredity* **35**, 182–189.

Lortie, G., Bouchard, C., Leblanc, C., *et al.* (1982) Familial similarity in aerobic power. *Human Biology* **54**, 801–812.

Lortie, G., Simoneau, J.A., Hamel, P., Boulay, M.R., Landry, F. & Bouchard, C. (1984) Responses of maximal aerobic power and capacity to aerobic training. *International Journal of Sports Medicine* **5**, 232–236.

Lucia, A., Gomez-Gallego, F., Chicharro, J.L., *et al.* (2005) Is there an association between ACE and CKMM polymorphisms and cycling performance status during 3-week races? *International Journal of Sports Medicine* **26**, 442–447.

Lucia, A., Gomez-Gallego, F., Santiago, C., *et al.* (2006) ACTN3 genotype in professional endurance cyclists. *International Journal of Sports Medicine* **27**, 880–884.

Luquet, S., Lopez-Soriano, J., Holst, D., *et al.* (2003) Peroxisome proliferator-activated receptor delta controls muscle development and oxidative capability. *FASEB Journal* **17**, 2299–2301.

Maekawa, M., Sudo, K., Kanno, T. & Li, S.S. (1990) Molecular characterization of genetic mutation in human lactate dehydrogenase-A (M) deficiency. *Biochemical and Biophysical Research Communications* **168**, 677–682.

Maes, H.H., Beunen, G., Vlietinck, R., *et al.* (1993) Heritability of health- and performance-related fitness: data from the Leuven Longitudinal Twin Study. In: *Kinanthropometry IV* (Duquet, W. & Day, J.A.P., eds.) Spon, London: 140–149.

Maes, H.H., Beunen, G.P., Vlietinck, R.F., *et al.* (1996) Inheritance of physical fitness in 10-yr-old twins and their parents. *Medicine and Science in Sports and Exercise* **28**, 1479–1491.

McArdle, B. (1951) Myopathy due to a defect in muscle glycogen breakdown. *Clinical Science* **10**, 13–33.

Mitchell, J.H. & Raven, P.B. (1994) Cardiovascular adaptation to physical activity. In: *Physical Activity, Fitness, and Health* (Bouchard, C., Shephard, R.Y. & Stephens, T., eds.) Human Kinetics, Champaign, IL: 286–301.

Montgomery, H.E., Marshall, R., Hemingway, H., *et al.* (1998) Human gene for physical performance. *Nature* **393**, 221–222.

Montoye, H.J. & Gayle, R. (1978) Familial relationships in maximal oxygen uptake. *Human Biology* **50**, 241–249.

Moran, C.N., Vassilopoulos, C., Tsiokanos, A., *et al.* (2006) The associations of ACE polymorphisms with physical, physiological and skill parameters in adolescents. *European Journal of Human Genetics* **14**, 332–339.

Moran, C.N., Yang, N., Bailey, M.E., *et al.* (2007) Association analysis of the ACTN3 R577X polymorphism and complex quantitative body composition and performance phenotypes in adolescent Greeks. *European Journal of Human Genetics* **15**, 88–93.

Myerson, S., Hemingway, H., Budget, R., Martin, J., Humphries, S. & Montgomery, H. (1999) Human angiotensin I-converting enzyme gene and endurance performance. *Journal of Applied Physiology* **87**, 1313–1316.

Niemi, A.K. & Majamaa, K. (2005) Mitochondrial DNA and ACTN3 genotypes in Finnish elite endurance and sprint athletes. *European Journal of Human Genetics* **13**, 965–969.

Ookawara, T., Dave, V., Willems, P., *et al.* (1996) Retarded and aberrant splicings caused by single exon mutation in a phosphoglycerate kinase variant. *Archives of Biochemistry and Biophysics* **327**, 35–40.

Pescatello, L.S., Kostek, M.A., Gordish-Dressman, H., *et al.* (2006) ACE ID genotype and the muscle strength and size response to unilateral resistance training. *Medicine and Science in Sports and Exercise* **38**, 1074–1081.

Prud'homme, D., Bouchard, C., Leblanc, C., Landry, F. & Fontaine, E. (1984) Sensitivity of maximal aerobic power to training is genotype-dependent. *Medicine and Science in Sports and Exercise* **16**, 489–493.

Rankinen, T., An, P., Perusse, L., *et al.* (2002) Genome-wide linkage scan for exercise stroke volume and cardiac output in the HERITAGE Family Study. *Physiological Genomics* **10**, 57–62.

Rankinen, T., Bouchard, C. & Rao, D.C. (2005) Corrigendum: Familial resemblance for muscle phenotypes: The HERITAGE Family Study. *Medicine and Science in Sports and Exercise* **37**, 2017.

Rankinen, T., Perusse, L., Gagnon, J., *et al.* (2000) Angiotensin-converting enzyme ID polymorphism and fitness phenotype in the HERITAGE Family Study. *Journal of Applied Physiology* **88**, 1029–1035.

Rankinen, T., Perusse, L., Rauramaa, R., Rivera, M.A., Wolfarth, B. & Bouchard, C. (2006a) The human gene map for performance and health-related fitness phenotypes: the 2005 update. *Medicine and Science in Sports and Exercise* **38**, 1863–1868.

Rankinen, T., Zuberi, A., Chagnon, Y.C., *et al.* (2006b) The human obesity gene map: the 2005 update. *Obesity (Silver Spring)* **14**, 529–644.

Rao, D.C. & Province, M.A. (2003) *Genetic Dissection of Complex Traits*. Academic Press, San Diego.

Rico-Sanz, J., Rankinen, T., Joanisse, D.R., *et al.* (2003) Familial resemblance for muscle phenotypes in the HERITAGE Family Study. *Medicine and Science in Sports and Exercise* **35**, 1360–1366.

Rico-Sanz, J., Rankinen, T., Rice, T., *et al.* (2004) Quantitative trait loci for maximal exercise capacity phenotypes and their responses to training in the HERITAGE Family Study. *Physiological Genomics* **16**, 256–260.

Rigat, B., Hubert, C., Alhenc-Gelas, F., Cambien, F., Corvol, P. & Soubrier, F. (1990) An insertion/deletion polymorphism in the angiotensin I-converting enzyme gene accounting for half the variance of serum enzyme levels. *Journal of Clinical Investigation* **86**, 1343–1346.

Roth, S.M., Ferrell, R.E., Peters, D.G., Metter, E.J., Hurley, B.F. & Rogers, M.A. (2002) Influence of age, sex, and strength training on human muscle gene expression determined by microarray. *Physiological Genomics* **10**, 181–190.

Saltin, B. & Strange, S. (1992) Maximal oxygen uptake: "old" and "new" arguments for a cardiovascular limitation. *Medicine and Science in Sports and Exercise* **24**, 30–37.

Scholte, H.R., Van Coster, R.N., de Jonge, P.C., *et al.* (1999) Myopathy in very-long-chain acyl-CoA dehydrogenase deficiency: clinical and biochemical differences with the fatal cardiac phenotype. *Neuromuscular Disorders* **9**, 313–319.

Secko, D. (2005) Genetics embraces expression. *The Scientist* **19**, 26–29.

Sherman, J.B., Raben, N., Nicastri, C., *et al.* (1994) Common mutations in the phosphofructokinase-M gene in Ashkenazi Jewish patients with glycogenesis VII: and their population frequency. *American Journal of Human Genetics* **55**, 305–313.

Simoneau, J.A. (1995) Adaptation of human skeletal muscle to exercise-training. *International Journal of Obesity and Related Metabolic Disorders* **19** (Supplement 4), S9–13.

Simoneau, J.A. & Bouchard, C. (1989) Human variation in skeletal muscle fiber-type proportion and enzyme activities. *American Journal of Physiology* **257**, E567–E572.

Simoneau, J.A. & Bouchard, C. (1995) Genetic determinism of fiber type proportion in human skeletal muscle. *FASEB Journal* **9**, 1091–1095.

Simoneau, J.A., Lortie, G., Boulay, M.R., Marcotte, M., Thibault, M.C. & Bouchard, C. (1986a) Inheritance of human skeletal muscle and anaerobic capacity adaptation to high-intensity intermittent training. *International Journal of Sports Medicine* **7**, 167–171.

Simoneau, J.A., Lortie, G., Boulay, M.R., Thibault, M.C. & Bouchard, C. (1986b) Repeatability of fibre type and enzyme activity measurements in human skeletal muscle. *Clinical Physiology* **6**, 347–356.

Sugie, H., Sugie, Y., Ito, M. & Fukuda, T. (1998) A novel missense mutation (837T → C) in the phosphoglycerate kinase gene of a patient with a myopathic form of phosphoglycerate kinase deficiency. *Journal of Child Neurology* **13**, 95–97.

Sundet, J.M., Magnus, P. & Tambs, K. (1994) The heritability of maximal aerobic power: a study of Norwegian twins. *Scandinavian Journal of Medicine in Science and Sports* **4**, 181–185.

Teran-Garcia, M., Rankinen, T., Koza, R.A., Rao, D.C. & Bouchard, C. (2005) Endurance training-induced changes in insulin sensitivity and gene expression. *American Journal of Physiology: Endocrinology and Metabolism* **288**, E1168–E1178.

Toscano, A., Tsujino, S., Vita, G., Shanske, S., Messina, C. & DiMauro, S. (1996) Molecular basis of muscle phosphoglycerate mutase (PGAM-M) deficiency in the Italian kindred. *Muscle Nerve* **19**, 1134–1137.

Tsujino, S., Servidei, S., Tonin, P., Shanske, S., Azan, G. & DiMauro, S. (1994a) Identification of three novel mutations in non-Ashkenazi Italian patients with muscle phosphofructokinase deficiency. *American Journal of Human Genetics* **54**, 812–819.

Tsujino, S., Shanske, S., Brownell, A.K., Haller, R.G. & DiMauro, S. (1994b) Molecular genetic studies of muscle lactate dehydrogenase deficiency in white patients. *Annals of Neurology* **36**, 661–665.

Tsujino, S., Shanske, S. & DiMauro, S. (1993a) Molecular genetic heterogeneity of myophosphorylase deficiency (McArdle's disease). *New England Journal of Medicine* **329**, 241–245.

Tsujino, S., Shanske, S., Sakoda, S., Fenichel, G. & DiMauro, S. (1993b) The molecular genetic basis of muscle phosphoglycerate mutase (PGAM) deficiency. *American Journal of Human Genetics* **52**, 472–477.

Tsujino, S., Tonin, P., Shanske, S., *et al.* (1994c) A splice junction mutation in a new myopathic variant of phosphoglycerate kinase deficiency (PGK North Carolina). *Annals of Neurology* **35**, 349–353.

Verhaaren, H.A., Schieken, R.M., Mosteller, M., Hewitt, J.K., Eaves, L.J. & Nance, W.E. (1991) Bivariate genetic analysis of left ventricular mass and weight in pubertal twins (the Medical College of Virginia twin study). *American Journal of Cardiolology* **68**, 661–668.

Vickers, M.H., Breier, B.H., McCarthy, D. & Gluckman, P.D. (2003) Sedentary behavior during postnatal life is determined by the prenatal environment and exacerbated by postnatal hypercaloric nutrition. *American Journal of Physiology Regulatory, Integrative and Comparative Physiology* **285**, R271–R273.

Vorgerd, M., Karitzky, J., Ristow, M., *et al.* (1996) Muscle phosphofructokinase deficiency in two generations. *Journal of Neurological Science* **141**, 95–99.

Wang, Y.X., Zhang, C.L., Yu, R.T., *et al.* (2004) Regulation of muscle fiber type and running endurance by PPARdelta. *PLoS Biology* **2**, e294.

Wehner, M., Clemens, P.R., Engel, A.G. & Kilimann, M.W. (1994) Human muscle glycogenosis due to phosphorylase kinase deficiency associated with a nonsense mutation in the muscle isoform of the alpha subunit. *Human Molecular Genetics* **3**, 1983–1987.

Williams, A.G., Day, S.H., Folland, J.P., Gohlke, P., Dhamrait, S. & Montgomery, H.E. (2005) Circulating angiotensin converting enzyme activity is correlated with muscle strength. *Medicine and Science in Sports and Exercise* **37**, 944–948.

Williams, A.G., Rayson, M.P., Jubb, M., *et al.* (2000) The ACE gene and muscle performance. *Nature* **403**, 614.

Wilmore, J.H., Stanforth, P.R., Gagnon, J., *et al.* (2001a) Cardiac output and stroke volume changes with endurance training: the HERITAGE Family Study. *Medicine and Science in Sports and Exercise* **33**, 99–106.

Wilmore, J.H., Stanforth, P.R., Gagnon, J., *et al.* (2001b) Heart rate and blood pressure changes with endurance training: the HERITAGE Family Study. *Medicine and Science in Sports and Exercise* **33**, 107–116.

Woods, D., Hickman, M., Jamshidi, Y., *et al.* (2001) Elite swimmers and the D allele of the ACE I/D polymorphism. *Human Genetics* **108**, 230–232.

Woods, D.R., World, M., Rayson, M.P., *et al.* (2002) Endurance enhancement related to the human angiotensin I-converting enzyme I-D polymorphism is not due to differences in the cardiorespiratory response to training. *European Journal of Applied Physiology* **86**, 240–244.

Yang, N., MacArthur, D.G., Gulbin, J.P., *et al.* (2003) ACTN3 genotype is associated with human elite athletic performance. *American Journal of Human Genetics* **73**, 627–631.

Zhao, B., Moochhala, S.M., Tham, S., *et al.* (2003) Relationship between angiotensin-converting enzyme ID polymorphism and Vo_{2max} of Chinese males. *Life Science* **73**, 2625–2630.

Chapter 13

Molecular Mechanisms of Adaptations to Training

FRANK W. BOOTH AND P. DARRELL NEUFER

Knowledge about changes in molecules as a result of physical training is increasing rapidly and will have an impact on training methods. The decision was made to limit this chapter to the interactions between nutrition and exercise as this topic is most relevant to optimal sports performance, which will likely be the interest of most readers of this chapter.

The timing and type of nutrition in relationship to an exercise bout has an impact on the resultant extent of the adaptation to training. In addition, the type of exercise (resistance or endurance) affects which genes interact with nutrition to produce the nature and magnitude of the training adaptation. Athletes are interested in superior physical performance so they wish to obtain every legal "edge." Only cellular and molecular studies of exercise and nutrition can provide the basic science which can then be applied to generate an "edge" in improved performance by means of the timing and quality of nutrition.

As every athlete knows, the ability to perform improves with training and declines when training ceases. The body senses exercise and signals changes to improve performance; likewise it senses abstinence from training. There are three major strategies the body uses to send messages (signals) after an exercise bout:

1 *Whole body messengers:* exercise releases hormones into the blood that signal all cells. For example, high

intensity exercise increases "stress hormones" such as catecholamines that enhance glycogen breakdown in contracting muscles.

2 *Signals released by the active muscle:* e.g., intense-resistance exercise increases the production of insulin-like growth factor 1 (IGF-1) in skeletal muscle cells. IGF-1 is released from the muscle cell and interacts with a receptor on the outer membrane of the same muscle cell. The binding of IGF-1 to its receptor (analogous to fitting a key [IGF-1] into a lock [IGF-1 receptor]) initiates a cascade of events leading to an increased size of the muscle cell (hypertrophy).

3 *Signals acting within active muscle cell:* the muscle cell can signal itself internally. Adenosine monophosphate kinase (AMPK) inside the muscle cell senses when the energy status of the muscle cell begins to drop during exercise and signals the same muscle cell to begin to oxidize greater amounts of fatty acids.

Transition from endurance to strength adaptations

Adaptations in skeletal muscle from endurance and strength training differ; endurance adaptations consist of minimal or no hypertrophy and large increases in mitochondrial density, while strength adaptations have hypertrophy with minimal or no increases in mitochondria. Recently, some of the cellular bases for these differential changes have been reported. AMPK senses cellular energy status. Increases in the AMP : ATP ratio during endurance and resistance types of muscle contraction activate AMPK, whose activation in skeletal muscle represses

The Olympic Textbook of Science in Sport, 1st edition. Edited by R.J. Maughan. Published 2009 by Blackwell Publishing. ISBN: 978-1-4051-5638-7.

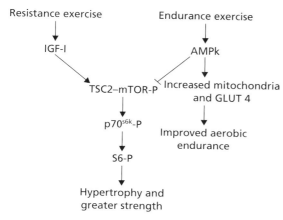

Fig. 13.1 An abbreviated view is shown for the differential signaling by two different exercise types that produce two different outcomes in physical performance. AMPK, adenosine monophosphate kinase; IGF-1, insulin-like growth factor 1; mTOR, mammalian target of rapamycin.

the growth-promoting mammalian target of rapamycin (mTOR) signaling pathway. A very simplified explanation is that endurance-type exercise may signal adaptations through the AMPK–PGC-1α pathway while hypertrophy-producing exercise may be signaling through the Akt (PKB)–TSC2–mTOR pathway (Fig. 13.1).

Forcing an increase in PGC-1α protein by genetic manipulation within non-exercising muscle causes increased mitochondrial density, which mimics an adaptation of endurance-type training. However, IGF-1, released locally within skeletal muscle as a result of mechanical overload, interacts with the IGF-1 receptor on the muscle's outer membrane and initiates signaling through Akt to increase the translation of mRNAs to make nascent proteins. Forcing an increase in Akt protein by genetic manipulation causes non-exercising muscles to hypertrophy, which mimics an adaptation of resistance-type training. A more in depth consideration of the two signaling pathways in response to endurance and strength exercises can be obtained from recent papers (Bolster *et al.* 2002; Atherton *et al.* 2005; Coffey *et al.* 2006).

The nutritional basis for resistance training is related more to the types and timing of amino acid availability, while for endurance training the timing of carbohydrate intake is more important.

Scientific basis for the timing of nutrition to enhance adaptations to resistance training

Response of protein synthesis and degradation to mechanically induced hypertrophy

GENERAL PRINCIPLES

Nutrients (amino acids as the building blocks of new protein as well as glucose and fatty acids as a source of ATP to fuel the assembly of amino acids into protein) are necessary to permit muscle growth in response to resistance exercise. The timing of nutrition in close relationship to the performance of the resistance exercise bout is necessary to enhance the potential for muscle growth.

PROTEIN SYNTHESIS INCREASES MORE THAN PROTEIN DEGRADATION IF MUSCLES HYPERTROPHY IN RESPONSE TO RESISTANCE TRAINING

In order to understand the concepts of timing and type of nutrition, the principles of the size of skeletal muscle mass need to be first presented. An increase in the mass of skeletal muscle can be caused by any of the following combinations:

• Protein synthesis increases while protein degradation decreases;
• Protein synthesis increases with no change in protein degradation;
• Protein synthesis is unchanged, but protein degradation falls;
• Percentage fall in protein degradation exceeds the percentage decline in protein synthesis;
• Percentage increase in protein synthesis greatly exceeds to the percentage increase in protein degradation.

The last of these seems to be what happens biologically, as first shown in living animals by Millward's laboratory with the model of stretch-induced hypertrophy of skeletal muscle in 1978 (Laurent, Sparrow & Millward 1978).

Wong and Booth (1990a) extended the stretch model of hypertrophy to actual resistance exercise by animals, and observed an increase in protein synthesis rates with resistance training. Because the percentage increase in protein synthesis greatly exceeded the percentage increase in muscle hypertrophy, they inferred that protein degradation must also have increased to eliminate the excess protein made. Similar observations were next made in human skeletal muscle by Chesley *et al*. (1992). Biolo *et al*. (1995) extended the findings by their direct determinations of muscle protein turnover; they found that an acceleration of both protein synthesis and degradation during recovery after resistance exercise. Biolo *et al*. (1995) employed stable isotopic tracers of amino acids, arteriovenous catheterization of the femoral vessels, and biopsy of the vastus lateralis muscle in human subjects.

Effect of nutrition timing in relation to resistance exercise time on protein synthesis

Studies have since refined these earlier observations by the important findings that the timing and type of nutrition affect the percentage increases in protein synthesis after resistance training.

PROTEIN MEAL

Biolo *et al*. (1997) found that infusing a balanced amino acid mixture immediately after resistance exercise in overnight fasted humans increased muscle protein synthesis to a greater extent than at rest, but did not affect protein degradation. An animal study extended the investigation of nutritional timing to resistance training. When a meal was ingested by animals in the hour immediately after resistance exercise during a 10-week training period, hind limb muscle weight was 6% higher than in a matched group eating in the fifth hour after the resistance exercise. Weights of abdominal fats were 24% lower in the animals fed immediately after exercise. These findings could be interpreted to suggest that the partitioning of calories between muscle and fat is dependent upon the timing of eating after resistance exercise. If muscles are primed by calories in the immediate period after resistance exercise, muscle protein synthesis can increase. These studies established that an edge in strength performance can be gained if food is ingested imme-

diately after resistance exercise. In conclusion, there is a small time window for nutrition to enhance protein synthesis when resistance exercise is performed; nutrition must be taken immediately before or after resistance exercise.

INCREASE IN PROTEIN TRANSLATION BY MECHANICALLY INDUCED HYPERTROPHY

To understand the scientific basis of how nutrition affects the magnitude of skeletal muscle hypertrophy it is necessary to present brief information on signaling to the translational regulation of protein synthesis. Protein translation is the amount of protein made from mRNA per unit of time. A guess that protein translation was increased by mechanical overload of muscle was already available in 1978 (Laurent, Sparrow & Millward 1978). Millward inferred that the increase in protein synthesis found in muscles undergoing stretch hypertrophy in the wings of chickens was mediated initially (after 1 day) by an increase in translation without any increase in RNA concentration. A few days of continued mechanical overload later, the increase in muscle protein synthesis reflected the higher RNA content. Wong and Booth (1990b) reported that as little as 8 min duration of total daily resistance-type exercise by animals increased gastrocnemius protein synthesis rates by nearly 50%, with minor effects on skeletal α-actin mRNA level, suggesting that translational and posttranslational mechanisms in the model of stimulated concentric resistance exercise likely were occurring. Later it was found that specific mRNAs are increased in muscle during recovery from resistance exercise.

BRANCHED-CHAIN AMINO ACIDS ENHANCE PROTEIN SYNTHESIS WHEN RESISTANCE EXERCISE OCCURS

In the 1970s, various investigators had already found that branched-chain amino acids (leucine, isoleucine, and valine), or leucine alone, stimulated protein synthesis rates in isolated or perfused skeletal muscles of animals. Almost two decades passed until similar experiments were performed in humans. Tipton *et al*. (1999) reported that comparable percentage enhancements in protein synthesis rates of skeletal muscle were obtained by oral solutions of either mixed (all) amino acids or of only essential amino acids (which include the branched-chain amino acids) after a bout of resistance exercise in men and women compared to an oral placebo solution. There was no significant difference between the treatments for the rate of protein breakdown. The amino acid effect on net muscle anabolism was also found not to be simply a caloric effect.

BRANCHED-CHAIN AMINO ACIDS ARE BEST CONSUMED IMMEDIATELY PRIOR TO RESISTANCE EXERCISE

The response of net muscle protein synthesis to consumption of an oral essential amino acid–carbohydrate supplement solution immediately before resistance exercise is greater than that when the solution is consumed after exercise in 30-year-old men and women. Tipton *et al.* (2001) suggest that this is primarily because of an increase in muscle protein synthesis as a result of increased delivery of amino acids to the legs during the exercise.

RECENT REVIEWS

There are numerous outstanding review articles with more detailed information on the effects of resistance exercise on muscle protein synthesis; the reader is encouraged to pursue them (Bolster *et al.* 2003a; Zambon *et al.* 2003; Phillips 2004; Norton & Layman 2006; Rennie *et al.* 2006; Wolfe 2006).

ALTERATIONS BY MECHANICALLY INDUCED HYPERTROPHY TO MOLECULES SIGNALING TO INCREASE PROTEIN TRANSLATION

One of the molecules activated downstream of Akt when Akt is activated by insulin or IGF-1 is mTOR. Bodine *et al.* (2001) showed that hypertrophy of skeletal muscle in adult animals seems to be crucially regulated by the activation of the Akt–mTOR pathway and its downstream targets, where mTOR phosphorylates the proteins $p70^{S6K}$ and 4E-BP1. When $p70^{S6K}$ and 4E-BP1 become phosphorylated, the translation of new proteins is increased. The post-exercise times of increases for the molecules

that increase protein translation in animal skeletal muscle in response to an acute bout of resistance exercise were first published by Bolster *et al.* (2003b). They are given in parenthesis after the molecule: Akt phosphorylation (5 and 10 min); mTOR (no change); 4E-BP1 phosphorylation (10, 15, and 30 min); eIF4E association to eIF4G (5 and 10 min); $p70^{S6K1}$ phosphorylation (no change); ribosomal protein S6 phosphorylation (10, 15, and 30 min); eIF2B activity (no change); and eIF2α phosphorylation (no change). Bolster *et al.* (2003a) interpreted their results as collectively providing strong evidence that events downstream of mTOR-mediating signaling are briefly upregulated during the first 30 min following an acute bout of resistance exercise and that this response may constitute the most proximal growth response of the muscle cell to resistance exercise. Phosphorylation of S6K1 is also increased 2- to 2.5-fold in human skeletal muscle during recovery from resistance exercise (Koopman *et al.* 2006). Because mTOR is a hub that integrates nutritional and mechanical signals, an implication is that the immediacy of the timing of nutrition to mechanical signals is related to the short window of time that Akt–mTOR pathway is increased by a mechanical signal. These observations have been extended to human skeletal muscle.

BRANCHED-CHAIN AMINO ACIDS INGESTED DURING AND AFTER RESISTANCE EXERCISE MAY MEDIATE SIGNAL TRANSDUCTION THROUGH $p70^{S6K}$ IN HUMAN SKELETAL MUSCLE

Activation of mTOR signals activation of $p70^{S6K}$ by phosphorylation. Resistance exercise leads to increased $p70^{S6K}$ phosphorylation at Ser^{424} and/or Thr^{421}, which continues for 1 and 2 h after exercise in 25-year-old male subjects (Karlsson *et al.* 2004) further observed that ingestion of branched-chain amino acids by the same subjects further increased $p70^{S6K}$ phosphorylation by 3.5-fold during recovery. $p70^{S6K}$ phosphorylation at Thr^{389} was unaltered directly after resistance exercise when subjects ingested only a placebo without branched-chain amino acids. However, the presence of branched-chain amino acids during recovery greatly enhanced Thr^{389} phosphorylation. The ribosomal protein S6 is activated by p70[S6K] phosphorylation. Phosphorylation of the ribosomal protein S6 was increased in the recovery period only when subjects ingested branched-chain amino acids (Karlsson *et al.* 2004).

MUSCLE GLYCOGEN CONCENTRATION PRIOR TO RESISTANCE EXERCISE AFFECTS SOME SIGNALING RESPONSES

While carbohydrate ingestion alone has a stimulatory effect on net muscle protein balance following resistance exercise, its effect is much less than the stimulation produced by amino acids (Miller *et al.* 2003). However, the concentration of glycogen within the muscle prior to the resistance exercise does affect the molecules that signal translational increases. In overnight fasted, well-trained cyclists performing resistance exercise, Akt phosphorylation was elevated 3.4-fold 10 min after resistance exercise when the muscle glycogen content was high, but was unaffected after exercise when the low muscle glycogen was low prior to exercise (Creer *et al.* 2005). p90 ribosomal S6 kinase phosphorylation was increased 10 min after exercise, regardless of muscle glycogen availability (Creer *et al.* 2005); however, mTOR protein concentration and phosphorylation were not significantly altered by the resistance exercise.

RESPONSE OF GENES DURING MECHANICALLY LOADED HYPERTROPHY OF SKELETAL MUSCLE

While great recent progress has occurred in understanding the translational mechanisms by which resistance exercise contributes to muscle growth, less emphasis has been placed upon the pre-translational responses of transcription, slicing, and mRNA stability. Carson *et al.* (1995) identified serum response factor (SRE) as a hypertrophy response element on the skeletal α-actin promoter during stretch hypertrophy. The hypertrophying muscles also had increases in ribosomal RNA per gram of muscle. While the concentration of skeletal α-actin mRNA per gram of muscle did not change, because the muscle hypertrophied, the amount of skeletal α-actin mRNA per whole muscle was greater.

The levels of hundreds of mRNAs in human skeletal muscle are altered by acute changes in nutrition and exercise. Insulin (a surrogate for nutrition) changes 800 mRNAs (Rome *et al.* 2003); 3 h of an exhaustive bout of high intensity cycling altered 126 mRNAs (Mahoney *et al.* 2005); 6 and 18 h after a bout of one-leg resistance exercise 704 and 1479 mRNAs, respectively, were different from those in the non-exercised leg (Zambon *et al.* 2003); and 600–1100 mRNAs changed 4–8 h after 300 eccentric contractions (Chen *et al.* 2003). Little is known about the interaction between the timing of food intake and a bout of resistance exercise on the timescale of changes in mRNA.

Scientific basis for the timing of nutrition to enhance adaptations to endurance training

In contrast to resistance exercise, the adaptive responses to endurance exercise in skeletal muscle center, not on contractile proteins, but on those proteins involved in the uptake and utilization of energy. The turnover rate of ATP in myofibers may increase by as much as 20-fold during endurance exercise, and these high rates of ATP synthesis and use must be sustained for prolonged periods. In order to meet this increased energy demand, the cell must undergo a corresponding increase the oxidation rate of substrates, the byproducts of which are used to drive the resynthesis of ATP. The rate at which those processes responsible for the provision and catabolism of substrates can operate ultimately sets the limit to the system (i.e., the intensity and/or duration at which an exercise bout can be sustained). From the muscle fiber's perspective, the objective is to meet the metabolic demand as efficiently as possible in an effort to minimize the disruption to overall cellular homeostasis. Once the activity is over, the priority shifts to replenishing metabolic reserves that have been depleted during exercise. At first, one might think that because the myofiber has no idea if another exercise bout will ever be performed again, there is no incentive to activate an adaptive response. However, as any endurance athlete will attest, skeletal muscle undergoes a remarkable adaptive response to endurance training, ultimately leading to increases in the efficiency of substrate utilization and, thus, the intensity and/or duration at which an exercise bout can be performed. The potential influence of nutrition during exercise recovery on the adaptive responses associated with endurance training is the topic of the following section.

Muscle glycogen resynthesis

During recovery from prolonged strenuous exercise, the resynthesis of muscle glycogen becomes the metabolic priority for skeletal muscle. Even in the absence of insulin, glucose uptake is elevated over basal levels. In addition, the sensitivity of muscle to insulin is increased to facilitate glucose uptake into muscle once carbohydrate is ingested. Glycogen synthase, the rate-limiting enzyme that catalyzes the deposition of glucosyl units on the glycogen molecule, is also activated in direct proportion to the level of muscle glycogen depletion. The activity of glycogen synthase is controlled primarily by phosphorylation at multiple regulatory sites within the enzyme. Dephosphorylation activates the enzyme, a process that is catalyzed by protein phosphatase 1G (PP1G), a glycogen-bound form of protein phosphatase that consists of a catalytic subunit targeted to the glycogen molecule via its interaction with a specific glycogen targeting protein. Interestingly, a number of enzymes (GSK3, PP1c) that interact with the glycogen targeting protein also bind to different types of targeting proteins that localize activity of the enzyme to other parts of the cell such as the sarcoplasmic reticulum, myofibrils, and the nucleus.

It is thus tempting to speculate that specific enzymes normally associated with the glycogen granule under resting conditions are released and targeted to other parts of the cell as glycogen content declines during exercise. These enzymes could then coordinate, for example, the transcriptional activation of specific genes related to metabolism. As glycogen content is restored, these enzymes would renew their interaction with glycogen targeting proteins and gradually become resequestered within the glycogen structure. Such a mechanism would serve to coordinate gene regulation with the intracellular energy status. In support of this hypothesis, transgenic mice harboring a genetically engineered defect in the glycogen synthase enzyme that renders the protein inactive fail to synthesize glycogen and develop nearly 10-fold greater percentage of type 1 myofibers, suggesting low glycogen content, serves as an intracellular signal to activate the expression of genes required to support oxidative-based metabolism.

Molecular basis for the adaptive responses to endurance exercise training

Any discussion of the mechanisms contributing to exercise training adaptations must take into account and be consistent with the principles of protein turnover kinetics. This is particularly challenging in the context of exercise because the stimulus experienced by the muscle is intermittent rather than continuous. In other words, the adaptive response to a single acute exercise bout, presumably in response to the disturbance to metabolic homeostasis, will be counterbalanced by the "de-exercise" response as the cell returns to and remains in the resting state until the next exercise bout occurs. In response to a single endurance exercise bout, a series of events take place that appear to lead ultimately to adaptations associated with exercise training. Using techniques to isolate nuclei in combination with reverse transcription polymerase chain reaction (RT-PCR) based nuclear run-on analysis, it has been demonstrated that the transcription of a number of genes is activated by exercise. This initial adaptive response of the muscle has a number of important features:

1 Although transcription is activated by some genes during the exercise bout, many genes are primarily not "turned on" until after exercise (Seip *et al.* 1997; Kraniou *et al.* 2000; Pilegaard *et al.* 2000, 2003; Hildebrandt *et al.* 2003).

2 The transcriptional activation of specific genes is transient, remaining elevated for a period of time during recovery before gradually returning to baseline (Pilegaard *et al.* 2000, 2003 Hildebrandt *et al.* 2003).

3 The magnitude and duration of increase in transcription varies tremendously between different genes.

4 The activation of transcription generates a corresponding increase in the mRNA for that gene and, although not as well studied, presumably an increase in the corresponding protein.

All mRNAs and proteins also undergo degradation at a certain rate (i.e., change in protein concentration and/or change in time) (O'Doherty *et al.* 1994; Seip *et al.* 1997; Kuo *et al.* 1999, 2004; Jones *et al.* 2003). Like the transcriptional activation of genes, the turnover rate of both mRNAs and proteins varies considerably between different genes. Thus, it should be apparent that the slower the turnover rate, the longer an adaptive increase in expression will persist during recovery from exercise. Only those mRNAs or proteins with a slow enough turnover rate will still be elevated by the time the next exercise bout is performed and, by extension, accumulate over the course of an exercise training program. A more detailed discussion of the kinetic principles of the adaptive response to exercise training is available (Booth & Neufer 2006).

Effect of timing and composition of meals on the adaptive responses to endurance exercise in skeletal muscle

The above discussion raises the question as to whether the control of exercise-responsive genes may be sensitive and/or associated with the metabolic state of the myofibers during recovery from exercise. To test this hypothesis, Pilegaard *et al.* (2002) had subjects perform one-legged cycling exercise to lower muscle glycogen content in one leg and, following a carbohydrate-restricted diet, the following day complete 2.5 h of two-legged cycling exercise. Although exercise induced a two- to threefold increase in transcription of the pyruvate dehydrogenase kinase 4 (PDK4) and uncoupling protein 3 (UCP3) genes in the reduced-glycogen leg only, interpretation of the results was somewhat complicated by the fact that the low-glycogen protocol increased the basal mRNA content for PDK4 and UCP3 as well as hexokinase II and lipoprotein lipase.

In a separate study, subjects completed two 3-h, two-legged knee-extensor trials (separated by 2 weeks) in which both muscle and liver glycogen content was either lowered or returned to control levels by an exercise and/or diet regimen the preceding day. Again, the induction of both PDK4 and UCP3 mRNA was significantly greater during the low glycogen trial. PDK4 encodes for a kinase that phosphorylates and inactivates pyruvate dehydrogenase, preventing entry of glycolytic products into the mitochondria for oxidation and thus, in theory, preserving glucose for muscle glycogen resynthesis (Pilegaard & Neufer 2004). UCP3 appears to be induced during recovery from exercise as a mechanism to protect against elevated mitochondrial reactive oxygen species (ROS) production (Anderson, Yamazaki & Neufer 2007).

The potential impact of glycogen content on genes that encode for mitochondrial enzymes has been more difficult to discern, presumably because of the generally low level of induction of these genes in response to exercise (Pilegaard *et al.* 2000, 2003, 2005; Hildebrandt *et al.* 2003). Clearly, more comprehensive research will be required to assess fully the impact of glycogen content on the regulation of metabolic gene expression in skeletal muscle. Perhaps the exercise-responsive gene most sensitive to glycogen content identified to date is the cytokine interleukin 6 (IL-6), the transcriptional activation and mRNA for which increase during exercise is far more dramatic when pre-exercise muscle glycogen content is low (Keller *et al.* 2001; Steensberg *et al.* 2001). Although it has been suggested that release of IL-6 from muscle may serve an interorgan signaling molecule to the liver to accelerate gluconeogenesis (Steensberg *et al.* 2000; Keller *et al.* 2001), direct evidence to support this hypothesis has been elusive, suggesting that IL-6 may have other biologic roles (Pedersen *et al.* 2004).

An alternative approach to test the potential influence of metabolic state on the regulation of exercise-induced gene expression is to manipulate the type of diet consumed during the recovery period after exercise. Indeed, restricting carbohydrate for as long as 66 h after exercise has been shown to elicit a sustained increase in muscle insulin sensitivity that appears to be mediated, at least in part, by a sustained increase in muscle GLUT4 transporter protein expression (Garcia-Roves *et al.* 2003). Muscle glycogen resynthesis after exercise is minimal in rats when carbohydrate intake is restricted (Richter *et al.* 2001). In addition, transitioning to a high-carbohydrate diet quickly reverses the exercise-induced increase in GLUT4 mRNA and protein (Garcia-Roves *et al.*

2003), again consistent with the notion that the adaptive response to exercise may be tied to the replenishment of glycogen reserves.

To test this hypothesis further in humans, Pilegaard *et al.* (2005) had subjects complete 75 min of cycling, consuming either a high- or low-carbohydrate diet during the ensuing 24 hours of recovery. Ingestion of carbohydrate reversed the exercise-induced transcriptional activation of several exercise-responsive genes (PDK4, UCP3, LPL, and carnitine palmitoyl transferase 1) within 5–8 h after exercise, whereas restricting carbohydrate intake resulted in a sustained activation of these genes through 8–24 h of recovery. It is important to note that many of the genes that respond to exercise and remain elevated under low carbohydrate intake are also upregulated in muscle by fasting and high-fat feeding (Tunstall *et al.* 2002; Cameron-Smith *et al.* 2003), raising the possibility that the increased reliance of skeletal muscle on lipid metabolism both during and after exercise, particularly when carbohydrate intake is restricted, may serve as the signaling mechanism to regulate exercise-responsive genes. Regardless of the exact molecular mechanisms leading to the transcriptional activation of genes in response to exercise, it is clear that substrate availability and/or cellular metabolic recovery (glycogen resynthesis) influence the magnitude and duration of metabolic gene activation. The extent to which the metabolic state of myofibers may affect the cumulative adaptive responses during exercise training requires further research.

Conclusions

While it has long been known that physical performance is limited by genes inherited from ancestors, it is now known that the level of expression by these genes can be modulated by environmental conditions. In 1967, Holloszy showed that the mitochondrial protein, cytochrome c, is increased by endurance training in rats, demonstrating that the protein level is not fixed. In the last decade it has now been demonstrated that nutrition interacts with both resistance and endurance types of exercise to adjust the degree of skeletal muscle's adaptation to exercise. The future will continue to explain, at the molecular level, how plastic and adaptable humans are to their level of physical activity. Such information on the molecular response of the body to exercise is not only of importance for those wishing maximal physical performance in sports, but also to the non-athlete who wishes to obtain maximal health benefits of a physically active lifestyle.

Acknowledgments

The authors thank Kevin Tipton for suggestions on the manuscript, which was written while supported by NIH grant AG18780.

References

Anderson, E.J., Yamazaki, H. & Neufer, P.D. (2007) Induction of endogenous uncoupling protein 3 suppresses mitochondrial oxidant emission during fatty acid-supported respiration. *Journal of Biological Chemistry* **282**, 31 257–31 266.

Atherton, P.J., Babraj, J., Smith, K., Singh, J., Rennie, M.J. & Wackerhage, H. (2005) Selective activation of AMPK–PGC-1α or PKB–TSC2–mTOR signaling can explain specific adaptive responses to endurance or resistance training-like electrical muscle stimulation. *FASEB Journal* **19**, 786–788.

Biolo, G., Maggi, S.P., Williams, B.D., Tipton, K.D., Wolfe, R.R. (1995) Increased rates of muscle protein turnover and amino acid transport after resistance exercise in humans. *American Journal of Physiology* **268**, E514–E520.

Biolo, G., Tipton, K.D., Klein, S. & Wolfe, R.R. (1997) An abundant supply of amino acids enhances the metabolic effect of exercise on muscle protein. *American Journal of Physiology* **273**, E122–E129.

Bodine, S.C., Stitt, T.N., Gonzalez, M., *et al.* (2001) Akt-mTOR pathway is a crucial regulator of skeletal muscle hypertrophy and can prevent muscle atrophy *in vivo*. *Nature Cell Biology* **3**, 1014–1019.

Bolster, D.R., Crozier, S.J., Kimball, S.R. & Jefferson, L.S. (2002) AMP-activated protein kinase suppresses protein synthesis in rat skeletal muscle through down-regulated mammalian target of rapamycin (mTOR) signaling. *Journal of Biological Chemistry* **277**, 23977–23980.

Bolster, D.R., Kimball, S.R. & Jefferson, L.S. (2003a) Translational control mechanisms modulate skeletal muscle gene expression during hypertrophy. *Exercise and Sport Sciences Reviews* **31**, 111–116.

Bolster, D.R., Kubica, N., Crozier, S.J., *et al.* (2003b) Immediate response of mammalian target of rapamycin (mTOR)-mediated signalling following acute resistance exercise in rat skeletal muscle. *Journal of Physiology* **553**, 213–220.

Booth, F.W. & Neufer, P.D. (2006) Exercise genomics and proteomics. In: *ACSM's Advanced Exercise Physiology* (Tipton,

C.M., ed.) Lippincott Williams & Wilkins, Philadelphia: 623–651.

Cameron-Smith, D., Burke, L.M., Angus, D.J., *et al.* (2003) A short-term, high-fat diet up-regulates lipid metabolism and gene expression in human skeletal muscle. *American Journal of Clinical Nutrition* **77**, 313–318.

Carson, J.A., Yan, Z., Booth, F.W., Coleman, M.E., Schwartz, R.J., Stump, C.S. (1995) Regulation of skeletal alpha-actin promoter in young chickens during hypertrophy caused by stretch overload. *American Journal of Physiology* **268**, C918–C924.

Chen, Y.W., Hubal, M.J., Hoffman, E.P., Thompson, P.D. & Clarkson, P.M. (2003) Molecular responses of human muscle to eccentric exercise. *Journal of Applied Physiology* **95**, 2485–2494.

Chesley, A., MacDougall, J.D., Tarnopolsky, M.A., Atkinson, S.A. & Smith, K. (1992) Changes in human muscle protein synthesis after resistance exercise. *Journal of Applied Physiology* **73**, 1383–1388.

Coffey, V.G., Zhong, Z., Shield, A., *et al.* (2006) Early signaling responses to divergent exercise stimuli in skeletal muscle from well-trained humans. *FASEB Journal* **20**, 190–192.

Creer, A., Gallagher, P., Slivka, D., Jemiolo, B., Fink, W. & Trappe, S. (2005) Influence of muscle glycogen availability on ERK1/2 and Akt signaling after resistance exercise in human skeletal muscle. *Journal of Applied Physiology* **99**, 950–956.

Garcia-Roves, P.M., Han, D.H., Song, Z., Jones, T.E., Hucker, K.A. & Holloszy, J.O. (2003) Prevention of glycogen supercompensation prolongs the increase in muscle GLUT4 after exercise. *American Journal of Physiology: Endocrinology and Metabolism* **285**, E729–E736.

Hildebrandt, A.L., Pilegaard, H. & Neufer, P.D. (2003) Differential transcriptional activation of select metabolic genes in response to variations in exercise intensity and duration. *American Journal of Physiology: Endocrinology and Metabolism* **285**, E1021–E1027.

Holloszy, J.O. (1967) Biochemical adaptations in muscle. Effects of exercise on mitochondrial oxygen uptake and respiratory enzyme activity in skeletal muscle. *Journal of Biological Chemistry* **242**, 2278–2282.

Jones, T.E., Baar, K., Ojuka, E., Chen, M. & Holloszy, J.O. (2003) Exercise induces an increase in muscle UCP3 as a component of the increase in mitochondrial biogenesis. *American Journal of Physiology: Endocrinology and Metabolism* **284**, E96–E101.

Karlsson, H.K., Nilsson, P.A., Nilsson, J., Chibalin, A.V., Zierath, J.R. & Blomstrand, E. (2004) Branched-chain amino acids increase p70S6k phosphorylation in human skeletal muscle after resistance exercise. *American Journal of Physiology: Endocrinology and Metabolism* **287**, E1–E7.

Keller, C., Steensberg, A., Pilegaard, H., *et al.* (2001) Transcriptional activation of the IL-6 gene in human contracting skeletal muscle: influence of muscle glycogen content. *FASEB Journal* **15**, 2748–2750.

Koopman, R., Zorenc, A.H., Gransier, R.J., Cameron-Smith, D. & van Loon, L.J. (2006) Increase in S6K1 phosphorylation in human skeletal muscle following resistance exercise occurs mainly in type II muscle fibers. *American Journal of Physiology: Endocrinology and Metabolism* **290**, E1245–E1252.

Kraniou, Y., Cameron-Smith, D., Misso, M., Collier, G. & Hargreaves, M. (2000) Effects of exercise on GLUT-4 and glycogenin gene expression in human skeletal muscle. *Journal of Applied Physiology* **88**, 794–796.

Kuo, C.H., Hunt, D.G., Ding, Z. & Ivy, J.L. (1999) Effect of carbohydrate supplementation on postexercise GLUT-4 protein expression in skeletal muscle. *Journal of Applied Physiology* **87**, 2290–2295.

Kuo, C.H., Hwang, H., Lee, M.C., Castle, A.L. & Ivy, J.L. (2004) Role of insulin on exercise-induced GLUT-4 protein expression and glycogen supercompensation in rat skeletal muscle. *Journal of Applied Physiology* **96**, 621–627.

Laurent, G.J., Sparrow, M.P. & Millward D.J. (1978) Turnover of muscle protein in the fowl. Changes in rates of protein synthesis and breakdown during hypertrophy of the anterior and posterior latissimus dorsi muscles. *Biochemical Journal* **176**, 407–417.

Mahoney, D.J., Parise, G., Melov, S., Safdar, A. & Tarnopolsky, M.A. (2005) Analysis of global mRNA expression in human skeletal muscle during recovery from endurance exercise. *FASEB Journal* **19**, 1498–1500.

Miller, S.L., Tipton, K.D., Chinkes, D.L., Wolf, S.E. & Wolfe, R.R. (2003) Independent and combined effects of amino acids and glucose after resistance exercise. *Medicine and Science in Sports and Exercise* **35**, 449–455.

Norton, L.E. & Layman, D.K. (2006) Leucine regulates translation initiation of protein synthesis in skeletal muscle after exercise. *Journal of Nutrition* **136**, 533S–537S.

O'Doherty, R.M., Bracy, D.P., Osawa, H., Wasserman, D.H. & Granner, D.K. (1994) Rat skeletal muscle hexokinase II mRNA and activity are increased by a single bout of acute exercise. *American Journal of Physiology* **266**, E171–E178.

Pedersen, B.K., Steensberg, A., Fischer, C., *et al.* (2004) The metabolic role of IL-6 produced during exercise: is IL-6 an exercise factor? *Proceedings of the Nutrition Society* **63**, 263–267.

Phillips, S.M. (2004) Protein requirements and supplementation in strength sports. *Nutrition* **20**, 689–695.

Pilegaard, H., Keller, C., Steensberg, A., *et al.* (2002) Influence of pre-exercise muscle glycogen content on exercise-induced transcriptional regulation of metabolic genes. *Journal of Physiology* **541**, 261–271.

Pilegaard, H. & Neufer, P.D. (2004) Transcriptional regulation of pyruvate dehydrogenase kinase 4 in skeletal muscle during and after exercise. *Proceedings of the Nutrition Society* **63**, 221–226.

Pilegaard, H., Ordway, G.A., Saltin, B. & Neufer, P.D. (2000) Transcriptional regulation of gene expression in human skeletal muscle during recovery from exercise. *American Journal of Physiology: Endocrinology and Metabolism* **279**, E806–E814.

Pilegaard, H., Osada, T., Andersen, L.T., Helge, J.W., Saltin, B. & Neufer, P.D. (2005) Substrate availability and transcriptional regulation of metabolic genes in human skeletal muscle during recovery from exercise. *Metabolism* **54**, 1048–1055.

Pilegaard, H., Saltin, B. & Neufer, P.D. (2003) Exercise induces transient transcriptional activation of the PGC-1α gene in human skeletal muscle. *Journal of Physiology* **546**, 851–858.

Rennie, M.J., Bohe, J., Smith, K., Wackerhage, H. & Greenhaff, P. (2006) Branched-chain amino acids as fuels and anabolic signals in human muscle. *Journal of Nutrition* **136**, 264S–268S.

Richter, E.A., Derave, W. & Wojtaszewski, J.F. (2001) Glucose, exercise and insulin: emerging concepts. *Journal of Physiology* **535**, 313–322.

Rome, S., Clement, K., Rabasa-Lhoret, R., *et al.* (2003) Microarray profiling of human skeletal muscle reveals that insulin regulates approximately 800 genes during a hyperinsulinemic clamp. *Journal of Biological Chemistry* **278**, 18063–18068.

Seip, R.L., Mair, K., Cole, T.G. & Semenkovich, C.F. (1997) Induction of human skeletal muscle lipoprotein lipase gene expression by short-term exercise is transient. *American Journal of Physiology* **272**, E255–E261.

Steensberg, A., Febbraio, M.A., Osada, T., *et al.* (2001) Interleukin-6 production in contracting human skeletal muscle is influenced by pre-exercise muscle glycogen content. *Journal of Physiology* **537**, 633–639.

Steensberg, A., van Hall, G., Osada, T., Sacchetti, M., Saltin, B. & Klarlund, P.B. (2000) Production of interleukin-6 in contracting human skeletal muscles can account for the exercise-induced increase in plasma interleukin-6. *Journal of Physiology* **529**, 237–242.

Tipton, K.D., Ferrando, A.A., Phillips, S.M., Doyle, D. Jr. & Wolfe, R.R. (1999) Postexercise net protein synthesis in human muscle from orally administered amino acids. *American Journal of Physiology* **276**, E628–E634.

Tipton, K.D., Rasmussen, B.B., Miller, S.L., *et al.* (2001) Timing of amino acid-carbohydrate ingestion alters anabolic response of muscle to resistance exercise. *American Journal of Physiology: Endocrinology and Metabolism* **281**, E197–E206.

Tunstall, R.J., Mehan, K.A., Hargreaves, M., Spriet, L.L. & Cameron-Smith, D. (2002) Fasting activates the gene expression of UCP3 independent of genes necessary for lipid transport and oxidation in skeletal muscle. *Biochemical and Biophysical Research Communications* **294**, 301–308.

Wolfe, R.R. (2006) Skeletal muscle protein metabolism and resistance exercise. *Journal of Nutrition* **136**, 525S–528S.

Wong, T.S. & Booth, F.W. (1990a) Protein metabolism in rat tibialis anterior muscle after stimulated chronic eccentric exercise. *Journal of Applied Physiology* **69**, 1718–1724.

Wong, T.S. & Booth, F.W. (1990b) Protein metabolism in rat gastrocnemius muscle after stimulated chronic concentric exercise. *Journal of Applied Physiology* **69**, 1709–1717.

Zambon, A.C., McDearmon, E.L., Salomonis, N., *et al.* (2003) Time- and exercise-dependent gene regulation in human skeletal muscle. *Genome Biology* **4**, R61.

Part 6

Biomechanics, Engineering, and Ergonomics

Chapter 14

Biomechanics of Human Movement and Muscle-Tendon Function

VASILIOS BALTZOPOULOS AND CONSTANTINOS N. MAGANARIS

Biomechanics (derived from the Greek words βίος/veos for life-living and μηχανική/mehaniki for mechanics) is the scientific discipline for the study of the mechanics of the structure and function of living biological systems. In the human biological system the application of the principles and methods of mechanics, and in particular the study of forces and their effects, has led to a significant advancement in our knowledge and understanding of human movement in a whole spectrum of activities ranging from pathologic conditions to elite sport actions.

The main aims of Biomechanics in the context of sports activities are:

1 To increase knowledge and understanding of the structure and function of the human musculoskeletal system;

2 To prevent injuries and improve rehabilitation techniques by examining the loading of specific structures in the human body during activity and their response; and

3 To enhance sports performance by analysing and optimising technique.

This chapter will examine recent developments in the above areas. In particular, given that the generation of movement *per se* and investigations into technique improvement or reduction in loading and prevention of injuries depend primarily on the mechanics and control of muscles and joints, special emphasis will be placed on issues relating to muscle-tendon and joint function. The chapter will also consider

The Olympic Textbook of Science in Sport, 1st edition. Edited by R.J. Maughan. Published 2009 by Blackwell Publishing. ISBN: 978-1-4051-5638-7.

future developments in equipment and techniques necessary to overcome existing measurement and modeling limitations. These will allow easier development and more widespread application of subject-specific models in order to improve the contribution of biomechanics research and support services to performance enhancement and injury prevention.

Biomechanical analysis of human movement

Performance in all locomotory activities, including sports, depends on a number of factors related to the function and control of all the systems in the human body. Biomechanics is only one of the scientific disciplines, in addition to physiology, biochemistry, neuroscience, psychology etc., that contribute to the understanding and enhancement of performance and the prevention of overloading and injuries. Given the multi-factorial nature of human performance, the contribution of biomechanics is crucial and is achieved using a combination of qualitative (Knudson & Morrison 1997) and quantitative (Payton & Bartlett 2008) experimental approaches, as well as theoretical approaches based on mathematical modeling and computer simulation (Yeadon & King 2008). Qualitative approaches have been developed in recent years and the processes involved in conducting an effective qualitative biomechanical analysis have been documented and described in great detail (Knudson & Morrison 1997). However, this approach essentially involves observation and subjective interpretation of the movement based on certain principles before any intervention. This chapter will concentrate on quantitative and theoretical approaches.

It is generally agreed (e.g., Lees 1999, 2002; Bahr & Krosshaug 2005; Elliott 2006) that biomechanical research and scientific support services, whether for the prevention of injuries or the improvement of technique to enhance performance, should follow a sequence of important steps to ensure that any interventions are appropriate and that the outcome is evaluated and contributes to evidence-based practice:

1 Analysis of the specific problem to establish the relevant context (technique and wider performance factors or the extent and epidemiologic evidence of the injury);

2 Establishment of the key techniques, variables, desired characteristics, faults, coordination mechanisms, or the mechanisms of injury and risk factors through observational, experimental, or theoretical approaches;

3 Design and implementation of an intervention; and

4 Evaluation of the intervention for improving performance or reducing injuries.

The multi-factorial and multi-disciplinary nature of sports performance and sports injuries means that it is very difficult to control all of the implicated factors and to study only one or a few in isolation, given their complex interactions. This is also one of the main reasons for the lack of well-controlled intervention and prospective evaluation studies or randomized control trials, especially in quantitative approaches. Furthermore, the design and implementation of an intervention necessitates collaboration with coaches or clinicians and other personnel. This highlights the need for effective communication with other professionals involved in athlete training or rehabilitation, and is another reason for the lack of interventional and evaluation studies. Although biomechanics has had a tremendous impact in sports, the difficulties of outcome intervention and well-controlled evaluation studies has lead to there being only a small evidence base for biomechanical support and injury prevention interventions and some unfounded criticisms for the contribution and influence of biomechanics. It is important that future work addresses these shortcomings, especially with the advent of sophisticated and versatile measurement, data collection, and analytical techniques.

Experimental approaches

Descriptive biomechanical analyses are usually based on the measurement of temporal (phase), kinematic, kinetic, or kinesiological/anatomical features of movement using the corresponding experimental techniques (Bartlett 1999). Although a descriptive analysis of movement may provide a useful starting point, it is important to understand the underlying mechanisms of coordination and control of movement, or the mechanisms of injuries. The determination of key technique variables related to movement control and coordination mechanisms, or the risk factors and the manner in which they are implicated in the mechanism of injury, is a very important step in any investigation, and in quantitative approaches these variables or factors are determined based on different methods that can be classified in general (e.g., Bartlett 1999; Lees 2002; Bahr & Krosshaug 2005) under the following headings:

1 Biomechanical principles of movement;

2 Hierarchical relationship (deterministic) diagrams; and

3 Statistical relationships.

Biomechanical principles of movement are formulated by applying some of the fundamental mechanical relations to the structural and functional characteristics of the neuromuscular system and to segmental motion and coordination. Although there is a general disagreement about the exact number, categorization, and even the definition and description of these principles (Bartlett 1999; Lees 2002), some of the more widely-accepted principles, such as the stretch-shortening cycle (SSC), the proximal to distal sequence of segmental action, and mechanical energy considerations have had a major impact on our understanding of the mechanisms of control and coordination during movement and injuries.

The SSC is explained in detail in Chapter 1, and it is important to emphasize that the main mechanism is based on the interaction between the muscle fascicles and the tendon in a muscle-tendon unit. During the preceding stretch or eccentric action phase, the muscle is activated so that elastic energy is stored in the tendon and is then released during the subsequent shortening phase, thus increasing the muscle force output (potentiation) above the level predicted by the isolated concentric force-velocity relationship alone, hence enhancing power production. In this way force production and timing in locomotory or throwing movements of short duration are optimized. However, the storage and utilization of elastic energy and the contribution of the stretch reflex to the potentiation of force depend on the muscles involved and their function (e.g., mono- or bi-articular), the intensity and the type of task or movement (e.g., the duration and optimal coupling between eccentric and concentric actions, or the contact phase) as they will influence fascicle-tendon interactions. It is therefore important to note that even universally accepted and well-defined biomechanical principles of movement require careful consideration when applied to different sports or activities. This is particularly relevant in jumping and throwing/hitting activities where the coupling (timing) between the stretch and shortening phases is crucial. In tennis, for example, the importance of a fast transition from the backswing to the forward swing of the racket or from knee flexion to extension during the serve is now clearly recognized (Elliott 2006).

The proximal to distal sequence of segmental action has been widely accepted in throwing and ballistic activities in general where the maximization of the endpoint velocity is the main aim, but it was originally developed for movement constrained mainly in two dimensions. According to this principle, the movement of each distal segment starts when the velocity of its proximal segment is near maximum. However, more recent studies have shown that this sequence is not followed in many throwing or hitting activities of three-dimensional nature where significant internal or external rotations of segments around their longitudinal axis are involved and contribute significantly to the end point or implement velocity (e.g., Marshall & Elliott 2000). These important rotations for the potentiation of muscle forces not only play an important role in

velocity generation, but also underline the important contribution of the SSC potentiation in muscles, which contributes to segment longitudinal rotation and the interaction between the different biomechanical principles.

Movement control and coordination analysis based on nonlinear dynamics and dynamical systems approaches and methodologies is one of the more recently emerging principles used to investigate the higher-order dynamics of movement (e.g., Hamill *et al.* 1999; Bartlett *et al.* 2007) and to establish the importance of variability for human movement and for the understanding of coordination and injury mechanisms. However, important questions, such as whether the complex variables used are the result or the cause of the injury, or whether they can be used for designing specific intervention measures to prevent the injury, are still unanswered; hence further work, including well-controlled prospective epidemiological and intervention studies, is required.

Mechanical energy and work principles are vital when examining the effects of not only the function of muscle-tendon units but also sports equipment in particular, because energy availability determines the ability to do work and increase performance, so the optimization of the energy transfer between athlete and equipment is crucial. This can be achieved by minimizing the energy lost, maximizing the energy returned, and optimizing the output of the musculoskeletal system (Nigg *et al.* 2000). Although any useful energy return is controversial given that it relies on certain conditions about the amount (if any), timing, location, and frequency of the energy return (Stefanyshyn & Nigg 2000), the optimization of muscle force and power output by operating the muscle-tendon complexes at optimum length and velocity conditions is an important determinant of increased performance (e.g., Herzog 1996).

Diagrammatic deterministic or conceptual models describe the hierarchical relationships of the various layers of factors that affect performance on the basis of temporal or mechanical principles (see Hay & Read 1982; Hay 1993). Assuming that certain criteria are satisfied when developing the model, these hierarchical relationships can then be useful in identifying important variables for biomechanical analysis, or they can form the basis of statistical models of performance (Bartlett 1999). In injury prevention applications, the identification of risk factors and mechanisms of injury is based on similar diagrammatic models. These models describe the conceptual interaction of intrinsic and extrinsic risk factors in causing an injury and acting through a specific mechanism that is suggested to include information on aspects of the inciting event at different levels, which can be classified into one of four categories: playing situation, athlete/opponent behavior, whole body biomechanics, and joint tissue biomechanics (Bahr & Krosshaug 2005).

The type and range of variables and factors resulting from the above approaches require instrumentation and techniques that can accurately measure a wide range of parameters. Such techniques include video and optoelectronic systems for kinematic (position, velocity, acceleration etc) parameters, force plates and pressure sensors for kinetic information, electromyographic (EMG) systems for the assessment of muscle activity (see Payton & Bartlett 2008), and ultrasound systems for the imaging of muscle fascicles and tendon function (Maganaris 2003). The biomechanical study of sports injuries requires additional techniques that include clinical investigations based on medical imaging (computed tomography (CT), magnetic resonance imaging (MRI), X-ray videofluoroscopy, arthroscopy etc.) and cadaveric studies (Krosshaug et al. 2005).

Mathematical modeling, computer simulation, and optimization

A theoretical approach is usually based on a simplified model of the essential aspects of the human body and can overcome some of the problems described above for experimental approaches. Mathematical modeling in sports biomechanics, e.g., prediction of jump distance or height (Hatze 1981; Alexander 2003), is a powerful research tool because it can simulate effects that are impossible to study experimentally in a systematic way, thus allowing us to understand which parameters are more important for improving athletic performance. This enables appropriate strategies to be adopted for executing the sporting task, and guides the design of training programs.

Modeling and computer simulation developments in human movement biomechanics have paralleled the technological development of computers and their processing power in the last few decades (Vaughan 1984), and there are now several dedicated computer software packages that allow mathematical modeling and simulation of human movement. However, despite predictions of widespread use, the number of studies using computer simulation is still limited because of the difficulties in modeling the human body accurately, thus limiting realistic applications, except in certain types of activities such aerial movements and throwing events (see Yeadon & King 2008), and some clinical applications (e.g., Neptune 2000; McLean et al. 2003, 2004). The models used range in complexity from single-point mass models of the athlete or the throwing implement, to rigid body models of the whole body, a single segment, or a series of linked segments, to very detailed models of the musculoskeletal system including all the essential elements of its structure and function (Blemker et al. 2007; Delp et al. 2007).

Given the complexity of the human body, all models are a simplification of the real structure and function of the modeled parts. The degree of simplification depends not only on the existing knowledge of the properties and function of the elements in the model, but also on the question to be answered. For example, in aerial sports movements rigid body models connected with pin joints are adequate for most questions, but in a model to study the loading in the knee joint during landings, a detailed model of the anatomical function of the patellar tendon is necessary as part of the knee joint kinematics modeling, including moment arms and geometrical data to allow accurate estimation of knee joint reaction forces and loading (e.g., Krosshaug et al. 2005). One of the other main problems in modeling and simulation is the development of models that are tailored to an individual athlete because of the difficulty in obtaining subject-specific data on the structure and properties of the modeled segments, joints, and muscle-tendon units (Yeadon & King 2008). These problems are further compounded by the difficulties of accurately measuring the joint moment under different segment configuration and velocity conditions (e.g., Baltzopoulos 2008). In inverse dynamics approaches specifically, the distribution of the calculated joint moment to the contributing muscles for the estimation of muscle-tendon forces and loading has been one of the fundamental problems of biomechanics research. Various optimization techniques have been applied in the past (for a review see Tsirakos *et al.* 1997), and more recent techniques show particularly promising results (Erdemir *et al.* 2007). However, these all rely on accurate subject specific information about muscle properties and moment arms which are either difficult or not possible to obtain *in vivo*. Activation criteria as opposed to optimization criteria for muscle force distribution have been proposed as the only way forward for this problem (Epstein & Herzog 2003).

Human movement and the mechanics of muscle-tendon and joint function

Human movement is the result of joint segment rotations generated by moments acting around the axes of rotations of joints. These moments result from muscle forces that are transmitted via tendons to the bones and in this way create rotation of the segment. Muscle force depends on the length, velocity, activation level, and previous activation state of the muscle (see Chapter 1 for further information). The function of the muscle in series with the tendon has important implications for their function because the mechanical properties of the tendon, in particular its viscoelastic, time-dependent properties, will affect the muscle length and velocity, and hence its force output. It is therefore clear that any attempt to optimize or change joint motion sequence (technique modification) will depend on the mechanical properties of muscle and tendon and their interaction during the particular activity. For this reason it is important to consider the architectural and mechanical properties of muscles, the mechanics of tendon function and force transmission and their interactions in order to understand the implications for human movement.

Muscle architecture

The term "muscle architecture" refers to the spatial arrangement of muscle fibers with respect to the

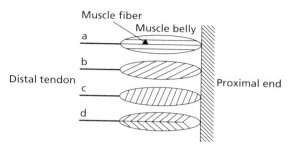

Fig. 14.1 The main muscle architectures. (a) Longitudinal muscle. (b, c) Unipennate muscles of different pennation angles. (d) Bipennate muscle.

axis of force generation in the muscle-tendon unit. Skeletal muscles may be categorized under two main types of architectural design – parallel-fibered and pennate. In parallel-fibered muscles, the muscle fibers run parallel to the action line of the muscle-tendon unit, spanning the entire length of the muscle belly (Fig. 14.1a). On the other hand, muscles with fibers arranged at an angle to the muscle-tendon action line are classified as pennate muscles. This specific angle is referred to as the pennation angle and necessitates that the fibers extend to only a part of the whole muscle belly length. If all of the fibers attach to the tendon plate at a given pennation angle, the muscle is termed unipennate (Figs. 14.1b,c). Multipennate structures arise when the muscle fibers run at several pennation angles within the muscle, or when there are several distinct intramuscular parts with different pennation angles (Fig. 14.1d). Out of approximately 650 muscles in the human body, most have pennate architectures with resting pennation angles up to ~30° (Wickiewicz *et al.* 1983; Friederich & Brand 1990).

From the above definitions and illustrations it soon becomes apparent that pennation angle affects muscle fiber length; i.e., for a given muscle volume or area (if volume is simplified by projecting the muscle in the sagittal plane), the larger the pennation angle the shorter the muscle fiber length relative to the whole muscle belly length. Since muscle fiber length is determined by the number of serial sarcomeres in the muscle fiber, the above relationship means that increasing pennation angle penalizes the speed of muscle fiber shortening and the excursion range of fibers. However, pennation

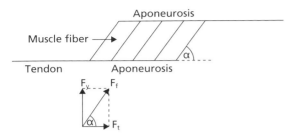

Fig. 14.2 Vectorial analysis of forces based on a simple 2-D muscle model with tendons and aponeuroses lying over straight lines. F_f is the fiber force, F_y is the component of F_f perpendicular to the tendon action line, F_t is the tendon force, and α is the pennation angle. From trigonometry it follows that $F_t = F_f \cdot \cos \alpha$.

and intramuscular tendons are in-line (Fig. 14.2), indicate that this is proportional to 1 – cosine of the pennation angle. Thus, despite the trade-off between the simultaneous force gain and loss by pennation angle, it seems that as long as the pennation angle does not exceed 45° (Alexander & Vernon 1975), the overall effect on the resultant tendon force remains positive.

The measurement that best describes the capacity of muscle to generate maximum contractile force is the physiological cross-sectional area (PCSA). This is because PCSA represents the sum of cross-sectional areas of all of the fibers in a muscle (Fig. 14.3), and it is therefore a measure of the number of in-parallel sarcomeres present (Fick 1911). PCSA can be calculated from the ratio of muscle volume over muscle fiber length, which highlights that muscles with larger volumes and anatomical cross-sectional areas (the area of a cross-section at right angles to the muscle-tendon line of action) may produce less force than smaller muscles, if they have longer muscle fibers.

angle also has the positive effect of allowing more muscle fibers to attach along the intramuscular tendon plate (also known as the aponeurosis). The existence of more in-parallel sarcomeres therefore means that the muscle can exert greater contractile forces. However, in contrast to the proportionally increasing penalizing effect of pennation angle on contractile speed and excursion range, the positive effect of pennation angle on maximum contractile force is not linear, because as pennation angle increases an increasing portion of the extra force gained in the direction of the fibers cannot be transferred through the muscle-tendon action line and thus effectively reach the skeleton and produce joint moment. The exact amount of this "force loss" is difficult to quantify realistically but simple planar geometric models, assuming that the extramuscular

Comparative results of muscle architecture based on anatomical dissection have been very useful in identifying and differentiating the distinct structural characteristics of muscles (Lieber & Friden 2000). Generally speaking, the antigravity extensor muscles have architectures that favor force production (i.e., large PCSA values). These muscles are crucial in sporting activities in which forces must be exerted against the ground to displace the body in a given direction. In contrast, the antagonistic flexors are

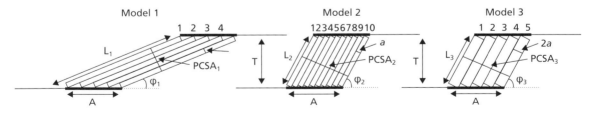

Fig. 14.3 Three muscle models in 2-D with different architectural characteristics. Hyperplasia and hypertrophy of the muscle in model 1 are represented by models 2 and 3, respectively. The muscle fibers are shown as a series of tilted parallelograms between the two tendons (horizontal thick line segments). A, total fiber attachment area on the tendon; L, fiber length; PCSA, muscle physiological cross-sectional area; φ, pennation angle; T, muscle thickness. Models 1 and 2 have the same fiber cross-sectional area (a), the same A, and the same T. However, $\varphi_2 > \varphi_1$ and $L_2 < L_1$. Note that although the two muscles occupy equal areas (A × T), the number of muscle fibers is 5 in model 1, and 10 and in model 2. Therefore, $PCSA_2$ (10) = $2PCSA_1$ (5a). Models 2 and 3 have the same A and T. Moreover, $L_3 = L_2$ and $\varphi_3 = \varphi_2$, but in Model 3 the fiber cross-sectional area is 2a and the number of fibers is 5; hence, $PCSA_3$ (5·2a) = $PCSA_2$ = $2PCSA_1$.

Fig. 14.4 *Top,* sagittal-plane ultrasound images of the gastrocnemius lateralis (GL) and soleus (SOL) muscles at rest (A), 20% (B), 40% (C), 60% (D), 80% (E), and 100% (F) of plantar flexion maximal voluntary contraction (MVC). The horizontal white stripes are ultrasonic waves reflected from the superficial and deep aponeuroses of each muscle and the oblique white stripes are echoes derived from fascia septas between muscle fascicles. *a* is the GL pennation angle and *b* is the SOL pennation angle. Note the gradual increase of *a*, *b* and muscle thickness in GL and SOL from A to F. *Bottom,* similar sonographs of the symmetric bipennate tibialis anterior muscle at rest and dorsiflexion MVC (reproduced with permission from Maganaris *et al.* 1998a; Maganaris & Baltzopoulos 1999).

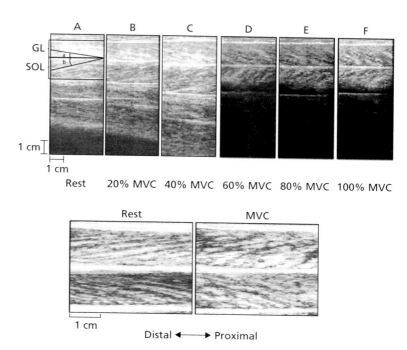

more appropriate for excursion and have longer muscle fibers. Based on such criteria, classification of cadaver muscles in a standardized and functionally relevant manner became possible (Lieber & Brown 1992; Lieber & Friden 2000). However, it must be recognized that preservation and fixation can cause substantial specimen shrinkage (Friederich & Brand 1990), and therefore cadaver-based measurements of muscle architecture are unlikely to accurately reflect the physiological state of a given muscle under *in vivo* conditions. This problem has recently been circumvented by advancements in the application of ultrasound imaging, which have enabled human muscle architecture *in vivo* to be quantified (e.g., Henriksson-Larsen *et al.* 1992; Rutherford and Jones, 1992; Kawakami *et al.* 1993; Narici *et al.* 1996; Maganaris *et al.* 1998a). The applicability of ultrasound scanning for muscle architecture measurements relates to the differential penetration of ultrasound waves to contractile and collagenous material. Fascicles of muscle fibers are more echo-absorptive and sagittal-plane scans recorded in real-time using B-mode ultrasound appear as oblique black stripes in relationship to the axis of the entire pennate muscle, with the white stripes in-between

showing the arrangement of the interfascicular more echo-reflective collagen (Fig. 14.4). Muscle fascicle length (which is assumed to also represent muscle fiber length) is measured as the length of the fascicular path between the two aponeuroses, usually in more than one site on the muscle, with or without accounting for any curvature present. If the muscle fascicles are longer than the scan window then a simplification that they extend linearly beyond the boundaries of the window has often been made without introducing large computational errors. The pennation angle is measured as the angle formed between the muscle fascicle trajectory and the aponeurosis visible on the scan, usually in proximity to the attachment points of the fascicle in the aponeurosis if curvature effects are not neglected for simplicity.

The first reports on *in vivo* human muscle architecture measurements using ultrasonography appeared in the early 1990s (Henriksson-Larsen *et al.* 1992; Rutherford & Jones 1992). Shortly after, this technique was validated through comparisons with direct anatomical measurements of muscle fascicle lengths and pennation angles on human cadaveric muscles (Kawakami *et al.* 1993; Narici *et al.* 1996). Since then, ultrasound scanning has been applied to study several human muscles and their adaptations to increased use and disuse. Both cross-sectional and longitudinal-design experiments confirm that muscle architecture displays considerable plasticity specific to the mechanical environment in which the muscle habitually operates. For example, it has been shown that the muscles of body-builders have a greater pennation angle than normal (Kawakami *et al.* 1993). Similarly, pennation angle increases have often been reported in sedentary individuals after several weeks of resistance training (Kawakami *et al.* 1995; Aagaard *et al.* 2001). As explained earlier, increases in pennation angle are expected in hypertrophied muscles (i.e., muscles that have undergone a PCSA increase). Interestingly, differences in pennation angle between populations/conditions have often been accompanied by differences in fascicle length in the same direction (Kearns *et al.* 2000; Blazevich *et al.* 2003), indicating that adaptations have occurred in the numbers of both in-parallel and in-series sarcomeres. Furthermore, leg muscle fascicle length in 100-m sprinters has been shown to correlate with sprinting performance (Kumagai *et al.* 2000), suggesting that differences between sprinters in the number of serial sarcomeres can partly account for the variation in their performance. Inter-population differences in the number of serial sarcomeres in a given muscle may also underlie a variation in the shape of the muscle's moment-angle relationship. For example, in one study it has been shown that cyclists exerted higher moments at shorter compared with longer rectus femoris muscle lengths, whereas the opposite was the case for runners (Herzog *et al.* 1991). An increased number of serial sarcomeres in the rectus femoris muscle of runners, who adopt an upright posture during running training (longer rectus femoris length), compared to cyclists, who adopt a flexed-hip posture during cycling training (shorter rectus femoris length), might explain this finding.

As opposed to training and physical activity, disuse reduces the PCSA, pennation angle, and fascicle length of muscles (Narici & Cerretelli 1998; Bleakney & Maffulli 2002). Disuse atrophy and the consequent changes in muscle architecture may partly explain the reduced muscle strength performance of athletes following discontinuation of their physical training due to an injury (e.g., Mandelbaum *et al.* 1995; St-Pierre 1995). Studies in which exercise training has been introduced in a controlled way during experimental disuse indicate that concurrent mechanical loading can partly prevent disuse muscle atrophy and architectural alterations, highlighting the importance of appropriate rehabilitation for early recovery in sporting activities after an injury (e.g., Mandelbaum *et al.* 1995; St-Pierre 1995). Similar muscle architecture changes with disuse are caused by ageing (Narici *et al.* 2003), which may partly explain the deterioration in muscle strength and power with age in master athletes (Wiswell *et al.* 2001).

Tendon mechanical properties and function

The primary role of tendons is to transmit contractile forces to the skeleton to generate joint movement. In doing so, however, tendons do not behave as rigid bodies but exhibit a time-dependent extensibility. This has important implications for muscle and joint function, as well as for the integrity of the tendon itself.

First, the elongation of a tendon during an *in situ* isometric muscle contraction will result in muscle shortening. For a given contractile force, a more extensible tendon will allow greater muscle shortening. The resultant extra sarcomeric shortening will affect the force that the muscle can generate and transmit to the skeleton. Whether the contractile force will be affected positively or negatively by the elasticity of the tendon depends on the region over which the sarcomeres of the muscle operate. If the sarcomeres operate in the descending limb of the force-length relationship (e.g., the extensor carpi radialis brevis muscle; Lieber *et al.* 1994), the more extensible tendon will result in greater contractile force. However, if the sarcomeres operate in the ascending limb of the force-length relationship (e.g., the gastrocnemius muscle; Maganaris 2003) then the more extensible tendon will result in less contractile force. This modulation of muscle force production by tendon elasticity needs to be accounted for in the design of athletic training and rehabilitation, since, as will be discussed later, chronic exercise and disuse may alter the mechanical properties of tendon tissue.

Second, a non-rigid tendon may complicate the control of joint position. For example, consider an external oscillating force applied to a joint at a certain angle. Trying to maintain the joint would still require the generation of constant contractile force in the muscle. If the tendon is very compliant, its length will be changed by the external oscillating load, even if the muscle length is held constant. This will result in the failure to maintain the joint steady at the desired angle. This specific interaction between muscle and tendon is relevant to sporting activities where small changes in joint positioning may affect performance, as is the case in events such as archery and shooting.

Third, the work done to stretch a tendon is stored as elastic energy, and most of this energy is recovered once the tensile load is removed and the tendon recoils. The passive mechanism of energy provision operates in the tendons of the lower extremity during application and release of ground reaction forces in locomotor activities, reducing the associated energy cost (for reviews see Alexander 1988; Biewener & Roberts 2000). This spring-like function of tendon is relevant to athletes involved in sporting events where metabolic energy supply is a limiting factor in performance, e.g., endurance activities. As a tendon recovers its length after the foot is released from the ground, some energy is also "dissipated" in the form of heat, evidenced by the presence of a loop between the loading and unloading directions in the tendon force-deformation curve (termed "mechanical hysteresis"). The amount of strain energy lost as heat is relatively small (i.e., the area of this loop) – ~10% of the total work done on the tendon by the ground reaction force to stretch it (Bennett *et al.* 1986) – and does not endanger the integrity of a tendon in a single stretch-recoil cycle. However, as a result of the repeated loading-unloading that tendons are subjected to during intense physical activities such as running, the heat lost may result in cumulative thermal damage and injury to the tendon, predisposing the tendon ultimately to rupture. Indeed, *in vivo* measurements and modeling-based calculations indicate that spring-like tendons may develop during exercise temperatures above the 42.5°C threshold for fibroblast viability (Wilson & Goodship 1994). These findings are in-line with the degenerative lesions often observed in the core of tendons acting as elastic energy stores, indicating that hyperthermia may be involved in the pathophysiology of exercise-induced tendon trauma.

To quantify the tensile behavior of tendons and assess the above effects, numerous *in vitro* studies have been performed. In such tests, an isolated tendon specimen is stretched by an actuator. The force and corresponding tendon deformation data recorded during the test are then combined to produce a force-deformation curve, from which structural stiffness (i.e., slope of the curve in $N \cdot mm^{-1}$) and energy (i.e. the area under the curve, in J or % values) can be calculated. Normalization of structural stiffness to the dimensions of the tendon gives Young's modulus (the units for which are GPa), which characterizes material stiffness.

Ultrasound scanning has recently made it possible to quantify the mechanical properties of human tendons *in vivo* (Maganaris & Paul 1999). By recording the displacement of anatomical markers along the tendon-aponeurosis unit during "isometric" muscle contractions and relaxations, we have been able to obtain realistic tendon force-deformation graphs, the Young's modulus values in the range 0.5–1.5 GPa, and hysteresis values in the range 10–25% (for a review see Maganaris *et al.* 2004). Moreover, the contribution of elastic energy returned by *in vivo* human tendon recoil to the total mechanical work in a locomotor task has been shown to increase with the intensity of the task. For example, the Achilles tendon contributes 6% of the total mechanical work in one step during walking (Maganaris & Paul 2002) and 16% of the total mechanical work in a one-legged hop (Litchwark & Wilson 2005). A common finding with important implications for sporting activities is that the stiffness of a tendon and the magnitude of its stretch-recoiling action in activities involving stretch-shortening cycles (e.g., counter-movement jumps in volleyball) positively affects the performance of activity (e.g., jump height; Kubo *et al.* 1999; Finni *et al.* 2003; Bojsen-Moller *et al.* 2005; Ishikawa *et al.* 2005; Fukashiro *et al.* 2006). This indicates that stiffer tendons may also be capable of returning more elastic energy on recoil, which in turn is used to produce mechanical work. Another common finding of *in vivo* human studies is the presence of a relationship between tendon stiffness and rate of torque development, highlighting the primary role of tendon as force transmitter, a function of crucial importance in sporting events where changes in posture need to be made rapidly – e.g., soccer and tennis. Somewhat surprising is the finding of a lack of association between human tendon stiffness and range of joint motion in one recent study (Bojsen-Moller *et al.* 2005), indicating that other anatomical structures in the joint (e.g., capsule and ligaments) may be more important limiting factors of joint extensibility.

Application of ultrasonography in sedentary individuals has shown that adaptability to mechanical loading is a feature not only of muscles, but also tendons. More specifically, resistance training for 12–14 weeks has been shown to increase tendon stiffness and Young's modulus (Kubo *et al.* 2001, 2006; Reeves *et al.* 2003), while stretching training for 3 weeks has been shown to reduce the mechanical hysteresis of tendons (Kubo *et al.* 2002). In one study, however, 9 months of habitual running in previously untrained individuals had no effect on the Achilles tendon mechanical properties (Hansen *et al.* 2003), indicating that a more intense mechanical stimulus was required to change the dimensions and/or material of the tendon. The concept of a threshold mechanical stimulus that needs to be exceeded to evoke tendon adaptations is also supported by a comparative study between sprinters, endurance runners, and sedentary individuals, showing an increased triceps surae tendon stiffness in the sprinters only (Arampatzis *et al.* 2007). Opposite to training, reports on disuse for periods ranging from several weeks (e.g., bed-rest; Reeves *et al.* 2005) to several years (e.g., paralysis due to spinal cord injury; Maganaris *et al.* 2006) indicate that the tendon's material undergoes substantial deterioration, rather rapidly, in the first few months or so. The findings on the plasticity of human tendons in response to disuse highlight the need for appropriate rehabilitation after injury to preserve the tendon's mechanical integrity and function.

Joint function and muscle-tendon moment arm

The muscle-tendon moment arm (d) is defined as the perpendicular from the axis of the joint that a muscle-tendon unit spans to the action line of this unit. This geometrical parameter is responsible for the transformation of:

1 Contractile force (F) to joint moment according to the equation

$$M = F \cdot d \qquad \text{(eqn. 1)}$$

and

2 Linear muscle-tendon displacement (Δx) to joint rotation ($\Delta \varphi$) according to the equation

$$M = \Delta x / \Delta \varphi \qquad \text{(eqn. 2)}$$

From eqn. 1 it becomes apparent that, for a given F, the greater the moment arm length d the greater the rotational outcome M of F. However, from eqn. 2, it also follows that, for a given dx, longer moment arms result in a smaller range of movements $\Delta \varphi$. This means that smaller muscles (i.e., muscles with smaller PCSA) may have an advantage over larger muscles in terms of "muscle strength", and longer muscles (subjected to greater Δx) may not correspond to wider ranges of joint movement than shorter muscles, if these smaller and shorter muscles cross joints with longer moment arms.

When applying eqn. 1 to calculate either M or F at a given joint angle, it is important to remember that the input d used should correspond not only to the joint angle in which M and F refer, but also to the contraction intensity examined. This is because d changes not only with joint angle, but also with the contractile force transmitted along the tendon. The latter effect is not trivial, as d has been reported to increase from rest to maximum intensity contractions by between 22 and 44% (Maganaris *et al.* 1998b, 1999; Tsaopoulos *et al.* 2007a). Clearly, failing to account for such sizeable changes will cause substantial errors in the outcome of eqn. 1. Changes in moment arm length with contraction at a given joint angle occur primarily because the tendon path may move away from the joint centre during exertion of muscle force against resistance. This is the case: (i) in tendons enclosed by retinacular sheaths extending on the application of muscle force (e.g., the tibialis anterior tendon; Maganaris *et al.* 1999); (ii) in tendons of muscles which thicken in the sagittal plane by contraction and cause a displacement of the tendon's origin in the muscle (e.g., the Achilles tendon; Maganaris *et al.* 1998b); and (iii) in situations where the bony insertion of a tendon is displaced because the distal bone is translated during contraction (e.g., the patellar tendon; Tsaopoulos *et al.* 2007a). Movement of the distal bone during muscle force application may also cause a shift of the joint centre away from the tendon (Maganaris *et al.* 1998b, 1999), further exacerbating the effect of contraction on the tendon moment arm.

The quantification of tendon moment arms has traditionally been based on morphometric analysis of joint images, recorded mainly in 2-D using expensive scanning techniques that enable identification of the tendon path and joint centre, for example MRI and X-ray fluoroscopy (e.g., Tsaopoulos 2007a,b). A more practical scanning method, which can be employed for estimating d values *in vivo*, is 2-D ultrasonography. Using this method, the muscle-tendon unit rather than the joint is scanned in the sagittal plane at different muscle lengths over a range of joint angles. By measuring the linear displacement Δx of a given anatomical marker on the muscle-tendon unit (e.g., the myotendinous junction or the insertion of an identifiable muscle fascicle in the aponeurosis) caused by a given joint rotation $\Delta\varphi$, d can be calculated according to eqn. 2. Moment arm measurements in 3-D require identification of the 3-D orientation of tendon paths and joint axes. Such measurements can now be made using MRI, but the long duration of scanning currently required (4–10 min; for a review see Maganaris 2004a) prevents the applicability of 3-D imaging for the quantification of tendon moment arms during continuous application of contractile forces.

The need for access to sophisticated scanning techniques when seeking to quantify the moment arm of a muscle-tendon unit could be circumvented if a relationship could be established with another easily measured anthropometric parameter, for example body segment dimensions. Recent studies show that moment arms do not scale linearly to basic anthropometric characteristics (Tsaopoulos *et al.* 2007b), but the possibility that more complex relationships exist, such as allometric scalings, cannot be excluded and requires systematic investigation in both skeletally mature individuals and in younger athletes during development and growth.

When considering the rotational outcome of muscular force about a joint, not only the muscle-tendon moment arm, but also the moment arm of the external force should be considered; i.e., the distance between the joint centre and the external force against which internal contractile force is produced. Two characteristics in the moment arm of the external resistance force are important: its length and its location relative to the muscle-tendon moment arm. If the joint centre is placed between the points of application of the external and muscular forces, then these forces must act in the same direction. An example of this type of lever is the elbow extension resistance exercise for triceps muscle strengthening (Fig. 14.5a). Because the triceps muscle-tendon moment arm is smaller than the external force moment arm, to achieve a moment equilibrium the triceps muscle must produce proportionally greater force than the resistance force. The antagonistic biceps flexion exercise is another type of lever in which the joint centre is at one end, the resistance force at the other end, and the muscular force in between the two ends but closer to the joint centre (Fig. 14.5b). Again, the muscular force applied in equilibrium conditions is greater than the external force. However, smaller muscle-tendon moment arms than external moment arms in the above examples also mean that the resultant distance traveled by the point of application of the external force during joint rotation is greater than the displacement of the muscle-tendon unit. Thus, although force production is penalized in these musculoskeletal lever types, effective external excursion and hence speed of movement are both favored.

Muscle-tendon modeling issues in computer simulation

Whole-body performance in sporting events results from the coordinated action of several muscle-joints systems. An important functional property in any muscle-joint system is its moment-angle relationship;

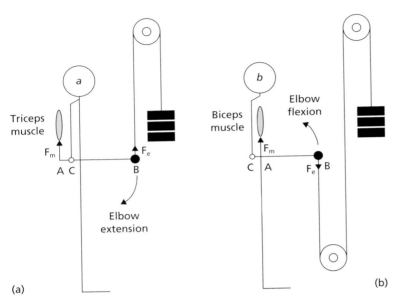

Triceps
muscle

F_m

A C   B F_e

Elbow
extension

(a)

Biceps
muscle

F_m

Elbow
flexion

C   A   B
        F_e

(b)

Fig. 14.5 An individual *a* on the left performs a "triceps push-down" exercise using a high pulley. Individual *b* on the right performs a "biceps-curl" exercise using a pulley system. C is the center of the elbow joint, A is the insertion point of the relevant agonist muscle-tendon in each case, and B is the point of application of the external force on the hands. (CA) is the muscle-tendon moment arm, (CB) is the external force moment arm, F_m is the muscle-tendon force, and F_e is the external force. In equilibrium conditions $F_m \cdot (CA) = F_e \cdot (CB)$. Because (CA) < (CB) it follows that $F_m > F_e$.

i.e., the capacity of a muscle to generate a moment about the joint it spans at different joint angles. In computer simulation applications of human movement, the motion of the model is driven by the application of muscle forces, or torques, around the joints. These are based on the output of theoretical muscle models using subject-specific scaling parameters whenever available, or on torque generator models using experimental measurements of the joint torque-angle-velocity relationship in a specific subject. However, both approaches have significant limitations (see Yeadon & King 2008). Models of moment-angle characteristics with high predictive accuracy have been reported (e.g., Hoy *et al.* 1990), but in most cases some of the input parameters in the models (e.g., maximum muscle force, tendon slack length, width of the muscle length-tension relationship) have been determined by tuning rather than measurement, with the aim being to fit the model's output with experimental results. A simple model for the prediction of moment-angle characteristics avoiding input parameter tuning can be based on the mathematical relationship between joint moment and force ($M = F \cdot d$; see eqn. 1), applied at different joint angles. The moment arm length d can be obtained *in vivo* using MRI or ultrasound, as described in the preceding section. The muscle force

F can also be obtained *in vivo* using strain gauges and optic fibers inserted surgically in the tendon of the muscle (e.g., Komi 1990; Finni *et al.* 2003). A less invasive and more practical approach is to calculate F based on the size (PCSA) and intrinsic force-generating potential (specific tension) of muscle (Maganaris 2004b). However, this approach requires muscle architecture measurements, which are currently limited to superficial muscles, mainly due to technical limitations in ultrasound penetration into deeper tissues.

Concluding comments and future challenges

This chapter examined some of the recent developments in the area of human movement biomechanics and the experimental and theoretical modeling approaches used for performance enhancement and injury prevention, with an emphasis on the issues of muscle-tendon mechanics and joint function. The biomechanical analysis of movement, especially in sporting activities, presents unique problems and challenges. Although sophisticated and accurate laboratory-based techniques have been developed, measurements in the field during actual competition are still limited. Real-time and minimal interference recording devices are especially useful once relevant parameters have been identified. Significant problems with accurate marker tracking and skin movement artifacts still remain, despite progress with calibration and correction algorithms. The measurement of subject-specific segmental and muscle-tendon mechanical parameters, together with appropriate optimization techniques, will allow further application of individualized modeling and computer simulation applications that are necessary for the modification of technique for the improvement of performance or prevention of injuries at an individual level.

References

Aagaard, P., Andersen, J.L., Dyhre-Poulsen, P., Leffers, A.M., Wagner, A., Magnusson, S.P., *et al.* (2001) A mechanism for increased contractile strength of human pennate muscle in response to strength training: changes in muscle architecture. *Journal of Physiology* **534**, 613–623.

Alexander, R.McN. (1988) *Elastic Mechanisms in Animal Movement*. Cambridge University Press, Cambridge, UK.

Alexander, R.McN. (2003) Modelling approaches in biomechanics. *Philosophical Transactions of the Royal Society B: Biological Sciences* **358**, 1429–1435.

Alexander, R.McN. & Vernon, A. (1975) The dimensions of knee and ankle muscles and the forces they exert. *Journal of Human Movement Studies* **1**, 115–123.

Arampatzis, A., Karamanidis, K., Morey-Klapsing, G., De Monte, G. & Stafilidis, S. (2007) Mechanical properties of the triceps surae tendon and aponeurosis in relation to intensity of sport activity. *Journal of Biomechanics* **40**, 1946–1952.

Bahr, R. & Krosshaug, T. (2005) Understanding injury mechanisms: a key component of preventing injuries in sport. *British Journal of Sports Medicine* **39**(6), 324–329.

Bartlett, R. (1999) *Sports Biomechanics: Reducing Injury and Improving Performance*. E. & F.N. Spon, London.

Bartlett, R., Wheat, J. & Robins, M. (2007) Is movement variability important for sports biomechanists? *Sports Biomechanics* **6**(2), 224–243.

Baltzopoulos, V. (2008) Isokinetic dynamometry. In: *Biomechanical Evaluation of Movement in Sport and Exercise* (Payton, C.J. & Bartlett, R.M., eds.) Routledge, London.

Bennett, M.B., Ker, R.F., Dimery, N.J. & Alexander, R.McN. (1986) Mechanical properties of various mammalian tendons. *Journal of Zoology, London A* **209**: 537–548.

Biewener, A.A. & Roberts, T.J. (2000) Muscle and tendon contributions to force, work, and elastic energy savings: a comparative perspective. *Exercise and Sport Sciences Reviews* **28**, 99–107.

Blazevich, A.J., Gill, N.D., Bronks, R. & Newton, R.U. (2003) Training-specific muscle architecture adaptation after 5-wk training in athletes. *Medicine and Science in Sports and Exercise* **35**, 2013–2022.

Bleakney, R. & Maffulli, N. (2002) Ultrasound changes to intramuscular architecture of the quadriceps following intramedullary nailing. *Journal of Sports Medicine and Physical Fitness* **42**, 120–125.

Blemker, S.S., Asakawa, D.S., Gold, G.E. & Delp, S.L. (2007) Image-based musculoskeletal modeling: Applications, advances, and future opportunities. *Journal of Magnetic Resonance Imaging* **25**(2), 441–451.

Bojsen-Møller, J., Magnusson, S.P., Rasmussen, L.R., Kjaer, M. & Aagaard, P. (2005) Muscle performance during maximal isometric and dynamic contractions is influenced by the stiffness of the tendinous structures. *Journal of Applied Physiology* **99**, 986–994.

Delp, S.L., Anderson, F.C., Arnold, A.S., Loan, P., Habib, A. & John, C.T., *et al.* (2007) OpenSim: Open-source software to create and analyze dynamic simulations of movement. *IEEE Transactions on Biomedical Engineering* **54**(11), 1940–1950.

Elliott, B. (2006) Biomechanics and tennis. *British Journal of Sports Medicine* **40**, 392–396.

Epstein, M. & Herzog, W. (2003) Aspects of skeletal muscle modelling. *Philosophical Transactions of the Royal Society B: Biological Sciences* **358**(1437), 1445–1452.

Erdemir, A., McLean, S., Herzog, W. & van den Bogert, A.J. (2007) Model-based estimation of muscle forces exerted during movements. *Clinical Biomechanics* **22**(2), 131–154.

Fick, R. (1911) *Spezielle Gelenk und Muskelmechanik* Vol. I. Gustav Fischer, Jena.

Finni, T., Ikegawa, S., Lepola, V. & Komi., P.V. (2003) Comparison of force-velocity relationships of vastus lateralis muscle in isokinetic and in stretch-shortening cycle exercises. *Acta Physiologica Scandinavica* **177**, 483–491.

Friederich, J.A. & Brand, R.A. (1990) Muscle fiber architecture in the human lower limb. *Journal of Biomechanics* **23**, 91–95.

Fukashiro, S., Hay, D.C. & Nagano, A. (2006) Biomechanical behavior of muscle-tendon complex during dynamic human movements. *Journal of Applied Biomechanics* **22**, 131–147.

Hansen, P., Aagaard, P., Kjaer, M., Larsson, B. & Magnusson, S.P. (2003) Effect of habitual running on human Achilles tendon load-deformation properties and cross-sectional area. *Journal of Applied Physiology* **95**, 2375–2380.

Hamill, J., van Emmerik, R.E.A., Heiderscheit, B.C. & Li, L. (1999) A dynamical systems approach to lower extremity running injuries. *Clinical Biomechanics* **14**(5), 297–308.

Hatze, H. (1981) A comprehensive model for human motion simulation and its application to the take-off phase of the long jump. *Journal of Biomechanics* **14**(3), 135–142.

Hay, J.G. (1993). Citius, altius, longius (faster, higher, longer): The biomechanics of jumping for distance. *Journal of Biomechanics* **26**(Suppl. 1), 7–21.

Hay, J.G. & Read, G. (1982) *Anatomy, Mechanics and Human Motion*. Prentice Hall, Englewood Cliffs.

Henriksson-Larsen, K., Wretling, M.L., Lorentzon, R. & Oberg, L. (1992) Do muscle fiber size and fiber angulation correlate in pennated human muscles? *European Journal of Applied Physiology* **64**, 68–72.

Herzog, W. (1996) Muscle function in movement and sports. *American Journal of Sports Medicine* **24**(6), S14–S19.

Herzog, W., Guimaraes, A.C., Anton, M.G. & Carter-Erdman, K.A. (1991) Moment-length relations of rectus femoris muscles of speed skaters/cyclists and runners. *Medicine and Science in Sports and Exercise* **23**, 1289–1296.

Hoy, M.G., Zajac, F.E. & Gordon, M.E. (1990) A musculoskeletal model of the human lower extremity: the effect of muscle, tendon, and moment arm on the moment-angle relationship of musculotendon actuators at the hip, knee, and ankle. *Journal of Biomechanics* **23**, 157–169.

Ishikawa, M., Niemelä, E. & Komi, P.V. (2005). Interaction between fascicle and tendinous tissues in short-contact stretch-shortening cycle exercise with varying eccentric intensities. *Journal of Applied Physiology* **99**, 217–223.

Kawakami, Y., Abe, T. & Fukunaga, T. (1993) Muscle-fiber pennation angles are greater in hypertrophied than in normal muscles. *Journal of Applied Physiology* **74**, 2740–2744.

Kawakami, Y., Abe, T., Kuno, S.Y. & Fukunaga, T. (1995) Training-induced changes in muscle architecture and specific tension. *European Journal of Applied Physiology and Occupational Physiology* **72**, 37–43.

Kearns, C.F., Abe, T. & Brechue, W.F. (2000) Muscle enlargement in sumo wrestlers includes increased muscle fascicle length. *European Journal of Applied Physiology* **83**, 289–296.

Knudson, D. & Morrison C. (1997) *Qualitative Analysis of Human Movement.* Human Kinetics, Champaign.

Komi, P.V. (1990) Relevance of *in vivo* force measurements to human biomechanics. *Journal of Biomechanics* **23**, 23–34.

Krosshaug, T., Andersen, T.E., Olsen, O.-O., Myklebust, G. & Bahr, R. (2005) Research approaches to describe the mechanisms of injuries in sport: Limitations and possibilities. *British Journal of Sports Medicine* **39**(6), 330–339.

Kubo, K., Kawakami, Y. & Fukunaga, T. (1999) Influence of elastic properties of tendon structures on jump performance in humans. *Journal of Applied Physiology* **87**, 2090–2096.

Kubo, K., Kanehisa, H., Ito, M. & Fukunaga, T. (2001) Effects of isometric training on the elasticity of human tendon structures *in vivo*. *Journal of Applied Physiology* **91**, 26–32.

Kubo, K., Kanehisa, H. & Fukunaga, T. (2002) Effect of stretching training on the viscoelastic properties of human tendon structures *in vivo*. *Journal of Applied Physiology* **92**, 595–601.

Kubo, K., Ohgo, K., Takeishi, R., Yoshinaga, K., Tsunoda, N., Kanehisa, H. & Fukunaga, T. (2006). Effects of isometric training at different knee angles on the muscle-tendon complex *in vivo*. *Scandinavian Journal of Medicine and Science in Sports* **16**, 159–167.

Kumagai, K., Abe, T., Brechue, W.F., Ryushi, T., Takano, S. & Mizuno, M. (2000) Sprint performance is related to muscle fascicle length in male 100-m sprinters. *Journal of Applied Physiology* **88**, 811–816.

Lees, A. (1999) Biomechanical assessment of individual sports for improved performance. *Sports Medicine* **28**(5), 299–305.

Lees, A. (2002) Technique analysis in sports: A critical review. *Journal of Sports Sciences* **20**(10), 813–828.

Lieber, R.L. & Brown, C.C. (1992) Quantitative method for comparison of skeletal muscle architectural properties. *Journal of Biomechanics* **25**, 557–560.

Lieber, R.L. & Friden, J. (2000) Functional and clinical significance of skeletal muscle architecture. *Muscle and Nerve* **23**:1647–1666.

Lieber, R.L., Loren, G.J. & Fridén, J. (1994) *In vivo* measurement of human wrist extensor muscle sarcomere length changes. *Journal of Neurophysiology* **71**, 874–881.

Lichtwark, G.A., Wilson, A.M. (2005) *In vivo* mechanical properties of the human Achilles tendon during one-legged hopping. *Journal of Experimental Biology* **208**, 4715–4725.

Maganaris, C.N. (2003) Force-length characteristics of the *in vivo* human gastrocnemius muscle. *Clinical Anatomy* **16**, 215–223.

Maganaris, C.N. (2004a) Imaging-based estimates of moment arm length in intact human muscle-tendons. *European Journal of Applied Physiology* **91**, 130–139.

Maganaris, C.N. (2004b) A predictive model of moment-angle characteristics in human skeletal muscle: application and validation in muscles across the ankle joint. *Journal of Theoretical Biology* **230**, 89–98.

Maganaris, C.N. & Paul, J.P. (1999). *In vivo* human tendon mechanical properties. *Journal of Physiology* **521**, 307–313.

Maganaris, C.N. & Paul, J.P. (2002) Tensile properties of the *in vivo* human gastrocnemius tendon. *Journal of Biomechanics* **35**,1639–1646.

Maganaris, C.N., Baltzopoulos, V. & Sargeant, A.J. (1998a) *In vivo* measurements of the triceps surae complex architecture in man: implications for muscle function. *Journal of Physiology* **512**, 603–614.

Maganaris, C.N., Baltzopoulos, V. & Sargeant, A.J. (1998b) Changes in Achilles tendon moment arm from rest to maximum isometric plantarflexion: *in vivo* observations in man. *Journal of Physiology* **510**, 977–985.

Maganaris, C.N., Baltzopoulos, V. & Sargeant, A.J. (1999) Changes in the tibialis anterior tendon moment arm from rest to maximum isometric dorsiflexion: *in vivo* observations in man. *Clinical Biomechanics* **14**, 661–666.

Maganaris, C.N., Narici M.V., Almekinders, L.C. & Maffulli, N. (2004) Biomechanics and pathophysiology of overuse tendon injuries: ideas on insertional tendinopathy. *Sports Medicine* **34**, 1005–1017.

Maganaris, C.N., Reeves N.D., Rittwege, J., Sargeant, A.J., Jones, D.A., Gerrits, K., et al. (2006) Adaptive response of human tendon to paralysis. *Muscle and Nerve* **33**, 85–92.

Mandelbaum, B.R., Myerson, M.S. & Forster, R. (1995) Achilles tendon ruptures: A new method of repair, early range of motion, and functional rehabilitation. *American Journal of Sports Medicine* **23**, 392–395.

Marshall, R.N. & Elliott, B.C. (2000) Long-axis rotation: The missing link in proximal-to-distal segmental sequencing. *Journal of Sports Sciences* **18**(4), 247–254.

McLean, S.G., Su, A. & van den Bogert, A.J. (2003) Development and validation of a 3-D model to predict knee joint loading during dynamic movement. *Journal of Biomechanical Engineering* **125**(6), 864–874.

McLean, S.G., Huang, X., Su, A. & van den Bogert, A.J. (2004) Sagittal plane biomechanics cannot injure the ACL during sidestep cutting. *Clinical Biomechanics* **19**(8), 828–838.

Narici, M.V., Binzoni, T., Hiltbrand, E., Fasel, J., Terrier, F. & Cerretelli, P. (1996) *In vivo* human gastrocnemius architecture with changing joint angle at rest and during graded isometric contraction. *Journal of Physiology* **496**, 287–297.

Narici, M.V. & Cerretelli, P. (1998) Changes in human muscle architecture in disuse-atrophy evaluated by ultrasound imaging. *Journal of Gravitational Physiology* **5**, P73–P74.

Narici, M.V., Maganaris, C.N., Reeves, N.D. & Capodaglio, P. (2003) Effect of aging on human muscle architecture. *Journal of Applied Physiology* **95**, 2229–2234.

Neptune, R.R. (2000) Computer modeling and simulation of human movement: Applications in sport and rehabilitation. *Physical Medicine and Rehabilitation Clinics of North America* **11**(2), 417–434.

Nigg, B.M., Stefanyshyn, D. & Denoth, J. (2000) Mechanical considerations of work and energy. In: *Biomechanics and Biology of Movement* (Nigg, B.M., MacIntosh, B.R. & Mester, J., eds.) Human Kinetics, Champaign: 5–18.

Payton, C.J. & Bartlett, R.M. (2008) *Biomechanical Evaluation of Movement in Sport and Exercise*. Routledge, London.

Reeves, N.D., Narici, M.V. & Maganaris, C.N. (2003) Strength training alters the viscoelastic properties of tendons in elderly humans. *Muscle and Nerve* **28**: 74–81.

Reeves, N.D., Maganaris, C.N., Ferretti, G. & Narici, M.V. (2005) Influence of 90-day simulated microgravity on human tendon mechanical properties and the effect of resistive countermeasures. *Journal of Applied Physiology* **98**, 2278–2286.

Rutherford, O.M. & Jones, D.A. (1992) Measurement of fiber pennation using ultrasound in the human quadriceps *in vivo*. *European Journal of Applied Physiology* **65**, 433–437.

Stefanyshyn, D.J. & Nigg, B.M. (2000) Work and energy influenced by athletic equipment. In: *Biomechanics and Biology of Movement* (Nigg, B.M., MacIntosh, B.R. & Mester, J., eds.) Human Kinetics, Champaign: 49–65.

St-Pierre. D.M. (1995) Rehabilitation following arthroscopic meniscectomy. *Sports Medicine* **20**, 338–347.

Tsaopoulos, D.E., Baltzopoulos, V., Richards, P.J. & Maganaris, C.N. (2007a) *In vivo* changes in the human patellar tendon moment arm length with different modes and intensities of muscle contraction. *Journal of Biomechanics* **40**, 3325–3332.

Tsaopoulos, D.E., Maganaris, C.N. & Baltzopoulos, V. (2007b) Can the patellar tendon moment arm be predicted from anthropometric measurements? *Journal of Biomechanics* **40**, 645–651.

Tsirakos, D., Baltzopoulos, V. & Bartlett, R. (1997) Inverse optimization: Functional and physiological considerations related to the force-sharing problem. *Critical Reviews in Biomedical Engineering* **25**(4–5), 371–407.

Vaughan, C.L. (1984) Computer simulation of human motion in sports biomechanics. *Exercise and Sport Sciences Reviews* **12**, 373–416.

Wickiewicz, T.L., Roy, R.R., Powell, P.L. & Edgerton, V.R. (1983) Muscle architecture of the human lower limb. *Clinical Orthopaedics and Related Research* **179**, 275–283.

Wilson, A.M. & Goodship, A.E. (1994) Exercise-induced hyperthermia as a possible mechanism for tendon degeneration. *Journal of Biomechanics* **27**, 899–905.

Wiswell, R.A., Hawkins, S.A., Jaque, S.V., Hyslop, D., Constantino, N., Tarpenning, K., *et al.* (2001) Relationship between physiological loss, performance decrement, and age in master athletes. *Journals of Gerontology. Series A, Biological Sciences and Medical Sciences* **56**, M618–M626.

Yeadon, M.R. & King, M.A. (2008) Computer simulation modelling in sport. In: *Biomechanical Evaluation of Movement in Sport and Exercise* (Payton, C.J. & Bartlett, R.M., eds.) Routledge, London: 103–128.

Chapter 15

Sports Ergonomics

THOMAS REILLY AND ADRIAN LEES

Ergonomists apply principles of the human sciences to individuals or groups in the working environment. This environment extends from the professional and occupational domains into domestic, leisure, and sports contexts. Ergonomics emerged as a technology from the realization during the World War II that performance of workers in munitions factories was variable, affected by environmental conditions, workplace design, hours of work, and the state of the individual. No single scientific discipline was capable of providing explanations for the errors, accidents, and fluctuations in output that were observed and it became evident that finding solutions to these problems called for an interdisciplinary approach. As a result of the wartime experiences, the Ergonomics Research Society was formed in 1949, later to become the Ergonomics Society as the applied focus became more clearly established. Its parallel in North America is the Human Factors Society and these bodies, together with a host of national and regional professional societies, are affiliated to the International Ergonomics Association. Both the Human Factors Society and the Ergonomics Society have their annual conferences and their own scientific journals whereas the International Ergonomics Association holds a triennial congress, the 16th event being held in Maastricht, the Netherlands in 2006. Since 1987, the Ergonomics Society has supported the International Conference on Sport, Leisure, and Ergonomics, the 6th event being held in 2007.

The Olympic Textbook of Science in Sport, 1st edition. Edited by R.J. Maughan. Published 2009 by Blackwell Publishing. ISBN: 978-1-4051-5638-7.

The scope of ergonomics is evident from the publication of special issues devoted to "sports ergonomics," first in the journal *Human Factors* in 1976 and later in *Applied Ergonomics* (Reilly 1984, 1991). The topics included, for example, novel techniques for measurement of motion (Atha 1984), the emerging uses of computers in sport (Lees 1985), the applications of hydrodynamics and electromyography to water-based sports (Clarys 1984), and controlling system uncertainty in sport and work (Davids *et al.* 1991). A breakdown of the material published in the proceedings of the first five conferences on Sport, Leisure, and Ergonomics shows the main areas of application of ergonomics to sport (Table 15.1). The material reviewed has been published in texts (Atkinson & Reilly 1995; Reilly & Greeves 2002) or in special issues of the journal *Ergonomics*. The areas of application range from health-related exercise to combinations of environmental conditions that pose challenges for elite performers (Table 15.1).

According to the International Ergonomics Association, "ergonomics (or human factors) is the scientific discipline concerned with the understanding of the interactions among humans and other elements of a system, and the profession that applies theoretical principles, data, and methods to design in order to optimize human well-being and overall system performance." This broad definition equally applies to the sports environment as to industrial circumstances. An interpretation restricted to occupational work would apply only to professional sport where talented individuals earn their livelihood by virtue of their specialized competitive competencies.

Table 15.1 Topics of reports in the five proceedings of Sport, Leisure, and Ergonomics and numbers for each category.

Aging	3
Body composition/functional anatomy	10
Circadian factors	6
Computers in sport	3
Corporate health and fitness	17
Disability	13
Environmental stress	10
Equipment design:	16
clothing	2
machines	5
protective devices	4
shoes/orthotics	5
Ergogenic aids/drugs	6
Fitness assessment	5
Injury	2
Measurement methods	14
Musculoskeletal loading	12
Pediatric ergonomics	4
Psychological stress	2
Sports coaching	4
Technique analysis	19
Training responses	7

Nevertheless, sport in general presents its participants with many of the conventional questions tackled in the pioneering years of ergonomics: examples include high levels of energy expenditure, thermoregulatory strain, pre-competition emotional stress, unique postural loadings, severe information processing demands, fatigue in sustained activities, and a myriad of other problems familiar to ergonomists. It has been suggested that, with the possible exception of military contexts, human limits are seldom so systematically explored and so ruthlessly exposed as they are in high-level sport (Reilly 1984). Indeed, the margin between success and failure is often less in sport than in warfare.

The human operator (the athlete) forms the centerpiece of a sports ergonomics model, the task or interface with machine or equipment being immediate connections. Then the environmental conditions can be considered, including workspace, temperature, pollution, and ambient pressure (Fig. 15.1). Finally, there are the more global parameters which

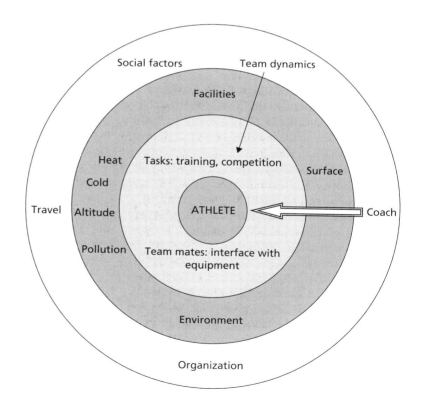

Fig. 15.1 The interface between the individual and the sports environment within an ergonomics framework.

embrace travel, social aspects, and organizational factors. The harmony with the coach and trainers may apply at this outer level, forming an aspect of team dynamics; alternatively it may have a more critical central role in the individual's well-being and motivation for performance.

In this chapter the more common concepts and principles of ergonomics are addressed and their applications to competitive sport are highlighted. These topics include the identification and monitoring of sources of competitive and training stress in its physiological, physical, and psychological forms. The phenomenon of fatigue is considered, as are safety principles and practices. The contributions of ergonomics to equipment design, in human–computer interaction and in different environments are exemplified. Finally, some predictions are made with respect to future developments in enhancing high performance sports.

Ergonomics model of the elite performer

Defining an ergonomics model for elite athletes is a matter of establishing coherence between the demands of the sport concerned and individual capabilities. These capabilities may be measured, improved by training, and form a consideration in selection. The demands may be expressed in quantifiable terms and lead to inclusion or exclusion according to fit, to counseling with respect to fitness, and to prescription of training (Fig. 15.2). Such regular assessments are implemented in a range of sports (Reilly & Doran 2003; Svensson & Drust 2005).

Team sports constitute complex systems from an ergonomist's perspective. Motion analysis, a classic technique in occupational ergonomics, may be employed in assessing the demands of the sport in team games (Reilly 2001). This approach allows feedback to participants of detailed aspects of their performance that might otherwise go undetected. Data on competitive activities can be complemented by physiological investigations, whether monitored unobtrusively (e.g., heart rate or gut temperature) or invasively during intermissions or at the end of the contest (e.g., blood sampling or muscle biopsies), although ergonomists generally prefer to use non-invasive methods, largely for fear of interfering

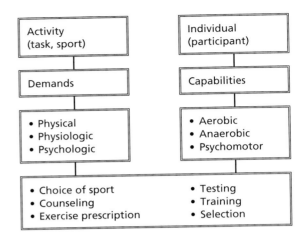

Fig. 15.2 Ergonomics model of the elite athlete.

with the activity being examined. More discrete information may be obtained from simulations of competition or in friendly contests where participants are less likely to be distracted and the rules for competition can be waived to allow for collection of data. A further opportunity for gaining insight into competitive demands is to conduct experimental studies; in this instance the non-competitive environment raises questions about ecologic validity.

The notion of "fitting the task to the person" is a fundamental principle of ergonomics and is characterized by a "user-centered" approach. While the sports participant may not have the freedom to redesign the task in hand, this goal can be reached in field games by altering the tactical role of specific individuals that render the team a more effective unit. In this way individuals can capitalize on their unique strengths and compensate for any deficiencies. A soccer mid-field player may, for example, be assigned a more defensive role when unable to match the work-rate requirements of both contributing to attacks and linking also to the defense. In many instances it is not practical to alter task characteristics, and specific training is necessary to improve those aspects of fitness in which defects have been exposed.

Assessment of physical and physiological capabilities is now a routine part of sports science support work. In order for these assessments to be of use to practitioners, fitness testing should be conducted on a regular basis, frequently enough to provide individual feedback but not so often that it disrupts ongoing training and becomes a chore. There are generic protocols for measurement of aerobic power, anaerobic capabilities, muscle performance, and other functional measures that employ standard ergometry. As these measures may lack specificity to the sport in question, a range of dedicated ergometers and tests has been designed to suit particular requirements. Exercise on these ergometers engages the most relevant muscle groups by mimicking the actions in the sport concerned. Consequently, it is possible to apply standard protocols for ski simulators, rowing and canoe ergometers, and other sports-specific devices. More sophisticated measurements may be obtained from exercise in water flumes for assessment of swimmers, kayakers, and rowers where biomechanical analysis can complement the recording of physiological responses.

Field-based tests have been employed to enhance the ecologic validity of fitness assessment and relate observations to competitive performance. Protocols have been designed that incorporate not only the locomotion patterns of the sport but also the essential skills (Reilly 2001). In these instances, the increased specificity is at a price of missing important physiological information. There are concessions for reliability in such tests when environmental and surface conditions vary with repeated measurements.

Assessments may embrace the range of scientific disciplines and include psychological as well as physical and physiological methods. Indeed, fitness requirements for most sports tend to be multidisciplinary. The predictive power of any multi-itemed test battery is low when the characteristics required for success are complex. Reilly *et al.* (2000) showed that young soccer players groomed for international level cannot be distinguished on the likelihood of future success, but they can be discriminated from subelite performers on a range of measures. Discriminant functions were found for aerobic power, speed and agility, and for anticipation and decision-making skills that characterize "game intelligence."

Monitoring and regulating loads

Physiological strain

A starting point in an ergonomics analysis is the quantification of load on the individual. The assumption is that the task imposes demands on the individual whose responses can be used as indicators of physiological strain. Physiological criteria corresponding to exercise intensity include energy expenditure, oxygen uptake, body temperature, heart rate, and blood metabolite concentrations. Such variables have been shown to be associated with subjective perceptions of exertion, task difficulty, and thermal comfort as well as with biomechanical measurements. Where chronic overloading is possible, endocrine responses and markers of immuno-suppression have been employed in attempts to explain underperformance (Gleeson *et al.* 1997).

Oxygen uptake and heart rate have traditionally been used in measuring physiological strain in heavy occupational work. The availability of short-range telemetric devices has made the continuous recording of these responses possible in a range of field settings. Monitoring of heart rate has conventionally been used to indicate physiological strain in occupational contexts and for estimating the energy cost of specific activities. While it can be maintained that these procedures are valid only in steady-rate exercise, the error in using heart rate to estimate energy expenditure during intermittent exercise of high intensity (such as soccer) is within acceptable limits (Bangsbo 1994). The recording of oxygen uptake during football training drills has yielded valuable information about metabolic loading related to competitive conditions (Kawakami *et al.* 1992). Continuous registration of heart rate during different training activities has generated information about their suitability for conditioning work or for "recovery training." Sassi *et al.* (2005) used blood lactate and heart rate responses to a range of football drills to identify those that could be employed as fitness stimuli and those that possessed purely tactical benefits. The physiological information can be used, not merely as descriptive feedback on training inputs, but also as a means of regulating the training intensity.

Forces

The measurement of force provides information on the interaction of an individual with the environment. There are several forces that act simultaneously on an individual to determine performance. While some of the forces are known (e.g., gravity) and some can be computed (e.g., air resistance), the force that has the greatest influence on performance is the contact force between the individual and the environment. This contact force, usually referred to as the "reaction force," often acts at the feet or hands but can, in principle, act at any point where the body makes contact with the surface. Specialized measurement equipment, referred to as a dynamometer, has evolved for monitoring the reaction force in specific situations.

The simplest form of dynamometer is one based on measuring the tension force in a wire and used when measuring isometric strength of a single joint. For example, when measuring the extension strength at the knee joint, the individual would normally be seated in a rigid chair with the ankle of the leg to be tested attached to a cuff, which in turn is attached via a cable to a strain gauge device. As the individual tries to extend the knee joint, the tension created in the cable is measured. Measurement of isometric force of a joint can provide useful data on strength capabilities of individuals, and on how strength is influenced by muscular fatigue and other factors such as diet and heat stress. The force data can be further processed to obtain variables such as the rate of force development and rate of force decay. These, together with the peak isometric force, represent a range of variables that can be used to monitor a wide variety of individual and muscle performance characteristics and the relationship between muscle groups.

More sophisticated muscle function dynamometers have been developed commercially (e.g., Kin-Com, Lido, Cybex, Biodex) whereby the angular velocity of movement can be pre-set. These devices are usually substantial pieces of equipment which were initially intended to provide a controlled environment for rehabilitation. Their measurement capability quickly led to their being used as a measurement tool. The measurement principle is similar to the strain gauge device mentioned above but they are capable of measuring muscle strength (usually expressed as joint torque) during isometric, concentric, and eccentric modes and can be configured to measure many of the body's joints in both flexion and extension. There are some measurement issues that users need to be aware of (Baltzopoulos & Gleeson 2003) but contemporary software enables these devices to be used widely in the evaluation of sports performers. For example, there has been much interest in evaluating the strength of soccer players at different levels (Rahnama et al. 2003), in terms of basic strength, bilateral strength, and strength asymmetries in these athletes as well as age-group soccer players (Iga et al. 2005) and the influences of match play in inducing fatigue (Rahnama et al. 2006).

Multijoint strength cannot be measured by the dynamometers reviewed above, and a force plate or platform is required. A force platform is a device that usually sits on the ground and can record the forces as contact is made on it, often with the feet but sometimes with the hands or other body part. The force platform is a sophisticated instrument that can directly measure up to six force variables (one vertical force, two horizontal friction force components, the friction torque, and two center of pressure locations). These force variables can be used directly or in combination to measure aspects of performance. The most informative force variable is the vertical force component as this usually is the largest. This force variable has been used to determine the forces brought about by walking (1.1 body weight) and running (up to 2.5 body weight) to the most demanding of sports such as triple jumping (up to 10 body weight; Hay 1992). The two horizontal friction forces can be used to record the frictional resistance as an athlete makes a change in direction during cutting or side stepping or the influence of shoe sole or stud design on the performance of sports footwear (Lake 2000). The friction torque is not widely used but has found some value in the etiology of injury in cyclists (Wheeler et al. 1992) where high rotational torques have been associated with knee injury. The center of pressure locations have been used to identify characteristics of running technique (Cavanagh & Lafortune 1980).

These force variables can assist in monitoring behavior in similar contexts, but the value of these force variables can be appreciated when they are combined with a motion analysis system to provide information on internal joint forces. Such a process is typified by "gait analysis" although it has been applied more widely to sports events. Data on joint moments and forces are now available in a variety of sports including running (Buzeck & Cavanagh 1990), cutting, jumping (Lees *et al.* 2004), and soccer kicking.

To gain an insight into the localized application of forces, a pressure-sensing device must be used. This is usually made of a series of small force-measuring cells (about 5 mm^2) which give the force acting over a small area. When several of these are put together as a mat, the device is able to measure the areas of high pressure; for example, under the foot as the heel makes initial contact with the ground, to toe-off where the pressure acts on the metatarsal heads. The regions of high pressure can lead to bruising and pressure sores, but can be prevented or alleviated with the use of custom-made orthoses, designed from the pressure data (Geil 2002). A pressure mat can also be placed in other body–environment interfaces; for example, in the stump of an amputee to monitor the fit of the prosthesis, or on the seat of a wheelchair athlete.

Electromyography

Electromyography (EMG) is a method for monitoring muscle activity by detecting the small electric field produced as muscle fibers are activated. The electrical field is detected either by surface electrodes placed on the surface of the skin over the muscle or by indwelling electrodes inserted into the muscle through a needle. The latter method of measurement is less popular because of its invasive nature and some element of risk that the fine wire making up the electrode may become detached during use. This risk is enhanced during vigorous muscle contractions where large changes in muscle fiber length occur. Nevertheless, in some cases this is the only way to monitor small or deep muscles (Morris *et al.* 1998). For these reasons, surface EMG is the most popular approach and there are now many commercial systems available that provide good quality pre-processed EMG signals for analysis.

The surface EMG signal can be used in a variety of ways but care must be taken in interpretation as the signal is susceptible to cross-talk from other active muscles. It is also necessary to know whether a muscle contraction is concentric, isometric, or eccentric as the EMG signal has a different appearance under these different contraction conditions. One of the more basic uses of surface EMG is to identify the muscles that are active in the performance of a task and their timing pattern relative to one another (for a review see Clarys & Cabri 1993). The surface EMG signal can be further processed to gain insights into muscle function. One method is to rectify the signal so that it has only positive components. Horita *et al.* (2002) used this method to detect the influence of muscle stretch on the stretch–shortening cycle in a jumping activity while the same group studied alterations in the lower limb muscles with increased running speed (Kyrolainen *et al.* 2005). More commonly, the EMG data are further smoothed to provide an "envelope" or "integrated" EMG signal which broadly reflects the action taking place. To relate the muscle activity to the motion, account must be taken of the electromechanical delay (i.e., the time from activation of the muscle fibers to the time when they develop maximum force), which is around 30–120 ms and is dependent on the level of pre-tension in the muscle. When relative activity between muscle groups is of interest, a method of normalization must be used. A maximum voluntary contraction (MVC) is often chosen, and while it too has some limitations, it does allow comparison between muscles and between individuals. Once the best processing method has been decided upon, surface EMG can be used in a variety of applications.

Sports equipment can be evaluated using EMG. For example, Robinson *et al.* (2005) investigated the efficacy of various commercial abdominal trainers in comparison to the traditional sit-up or "crunch" method of performing this task. They monitored the lower rectus abdominis, upper rectus abdominis, and external obliques muscles over five different types of abdominal exercise including a commercially manufactured device. They reported significant differences between exercises with three exercises (one involving a "gym ball," another using raised legs and another using a weight behind the head) showing greater muscle activity, while the commercially available abdominal roller showed less muscle activity than the standard sit-up. These data suggest that the commercially available device should be used with inexperienced individuals who may be able to perform a greater number of repetitions using the device than they otherwise would, which in turn may help their motivation to exercise. For maximal loading, exercises other than the standard sit-up can be chosen. It is also apparent that the exercise involving the gym ball is an advanced exercise suitable only for those already with a high level of training experience or requiring a high level of muscle training.

The effects of fatigue can be monitored using surface EMG. In the study by Robinson *et al.* (2005), the influences of a typical 30-min circuit training program on muscle activity were investigated. In the fatigued state, the normalized mean EMG for both exercises increased for lower and upper rectus abdominis, but not for the external obliques. This differential result illustrated that the external obliques were not highly used during the "fatigue condition." The increase in EMG signal because of fatigue is thought to reflect the greater central effort made or the different muscle recruitment pattern used when muscles become fatigued. Not all fatigue leads to a greater EMG signal. In a study of the effect of match fatigue in a simulation of the exercise intensity of soccer, Rahnama *et al.* (2006) reported an increase in EMG due to running speed (at 6, 9, 12, and 15 km·h^{-1}) but a reduction from the start of activity to the end of a 90-min soccer simulation protocol in some of the muscles monitored. This reduction was deemed to reflect the decline in strength found in players as a result of game play (Rahnama *et al.* 2003).

Stress and fatigue

The concepts of stress and fatigue are central in the applications of ergonomics. Agents of stress are referred to as stressors, and the main objective of an ergonomics intervention is to reduce their impact on the individual. This goal can be achieved by increasing stress tolerance or by reducing the strength of the stressor. Environmental sources of stress are dealt with separately in a later section and in more detail elsewhere in this volume.

Stress represents an internal response and its effects are dependent on individual reactions. Acute responses may include changes in endocrine secretions such as increases in circulating epinephrine and norepinephrine, whereas more long-term responses are reflected in cortisol levels or metabolites of adrenocorticotropic hormone. Sustained stress reactions may lead to a suppression of immune function and the syndrome of underperformance (Gleeson *et al.* 1997; Halson *et al.* 2003).

Various methods have been proposed to counter the adverse effects of stress on performance. These methods include preparing athletes through mental rehearsal prior to encountering stressful events or designing appropriate coping strategies. Stress inoculation techniques, for example, have proved to be effective in optimal mental preparation for activities that induce anxiety (Mace & Carroll 1989).

Alternative strategies are needed to offset fatigue. This concept refers to a reduction in performance in spite of attempts to maintain the level of competitive activity. Fatigue can therefore occur relatively quickly in all-out activities because of inadequate metabolic substrate to sustain peak power output or to the accumulation of metabolites associated with all-out efforts. In prolonged activity a fall in work rate may be attributable to a reduction in muscle glycogen, especially its depletion in some muscle fibers (Bangsbo *et al.* 2006). There may also be a downregulation of exercise intensity as a result of hyperthermia (Reilly *et al.* 2006). The onset of fatigue may be delayed by endurance training, by nutritional strategies that boost glycogen stores prior to exercise, or by a more appropriate pacing strategy for competitive performance (Atkinson *et al.* 2003). Transient fatigue during games may occur after a brief period of repetitive high-intensity efforts and normal capability can be restored when rest periods after such bouts are adequate for full recovery.

Whether fatigue results from a failure of peripheral or central mechanisms is subject to continuing debate. This question has been addressed in some studies (Giacomoni *et al.* 2005) by using twitch-interpolation whereby the fatigued muscle is presented directly with an electrical stimulus. When the electrical stimulation causes an increase in the tension evoked compared with a maximal voluntary effort, this observation is interpreted as evidence of central fatigue.

Mental fatigue is reflected in errors of attention, slowing of choice reactions, and faulty decision making. The conventional approach to examine effects of exercise on cognitive function is to monitor mental performance by administering standard or sports-specific tests during concomitant exercise. This type of protocol has been successful in establishing the effects of exercise intensity on psychomotor and decision-making tasks (Reilly & Smith 1986). Contemporary research techniques permit exploration of the cerebral mechanisms involved in the maintenance of mental performance. Functional magnetic resonance imaging has made it possible to register the amounts of glycogen stored in the brains of individuals who reach volitional fatigue and laser Doppler systems enable researchers to monitor cerebral blood flow changes as fatigue is approached (Dalsgaard 2006). Electroencephalography is another tool that has potential for investigating the phenomena associated with mental fatigue. The dopamine–serotonin neurotransmitter system and its substrates have been implicated in the phenomenon of mental fatigue and circulating prolactin, a posterior pituitary hormone, has been employed as a surrogate measure of serotonergic activity in attempts to highlight the role of this system in fatigue (Low *et al.* 2005). Because cerebral mechanisms regulate the self-chosen exercise intensity in competitive situations, understanding how the various factors initiating and offsetting fatigue are integrated awaits a resolution. Similarly, there is a need for more sensitive measures of mental performance that can be utilized in a practical setting, to complement the laboratory-based work.

Safety

An appreciable amount of research effort has been put into the calculation of risk in sport in order to quantify the likelihood of injury occurring to participants. These studies have been based on epidemiologic designs; typically causes of injury have been attributed to intrinsic and extrinsic factors, and preventive measures recommended where possible. Depending on the sport, these recommendations are directed towards using or improving protective equipment, improving fitness of the participants, isolating the hazards to the individual, and identifying the rule changes that might reduce risk. Redesigning the stadium lay-out has been suggested in some cases (Fuller & Drawer 2004) but formal risk assessment, as is obligatory in most industrialized settings, is only rarely utilized.

Injuries occur last in a change of events and are mostly the result of accidents. Assuming accidents are unplanned events, these arise from human error and so concentrating on the precursors of error is a potential means of preventing or reducing injuries. The "critical incident technique" has been applied to the study of safety in air flight and vehicular traffic by focusing on events in which an accident almost occurred. Jones *et al.* (1999) stated that a near-miss should be treated as an important warning that an accident may occur and that an internal investigation of near-misses should be an integral part of a safety management system. They found an inverse relationship between the number of reported near-misses and the incidence of accidents. These observations suggest that an awareness of safety can help reduce the number of accidents likely to cause injury.

Rahnama *et al.* (2002) applied a critical incident technique to study injury risk in soccer. Key incidents were monitored by means of a computerized notation analysis system with respect to the degree of injury potential (Fig. 15.3), location on the pitch, home and away, and other factors. Altogether about 18 000 playing actions were analyzed, and players were found to be most at risk when being tackled or charged, or when making a tackle. The risk was highest during the first and the last 15 min of the game, reflecting the intense contest for possession in the opening period and the possible effect of fatigue towards the end of the match. It was recommended that trainers and coaches as well as medical support staff should take the trends observed into consideration when preparing their players for action.

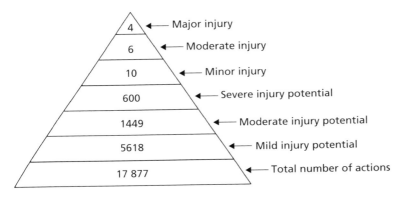

Fig. 15.3 Categories of injury potential for playing actions during soccer. From Rahnama *et al.* (2002). Reproduced with permission from the BMJ Publishing Group.

The risk inherent in sport may itself be an attraction for some participants, especially in the winter sports such as ski-jumping and the sliding events (bobsleigh and skeleton). The thrill of adventure activities such as parachuting and "extreme sports" may lie in the experience of risk exposure and overcoming it. In an effort to understand the paradox of simultaneously experiencing anxiety and exhilaration, Reilly *et al.* (1985) studied participants in a high-acceleration ride in a leisure park. Heart rate varied among individuals from 150 to 186 beats·min^{-1} while stationary during the 95-s ride, changes being associated with abrupt alterations in G forces and body orientation as the car being ridden went through spiral and helical sections of the electromechanical track. Epinephrine and norepinephrine concentrations were more highly correlated with anxiety than with feelings of thrill. Habituation to the experience was demonstrated by an average fall of 15 beats·min^{-1} when the ride was repeated, an adaptation likely to occur in those seeking excitement in such activities and in sports with high elements of risk.

Participation in high-risk activities, in training or competition, raises ethical issues for organizers of events and for mentors of participants. Risk is accepted in mountain sports including those of the Winter Olympics, in human-machine sports, and in quests for World Records or endurance achievements. McCrory (2003) described the case of an assisted "free" diver who died in an attempt to extend her newly acquired World Record of 171 m depth. Such endeavors are documented in other adventure sports but will not deter those who challenge to reach new heights or depths.

In sports where risk is deemed to be within acceptable limits, injury may occur as a result of intrinsic or extrinsic factors. Intrinsic factors might include poor joint flexibility, lack of musculoskeletal strength, biomechanical deficiencies in gait, and poor technique. Asymmetrical physical development is often implicated, either as differences between left and right sides of the body or an inappropriate flexor : extensor ratio. An example of the latter is where the quadriceps muscle group is trained to the exclusion of the hamstrings which then become liable to injury, especially during an enforced eccentric muscle action. For this reason, the dynamic control ratio, in which the peak eccentric torque of the hamstrings is expressed relative to the peak concentric torque of the quadriceps, is considered to be the most appropriate index of muscle balance.

Extrinsic factors associated with sports injuries include unintentional contact with opposing competitors, surface characteristics, and weather conditions. Clothing and equipment offer a measure of protection to participants, as for example the apparel and protective equipment worn by American footballers. In such cases, clothing and helmets must fit the user to be effective. Protective features may be designed into sports equipment on a user-centered philosophy, the safe release bindings on skis and ski boots being determined according to the mass of the individual.

Equipment design

Equipment is used in sport as an integral part of the challenge provided to players and performers (such as the ball in football, the stick in hockey, or the racket in tennis), to enhance performance (such as the "aero frame" cycle in cycling, the driver in golf, or the swimsuit in swimming) and to enhance safety (such as the helmet in horse riding, the shoulder pads in football, or the arm guard in archery). Where equipment is an essential part of play, the design principles that have governed its evolution have generally been related to functionality (including comfort), performance, and safety. Evolution of equipment has been restricted by the rules of the game. Economic considerations also determine the extent to which highly evolved equipment is available to players across a wide ability range.

It is essential that sports equipment is functional if players are to enjoy their sport and develop the skills necessary to compete at high levels. Physical size and strength differences between population groups have influenced equipment design, enabling it to be fit for purpose. For example, while it has always been possible to purchase sports shoes designed specifically for children, it is now quite common to be able to find sports shoes that are fabricated exclusively for females. There are also ethnic differences in foot shape that have been reflected in the manufacture of footwear for different ethnic groups. Sports equipment sized to the individual is common in sports such as golf, tennis, cycling, and soccer as well as for generic equipment such as headgear and footwear. In these sports, manufacturers have relied on anthropometric databases that use one or more of segment lengths, girths, joint mobility, reach, strength, handedness, and comfortable exertion to design their products. For high-level performance it is more normal to "custom fit" equipment to suit the requirements of the player and, sometimes, the sponsor. Skill development can be influenced by equipment design. In tennis, children learn through "short tennis" (Coldwells & Hare 1994), which goes further than just scaling down the traditional tennis racket and ball, by creating a shorter larger headed racket and softer, slower ball so that young children gain early success in the hand–eye coordination skills that underpin the adult game. These aids to skill development continue into the adult game, where some years ago the "jumbo" racket evolved with a greater

head size than that of the conventional racket available at the time. The larger hitting area benefited the less skilled player, not only because the hitting area was larger, allowing for a greater margin of error, but the rebound power and directional control of the racket were greater, both features assisting the less skilled player. The rules of the game were subsequently changed to prevent racket heads from becoming any larger than the "jumbo" racket. The rules of tennis have been changed more recently to allow for three different types of ball in professional play. These ball types have different diameters and internal pressures and are characterized by their rebound characteristics. The rationale for their introduction was to slow down performance on fast grass courts and speed it up on slow clay courts in an attempt to make the transition from one surface to the other easier for players, and more enjoyable for spectators. The specific influence of these ball types is a current research topic (Blackwell et al. 2004). Similar developments have occurred in golf where the shaft flexibility has been matched to the length of club and speed of swing of the player so as to retain a consistency in the "feel" players experience as they make a drive.

Comfort is an important consideration for some equipment and this property can be enhanced by design. In running, the shock experienced during heel strike can be reduced by the inclusion of an air cell or other viscoelastic material under the heel of the shoe (Lake 2000). Studded footwear is another good example of where comfort can be affected by the protrusion that studs make into the foot-bed of the shoe. Careful location of the studs, pressure distribution of the studs on the sole, and insole profiling are methods that have been used to minimize the build-up of pressure points in the shoe (Rodano et al. 1988; Lees & Lake 2002).

Performance can be aided by appropriate functionality as described above, but has always been a major design focus in its own right. In racket sports, great attention has been paid, not only to the shape of the racket head, but also to racket head width, cross-sectional profiles, materials for racket, and string construction influencing flexibility and vibrational effects (Cross & Bower 2006). Computer-aided design, following engineering principles, has allowed the performance features of the racket to be enhanced. Modern rackets have a larger "sweet spot" and greater power rebound than their predecessors. Similar developments have occurred in golf, with the larger headed "metal wood" being designed hollow to reduce weight, increase ball impact area, and take advantage of the trampoline effect of the club head impact surface (Farrally *et al.* 2003). These authors have also reported that the golf ball has evolved in design, in order to fly further, by improvements in ball construction methods, materials, and aerodynamic design. Players should be cautious though, as the performance benefits claimed by manufacturers are usually optimistic.

Other "striking" sports have seen similar developments such as the baseball (Penrose & Hose 1999), cricket (Bartlett 2003), and table tennis bats (Major & Lang 2004). High-speed sports, such as cycling, have benefited from ergonomic design to reduce the effects of air resistance. Wind tunnel testing has shown that elliptical shapes possess better air flow properties than circular shapes, an observation now reflected in the frame design of high-performance cycles. The design can also achieve lightness while retaining strength. This principle has been extended to the bicycle wheels of a disc or tri-spoke design to reduce the air drag acting on them (Fig. 15.4). The cycling helmet, principally used for safety, has also evolved an aerodynamic shape to reduce the drag it would otherwise cause. The performance of footwear can similarly be enhanced by careful design. The

soccer boot protects the foot and the studs allow players better traction with the turf surface on which they play. The boot is also the means by which the ball is propelled and the boot can be constructed so as to enhance the player's kicking performance. This is particularly important in situations where spin is applied to the ball to deceive opponents. Ball spin is created by striking the ball obliquely so that the foot moves over the surface of the ball so to enhance the grip between foot and ball some manufacturers have placed high grip surfaces on the toe box and side panels of the boot. This modification enables more spin to be produced which in turn causes the ball, if struck correctly, to deviate in flight so as to deceive opponents.

Safety is also a key issue in the design of sports equipment. The running shoe has been the subject of investigation for many decades and its protective characteristics have dominated any performance characteristics the shoe might have. In most runners, the heel usually makes first contact with the ground and this generates a high rise shock force. This force is transmitted through the skeletal structure and can be the cause of overuse injuries at the lower limb joints and spine. This shock force is minimized by including some shock-absorbing material in the heel of the shoe. Early materials used included ethylene vinyl acetate (EVA) and closed cell polymer which has considerable shock-absorbing properties. This material can be easily manufactured in different densities and thicknesses, but the EVA was found to compress with use (McCullagh & Graham 1985) and so becomes ineffective after a short period of use. Subsequent design evolutions included the use of other viscoelastic materials inserted into the heel space or an air cell; the latter has proven to be particularly effective by combining shock absorption with low weight. The characteristics of the material that allow shock to be absorbed also cause the foot to be unstable and encourage the foot to pronate during mid-stance. The control of rear-foot pronation and construction of various antipronation devices have progressed in concert with the developments in shock absorption. With these design innovations the running shoe has evolved into a sophisticated piece of sports equipment.

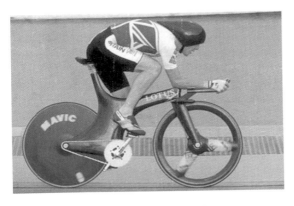

Fig. 15.4 Helmeted cyclist in aerodynamic posture on a purpose designed bicycle.

Helmets are used to protect the head in various high-risk sports. In some of these sports, the helmet has been designed with regard to the nature of risk. For example, in considering design criteria for cycling helmets, the most dangerous type of fall was deemed to be from a collision with a car where the cyclist is thrown to the ground landing on the head. In this type of contact the helmet has to absorb energy so the helmet is made of thick and stiff material (e.g., polystyrene). Some debate has existed regarding the nature of the covering surface. If this is a "soft" material, the helmet can grip the ground causing the head to roll as it makes contact, hyperflexing the neck and potentially causing neck injuries. If the material is "hard," the head will have a tendency to bounce on contact and lead to a second landing on the face, likely causing facial injuries (Swart 1990). Helmets in ice-hockey have different requirements. In this sport the main danger comes from an object (the stick, puck, or blade) penetrating the skull. Consequently, the helmet has a thick rigid exterior to protect from the penetration with an inner liner of medium-density resilient foam. While this helmet can receive multiple blows of moderate intensity and still provide a protective function, the cycling helmet must be discarded after one protective use.

Various examples have been given where ergonomic design principles have been applied to sports equipment. The efficacy of designs needs to be evaluated and this is usually an iterative process against criteria that are based on performance metrics. In many cases these are undertaken through mechanical testing, but in the later stages, and if practical, the usability of equipment is evaluated through "human response" testing. Mechanical testing also provides a means for setting standards, often controlled by national agencies. For cycling helmets for example, the American National Standards Institute (ANSI) requires the peak acceleration on impact on to a flat anvil from 1.5 m to be under 300 g, while the Snell (Snell Memorial Foundation) standard requires the same acceleration limit but when the helmet is dropped from 2 m on to a rounded anvil. While the Snell standard is more difficult to meet than the ANSI standard, it can be appreciated that this is not the type of evaluation that humans would risk taking part in!

Human–computer interaction

Computers have pervaded most aspects of modern life and it is now common to see computers controlling displays that enliven and make more realistic the experience of a sports participant. Perhaps of particular note are the various training devices that monitor performance and give feedback to the participant. This feedback is often in the form of a visual display which can contain other information. A typical example is a "cycle trainer," which is based on a cycle ergometer which can monitor speed and load and change these according to a predefined program. As a part of this system there is a visual display which shows the road the cyclist is on and other information in numerical form on distance travelled, speed, incline, and so on. As the cyclist speeds up, the movement along the road appears to get faster and the background changes to reflect cycling through the countryside. A computer program enables the ergometer to add or subtract load to simulate going up or down hills and the view changes appropriately. Competitors can be programed in so that the cyclist has an opponent to chase, and physiological variables such as heart rate and oxygen uptake can be monitored simultaneously.

Improving the quality of display leads to a more realistic experience and if that display is sufficiently large to fill a person's field of view it is possible to get the experience of being immersed in the environment. If the visual field can be manipulated in response to a person's movements then a virtual reality environment can be created. A virtual reality environment can be very sophisticated but the sensation of reality is based on the quality of display and speed with which movements are detected and simulated environmental responses are noted. Many virtual reality systems are used for familiarizing a person with a new environment or for training movements in a specific context. The system usually uses a head-mounted display and works by recording the position in space of the head and changing the visual display according to the movement of the head. Yeadon and Knight (2006) have developed a system to train gymnasts to pick up visual cues in the environment as they are performing various twisting somersaults. The system was well received by elite gymnasts who rated it helpful, realistic, and useful.

A novel application of virtual reality is from a new device known as CAREN (Barton *et al.* 2006) which is based on a computer-controlled moveable platform within a virtual reality environment. This system records movements of the body (the center of gravity, segment or other point attached to the body using an optoelectronic motion analysis system) and uses this information to drive the visual display and the movement of the platform in six degrees of freedom. Environments can be configured that reflect, for example, the experience of standing on a moving surface such as a bus, boat, or train. A more ambitious reconstruction is the replication of a rollercoaster ride. Developing the scene is time consuming and complex and requires specialist skills, but the result is a more realistic simulation of the environment, and an opportunity to train, habituate, rehabilitate, or monitor individuals and their responses. There is also the opportunity for individuals to engage in computer games whereby their responses are driven by activating specific muscles; in this way muscles that determine "core stability" can be targeted and trained.

Characteristic patterns of movement during games may be observed and used to generate physiological responses in a laboratory setting that correspond to those in competition. Drust *et al.* (2000) described how match-play characteristics in soccer could be designed into software that controlled exercise protocols on a motor-driven treadmill in order to facilitate experimental work relevant to the game. Despite the correspondence of physiological responses, ecologic validity is limited by the absence of game skills, a partisan audience, and the competitive context.

In an earlier publication by Lees (1985), the increasing impact of computers within sport was acknowledged. Computers are now recognized as an integral part of contemporary lifestyle, and are pervasive within sport and leisure. Their applications extend throughout the domains of sport from Internet access to sports news to the design of optimal strategies for success in competition. Computer-led feedback on performance is presented after the event in a user-friendly mode and with attractive displays. This form may be a highly selective DVD, the content being designed for the team coach or individual athletes. Without this expert selective screening, the amount of data available might be bewildering rather than helpful to practitioners.

Engineering the environment

The environment in which individuals train and compete may impose extra demands on sports participants. Environmental stressors include heat and cold, altitude and hyperbaric pressure, noise, and air pollution. Air conditioning provides thermal comfort for individuals in indoor arenas, although the humidity in swimming pools is not ideal for spectators and swimmers alike at the same time. Athletes may transfer quickly between entirely different environments and climates, encountering the disturbances associated with multiple time-zone transitions. While specific environments are considered in detail elsewhere in this volume, the present emphasis is on designing methods and strategies for monitoring and aiding coping mechanisms.

Ambient temperature is measured with a dry-bulb thermometer but wet-bulb temperature is especially relevant when exercise is undertaken in conditions of high relative humidity. Both measures are combined in guidelines for coping with likely heat stress levels encountered in outdoor sports. Globe temperature indicates the prevailing radiant heat load and is incorporated in the wet bulb and globe temperature (WBGT) index (Reilly & Waterhouse 2005). The cooling effect of air is dependent on the velocity of flow over the body's surface and cloud cover can also reduce heat load when exercising outdoors.

Tolerance to heat can be improved by means of acclimatization. This process is most effective when exercise is conducted in hot conditions that raise body temperature and activate sweating mechanisms. Physiological adaptation leads to an expansion of plasma volume, an elevation of the core temperature at which hyperthermic fatigue occurs (Patterson *et al.* 2004), a reduction in core temperature at a fixed submaximal exercise, a more effective distribution of blood for peripheral cooling, and hypertrophy of sweat glands. The eccrine glands also become more responsive to a rise in internal temperature and are activated at a lower threshold than before acclimatization. These adaptations may be secured by exercising in an environmental chamber where heat and humidity may be controlled, and some measure of adaptation occurs when extra "sweat clothing" is worn during training (Dawson *et al.* 1989). Physiological adaptation to heat can be achieved relatively quickly, the major adjustments being complete with 10–14 days of initial exposure.

Acute exercise performance in the heat can be improved by pre-cooling the body prior to starting. This alteration can be realized by wearing iced jackets, cooling vests, or partial immersion in iced water. Cooling core temperature by about 0.6°C has been shown to delay the subsequent rise to a fixed level and to improve performance (Reilly *et al.* 2006). The cooling maneuver does not negate the need for conducting warm-up practices. Cooling methods can also be employed in sports with half-time intermissions, combined with strategies to replace fluid lost through sweating. Hand cooling may also have value in reducing whole-body temperature, especially in locomotor sports where the lower limb muscles are actively engaged (Grahn *et al.* 2005). The various factors by which pre-cooling increases the capability to tolerate heat stress are included in Fig. 15.5 (Reilly *et al.* 2006).

The opposite scenario applies to cold conditions when the emphasis is placed on avoidance of undue heat loss. Clothing technology has advanced to provide wind- and wet-proof characteristics and layered clothing ensembles that protect the microclimate next to the skin's surface. The wind-chill index (Siple & Passel 1945) has been adopted to

indicate indirectly the risk of hyperthermia in cold weather and is used in many outdoor activities in winter months. Weather conditions can change abruptly in wilderness environments and changes in behavior can also lead to rapid loss of heat from the body. Ainslie and Reilly (2003) reported an alteration in body temperature towards hypothermia when hill-walkers rested outdoors for lunch during their activities. A behavioral strategy to deal with cold protection should include appropriate clothing with good insulative properties and taking shelter when necessary. Gloves and headware safeguard against excessive heat loss through these routes and can prevent errors and potential accidents by preserving thermal comfort and manual dexterity.

The mountainous environment provides additional extraneous stresses on those who use it for sport, training, or leisure purposes. Treacherous weather conditions accentuate the difficulties of coping with the reduced partial pressure of oxygen in inspired air that is associated with altitude. The prevailing hypoxia causes performance to be impaired, and this effect becomes more apparent with increasing altitude above 2000 m. In order to prepare for competition at altitude, athletes benefit from prior acclimatization. This procedure improves physiological responses to exercise at altitude but those dwelling at sea level are still at a disadvantage compared to natives.

A relatively novel development has been the introduction of altitude simulators to provide a physiological adaptation that would benefit performance at sea level. The oxygen content of ambient air may be reduced by partially replacing oxygen with nitrogen, while keeping the ambient air pressure constant. Athletes who train in normobaric hypoxia for 2–3 sessions per week may gain benefit without necessarily achieving the elevations in red blood cells stimulated by erythropoietin that are found when athletes have a prolonged stay at altitude. Dufour *et al.* (2006) showed that training at a high intensity for 40 min twice a week at a simulated altitude (inspired O_2 fraction: 14.5%) was successful in raising $\dot{V}O_{2max}$ by 6%. The improvement was linked to changes in muscle mitochondrial activity that more tightly integrated the fuel supply and demand at cellular level. In use of normobaric hypoxia, the

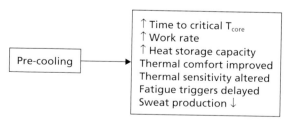

$\uparrow$ Time to critical T_{core}
$\uparrow$ Work rate
$\uparrow$ Heat storage capacity
Thermal comfort improved
Thermal sensitivity altered
Fatigue triggers delayed
Sweat production $\downarrow$

Pre-cooling

Fig. 15.5 The proposed mechanisms for the effectiveness of pre-cooling.

athlete can train periodically in conditions that simulate medium to high altitude while sleeping at sea level. An alternative ploy is to use altitude huts for sleeping to stimulate renal production of erythropoietin, in accordance with the "live high, train low" philosophy proposed by Levine (1995).

Noise and environmental pollution can challenge both the health and the performance of athletes during training and competition. Noise can have emotional as well as physical effects, depending on its characteristics. Crowd noise can influence the motivation of participants or antagonize them; music can engage individuals when exercising or preparing mentally for competition, or become an irritant to others. External noise can hinder sleep, while impact or sustained intermittent noise can cause auditory threshold shifts that may be temporary or become permanent.

Sports such as shooting expose participants to risk of hearing damage. In motor racing, technicians and spectators may also be subject to high noise levels. The addition of noise in do-it-yourself activities or listening to highly amplified music may take the noise dose to a damaging level. The range of sport and recreational activities where high decibel levels are experienced has been outlined by Reilly and Waterhouse (2005). Remedial behavior takes the form of noise reduction by use of appropriate protective devices. It is important that ear protectors are fit for purpose and produce attenuation of noise levels to below risk thresholds.

The quality of environmental air is also a factor in optimizing the environment for exercise performance. Major tournaments have been held in cities with high levels of pollution which were a source of concern to participants in advance of the competition but were not as extreme as feared. Pollutants can also affect training responses and cause discomfort to susceptible individuals. These include asthmatics, those prone to allergies, and those with pulmonary defects. The main primary pollutants outdoors include sulfur dioxide, carbon monoxide, nitrogen oxides, benzene, particulate matter (PM-10s); secondary pollutants include ozone and peroxyacetyl nitrate. Their effects and countermeasures have been reviewed elsewhere (Florida-James et al. 2004; Reilly & Waterhouse 2005). Pollution can also occur in indoor environments (e.g., as a result of cleansing agents in ice rinks).

Traveling athletes may be exposed to variations in climatic features when going overseas to attend training camps or take part in competition. Such long-haul flights are now commonplace among professional athletes. Those traveling from north to south or in the reverse direction experience travel fatigue and seasonal variations in climate. Travel fatigue is easily overcome; for example, with a shower or a good night's sleep. Those traveling across multiple time zones are subject to disruption of the circadian body clock and experience the syndrome known as jet-lag. Its symptoms include disorientation, difficulties in sleeping at the correct time, digestive disturbances, and a general feeling of being below par.

Jet-lag is caused by a desynchronization of circadian rhythms as the body clock is out of harmony with local time. The body clock adjusts slowly to the new environment, the main external signal facilitating the adjustment being natural daylight. While commercial "light boxes" have been effective in alleviating jet-leg symptoms, the more appropriate strategy is to seek out and avoid natural light at the appropriate times. These times are determined by the phase–response curve to light and have been listed for different directions of travel and time zones crossed (Reilly et al. 2005).

In its position statement on sleeping pills and chronobiotic drugs, the British Olympic Association advocated a behavioral strategy rather than drugs to accelerate adjustment to the new time zone (Reilly et al. 1998). Exercise can be effective after traveling westwards but morning exercise after traveling eastwards should be avoided for the first few days; the combination of exercise and light could promote a delay rather than the required advance of the body clock, in accordance with the phase–response curve to light. Drugs such as melatonin (Arendt 1992) and temazepam have been advocated, but for long-haul flights the phase–response curve of melatonin – which is opposite to that of light – makes its proper timing difficult to administer. The lag in adjusting to the new time zone should be taken into account when planning the itineraries of athletes competing overseas.

While isolation units may be employed to simulate time zone transitions, their uses are limited to research rather than practical applications. It is possible to protect traveling teams against circadian desynchronization by adhering to sleep–wake cycles of the home location just deserted. This strategy is only effective if travel is across no more than 2–3 meridians, the visit is for no longer than 2 days, and competition is not too late in the evening after the downturn of the circadian curve in body temperature (Reilly *et al.* 2005). Similarly, sports participants may be protected from inclement weather in roofed stadia. An impressive novel feature of the FIFA World Cup venue in Sapporo in 2002 (replicated in Germany, 2006) was that the entire playing surface was placed on a hydraulic bed that could be moved into the interior of the stadium hours before the appointed start time. This adaptability of the current generation of sports arenas means that their designs can accommodate different sports and crowd sizes while a common infrastructure for spectator comfort can be maintained. This facility can also assist in maintaining the integrity of the playing surface by exposing it to natural conditions in between the periods it is in place within the roofed stadium.

Future scenarios

The systemization of support mechanisms for enhancement of sports performance is likely to continue into the future. At elite level of performance, athletes will endeavor to stretch their capabilities to their limits and extend those limits by optimizing their training programs. The monitoring of physiological responses by means of miniaturized recording devices and movement and navigational information by means of global positioning systems yield layers of feedback to participants about their training and competitive targets. As feedback from performance analysis, training responses, and fitness assessments becomes ever more refined, the uncertainties about ultimate ceilings of achievement are reduced. The result is likely to be a greater consistency of performance level among the top performers. Another outcome may be a greater match between training input and physiological response so that injuries brought about by training error or accumulated overload are decreased.

In view of the range of individual differences that exist, there is still opportunity for designing sports equipment and apparel to suit the participant, especially where special populations are concerned. This process may engage multivariate accommodation rather than design for all, using sophisticated anthropometric databases to cover a range of sizes and ability levels. The greatest developments are likely in human-machine sports by utilizing computer-aided designs alongside formative and summative evaluations of existing equipment. While comfort and efficiency may be promoted as a result, the human urge to break through perceived and accepted boundaries means that risk is an inevitable part of human endeavor, especially in high-performance sports.

References

Ainslie, P.N. & Reilly, T. (2003) Physiology of accidental hypothermia in the mountains: a forgotten story. *British Journal of Sports Medicine* **37**, 548–550.

Arendt, J. (1992) The pineal. In: *Biological Rhythms in Clinical and Laboratory Medicine* (Touitou, Y. & Haus, E., eds.) Springer, Berlin: 348–362.

Atha, J. (1984) Current techniques for measuring motion. *Applied Ergonomics* **15**, 245–257.

Atkinson, G. & Reilly, T. (1995) *Sport, Leisure and Ergonomics*. E. & F.N. Spon, London.

Atkinson, G., Davison, R., Jeukendrup, A. & Passfield, L. (2003) Science and cycling: current knowledge and future directions for research. *Journal of Sports Sciences* **21**, 767–787.

Baltzopoulas, V. & Gleeson, N.P. (2003) Skeletal muscle function. In: *Kinanthropometry and Exercise Physiology Laboratory Manual: Tests, Procedures and Data*, Vol. 2 (Eston, R. & Reilly, T., eds.) 2nd edn. Routledge, London: 7–35.

Bangsbo, J. (1994) The physiology of soccer: with special reference to intense intermittent exercise. *Acta Physiologica Scandinavica* **151** (Supplement 619), 1–155.

Bangsbo, J., Mohr, M. & Krustrup, P. (2006) Physical and metabolic demands of training and match-play. *Journal of Sports Sciences* **24**, 665–674.

Bartlett, R. (2003) The science and medicine of cricket: an overview and update. *Journal of Sports Sciences* **21**, 733–752.

Barton, G., Vanrenterghem, J., Lees, A. & Lake, M. (2006) A method for manipulating a moveable platform's axes of rotation: A novel use of the CAREN system. *Gait and Posture* **24**, 510–514.

Blackwell, J.R., Heath, E.M. & Thompson, C.J. (2004) Effect of the Type 3 (oversize, slow speed) tennis ball on heart rate, activity level and shots per point during tennis play. In: *Science and Racket Sports*

Vol. III (Lees, A., Kahn, J.F. & Maynard, I., eds.) Routledge, London: 37–42.

Buzeck, F.L. & Cavanagh, P.R. (1990) Stance phase knee and ankle kinematics and kinetics during level and downhill running. *Medicine and Science in Sports and Exercise* **22**, 669–677.

Cavanagh, P.R. & Lafortune, M.A. (1980) Ground reaction forces in distance running. *Journal of Biomechanics* **13**, 397–406.

Clarys, J. (1985) Hydrodynamics and electromyography: ergonomic aspects in aquatics. *Applied Ergonomics* **16**, 11–24.

Clarys, J.P. & Cabri, J. (1993) Electromyography and the study of sports movements: A review. *Journal of Sports Sciences* **11**, 379–448.

Coldwells, A. & Hare, M.E. (1994) The transfer of skill from short tennis to lawn tennis. *Ergonomics* **37**, 17–22.

Cross, R. & Bower, R. (2006) Effects of swing weight on swing speed and racket power. *Journal of Sports Sciences* **24**, 23–30.

Dalsgaard, M.K. (2006) Fuelling cerebral activity in exercising man. *Journal of Cerebral Blood Flow and Metabolism* **26**, 731–750.

Davids, K., Smith, L. & Martin, R. (1991) Controlling system uncertainty in sport and work. *Applied Ergonomics* **22**, 312–315.

Dawson, B., Pyke, F.S. & Morton, A.R. (1989) Improvements in heat tolerance induced by interval running training in the heat and in sweat clothing in cool conditions. *Journal of Sports Sciences* **7**, 189–203.

Drust, B., Reilly, T. & Cable, N.T. (2000) Physiological responses to laboratory-based soccer-specific intermittent and continuous exercise. *Journal of Sports Sciences* **18**, 885–892.

Dufour, S.P., Ponsot, E., Joffrey, Z., *et al.* (2006) Exercise training in normobaric hypoxia in endurance runners. I. Improvement in aerobic performance capacity. *Journal of Applied Physiology* **100**, 1238–1248.

Farrally, M.R., Cochran, A.J., Crews, D.J., *et al.* (2003) Golf science research at the beginning of the twenty-first century. *Journal of Sports Sciences* **21**, 753–765.

Florida-James, G., Donaldson, K. & Stone, V. (2004) Athens 2004: the pollution climate and athletic performance. *Journal of Sports Sciences* **22**, 967–980.

Fuller, C.W. & Drawer, S.D. (2004) The application of risk management in sport. *Sports Medicine* **34**, 349–356.

Geil, M.D. (2002) The role of footwear on kinematics and plantar foot pressure in fencing. *Journal of Applied Biomechanics* **18**, 155–162.

Giacomoni, M., Edwards, B. & Bambaeichi, E. (2005) Gender differences in the circadian variation in muscle strength assessed with and without superimposed electrical twitches. *Ergonomics* **48**, 1473–1487.

Gleeson, M., Blannin, A. & Walsh, N.P. (1997) Overtraining, immunosuppression, exercise-induced muscle damage and anti-inflammatory drugs. In: *The Clinical Pharmacology of Sport and Exercise* (Reilly, T. & Orme M., eds.) Elsevier, Amsterdam: 47–57.

Grahn, D.A., Cao, V.H. & Heller, C. (2005) Heat extraction through the palm of one hand improves aerobic endurance in a hot environment. *Journal of Applied Physiology* **99**, 972–978.

Halson, S.L., Lancaster, G.I., Jeukendrup, A. & Gleeson, M. (2003). Immunological responses to overreaching in cyclists. *Medicine and Science in Sports and Exercise* **35**, 854–861.

Hay, J.G. (1992) The biomechanics of the triple jump: A review. *Journal of Sports Sciences* **10**, 343–378.

Horita, T., Komi, P.V., Nicol, C. & Kyrolainen, H. (2002) Interaction between pre-landing activities and stiffness regulation of the knee joint musculoskeletal system in the drop jump: implications to performance. *European Journal of Applied Physiology* **88**, 76–84.

Iga, J., Reilly, T., Lees, A. & George, K. (2005) Bilateral isokinetic knee strength profiles in trained junior soccer players and untrained individuals. In: *Science and Football*, Vol. V (Reilly, T., Cabri, J. & Araujo, D., eds.) Routledge, London: 442–447.

Jones, S., Kirchsteiger, C. & Bjerke, W. (1999) The importance of near miss reporting to further improve safety performance. *Journal of Loss Prevention in the Process Industries* **12**, 59–67.

Kawakami, Y., Nozaki, D., Matsuo, A. & Fukunaga, T. (1992) Reliability of measurement of oxygen uptake by a portable telemetric system. *European Journal of Applied Physiology* **65**, 409–414.

Kyrolainen, H., Avela, J. & Komi, P. (2005) Changes in muscle activity with increasing running speed. *Journal of Sports Sciences* **23**, 1101–1109.

Lake, M. (2000) Determining the protective function of sports footwear. *Ergonomics* **43**, 1610–1621.

Lees, A. (1985). Computers in sport. *Applied Ergonomics* **16**, 3–10.

Lees, A. & Lake, M. (2002) Biomechanics of soccer surfaces and equipment. In: *Science and Soccer*, 2nd edn. (Reilly, T., ed.) E. & F.N. Spon, London: 135–150.

Lees, A., Vanrenterghem, J. & de Clercq, D. (2004) Understanding how an arm swing enhances performance in the vertical jump. *Journal of Biomechanics* **37**, 1929–1940.

Levine, B. (1995) Training and exercise at high altitudes. In: *Sport, Leisure and Ergonomics* (Atkinson, G. & Reilly, T., eds.) E. & E.F. Spon, London: 74–92.

Low, D., Purvis, A., Reilly, T. & Cable, N.T. (2005) Prolactin responses to active and passive heating in man. *Experimental Physiology* **90**, 909–917.

Mace, R.D. & Carroll, D. (1989) The effect of stress inoculation training on self-reported stress, observer's rating of stress, heart rate and gymnastics. *Journal of Sports Sciences* **7**, 257–266.

Major, Z. & Lang, R.W. (2004) Characterization of table tennis racket sandwich rubbers. In: *Science and Racket Sports*, Vol. III (Lees, A., Kahn, J.-F. & Maynard, I., eds.) Routledge, London: 146–152.

McCrory, P. (2003) The big blue. *British Journal of Sports Medicine* **37**, 1.

McCullagh, P.J.J. & Graham, I.D. (1985) A preliminary investigation into the nature of shock absorption in synthetic sports materials. *Journal of Sports Sciences* **3**, 103–114.

Morris, A.D., Kemp, G.J., Lees, A. & Frostick, S.P. (1998) A study of the reproducibility of three different normalisation methods in intra-muscular dual fine wire electromyography of the shoulder. *Journal of Electromyography and Kinesiology* **8**, 317–322.

Patterson, M.J., Stock, J.M. & Taylor, N.A. (2004). Sustained and generalized extracellular fluid expansion following heat acclimation. *Journal of Physiology* **559**, 327–334.

Penrose, J.M.T. & Hose, D.R. (1999) An impact analysis of a flexible bat using an iterative solver. *Journal of Sports Sciences* **17**, 677–682.

Rahnama, N., Lees, A. & Reilly, T. (2006) Electromyography of selected lower-limb muscles fatigued by exercise at the intensity of soccer match-play. *Journal of Electromyography and Kinesiology* **16**, 257–263.

Rahnama, N., Reilly, T. & Lees, A. (2002) Injury risk associated with playing actions during competitive soccer. *British Journal of Sports Medicine* **36**, 354–359.

Rahnama, N., Reilly, T., Lees, A. & Graham-Smith, P. (2003) A comparison of musculoskeletal function in elite and sub-elite English soccer players. In: *Kinanthropometry*, Vol. VIII (Reilly, T. & Marfell-Jones, M., eds.) Routledge, London: 155–164.

Reilly, T. (1984) Ergonomics in sport: an overview. *Applied Ergonomics* **15**, 243.

Reilly, T. (1991) Ergonomics and sport. *Applied Ergonomics* **22**, 290.

Reilly, T. (2001) Assessment of performance in team sports. In: *Kinanthropometry and Exercise Physiology Laboratory Manual: Tests, Procedures and Data*, Vol. 1 (Eston, R. & Reilly, T., eds.) Routledge, London: 171–182.

Reilly, T. & Doran, D. (2003) Fitness assessment. In: *Science and Soccer* (Reilly, T. & Williams, A.M., eds.) Routledge, London: 21–46.

Reilly, T. & Greeves, J. (2002) *Advances in Sport, Leisure and Ergonomics*. Routledge, London.

Reilly, T. & Smith, D. (1986) Effect of work intensity on performance of a psychomotor task during exercise. *Ergonomics* **29**, 601–606.

Reilly, T. & Waterhouse, J. (2005). *Sport, Exercise and Environmental Physiology*. Elsevier, Edinburgh.

Reilly, T., Drust, B. & Gregson, W. (2006) Thermoregulation in elite athletes. *Current Opinions in Clinical Nutrition* **9**, 666–671.

Reilly, T., Maughan, R. & Budgett, R. (1998) Melatonin: a position statement of the British Olympic Association. *British Journal of Sports Medicine* **32**, 99–100.

Reilly, T., Waterhouse, J. & Edwards, B. (2005) Jet lag and air travel: implications for performance. *Clinics in Sports Medicine* **24**, 367–380.

Reilly, T., Lees, A., MacLaren, D. & Sanderson, F.H. (1985) Thrill and anxiety in adventure leisure parks. In: *Contemporary Ergonomics* (Oborne, D.J., ed.) Taylor & Francis, London: 210–214.

Reilly, T., Williams, A.M., Nevill, A. & Franks, A.M. (2000) A multidisciplinary approach to talent identification in soccer. *Journal of Sports Sciences* **18**, 695–702.

Robinson, M., Lees, A. & Barton, G. (2005) An electromyographic investigation of abdominal exercises and the effects of fatigue. *Ergonomics* **48**, 1604–1612.

Rodano, R., Cova, P. & Vigano, R. (1988) Designing a football boot: a theoretical and experimental approach. In: *Science and Football* (Reilly, T., Lees, A., Davids, K. & Murphy, W.J., eds.) E. & F.N. Spon, London: 416–425.

Sassi, R., Reilly, T. & Impellizeri, F. (2005) A comparison of small-sided games and interval training in elite professional soccer players. In: *Science and Football V* (Reilly, T., Cabri, J. & Araujo, D., eds.) Routledge, London: 341–343.

Siple, P.A. & Passel, C.F. (1945) Measurement of dry atmosphere cooling in sub-freezing temperatures. *Proceedings of the American Philosophic Society* **89**, 177–199.

Svensson, M. & Drust, B. (2005) Testing soccer players. *Journal of Sports Sciences* **23**, 601–618.

Swart, R. (1990) Soft shell versus hard shell helmets. *Cycling Science* **Dec**, 13–16.

Wheeler, J.B., Gregor, R.J. & Broker, J.P. (1992) A duel piezoelectric bicylcle pedal with multipleshoe/pedal interface capability. *International Journal of Sport Biomechanics* **8**, 251–258.

Yeadon, M.R. & Knight, J.P. (2006). Interactive viewing of simulated aerial movements. Proceedings of XVII International Symposium on Biomechanics in Sports, Saltzburg, July 14–18: 438–441.

Part 7

Psychology

Chapter 16

Exercise and Psychological Well-being

PANTELEIMON EKKEKAKIS AND SUSAN H. BACKHOUSE

Although anecdotal reports praising the benefits of exercise not only for the soma but also for the psyche date back to antiquity, the systematic investigation of these effects began no earlier than the 1960s. Particularly in the last decade or so, this research area has witnessed explosive growth, spurred by several factors. First, there has been an overall increase of interest in health-oriented exercise, culminating in the promotion of exercise being one of the cardinal objectives of public health efforts in many industrialized countries. The Surgeon General in the USA and the Chief Medical Officer in the UK published landmark documents outlining the health benefits of exercise, including its psychological benefits. Second, the notion that health is not merely the absence of disease but rather the lifelong active pursuit of a holistic sense of well-being went from a fringe "new age" idea to a widely accepted guiding principle for health professionals. This is evidenced in the development and maturation of such scientific areas as behavioral and preventive medicine. Third, the high-pressure conditions of modern living have led to an increase in the number of individuals suffering from mental health problems such as anxiety and depression. The high cost and side effects of traditional forms of therapy (i.e., pharmacotherapy and psychotherapy) have left researchers, mental health professionals, and patients seeking effective and well-tolerated methods not only of treatment but also of prevention. These conditions have created

a fertile ground for the development of the field of "exercise psychology," the scientific discipline concerned with investigating the psychological effects of exercise, as well as the psychological factors that underlie the processes of engaging in, adhering to, and disengaging from regular exercise participation.

The purpose of this chapter is to provide an overview of what exercise psychology research has uncovered about the benefits of exercise for psychological well-being. This survey will span various aspects of well-being, reflecting both the breadth of this concept and the diverse research foci that have emerged within exercise psychology. In discussing the evidence, it is important, rather than portraying exercise as a universally accepted panacea, to acknowledge that not everyone finds the evidence compelling. In fact, whether exercise can truly benefit some aspects of well-being continues to be viewed as an open, if not controversial, question. Even reviewers who have endorsed exercise have pointed out that, in many cases, statements about the psychological benefits of exercise seem to "anticipate rather than reflect the accumulation of strong evidence" (Salmon 2001). An insurmountable stumbling block is the fact that there can be no placebo exercise intervention. Therefore, the element of expectancy, which can be very influential, particularly considering that most well-being-related outcomes are self-reported (in the form of questionnaires or interviews), cannot be fully controlled. In this sense, the methodological rigor of exercise trials, although greatly improved over the years, cannot satisfy the most stringent of criteria, such as those established for evaluating the effectiveness of prescription drugs.

The Olympic Textbook of Science in Sport, 1st edition. Edited by R.J. Maughan. Published 2009 by Blackwell Publishing. ISBN: 978-1-4051-5638-7.

This problem has led to the phenomenon of different authors examining the same literature and reaching different conclusions. In the early 1980s, based on the few preliminary studies that were available at the time, Morgan (1981) asserted that "the 'feeling better' sensation that accompanies regular physical activity is so obvious that it is one of the few universally accepted benefits of exercise." However, examining this literature at approximately the same time, Hughes (1984) concluded that "the enthusiastic support of exercise to improve mental health has a limited empirical basis and lacks a well-tested rationale." Although the amount of evidence increased and the quality improved, the disagreement among reviewers continues. Following a systematic and in-depth review of the evidence on the effects of exercise on depression, Biddle *et al.* (2001) stated that "overall, the evidence is strong enough for us to conclude that there is support for a causal link between physical activity and reduced clinically defined depression. This is the first time such a statement has been made." At the same time, Lawlor and Hopker (2001), based on a meta-analysis on the same topic, concluded that "the effectiveness of exercise in reducing symptoms of depression cannot be determined because of a lack of good quality research on clinical populations with adequate follow up."

Interestingly, conflicting messages can also be found in official documents, even from the same source. In 1996, the report of the Surgeon General of the USA on the relationship between physical activity and health included the following statement:

> The literature suggests that physical activity helps improve the mental health of both clinical and nonclinical populations. Physical activity interventions have benefitted persons from the general population who report mood disturbance, including symptoms of anxiety and depression, as well as patients who have been diagnosed with nonbipolar, nonpsychotic depression. These findings are supported by a limited number of intervention studies conducted in community and laboratory settings . . . The psychological benefits of regular physical activity for persons who have relatively good physical and mental health are less clear (US Department of Health and Human Services 1996).

However, in 1999, the 458-page report of the Surgeon General on mental health did not mention physical activity among the recognized methods of treatment for anxiety and depression, focusing instead on psychotherapy and pharmacotherapy. Physical activity was only mentioned as one of an "ever-expanding list" of "informal" interventions for coping with stressful life events, alongside "religious and spiritual endeavors" and "complementary healers" (US Department of Health and Human Services 1999). Some possible benefits were acknowledged, echoing the earlier report, but this was followed by the caveat of poor methodological quality:

> Physical activities are a means to enhance somatic health as well as to deal with stress. A recent Surgeon General's Report on Physical Activity and Health evaluated the evidence for physical activities serving to enhance mental health. Aerobic physical activities, such as brisk walking and running, were found to improve mental health for people who report symptoms of anxiety and depression and for those who are diagnosed with some forms of depression. The mental health benefits of physical activity for individuals in relatively good physical and mental health were not as evident, but the studies did not have sufficient rigor from which to draw unequivocal conclusions (US Department of Health and Human Services 1999).

Although a certain dose of disciplinary bias on both sides cannot be ruled out as a possible explanation for these discrepant assessments, a balanced evaluation of the literature would probably lead to the conclusion that, although the extant evidence is promising, there are simply not enough high-quality and large-scale randomized clinical trials of exercise to justify definitive statements about the effects of exercise on most aspects of well-being (Brosse *et al.* 2002). Therefore, perhaps the most appropriate approach at the present juncture is one characterized by careful, cautious, critical, and systematic review of the evidence. Although all scientists strive for objectivity, deciding whether a piece of evidence can be deemed compelling or not has an inherent element of subjectivity that can occasionally blur the line between strict impartiality and advocacy for the presumed good cause of promoting physical activity.

In this review, we focus on anxiety, depression, mood and affect, health-related quality of life, cognitive function, and self-esteem. Because of space limitations, this cannot be an exhaustive list. The research literature also contains interesting studies on the role of physical activity in a wide range of additional parameters of well-being, including sleep (Youngstedt & Freelove-Charton 2005), stress reactivity (Sothmann 2006), and relief from addictions (Donaghy & Ussher 2005). Also because of space constraints, in this broad-scope overview of the field, we focus on meta-analyses and recent systematic reviews of the literature.

Anxiety

Construct description

Anxiety is the negative emotional state that results from the cognitive appraisal of a situation as threatening. This cognitive appraisal, which is considered its essential eliciting mechanism, mainly involves the comparison of two subjectively estimated quantities: the degree of threat (to one's physical self, interpersonal status, or goals) that the situation poses and the capabilities or coping resources of the individual. This is a quintessentially subjective process that is under the influence of the individual's life experiences and personality traits. One of these traits, in particular, called trait anxiety, tends to bias the appraisal process in the direction of consistently minimizing one's perceived capabilities and exaggerating the degree of threat. The anxiety response consists of several clusters of symptoms, including cognitive (worry, apprehension, fear of failure and future consequences), emotional (negative affect), behavioral (nervousness, exaggerated mannerisms, tics), and physiological (increases in heart rate, blood pressure, muscle tension, perspiration, stress hormone levels).

Although a certain degree of anxiety is a common part of everyday life (as we take exams, undergo interviews, or speak in public), anxiety disorders can be extremely disruptive. An anxiety *disorder*, such as Generalized Anxiety Disorder, one of the most common diagnostic classifications according to the *Diagnostic and Statistical Manual* of the American Psychiatric Association, is distinguished by such criteria as the persistence of the symptoms (e.g., at least 6 months), the excessive frequency and intensity of worry, the difficulty or inability to control the worry, and the impairment of social or occupational functioning. Other types of anxiety are distinguished by the specific object of the anxiety, such as anxiety about having a panic attack (as in a Panic Disorder), being embarrassed in public (as in Social Phobia), being contaminated (as in Obsessive–Compulsive Disorder), being away from home or close relatives (as in Separation Anxiety Disorder), gaining weight (as in Anorexia Nervosa), having multiple physical complaints (as in Somatization Disorder), or having a serious illness (as in Hypochondriasis).

Societal importance

Exact estimates of the prevalence of mental health problems in general, and anxiety in particular, are difficult to obtain and different surveys often yield different numbers. Moreover, it is believed that the majority of people who need help do not seek help because they prefer to try to address the problems on their own, because of fears about the high cost of diagnosis and treatment, or because of the social stigma that is still attached to mental health problems. Therefore, it is accepted that prevalence figures most likely underestimate the actual prevalence. In the USA, the 1-year prevalence for all anxiety disorders among adults exceeds 16%. Importantly, anxiety is often accompanied by so-called "comorbid" conditions, including depression (at rates of 50% or even higher) and substance abuse.

Construct assessment

Theoreticians make a distinction between anxiety as a state and anxiety as a trait. State anxiety is the acute (or short-term) emotional response that follows the appraisal of threat. Trait anxiety, as noted earlier, is the predisposition to interpret a variety of situations as threatening and to respond to them with increases in state anxiety. The assessment of anxiety in intervention studies usually follows this important theoretical distinction. Thus, studies of the effects of "acute exercise" (i.e., a single bout of exercise) typically focus on changes in state anxiety, whereas studies of the effects of "chronic exercise" (i.e., a program of exercise lasting for several weeks or months) typically focus on changes in trait anxiety. State and trait anxiety are usually assessed by self-report questionnaires. In responding to an item from the state anxiety portion of a commonly used questionnaire, the State-Trait Anxiety Inventory, an individual would be asked to report to what extent he or she feels "anxious" or "worried" at that moment (not at all, somewhat, moderately so, very much so). On the other hand, an item from the trait anxiety portion of the questionnaire would inquire how frequently the respondent "feels that difficulties are piling up so that he or she cannot overcome them" (almost never, sometimes, often, almost always).

Role of exercise

An extensive, although somewhat dated, meta-analytical review reported that bouts of exercise reduced state anxiety, on average, by approximately one-quarter of a standard deviation (0.24 SD) (Petruzzello et al. 1991; Landers & Petruzzello 1994) and were no different in lowering state anxiety from other treatments with known anxiety-reducing effects (meditation, relaxation, quiet rest). Factors such as the self-report questionnaire used, the age and health status of the participants and even the intensity of exercise, did not seem to make a difference. On the other hand, aerobic forms of activity (e.g., walking, jogging, swimming, cycling) were found to be effective, whereas non-aerobic modes (e.g., strength or flexibility training) were not. However, non-aerobic modes were vastly underrepresented in the analysis (only 13 effect sizes, compared to 173). Although an initial analysis indicated that activities lasting less than 20 min were not effective in lowering state anxiety, the authors noted that almost half of the effect sizes in that category were derived from studies that compared the effects of exercise to those of known anxiety-reducing treat-

ments. When only the effect sizes from studies involving other comparison groups or conditions were taken into account, activity bouts lasting less than 20 min were just as effective as longer ones.

The same meta-analytic review also showed that long-term exercise interventions were associated, on average, with reductions in trait anxiety by 0.34 SD (Petruzzello et al. 1991). Again, factors such as the self-report questionnaire used, the age and health status of the participants, and even the intensity of exercise did not make a difference. The presence of only two effect sizes from studies involving non-aerobic modes of activity did not permit a meaningful comparison of their effectiveness compared with aerobic activities. An interesting finding was that longer activity programs were generally associated with larger effects. Short programs of 9 weeks or less were associated with small effect sizes (0.14–0.17), those lasting between 10 and 15 weeks yielded medium effect sizes (0.36–0.50), and programs lasting 15 or more weeks produced large effect sizes (0.90).

Other meta-analyses examined smaller samples of studies and have led to some contradictory conclusions, although not different numerical findings, because the average effect sizes appear to be in the 0.25–0.35 range, consistently pointing to reductions in anxiety. McDonald and Hodgdon (1991) conducted a meta-analysis focusing specifically on exercise interventions designed to improve aerobic fitness and therefore followed established training guidelines and included assessments of fitness at the beginning and end of the program. The 13 studies on state anxiety yielded an average effect size of 0.28, whereas the 20 studies on trait anxiety yielded an average effect size of 0.25. Importantly, however, although several of the studies examined women, the average effect size for women was not significantly different from zero.

Long and van Stavel (1995) examined 40 studies on the effects of exercise interventions on state and trait anxiety in adults. The average effect size for within-subject contrasts was 0.45, indicating a decrease in anxiety by almost half of a standard deviation, whereas the average effect size for between-subject contrasts (e.g., experimental versus control) was 0.36, indicating a decrease in anxiety by approximately one-third of a standard deviation. The effect was similar for state and trait anxiety. Importantly, in between-subject contrasts, the effect was significantly larger for high-anxious samples (0.51) than low-anxious ones (0.28).

Schlicht (1994) conducted a meta-analysis of 20 studies, published between 1980 and 1990, examining anxiety changes in non-clinical (healthy) samples associated with leisure-time physical activity (not sports training). The average effect size, expressed as a correlation coefficient, was only −0.15, corresponding to a decrease in anxiety by 0.29 SD. This effect was not significantly different from zero and was found to be heterogeneous. The small number of studies included in the analysis, however, did not permit a meaningful test of mediators. Schlicht (1994) concluded that the literature "provides only little support for the hypothesis that physical exercise reduces anxiety."

Finally, Kugler et al. (1994) examined 13 studies on the effects of exercise cardiac rehabilitation programs on anxiety. The average effect size (0.31) suggested a decrease in anxiety by almost one-third of a standard deviation. Kugler et al. commented that, particularly in light of the increases in anxiety (and depression) commonly experienced by cardiac patients, exercise programs "appear markedly less effective than psychotherapy, for which average effect sizes of more than 0.80 are reported."

The magnitude and consistency of the anxiety-reducing effects, however, is only one aspect of the story. The methodological quality of the studies is another and this is clearly where the challenge lies for future research. There are presently no large-scale, high-quality, randomized clinical trials on the effects of exercise on anxiety. The bulk of the evidence reviewed in the aforementioned meta-analyses comes from small-scale studies with a host of methodologic limitations. According to Salmon (2001), "Many positive reports were uncontrolled or inadequately controlled by procedures which were less involving or less plausible than exercise." According to Scully et al. (1998), "Explicating the variables that mediate the relation between exercise and anxiety reduction has proved problematic, a task made doubly difficult because so few studies specify levels of intensity, duration, and/or length of exercise program." Besides

such design and methodological issues, authors in recent years have also raised concerns about the validity of some self-report questionnaires commonly used to assess state anxiety in the context of exercise. These questionnaires do not distinguish cognitive symptoms of anxiety (worry, apprehension) from somatic symptoms (tension, nervousness), based on the assumption that these usually occur in unison, as parts of an integrated state anxiety response. However, exercise is a special case in which some of the psychophysiological responses that might otherwise be attributed to anxiety (e.g., increased heart rate, blood pressure, muscle tension) are in fact brought about by the metabolic demands of the activity. In the absence of the defining element of anxiety, namely the perception of threat, the occurrence or dissipation of such somatic symptoms may be unrelated to fluctuations in anxiety (Ekkekakis et al. 1999). However, other reviewers tend to discount these concerns. For example, according to Landers and Arent (2001), "It is highly unlikely that this relationship is due to a behavioral artifact," such as expectancy or response distortions.

In summary, the extant evidence indicates that exercise is associated with small to moderate decreases in anxiety. However, in the continued absence of large-scale, carefully controlled, randomized clinical trials with multiple outcome assessments and adequate follow-up, the quality of this evidence remains in question. The views, even within exercise psychology and exercise science, remain divided, a reminder of the subjectivity inherent in evaluating the quality of research.

Depression

Construct description

Depression is one of a group of "mood disorders" that also includes mania, bipolar disorder, cyclothymic disorder, and dysthymic disorder. Although depression tends to co-occur with anxiety and some medications that are effective for one are also effective for the other, the two conditions have several distinct features (antecedents, correlates, experiential characteristics, and other consequences). A primary difference is that, although anxiety is often associated with active forms of coping and the eliciting stimulus is still perceived as something that, at least to some extent or with some difficulty, could be dealt with, depression is often characterized by passivity and withdrawal. A common cognitive feature of depression is a pattern of appraisal called "learned helplessness," the persistent belief that one has no viable response options available and that the negative situation one finds oneself in is under the control of external and uncontrollable factors. As a result, the situation is seen as unavoidable, inescapable, or inevitable. The vulnerability to depression is increased by the tendency to make cognitive appraisals characterized by a strong negative bias or irrationality. Specifically, the scope of problems is exaggerated, such that they are seen as having a global impact (e.g., believing that a failure in one domain of life is evidence of failure in one's life overall); the causes are consistently attributed to oneself rather than to others; and negative outcomes are seen as permanent and irreversible.

A diagnosis of Major Depressive Disorder is based on evidence that the symptoms are frequent and severe enough to cause significant distress or impairment in social or occupational function. According to the *Diagnostic and Statistical Manual* of the American Psychiatric Association, an individual must report at least five of the following symptoms during a 2-week period:

1 Presence of symptoms on a nearly daily basis;
2 Depressed mood most of the day;
3 Markedly diminished interest or pleasure in almost all activities;
4 Weight loss;
5 Sleep disturbances (insomnia or hypersomnia);
6 Psychomotor agitation or retardation;
7 Feelings of fatigue or diminished energy;
8 Feelings of worthlessness or excessive guilt;
9 Inability to concentrate or make decisions; or
10 Recurrent thoughts of death or suicide.

Societal importance

Major Depressive Disorder (also known as unipolar major depression), the most common mood disorder, ranks as the leading cause of disability worldwide.

In the USA, the 1-year prevalence is approximately 10% but there is a clear gender effect, with women exhibiting a prevalence almost twice as high as that in men. When the costs of diagnosis, treatment, and productivity losses are taken into account, the total economic cost associated with depression is staggering. In the USA, this figure is approximately 20% of the total health care costs, but obviously the problems extend well beyond the economic sphere. Besides having a devastating effect on quality of life, depression is accompanied by a host of other problems, including anxiety, addictions, suicide, and increased risk for chronic, life-threatening physical diseases such as cardiovascular disease and cancer. Friends and family members of depressed patients also suffer consequences, including guilt, frustration, economic burden, and even physical abuse.

Construct assessment

In intervention studies, depression is typically quantified by self-report questionnaires, ratings made by a clinician on the basis of an interview and a standard protocol, or both. For example, an item from a commonly used depression questionnaire, the Beck Depression Inventory, includes four alternatives from which the respondent is asked to choose:

1 I do not feel sad.
2 I feel sad.
3 I am sad all the time and I can't snap out of it.
4 I am so sad or unhappy that I can't stand it.

These alternative statements count for 0, 1, 2, or 3 points toward the total depression score. Similarly, in a commonly used clinical assessment method, the Hamilton Depression Rating Scale, the interviewer has to decide whether a key symptom, such as depressed mood (feelings of sadness, hopelessness, helplessness, or worthlessness) is absent, is reported only upon questioning, is reported spontaneously, is communicated not only verbally but also non-verbally (by facial expressions, posture, or weeping), or is the only kind of mood that the patient reports during the interview. These different assessments then receive 0, 1, 2, 3, or 4 points, respectively, toward the total depression score.

Role of exercise

In the first meta-analysis on this topic, North *et al.* (1990) located 80 studies examining the effects of exercise on depression. Of these, 76 examined the effects of exercise programs, 7 included follow-ups, and 10 examined the effects of single bouts of activity. The overall effect size was 0.53, indicating a decrease in depression by approximately half of a standard deviation. The effect was significantly higher for the 21 studies involving medical or psychological patients (0.94) and the 13 studies in which participation in exercise programs was aimed as a mode of medical rehabilitation (0.97). Although the studies examining changes in trait depression were the minority (16 studies), they yielded larger effects (0.91) compared to those examining changes in state depression (0.45). Age, gender, and mode of activity were not significant mediators. Aerobic forms of activity had antidepressant effects similar to those of anaerobic forms. Likewise, the effects of exercise did not appear to be different from those of psychotherapy. Importantly, the length of the program was shown to be a strong mediator, with longer programs being associated with larger decreases in depression. However, it should be pointed out that there were relatively few long-term studies (lasting for more than 16 weeks). The meta-analysis also found that the effect was larger for published than unpublished studies (possibly suggesting publication bias), for studies using random assignment of participants to conditions, and studies characterized by a medium (as opposed to low or high) degree of internal validity.

McDonald and Hodgdon (1991) examined 15 studies on the effects of aerobic fitness training (running or jogging) on depression. The average effect size was 0.97, indicating a decrease in depression of approximately one standard deviation. Among the 10 studies that identified the gender of the participants, the effect appeared larger for men (1.1) than women (0.66). Furthermore, the effects of age, survey vs. experimental studies, or self-report measure of depression used were not significant. Depressed patients showed larger decreases in depression (1.17) than individuals who were not depressed at baseline (0.83), although this difference was again not statistically significant. McDonald and Hodgdon, who also examined the effects of aerobic fitness training on anxiety, noted that "the decrease in depression scores was greater than the decrease in anxiety-state and anxiety-trait scores."

Kugler *et al.* (1994) identified 15 studies examining the effects of exercise on depression among coronary heart disease patients. The average effect size was 0.46, almost one-half of a standard deviation. As noted in the section on anxiety, Kugler *et al.* expressed some surprise that the effect was less-than-medium, given the fact that heart disease is typically associated with increased levels of depression, thus also increasing the possible margin of improvement.

Craft and Landers (1998) focused on 30 studies examining the exercise–depression relationship among individuals who were clinically depressed or were diagnosed with depression as a result of a medical illness. Nineteen of these studies were different from those included in the North *et al.* (1990) meta-analysis. They reported a large effect size of 0.72, a decrease of nearly three-quarters of a standard deviation. Importantly, different types of exercise (e.g., running, walking, non-aerobic activities) did not differ in terms of effectiveness. Moreover, exercise was not different from other comparison interventions, such as therapy or behavioral interventions but these modalities were represented by a very small number of studies (three and five, respectively). Longer activity programs (9–12 weeks) were more effective (1.18) than shorter programs (8 weeks or less; 0.54). Also, patients who were moderately to severely depressed showed larger decreases (0.88) than those who were mildly to moderately depressed at the beginning of the program (0.34).

Lawlor and Hopker (2001) conducted a targeted meta-analysis, focusing only on randomized controlled trials (i.e., involving random allocation of participants to treatment and comparison groups) that involved adults (over 18 years of age) who had been diagnosed with depression (regardless of severity or method of diagnosis). Importantly, emphasis in this analysis was placed on the quality of experimental evidence, concentrating on three key issues:

1 Whether allocation was concealed (whether randomization took place at a site remote from the study and the records were secured);

2 Whether intention-to-treat analysis was undertaken (i.e., whether all the patients were analyzed in the groups to which they were randomly allocated, rather than including only those who started or completed treatment); and

3 Whether there was blinding (i.e., whether the main outcome was evaluated by an assessor who was blind to treatment allocation).

Of 72 publications identified as potentially relevant, 29 were reviews or commentaries, 15 were non-randomized controlled trials, three involved psychiatric patients with mixed diagnoses, five did not have an outcome measure of depression, and four compared different types of exercise but no non-exercise group, leaving 16 articles describing 14 eligible studies. Ten studies in which exercise was compared to a "placebo" intervention (e.g., lectures, home visits for "chats," occupational therapy) or was used as an adjunct to standard treatment (e.g., counseling, cognitive therapy) included adequate data for quantitative analysis. The average effect size was 1.1, indicating that the depression scores of physically active individuals were lower by slightly more than one standard deviation compared to physically inactive individuals. Contradicting the results of other analyses, the duration of exercise programs was inversely related to effectiveness, with programs lasting less than 8 weeks yielding the largest effect (1.8), and programs lasting more than 8 weeks yielding the smallest effect (0.6). An examination of the six studies that compared exercise with standard interventions for depression produced a non-significant effect size of 0.3, suggesting that exercise was no less effective than standard forms of therapy. Also, aerobic and non-aerobic types of exercise did not differ in their effectiveness.

Although this meta-analysis showed that exercise interventions produce large effects, it has drawn some criticisms from reviewers within exercise science for what was perceived as an overly critical tone. Specifically, Lawlor and Hopker (2001) concluded that "The effectiveness of exercise in reducing symptoms of depression cannot be determined because of a lack of good quality research on clinical populations with adequate follow-up." For example, they noted that the absence of a difference between aerobic and non-aerobic forms of activity might indicate that "The effect is due to psychosocial factors, such as learning a new skill or socializing, rather than to the exercise itself." After all, none of the studies involved exercise performed in social isolation and one study that directly compared exercise to a social-contact control group found that these treatments were equally effective in reducing depression. Of the 14 studies that were examined, randomization was concealed in only three, intention-to-treat analyses were undertaken in only two, and assessment of outcome was blinded in only one. None of the 14 studies satisfied all three of these quality criteria, leading the authors to state that "most studies were of poor quality." These words have been characterized as "a bit harsh" despite acknowledging that "if the prescription of exercise for [major depressive disorder] required approval from the Food and Drug Administration, it probably would not pass current standards" (Brosse *et al.* 2002). Other authors have been more dismissive of the concerns expressed by Lawlor and Hopker, questioning whether such factors as conducting outcome assessments with a blinded assessor, as opposed to self-reports, would make an important difference (Landers & Arent 2007).

An examination of the meta-analytical findings indicates that exercise is associated with lower depression scores. The magnitude of the effect is moderate to large and the effects seem consistent. There is also agreement that, although there are numerous studies, only a few can withstand any serious methodological scrutiny. The question then becomes whether more emphasis and faith can be placed on the fact that most studies, regardless of quality, show substantial and consistent benefits or on the fact that the body of evidence overall would not pass muster against established and time-honored criteria for evaluating the quality of experimental research. This is not an easy question, as is evident from the ongoing controversy in the literature. What is clear is that this is not a "black or white" issue and the criticisms, "harsh" or not, warrant serious consideration.

As a case in point, let us consider the arguably most complete study on the effects of exercise on depression conducted to date (Blumenthal *et al.* 1999). In this study, 156 men and women, 50 years of age or older, who had been diagnosed with major depressive disorder, were randomly assigned to one of three 16-week treatment conditions:

1 Exercise (three sessions per week, lasting for 45 min each, at 70–85% of heart rate reserve);

2 Antidepressant medication (using the popular serotonin reuptake inhibitor sertraline hydrochloride or Zoloft™); or

3 A combination of the exercise and antidepressant treatments.

At the end of the treatment period, both clinician-rated and self-reported levels of depression were reduced compared to baseline, with no significant differences between the groups. At the 10-month follow-up (6 months after the conclusion of treatment), self-reported depression scores were also not different across the three groups. However, the participants in the exercise group had a lower rate of depression (30%) than those in the medication (52%) and combined-treatment groups (55%). Furthermore, of the participants who were in remission after the initial 16-week treatment period, those who had been assigned to the exercise-only group were more likely to have partly or fully recovered after 6 months than those in the medication and combined (exercise plus medication) groups (Babyak *et al.* 2000). This somewhat puzzling finding was interpreted by the authors as possibly indicating that exercise helps participants develop "a sense of personal mastery and positive self-regard," whereas the exclusive reliance on or the inclusion of medication "may undermine this benefit by prioritizing an alternative, less self-confirming attribution for one's improved condition" (Babyak *et al.* 2000).

On the one hand, this study overcame several of the methodological shortcomings of earlier studies, having an adequate sample size, including both men and women, and examining individuals who were depressed at baseline rather than a convenience sample. Furthermore, the study involved reasonably long treatment and follow-up periods, two comparison conditions, and more than one standard measure of the main outcome variable (i.e., both self-reports and clinician ratings of depression). Finally, the study did involve an "intention-to-treat" analysis,

thus accounting for the possible biasing effects of the less than perfect adherence and often substantial dropout rates commonly associated with exercise and medication interventions.

However, this study could not address other potentially important problems. First, there was a selection bias, because the participants were all volunteers who responded to advertisements for a research study of "exercise therapy for depression." Thus, as discussed by Babyak *et al.* (2000), it is possible that an "antimedication" bias among some participants might have influenced the results. Perhaps associated with volunteerism, the participants were also highly educated and physically healthy. Furthermore, the possibility of "spontaneous recovery" cannot be excluded as there was no no-treatment control condition. Because there can be no true "placebo" exercise intervention, many control interventions (e.g., wait list) are really of questionable meaningfulness, because they fail to control for expectancy. Moreover, because the exercise was conducted in a group environment, it is possible that the beneficial effects of exercise were partly or fully mediated by social interaction. Finally, there is no way to fully account for treatment crossovers that can take place during the follow-up period (e.g., participants opting to switch or discontinue treatments). These limitations, which are clearly not trivial, underscore the fact that even large, costly, and well-designed studies that produce seemingly robust results supporting the beneficial role of exercise should be viewed cautiously.

Besides studies examining the strength of the association between exercise and depression, or reviews focusing on the consistency and quality of the experimental evidence, research is also focusing on such critically important questions as the dose–response relationship and the biological mechanisms that might underlie the beneficial effects of exercise on depression. On the issue of dose–response, there is consensus that "There is little evidence for dose–response effects, though this is largely because of a lack of studies rather than a lack of evidence" (Dunn *et al.* 2001). A recently published randomized clinical trial with adults diagnosed with mild to moderate major depressive disorder compared four 12-week exercise conditions, crossing two levels of energy expenditure (7.0 or 15.5 kcal·kg^{-1}·week^{-1}) and two frequencies (3 or 5 days per week), and a "placebo exercise" intervention consisting of flexibility exercises performed 3 days per week. At the end of the programs, the effect of frequency was not significant but that of energy expenditure was, with the higher dose leading to lower clinician ratings of depression than the lower dose and "placebo," the latter two being no different from each other (Dunn *et al.* 2005).

On the issue of biological mechanisms, research is focusing mainly on the apparent ability of exercise to act as a natural analog of pharmacological interventions by correcting deficiencies in serotonin and norepinephrine neurotransmission (Meeusen 2006). Such deficiencies are considered hallmarks of clinical depression and anxiety and, consequently, have been the targets of antidepressive and antianxiety medications (i.e., serotonin- and norepinephrine-specific reuptake inhibitors).

Mood and affect

Construct description

Anxiety and depression are subjective states that generally follow specific patterns of cognitive appraisals (threat or helplessness, respectively). However, there are other salient subjective states that either have a loose connection to a cognitive appraisal or can even occur in the absence of a cognitive appraisal. "Moods" are believed to be linked to certain patterns of thought. However, unlike emotions, the target or eliciting stimulus might not be something obvious or specific. On the contrary, it could be something that happened a long time ago (e.g., a recollection of an unpleasant childhood event), something that could potentially occur in the distant future (e.g., that one's child might grow up to be a criminal), or even a large, existential question (e.g., wondering whether one's life has meaning or is consistent with what one had envisioned). Thus, moods are often "diffuse" and long-lasting, associated with a low tendency to act in response (i.e., "do something about it"), and even an inability to identify precisely why one feels the way that one does at a given moment. Moods are related to emotions in several ways. For example, one can be in an

"anxious mood" or a "depressed mood" when one is bothered by persistent or ruminating thoughts of threat or inevitability not necessarily linked to a specific recent or impending situation or event. Furthermore, being in a certain mood lowers the threshold for the induction of the consonant emotion. For example, waking up in a worrisome or nervous mood might predispose one to evaluate many situations arising that day as posing a threat and, thus, respond with frequent state anxiety reactions.

"Affect" is an even more general term that refers to the defining subjective quality of all valenced (pleasant or unpleasant) states, including moods and emotions (Ekkekakis & Petruzzello 2000). Affect is an inherent component of all emotions and moods (it is what makes them "feel" pleasant or unpleasant) but can also occur independently of these, as in the case of the strong unpleasant sensations that accompany pain and injury or the sense of exhaustion that accompanies strenuous exercise on a hot, humid day. Affect is distinct from emotion and mood in that, as concepts, they also include several additional components such as cognitive appraisals, attributions to (proximal or distal) eliciting stimuli, and behavioral reactions (e.g., facial expressions or postural adjustments). In other words, moods and emotions are considerably more complex and multifaceted constructs than affect. Affect is commonly viewed as varying in terms of two key underlying dimensions: valence (pleasure vs. displeasure) and perceived activation or arousal. The combination of these two dimensions, which are theorized to be orthogonal to each other, produces four main variants of affective experience:

1 High-activation pleasant affect, characterized by energy, vigor, or excitement;

2 High-activation unpleasant affect, characterized by tension or distress;

3 Low-activation unpleasant affect, characterized by fatigue, boredom, or depression; and

4 Low-activation pleasant affect, characterized by calmness or relaxation.

Societal importance

Numerous exercise studies have examined changes in mood or affect. One category of studies has focused on the effects of regular exercise or physical activity participation on "baseline" or average levels of mood and affect. Another category of studies has examined whether single bouts of exercise can "make people feel better" in a transient sense (during exercise, as well as in the minutes and hours following the exercise bout). Of particular interest for the studies in the latter category is the question of dose–response, which includes questions pertaining to the lowest "dose" (intensity, duration) that can improve affect, the dose that can optimize affective change, and the dose that might induce a deterioration, instead of an improvement, in affect. Besides the relevance of dose–response research to the issue of well-being, it is also believed that it might shed light on the severe public health problem of physical inactivity. Simply put, because humans generally tend to do what makes them feel better but avoid what makes them feel worse, it is reasonable to assume that they would avoid those doses of exercise that consistently make them feel worse.

Construct assessment

Mood and affect are typically assessed by questionnaires or rating scales. Mood questionnaires focus on either a single mood state (e.g., euphoria) or various assortments of mood states, most commonly the six mood states contained in the 65-item questionnaire entitled the Profile of Mood States (tension, depression, anger, vigor, fatigue, and confusion). These questionnaires can be administered with different time-frame instructions, ranging from "How do you feel right now?" to "How have you felt during the past month, including today?" depending on the purpose of the study. Measures of affect, given the broad scope of this construct, tend to focus on a few key dimensions that are believed to underlie the domain of affect. Thus, the Positive and Negative Affect Schedule questionnaire includes one scale measuring high-activation pleasant affect (termed "Positive Affect" or "Positive Activation") and another measuring high-activation unpleasant affect (termed "Negative Affect" or "Negative Activation"). The Activation Deactivation Adjective Check List questionnaire includes one bipolar scale

measuring "Energetic Arousal" (ranging from Energy, or high-activation pleasant affect, to Tiredness, or low-activation unpleasant affect) and another measuring "Tense Arousal" (ranging from Tension, or high-activation unpleasant affect, to Calmness, or low-activation pleasant affect). Alternatively, responses during bouts of exercise, when the use of multi-item questionnaires would be impractical, can be assessed by single-item rating scales, such as a scale that measures affective valence (ranging from pleasure to displeasure) and a scale that measures perceived activation or arousal (ranging from low arousal to high arousal). The combination of these two scales can produce a two-dimensional "map" of affective space, on which researchers can plot the trajectory of affective changes during an exercise bout and subsequent recovery period.

Role of exercise

One meta-analysis examined the effects of chronic exercise on mood in older adults, over 65 years of age (Arent *et al.* 2000). The 32 relevant studies that were retrieved were divided into three groups:

1 Experimental vs. control group comparisons;
2 Pre- to post-treatment comparisons; and
3 Correlational studies.

The average effect size from experimental vs. control group comparisons was 0.24. However, after studies in which experimental and control groups differed at baseline were removed, the average effect size rose to 0.34, or approximately one-third of a standard deviation. The effects were similar for increasing scores on "positive" (0.33) and reducing scores on "negative" (0.35) mood variables. The effects were larger for exercise performed on fewer than 3 days per week (0.69) than 3 or more days per week (0.28), when the duration per session was self-selected (0.86), when the duration of the program was up to 12 weeks (0.45–0.48) but no longer (0.19), and when the intensity of exercise was low (0.58) rather than medium (0.26) or high (0.29). The average effect size from pre- to post-treatment comparisons was 0.38. Again, there was no difference in the extent to which exercise was associated with increases in "positive" (0.35) and decreases in "negative" (0.39) mood variables. Finally, the average effect size from correlational studies was 0.46, and this was again similar for increases in "positive" (0.42) and decreases in "negative" (0.47) mood variables. Although certainly informative, this meta-analysis was limited by the fact that mood and affect were considered interchangeable constructs and no information was provided as to exactly which "positive" and "negative" mood variables were included (other than to say that the studies that were selected assessed "some construct of mood").

A recent meta-analysis targeted 158 studies on the effects of aerobic exercise on changes in high-activation pleasant affect from before to after a bout (Reed & Ones 2006). Effect sizes were weighted for sample sizes and corrected for the unreliability of measurement and other possible sources of bias. Overall, the analysis indicated that exercise treatments were associated with an increase in high-activation pleasant affect by almost one-half of a standard deviation (average effect size of 0.47), whereas control or comparison treatments were associated with a small decrease (0.17). The positive effect of exercise was larger for individuals who had the lowest pre-exercise scores (0.63), for exercise of low intensity (0.57), for exercise duration up to 35 min (0.46–0.57), for low and moderate "doses" of exercise (product of intensity and duration, 0.45–0.46), and for assessments taken up to 5 min post-exercise (0.61). Interestingly, studies that attempted to control three or more threats to internal validity were associated with larger effect sizes (0.49–0.50) than less well-controlled studies (0.30).

A series of recent studies has started to delineate the important relationship between the intensity of exercise and the affective responses that occur during and after an exercise bout. The picture that is emerging at this early stage is that at:

1 *Low levels of intensity:* during-exercise changes tend to be mostly positive, characterized primarily by shifts toward a high-activation pleasant affective state;

2 *High and near-maximal levels of intensity:* during-exercise changes are negative in most participants; and

3 *Mid-range intensities:* during-exercise changes tend to vary from individual to individual, with some reporting increases and other reporting decreases in pleasure.

It also appears that the intensity associated with the ventilatory or lactate threshold is the "turning point," beyond which the declines in pleasure begin. Depending on whether the affective changes that occur during exercise are positive or negative, the typically positive changes observed after exercise may represent either the continuation of a positive during-exercise trend or the result of a rapid post-exercise rebound, which tends to be proportional in magnitude to the during-exercise decline. According to a "dual-mode" theoretical model, the affective responses to exercise are the result of the continuous interplay between two general factors:

1 *Cognitive variables:* e.g., self-efficacy, self-presentational concerns, or attributions; and

2 *Interoceptive variables:* e.g., respiratory or muscular cues.

The relative salience of these two factors is expected to vary systematically as a function of exercise intensity, with cognitive variables being the dominant determinants of affect at intensities below and proximal to the ventilatory threshold and interoceptive variables gradually increasing their influence at intensities above the ventilatory threshold and until the point of maximal capacity (Ekkekakis 2003; Ekkekakis *et al.* 2005). This model has implications for the extent to which cognitive techniques that are commonly used to control affective responses to exercise (e.g., attentional dissociation, cognitive reframing, or boosting self-efficacy), particularly among novice exercisers, can remain effective as the intensity rises. The dual-mode theory suggests that, as the intensity of exercise begins to exceed the level associated with the ventilatory threshold, the role of cognition in controlling affect is reduced, as a barrage of inherently unpleasant interoceptive cues flood consciousness. Therefore, interventions designed to improve the ability of novice exercisers to self-monitor and self-regulate their exercise intensity may be warranted.

Cognitive function

Construct description

Cognitive function depends on such critically important abilities as perceiving, recognizing, and interpreting sensory stimuli, storing information in memory and retrieving it when needed, and using these data to make appropriate behavioral decisions. Some cognitive abilities are based on knowledge (such as verbal fluency and comprehension or wealth of vocabulary) and are termed "crystallized" abilities. These typically continue to improve over the course of one's lifetime and tend to resist the effects of aging. However, other cognitive abilities, which are process-based (e.g., the speed and accuracy of perception and decision making), termed "fluid" abilities, seem to be susceptible to aging-related declines. The decline in such abilities can begin as early as the third decade of life and is typically accelerated after the age of 70 years. On average, between 30 and 90 years of age, humans lose approximately 15% of their cerebral cortex and 25% of their cerebral white matter, with the frontal, parietal, and temporal cortices being affected the most. Not surprisingly, the loss of brain tissue and the decline in cognitive function parallel each other.

Societal importance

Although a certain degree of cognitive decline is often seen as a normal part of the aging process, there appear to be some striking interindividual differences, with some individuals maintaining seemingly perfect mental sharpness and clarity well into old age. Although most individuals experiencing cognitive decline preserve adequate function to stay independent, in some cases the decline is such that it is recognized as a clinical condition, known as dementia. The most common cause of dementia is Alzheimer's disease, currently afflicting 2–4 million people in the USA alone. In turn, old age, family history of dementia, low levels of educational and occupational attainment, and the apolipoprotein E genotype ε4 allele are the only known risk factors for Alzheimer's disease. Dementia and Alzheimer's disease have a devastating effect on quality of life. They gradually rob patients of their intellectual faculties, eventually making even the most basic forms of self-care and social interaction impossible. Besides increasing the risk of loss of independence, hospitalization, or institutionalization, Alzheimer's disease is associated with life-threatening physical comorbidities, such as stroke, and can ultimately lead to death.

Construct assessment

Cognitive function is multifaceted and, accordingly, can be evaluated in a variety of ways. The simplest tool, used extensively in epidemiological research, is a short survey called the Mini Mental State Examination. During a short conversation, the patient is asked questions designed to assess basic orientation (identify the time and place), memory (name and later recall certain items), attention and calculation (count by seven), and language (follow a three-stage command). Other assessment options include standardized tests designed to assess diverse abilities (e.g., perceptual speed, working memory, tracking, decision making, multitasking), most of which are computerized. Furthermore, cognitive processing is often evaluated by psychophysiological indices. Specifically, in a technique called Event Related Potentials, the electroencephalographical traces following the presentation of several target (uncommon) and non-target (common) stimuli are averaged and compared. A particular element of the waveform, a positive voltage change occurring approximately 300 ms after the presentation of the stimulus (hence named P300 or P3), is examined in terms of its amplitude (which is interpreted as an indication of the extent of recruitment of cognitive resources) and latency (which is interpreted as an indication of the speed of cognitive processing). Finally, given the close correspondence between structural or anatomical changes in the brain and cognitive performance, brain imaging methods, such as magnetic resonance imaging, have also been used.

Role of exercise

The role of exercise in promoting and preserving cognitive function was originally examined based on the rationale that the beneficial effects of exercise on the cardiovascular system might also be reflected in a healthy blood supply to and therefore ample oxygenation of the brain. Over the years, this rationale has been extended and strengthened, as additional mechanisms for a possible beneficial effect on cognitive function have been uncovered. Specifically, exercise has been shown to promote synaptogenesis (the formation of new synapses), neurogenesis (the formation of new neurons), and the upregulation of growth factors that are important to the healthy development and preservation of neural tissue, such as Brain Derived Neurotrophic Factor (van Praag 2006).

The first meta-analysis on the link between exercise and cognitive function examined 134 studies (Etnier *et al*. 1997). The average effect size was small (0.25), indicating an improvement in cognitive performance by one-quarter of a standard deviation. Cross-sectional or correlational designs yielded higher effects (0.53) than chronic (0.33) or acute (0.16) designs. This finding cannot be interpreted in an unequivocal fashion. One possible interpretation is that cross-sectional studies generally have more power, since "fit" or "active" and "unfit" or "inactive" participants generally differ more in terms of fitness compared to how much participants can improve over the course of an exercise training program lasting for a few weeks or months. Another way to approach this finding, however, is by recognizing that the quasi-experimental nature of this evidence does not permit any inferences about causation to be made. In studies of acute exercise, age, mental ability, the intensity and duration of the bout, and the interaction of intensity and duration were not found to moderate the results. Surprisingly, measures of simple reaction time were associated with larger effect sizes than measures of choice reaction time, despite the larger cognitive component of the latter. In chronic exercise studies, although the mental ability of the participants did not moderate the results, their age did. Specifically, the effects were larger for participants aged 46–60 years (1.02) and 18–30 years (0.64), whereas there was no apparent benefit for individuals aged 31–45 years (0.06) or 61–90 years (0.19). The duration of exercise sessions, the days of exercise per week, the total number of exercise sessions, and the changes in fitness were not associated with the size of the effect. In cross-sectional or correlational studies, the age and mental ability of the participants were not significant moderators. However, the effects were again found to be larger for measures of simple than choice reaction time. The authors emphasized that, in both acute and chronic exercise studies, as the number of

threats to internal validity increased, so did the effect sizes. This finding underscores the importance of conducting studies characterized by the highest degree of methodological rigor. When only the 17 randomized clinical trials were examined, the average effect size was 0.18, which, although positive and significantly different from zero, was small and of questionable practical importance.

A subsequent meta-analysis of 44 studies focused on the effects of exercise on cognitive performance among children (Sibley & Etnier 2003). The average effect size was 0.32, indicating that children who exercised outperformed children who did not by approximately one-third of a standard deviation. The effect sizes derived from true experiments (0.29), quasi-experiments (0.37), and cross-sectional or correlational studies (0.35) did not differ significantly. Likewise, whether the children were healthy, mentally impaired, or physically disabled, as well as the type of exercise used, were not significant moderators. Middle-school (11–13 years; 0.48) and young elementary school children (4–7 years; 0.40) showed the largest effects. Tests of perceptual skills yielded the largest effects (0.49), whereas math tests (0.20), verbal tests (0.17), and memory tests (0.03) yielded the smallest.

At the other end of the developmental spectrum, in older adults, there has been a history of mixed results. The cause of the inconsistency was elucidated recently, following a proposal that the effects of exercise in older adults do not manifest themselves across the entire range of cognitive abilities but are rather selective, benefiting primarily functions that depend on executive control. This proposal makes logical sense because cognitive skills that have a large executive-control component, and the brain regions that control them, appear to be selectively impacted by aging. This idea was tested in a meta-analysis of 18 randomized fitness intervention trials that involved adults aged 55–80 years (Colcombe & Kramer 2003). Studies were excluded if the design was cross-sectional, the participants were not randomly assigned, the exercise program was unsupervised, or the exercise program did not include an aerobic fitness component. The meta-analysis examined four competing theoretical predictions; namely, that the effects of exercise or fitness would be specific to:

1 *Speed:* tasks representing low-level neurologic functioning, such as simple reaction time;

2 *Visuospatial ability:* ability to transform or remember visual and spatial information, such as redrawing shapes from memory;

3 *Controlled processes:* tasks requiring some cognitive control, such as simple rule-based decision-making or choice reaction time tasks; and

4 *Executive control:* planning, inhibition, and scheduling, such as responding to one cue while suppressing other, simultaneously presented, conflicting, or irrelevant cues.

Exercise training groups showed an average effect size of 0.478, whereas control groups showed an average effect size of 0.164. In other words, exercise training was associated with almost an improvement of one-half of a standard deviation in cognitive performance, regardless of the nature of the task. Importantly, however, the effect was found to be the largest for executive-control tasks (0.68), followed by controlled processes (0.46), visuospatial tasks (0.43), and speed tasks (0.27), thus providing support to the hypothesis that the effects of exercise are selective. Individuals who were trained using a combination of aerobic and strength-training exercises improved significantly more (0.59) than those who used aerobic exercise alone (0.41). Short training programs, lasting 1–3 months, were shown to be effective (0.52), although not as much as programs lasting more than 6 months (0.67). However, programs consisting of short exercise bouts, lasting 30 min or less, were not effective (0.18); bouts lasting 31–45 min (0.61) or 46–60 min (0.47) were necessary for significant effects. Samples consisting mostly of women were associated with a clearly larger effect (0.60) than samples consisting mostly of men (0.15), the latter being only borderline significant. Also, individuals aged 66–70 years reaped the largest benefit (0.69), followed by those aged 71–80 years (0.55) and those aged 55–65 years (0.30).

Finally, a recent meta-analysis focused on what has been termed the "cardiovascular fitness hypothesis," or the idea that the beneficial effect of exercise on cognitive function is mediated by improvements in aerobic capacity (Etnier *et al.* 2006). The average effect size was 0.34, indicating that aerobic training and fitness were associated with approximately

one-third of a standard deviation improvement in cognitive performance. The 37 studies that were identified were divided into four groups:

1 Cross-sectional designs (mean effect size 0.40);
2 Post-test comparisons (mean effect size 0.27);
3 Pre-post comparisons (mean effect size 0.25); and
4 Correlational studies (mean correlation 0.29).

Within category 1, fitness was not related to cognitive performance overall but only among middle-aged adults; in fact, it was a negative predictor of cognitive performance among children and young adults and was unrelated to cognitive performance among older adults. Within category 2, fitness and cognitive performance were unrelated. Within category 3, gains in aerobic fitness were negatively correlated with improvements in cognitive performance. Age interacted with fitness, in that fitness was a significant negative predictor of cognitive performance only among older adults, and was unrelated to cognitive performance among children, young adults, and middle-aged adults. Health status or the type of cognitive test involved were not shown to be significant mediators in any of the analyses. The clear lack of support for the cardiovascular fitness hypothesis in this analysis opens the door to other explanations for the beneficial effects of exercise on cognitive function, including improved cerebral oxygenation, improved neurotransmitter availability, synaptogenesis, neurogenesis, and upregulation of brain neurotrophic factors.

Self-esteem

Construct description

Self-concept and self-esteem are two constructs at the core of our self-perceptions. They refer to how people see themselves and how they evaluate their worth, their capabilities, and their limitations. Although the two terms are often used interchangeably, self-concept refers to one's self-description and is therefore more "cognitive" in nature, whereas self-esteem refers primarily to the positivity or negativity of these self-perceptions and is therefore more "affective" in nature. Self-concept and self-esteem are believed to have a multidimensional and hierarchical structure. The term "hierarchical" is meant to convey that these constructs have a pyramid-like structure, with multiple domain-specific self-appraisals at the bottom of the hierarchy (i.e., how we see and evaluate ourselves in terms of our physical appearance or capability, in terms of our academic or occupational achievements, in terms of the breadth and quality of our social relationships, and so on) and a global, over-arching self-appraisal at the top. Each domain can also have additional subdivisions. For example, the academic domain can be further divided into math, history, science, language, and other subdomains. The term "multidimensional" is meant to convey that our domain-specific (and subdomain-specific) self-appraisals can vary, to some degree, independently of each other. For example, although we may think that we have done a great job in the professional arena, this does not necessarily entail that we must have an equally positive view of our performance as spouses or parents. Likewise, although we may think of ourselves as exceptionally strong in math, we may view our historical knowledge as weak.

Societal importance

The physical aspect of the self is one of its essential components, although the importance assigned to it can clearly vary from one individual to the next. For some, it may acquire central importance, to the extent that global self-worth hinges almost entirely upon one's view of one's body and physical appearance. This unbalanced view of the self is often associated with such serious problems as body dysmorphic disorder, eating disorders (anorexia, bulimia), or obsessive exercise. In turn, these conditions are frequently comorbid with other psychological problems, such as major depressive disorder, social anxiety or phobia, and obsessive–compulsive disorder. Dissatisfaction with a certain aspect of one's physical appearance or with one's overall physical appearance can lead to avoidance of usual activities, development of problems in interpersonal behavior, and social isolation. At the other end of the spectrum, some individuals pay very little attention to their body, viewing it more or less as a vehicle for getting around and as having a negligible role in determining their self-worth. In these cases, overeating and underexercising, or an overall neglect of one's health can occur, often with negative consequences for health and well-being.

It is also important to point out that the physical domain is not unitary. It can consist of several appearance-related aspects (e.g., tallness, leanness, muscularity) and several performance-related aspects (e.g., strength, endurance, flexibility), including general skills (e.g., dexterity, grace, speed) and sport-specific skills (e.g., in basketball or swimming). Given the multidimensional nature of such self-appraisals, these can vary, to some degree, independently. For example, a man might see himself as impressively muscular but lacking in endurance.

Construct assessment

Because self-concept and self-esteem are quintessentially subjective constructs, the typical method used for their assessment is the questionnaire. In recent years, there has been a shift from viewing the self as a unitary construct to conceptualizing the self as multifaceted and context-dependent. Global self-esteem is generally measured by unidimensional inventories, one of the most popular being the Rosenberg Self-Esteem scale. It consists of 10 items, some of which are worded positively (e.g., "I feel that I am a person of worth, at least on an equal plane with others") and some worded negatively (e.g., "I certainly feel useless at times"). Another approach to measurement focuses on domain-specific self-appraisals. In the case of the physical domain, one of the most popular measures is the Physical Self Perception Profile, a multidimensional questionnaire that includes scales measuring perceptions of physical strength, physical condition, sport competence, body attractiveness, and overall self-worth. Additional measures are also available that tap the physical domain such as body image, body satisfaction, and social physique anxiety.

Role of exercise

Given the impact of physical activity on the body, it is reasonable to assume that physical self-esteem can change as a consequence of exercise participation.

Given the hierarchical structure of this construct, domain-specific change may in turn serve to modify global self-esteem. This relationship could prove beneficial because research suggests that self-esteem occupies a central position in the psychology of health and well-being and is related to choice and persistence in a range of achievement and health behaviors (Fox 2000). Indeed, one way that exercise activity may help people "feel better" is through enhanced self-perceptions (such as physical self-worth, physical condition, and physical health) and improved self-esteem.

A number of narrative reviews on the relationship between exercise and self-esteem have concluded that the weight of the evidence supports a positive link between the two. Fox's review (2000), which examined 36 randomized clinical trials, noted that 78% of studies observed positive changes in some aspect of physical self-esteem or self-concept as a result of exercise. However, the strength of the association between exercise and global self-esteem has been questioned.

A recent meta-analysis by Spence et al. (2005) on adults over 18 years found an average effect size of 0.23, suggesting that exercise is associated with an increase in global self-esteem of approximately one-quarter of a standard deviation, a small effect. Significant changes in physical fitness were associated with greater changes in global self-esteem (0.32) than exercise that did not elicit such changes (0.15, not significantly different from zero). Initial level of self-esteem, exercise intensity, and length of the program were not significant moderators of the exercise effects. The effects were larger when the program was exercise-based (0.26) or lifestyle-based (0.36) than on programs involving training in skill-based activities, which had no effect (−0.03).

Ekeland et al. (2005) focused their systematic review on the effects of exercise on global self-esteem in children and youth. The 23 included studies were divided into two groups which focused either only on exercise or on skill training, counseling, the social setting, or other motivational factors that were part of the exercise intervention. The overall standardized mean difference between the exercise and control group was 0.49, equating to a 10% difference between the groups in favor of the intervention.

However, a sensitivity analysis showed that this effect was not significant when the data were re-examined after excluding studies of healthy children, strength-training studies, programs lasting less than 10 weeks, or studies with large baseline differences. When exercise as part of a holistic program was compared with no-intervention, a similar difference emerged (0.51, equating to a 10% difference between the intervention and control group). However, this finding should be interpreted cautiously as only four studies were included in the analysis. What emanates from the meta-analyses that span gender, age, and physical activity domains is the conclusion that physical activity brings about statistically significant increases in global self-esteem, but the effects are small. Indeed, Spence et al. (2005) assert that the effects of exercise on global self-esteem have been overstated in the literature.

The only medium-sized effect (−0.41) was reported in the meta-analytical review of McDonald and Hodgdon (1991). This discrepancy may relate to the extent to which the reviewed literature focuses on global self-esteem or on domain-specific components. This is important because, not surprisingly, the magnitude of change brought about by exercise within the specific domain of physical self-perceptions has been found to be larger than changes at the global level (Fox 2000). A recent meta-analysis targeted 121 studies on the effects of exercise on body image (Hausenblas & Fallon 2006). The studies were divided into three groups:
1 Experimental vs. control group studies;
2 Single-group studies; and
3 Correlational studies.
The overall mean effect size from experimental vs. control group comparisons was 0.28, with women reporting a significantly larger effect (0.43) than men (0.39). Similar effects were also found across all the study groupings. In terms of exercise mode, combined aerobic and anaerobic exercise elicited a larger effect (0.45) compared with aerobic (0.25) or anaerobic (0.27) exercise alone. Further, in this study grouping, adolescents had a significantly larger effect (0.71) than university students (0.25) and adults (0.46). However, although the overall mean effect size was larger for the correlational (0.41) studies, this age effect was not replicated, with adolescents in this

group of studies reporting significantly smaller effect sizes (0.18) than college-age (0.53) and adult populations (0.59). The use of age categories, rather than mean age, is offered as a possible explanation for these varying results. The overall conclusion of this analysis was that exercise is associated with a more positive body image, but the effects are, once again, small. Furthermore, the extent to which changes in physical self-perceptions are accompanied by improvements in the overall sense of worth or general self-esteem, appears equivocal.

The absence of systematic exercise effects on global self-esteem has been attributed to the fact that such effects are mediated by psychosocial rather than physiologic mechanisms (Fox 2000). The subjective nature of the self means that the mechanisms accounting for change are variable and will depend on the individual's subjective experience of the activity and the setting in which it takes place. Although many mechanisms have been proposed, including change in physical fitness, goal achievement, and social experiences, little evidence exists supporting their efficacy for eliciting change. Finally, it is important to contextualize physical activity. Individuals do not partake in this behavior in a vacuum, so many moderating variables likely exist. Given the highly idiosyncratic nature of the self, the challenge ahead lies in unravelling this complex relationship. In the future, studies may be complemented by idiographic research to explore the different ways that individuals interpret the importance placed on exercise in their everyday lives.

Health-related quality of life

Construct description

Despite the average life expectancy for both men and women continuing to rise in the developed world, *healthy life* expectancy, although increasing, has not matched the pace of total life expectancy. Before the 1970s, the concept of "quality of life" had received little attention in the fields of medicine and public health. However, much has changed since then. Today, according to the World Health Organization, health is not viewed merely as the absence of disease but as a state of complete physical, mental, and social well-being. Attention to quality of life emerged as a natural consequence of this new perspective. The term "quality of life" refers to an individual's perception of his or her position in life, within the context of the surrounding culture and value systems and in relation to the individual's goals, expectations, standards, and concerns. Clearly, this is a multifaceted construct. It is believed to be the product of a complex interaction between the individual's physical health, psychological health, independence, personal beliefs, social relationships, and the physical, social, cultural, political, or economic environment.

Societal importance

The domain of physical health includes such components as perceived levels of energy or fatigue, pain, and discomfort. The domain of psychological health encompasses such elements as body image, emotions, self-esteem, and cognitive vitality. Independence refers to mobility, the ability to carry out activities of daily living, the degree of dependence on medicinal substances or medical aids, and the ability to work. The domain of personal beliefs refers to religion and spirituality. The domain of social relationships includes such notions as social support, human contact, and sexuality. Finally, the environment encompasses a broad array of elements that have direct or indirect relevance to the quality of life, including financial resources, freedom and security, access to high-quality health and social care, opportunities for education and self-improvement, opportunities for recreation and leisure, and an unpolluted and non-congested physical environment.

Of these components of quality of life, the ones that are of particular relevance to exercise and physical activity are the first three: the domains of physical and psychological health, and independence. Collectively, these can be categorized under the rubric of health-related quality of life (HRQL). According to the World Health Organization, this notion refers to the impact of treatments and disease processes on the overall satisfaction with life or, more specifically, with physical, emotional, and social functioning. A paradoxical outcome of medical treatments is that they often reduce morbidity or mortality but they do not always improve the quality of a person's everyday life. Therefore, improvements in physiologic condition or even physical function are not necessarily associated with improvements in HRQL.

Construct assessment

Overall quality of life and HRQL are assessed at a global level (i.e., with measures that tap overall life satisfaction), at the level of specific domains (i.e., with multidimensional measures that assess satisfaction with social relationships, physical health, etc.), or with measures specific to the unique conditions resulting from a certain disease (e.g., measures specific to arthritis, diabetes, or parkinsonism). A measure of global quality of life, the unidimensional Satisfaction with Life Scale, includes questions asking respondents whether or not they agree with the statement that "In most ways, my life is close to my ideal" or "If I could live my life over, I would change almost nothing." A popular multidimensional measure of quality of life, called SF-36, includes 36 items divided into the following eight scales:

1 Physical function;
2 Role limitations resulting from physical problems;
3 General health;
4 Bodily pain;
5 Social function;
6 Role limitations resulting from emotional problems;
7 Mental health; and
8 Vitality.

Role of exercise

A relatively small but growing research literature suggests that physical activity and regular exercise can lead to improvements in HRQL. Rejeski et al. (1996) were the first to undertake an extensive review of the literature on physical activity and HRQL. This review was updated recently (Rejeski & Mihalko 2001). Collectively, these reviews examined 45 studies of the relationship between physical activity and HRQL. The overall conclusion was that physical activity is *associated* with improvements in various aspects of HRQL, regardless of age, activity status,

or the health of the participants. Yet, Rejeski and Mihalko (2001) acknowledged that a confusing picture emerged when the latest randomized clinical trials were examined. Specifically, half of the studies reported an improvement in HRQL but the other half failed to show a beneficial effect compared to control or comparison treatments. Methodological differences, including varying activity prescriptions, appear to be the root of these disparities. Rejeski and Mihalko commented that there is "little hope of ever integrating extant research, because quality of life has no consistent meaning across studies."

Recently, Netz et al. (2005) conducted a meta-analysis on organized physical activity and well-being in older adults without clinical disorders. Although this meta-analysis did not examine HRQL per se, well-being was defined as a multifaceted construct, with emphasis on four general components closely related to HRQL:

1 Emotional well-being;
2 Self-perceptions;
3 Bodily well-being; and
4 Global perceptions, such as life-satisfaction.

Overall, the weighted mean effect size for the physical activity intervention groups (0.24) was almost three times larger than the mean for control groups (0.09). In terms of the constructs assessed, self-efficacy (0.38), overall well-being (0.37), and view of self (0.16) were all positively affected by physical activity and showed the largest treatment–control differences. The same significant difference, however, was not found for life satisfaction, depression, anger, and confusion. Moderator variables were examined, and aerobic exercise (0.29) and moderate intensity exercise (0.34) were found to be the most beneficial for improving well-being. Additional moderators included improvements in cardiovascular capacity (0.32), strength (0.20), and functional capacity (0.32). Overall, based on the findings of this analysis, there appears to be a significant relationship between physical activity and well-being enhancement in older adults. Netz et al. (2005) concluded that the small overall effect size could be a result of the fact that no samples with clinical disorders were included in this analysis.

Even though the weight of direct and indirect evidence available at this time supports a positive association between physical activity and HRQL, it should be kept in mind that this line of research is still in its infancy. Strong evidence for a causal relationship is lacking. Although it is plausible that physical activity could improve HRQL, particularly given its established role in preserving health and function, at this point it is also plausible that the observed positive association might be influenced by such factors as volunteerism or expectancy bias. Also, deciphering the influence of mediating and moderating variables is going to be a long and challenging process (Rejeski & Mihalko 2001). Such factors as optimism, health locus of control, hardiness, or the importance placed upon HRQL among different individuals might be influential but their role remains to be clarified.

Conclusions

Having completed this selective survey of the literature on the role of exercise and physical activity in several key components of psychological well-being, let us return to the issue raised in the introduction. At least some of the reasons behind the divergent assessments of the role of exercise are hopefully a little more apparent. On the one hand, there is a remarkable consistency in the evidence for a positive association between exercise and a broad range of components of well-being. Most meta-analyses and systematic reviews agree that there is at least a statistically reliable association and this is clearly not a finding that can be easily ignored. However, there is also the other side. First, most of the effects are small to medium in magnitude. Second, and most importantly, the quality of the evidence, for the most part, is not optimal. Authors both within and outside the exercise sciences have raised some serious concerns, which are highlighted here. Large-scale, randomized clinical trials are a recent development and even these are bound to face challenges. The fact that participants are volunteers and most psychological outcomes are self-reported and therefore subject to expectancy bias, in conjunction with the inability to implement a "placebo" exercise control, make it practically impossible to design a "definitive" exercise intervention study. Despite this, there are methodological steps that can bring future studies at least closer to this untenable ideal: randomization; blinding of outcome assessors; careful selection of outcome measures and protocols; adequate intervention and follow-up periods; and intention-to-treat analyses.

References

Arent, S.M., Landers, D.M. & Etnier, J.L. (2000) The effects of exercise on mood in older adults: A meta-analytic review. *Journal of Aging and Physical Activity* **8**, 407–430.

Babyak, M., Blumenthal, J.A., Herman, S., *et al.* (2000) Exercise treatment for major depression: Maintenance of therapeutic benefit at 10 months. *Psychosomatic Medicine* **62**, 633–638.

Biddle, S.J.H., Fox, K.R., Boutcher, S.H. & Faulkner, G.E. (2000) The way forward for physical activity and the promotion of psychological well-being. In: *Physical Activity and Psychological Well-being* (Biddle, S.J.H., Fox, K.R. & Boutcher S.H., eds.) Routledge, London: 154–168.

Blumenthal, J.A., Babyak, M.A., Moore, K.A., *et al.* (1999) Effects of exercise training on older patients with major depression. *Archives of Internal Medicine* **159**, 2349–2356.

Brosse, A.L., Sheets, E.S., Lett, H.S. & Blumenthal, J.A. (2002). Exercise and the treatment of clinical depression in adults. Recent findings and future directions. *Sports Medicine* **32**, 741–760.

Colcombe, S. & Kramer, A.F. (2003) Fitness effects on the cognitive function of older adults: A meta-analytic study. *Psychological Science* **14**, 125–130.

Craft, L.L. & Landers, D.M. (1998) The effect of exercise on clinical depression and depression resulting from mental illness: A meta-analysis. *Journal of Sport and Exercise Psychology* **20**, 339–357.

Donaghy, M.E. & Ussher, M.H. (2005) Exercise interventions in drug and alcohol rehabilitation. In: *Exercise, Health, and Mental Health: Emerging Relationships* (Faulkner, G.E.J. & Taylor, A.H., eds.) Routledge, London: 48–69.

Dunn, A.L., Trivedi, M.H., Kampert, J.B., Clark, C.G. & Chambliss, H.O. (2005) Exercise treatment for depression: Efficacy and dose–response. *American Journal of Preventive Medicine* **28**, 1–8.

Dunn, A.L., Trivedi, M.H. & O'Neal, H.A. (2001) Physical activity dose–response effects on outcomes of depression and anxiety. *Medicine and Science in Sports and Exercise* **33**, S587–S597.

Ekelund, E., Heian, F. & Hagen, K.B. (2005) Can exercise improve self-esteem in children and young people? A systematic review of randomized clinical trials. *British Journal of Sports Medicine* **39**, 792–798.

Ekkekakis, P. (2003) Pleasure and displeasure from the body: Perspectives from exercise. *Cognition and Emotion* **17**, 213–239.

Ekkekakis, P., Hall, E.E. & Petruzzello, S.J. (1999) Measuring state anxiety in the context of acute exercise using the State Anxiety Inventory: An attempt to resolve the brouhaha. *Journal of Sport and Exercise Psychology* **21**, 205–229.

Ekkekakis, P., Hall, E.E. & Petruzzello, S.J. (2005) Variation and homogeneity in affective responses to physical activity of varying intensities: An alternative perspective on dose–response based on evolutionary considerations. *Journal of Sports Sciences* **23**, 477–500.

Ekkekakis, P. & Petruzzello, S.J. (2000) Analysis of the affect measurement conundrum in exercise psychology: I. Fundamental issues. *Psychology of Sport and Exercise* **1**, 71–88.

Etnier, J.L., Salazar, W., Landers, D.M., Petruzzello, S.J., Han, M. & Nowell, P. (1997) The influence of physical fitness and exercise upon cognitive functioning: A meta-analysis. *Journal of Sport and Exercise Psychology* **19**, 249–274.

Etnier, J.L., Nowell, P.M., Landers, D.M. & Sibley, B.A. (2006) A meta-regression to examine the relationship between aerobic fitness and cognitive performance. *Brain Research Reviews* **52**, 119–130.

Fox, K.R. (2000) The effects of exercise on self-perceptions and self-esteem. In: *Physical Activity and Psychological Well-being* (Biddle, S.J.H., Fox, K.R. & Boutcher, S.H., eds.) Routledge, London: 88–117.

Hausenblas, H.A. & Fallon, E.A. (2006) Exercise and body image: A meta-analysis. *Psychology and Health* **21**, 33–47.

Hughes, J.R. (1984) Psychological effects of habitual aerobic exercise: A critical review. *Preventive Medicine* **13**, 66–78.

Kugler, J., Seelbach, H. & Krüskemper, G.M. (1994) Effects of rehabilitation exercise programmes on anxiety and depression in coronary patients: A meta-analysis. *British Journal of Clinical Psychology* **33**, 401–410.

Landers, D.M. & Arent, S.M. (2001) Physical activity and mental health. In: *Handbook of Sport Psychology*, 2nd edn. (Singer, R.N., Hausenblas, H.A. & Janelle, C.M., eds.) John Wiley and Sons, New York: 740–765.

Landers, D.M. & Arent, S.M. (2007) Physical activity and mental health. In: *Handbook of Sport Psychology*, 3rd edn. (Tenenbaum, G. & Eklund, R.C., eds.) John Wiley and Sons, New York.

Landers, D.M. & Petruzzello, S.J. (1994) Physical activity, fitness, and anxiety. In: *Physical Activity, Fitness, and Health:*

International Proceedings and Consensus Statement (Bouchard, C., Shephard, R.J. & Stephens T., eds.) Human Kinetics. Champaign, IL: 868–882.

Lawlor, D.A. & Hopker, S.W. (2001) The effectiveness of exercise as an intervention in the management of depression: Systematic review and meta-regression analysis of randomised control trials. *British Medical Journal* **322**, 1–8.

Long, B.C. & van Stavel, R. (1995) Effects of exercise training on anxiety: A meta-analysis. *Journal of Applied Sport Psychology* **7**, 167–189.

McDonald, D.G. & Hodgdon, J.A. (1991) *The Psychological Effects of Aerobic Fitness Training: Research and Theory.* Springer Verlag, New York.

Meeusen, R. (2006) Physical activity and neurotransmitter release. In: *Psychobiology of Physical Activity* (Acevedo, E.O. & Ekkekakis, P., eds.) Human Kinetics, Champaign, IL: 129–143.

Morgan, W.P. (1981) Psychological benefits of physical activity. In: *Exercise in Health and Disease* (Nagle, F.J. & Montoye, H.J., eds.) Charles C. Thomas, Springfield, IL: 299–314.

Netz, Y., Wu, M.J., Becker, B.J. & Tenenbaum, G. (2005) Physical activity and psychological well-being in advanced age: A meta-analysis of intervention studies. *Psychology and Aging* **20**, 272–284.

North, T.C., McCullagh, P. & Tran, Z.V. (1990) Effect of exercise on depression. *Exercise and Sport Science Reviews* **18**, 379–415.

Petruzzello, S.J., Landers, D.M., Hatfield, B.D., Kubitz, K.A. & Salazar, W. (1991) A meta-analysis on the anxiety-reducing effects of acute and chronic exercise. *Sports Medicine* **11**, 143–182.

Reed, J. & Ones, D.S. (2006) The effect of acute aerobic exercise on positive activated affect: A meta-analysis. *Psychology of Sport and Exercise* **7**, 477–514.

Rejeski, W.J., Brawley, L.R. & Shumaker, S.A. (1996) Physical activity and health-related quality of life. *Exercise and Sport Sciences Reviews* **24**, 71–108.

Rejeski, W.J. & Mihalko, S.L. (2001) Physical activity and quality of life in older adults. *Journals of Gerontology* **56**, 23–35.

Salmon, P. (2001) Effects of physical exercise on anxiety, depression, and sensitivity to stress: A unifying theory. *Clinical Psychology Review* **21**, 33–61.

Schlicht, W. (1994) Does physical exercise reduce anxious emotions? A meta-analysis. *Anxiety, Stress, and Coping* **6**, 275–288.

Scully, D., Kremer, J., Meade, M.M., Graham, R. & Dudgeon, K. (1998) Physical exercise and psychological well-being: A critical review. *British Journal of Sports Medicine* **32**, 111–120.

Sibley, B.A. & Etnier, J.L. (2003) The relationship between physical activity and cognition in children: A meta-analysis. *Pediatric Exercise Science* **15**, 243–256.

Sothmann, M.S. (2006) The cross-stressor adaptation hypothesis and exercise training. In: *Psychobiology of Physical Activity* (Acevedo, E.O. & Ekkekakis, P., eds.) Human Kinetics, Champaign, IL: 149–160.

Spence, J.C., McGannon, K.R. & Poon, P. (2005) The effect of exercise on global self-esteem: A quantitative review. *Journal of Sport and Exercise Psychology* **27**, 311–334.

US Department of Health and Human Services (1996) *Physical Activity and Health: A report of the Surgeon General.* US Department of Health and Human Services, Centers for Disease Control and Prevention, National Center for Chronic Disease Prevention and Health Promotion, Atlanta, GA.

US Department of Health and Human Services (1999) *Mental Health: A report of the Surgeon General.*, US Department of Health and Human Services Substance Abuse and Mental Health Services Administration, Center for Mental Health Services, National Institutes of Health, National Institute of Mental Health, Rockville, MD.

van Praag, H. (2006) Exercise, neurogenesis, and learning in rodents. In: *Psychobiology of Physical Activity* (Acevedo, E.O. & Ekkekakis, P., eds.) Human Kinetics, Champaign, IL: 61–73.

Youngstedt, S.D. & Freelove-Charton, J.D. (2005) Exercise and sleep. In: *Exercise, Health, and Mental Health: Emerging Relationships* (Faulkner, G.E.J. & Taylor, A.H., eds.) Routledge, London: 159–189.

Chapter 17

Psychological Characteristics of Athletes and their Responses to Sport-Related Stressors

JOHN S. RAGLIN AND GREGORY WILSON

The notion that psychological factors play a role in sport performance is not new; over a century ago Dudley (1888) stated that the difference between winning or losing in sport often depends on the "mental qualities" of athletes. Only recently, however, has the impact of psychology been examined through controlled experimentation. Although this work has revealed an association between selected psychological variables and athleticism, some research has yielded contradictory results. More perplexing are studies indicating that under specific circumstances negative emotions such as anxiety paradoxically exert beneficial effects on performance, an observation that calls into question the uniform application of stress-reducing techniques such as relaxation by sport psychologists.

This chapter will summarize findings regarding the psychological characteristics that occur in athletes at the group (i.e., nomothetic) and individual (i.e., ideographic) level, as well as results comparing the psychological profiles of successful and unsuccessful competitors. Research will also be presented describing the psychological consequences of sport-related stressors that occur: (i) during training; (ii) before competition, and (iii) during competition, and their impact on performance. Methodological and theoretical issues will be discussed in an attempt to rectify conflicting conclusions where findings have been contested within the field

of sport psychology. Because many of the psychological concepts employed in this chapter (e.g., personality) are used in a variety of contexts and meanings in everyday language, standard definitions established within academic psychology will be provided.

Personality characteristics and athletic performance

Psychologists have defined personality traits as "relatively enduring differences among people in specifiable tendencies to perceive the world in a certain way and in dispositions to react or behave in a specified manner with predictable regularity" (Spielberger *et al.* 1983), and the link between personality traits and sport performance is one of the oldest topics in sport psychology. While most coaches and athletes have long believed that an athlete's personality plays at least some role in sporting success, the empirical evidence for this relationship has at times been conflicting and hotly debated.

Research into the association between personality traits and athleticism began in earnest in the 1960s, and by the end of the decade the first summaries of the empirical literature appeared. These reviews concluded that athletes did indeed differ psychologically from non-athletes. Specifically, it was found that athletes were typically more extroverted and less neurotic than non-athletes, with the exception of some individual sports (e.g., pistol shooting) where introversion was a more common trait (Warburton & Kane, 1966; Cooper 1969). Little evidence was found for other sport-specific personality profiles. A problem of much of this early research, however, was

The Olympic Textbook of Science in Sport, 1st edition. Edited by R.J. Maughan. Published 2009 by Blackwell Publishing. ISBN: 978-1-4051-5638-7.

that it was cross-sectional and precluded tests to determine whether the psychological characteristics of athletes were innate or a consequence of sport participation. As a result, some researches employed longitudinal designs where participants completed psychological questionnaires before and following their initial involvement in organized sport. The findings of this work reveal that the unique personality characteristics found in athletes are present prior to involvement in sport and do not emerge as a consequence of participation. These results imply that specific psychological factors such as extroversion may predispose individuals to become physically active or to participate in sports, and conversely the absence of these traits could work to deter sport participation.

Reviews published the following decade, however, often reached very different conclusions, declaring either that personality traits exerted little or no impact on athletic performance (Rushall 1970), or that the influence of personality could not be ascertained until appropriate sport-specific psychological questionnaires were developed (Martens 1975). These antithetical perspectives on personality and athleticism were rectified in landmark reviews by William Morgan (1978, 1980) who noted that most of the research rejecting the role of personality in sport was marred by one or more methodological flaws that could have resulted in null findings. Many of these problems centered on the inappropriate use of psychological questionnaires, including the misinterpretation of the theories underlying these measures or the data yielded by them. A specific concern common to many studies was the failure to test for response distortion, a phenomenon whereby individuals fake their responses to psychological questionnaires, most often in a uniformly positive manner. Cases of response distortion can be detected by using so-called "lie scales" and the failure to do so can result in accepting falsified data that could invalidate findings. In examining studies that carefully controlled for this and other experimental containments, Morgan concluded that athletes did indeed exhibit unique personality traits when compared with the published norms for non-athletes, although these differences were sometimes found to be small (Eysenck *et al.* 1982).

These findings were further developed by Morgan (1985) in a subsequent review summarizing results from his own studies and related work by others. These studies assessed personality traits and other psychological variables in Olympic and collegiate athletes and then determined the accuracy by which psychological information alone could identify successful and unsuccessful competitors. With some exceptions, it was found that 70–85% of athletes could be correctly identified as either successful or unsuccessful (e.g., making an Olympic squad or not), a range of accuracy that was statistically better than chance levels of prediction. As the case with the earliest reviews, successful athletes tended to be more extroverted and emotionally stable than their less successful competitors, but Morgan concluded that the more crucial factor in athletic success was the absence of pronounced introversion rather than the presence of extroversion. Among the most consistent findings were results based on the Profile of Mood States (POMS; McNair *et al.* 1992) – a 65-item Likert format questionnaire that yields measures of general and specific moods. POMS data indicated that successful athletes in a variety of sports scored significantly lower than the published norms for undesirable mood factors (i.e., tension, depression, anger, fatigue and confusion) and higher in the desirable mood state of vigor compared to unsuccessful athletes. This was labeled the "Iceberg Profile" because of the unique pattern these scores form (Morgan 1985; Fig. 17.1).

On the basis of these and similar results yielded by others, Morgan (1985) developed a 'Mental Health Model' of sport performance that posited the existence of a negative relationship between psychopathology and athletic capability. The model predicts that athletes who are depressed, anxious, or possess other forms of mental illness would be less successful than individuals with average or above-average mental health. Support for the Mental Health Model has also been found in other carefully conducted research that utilized valid psychological measures (Mahoney 1989; Vanden Auweele *et al.* 1993) and tested for cases of response distortion (Newcombe & Boyle 1995). Moreover, the desirable psychological characteristics associated with success have been found to be quite stable over time. Morgan and

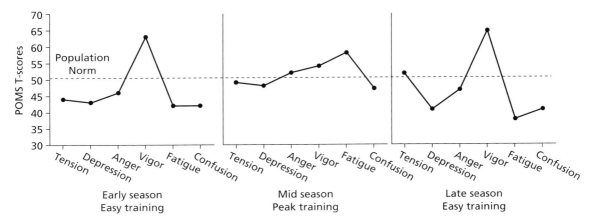

Fig. 17.1 Profile of mood states (POMS) T-scores at three training phases in 35 female and male collegiate swimmers. (Adapted with permission from Raglin 1993.)

Costill (1996) conducted a longitudinal study with a sample of elite long-distance runners and found remarkably little deviation in the athletes' positive mood profiles over a 20-year period.

Despite the predictive efficacy of the Mental Health Model, Morgan (1985) cautioned against using it to choose individuals for athletic competition. Predictions based on the model typically result in misclassifications (i.e., false positives and negatives), and some athletes possess intermediate psychological profiles that preclude categorization as either successful or unsuccessful. Furthermore, the level of accuracy achieved with mental health model research is not in itself sufficient to select athletes for teams or competitions, and there is no evidence that other psychological identification strategies are any more precise (Raglin 2001). Nonetheless, the findings of this research do have practical implications for athletes. The field of sports medicine has long focused the bulk of its resources and efforts toward maintaining the physical health of the athlete with little attention to emotional health, despite the fact that athletes suffer from psychological disorders at a similar rate to the general population. Because the findings of the mental health model demonstrate that psychopathology has a significant impact on the playing field, it is imperative that mental health services be made available to athletes, whether out of a humanitarian concern for their general welfare or for the specific goal of optimizing performance.

Motivational characteristics of athletes

Motivation is a psychological topic of obvious interest to any coach concerned with getting the utmost out of an athlete. However, insight into its role in sport has been clouded by the use of widely divergent definitions and models of motivation as well as the availability of a dizzying number of motivational questionnaires, many of which have not been properly validated. In its broadest sense, motivation is commonly defined as the effort with which a person works towards achieving goals. For instance, Sage (1977) defined this concept as the direction and intensity of one's efforts, while Ryan and Deci (2000) stated motivation to be the energy, direction, and persistence of an individual's actions. Early researchers on this topic believed that humans are motivated primarily by efforts to seek pleasure and to avoid pain (Thorndike 1935). McClelland and colleagues (1953) furthered this concept by developing the McClelland–Atkinson model of motivation based on two central principles: internal motivation and fear of failure. The first principle refers to the extent to which an individual desires to achieve success, while the latter reflects the degree to which fear of failure affects an individual's decision to participate in an activity or not. McClelland (1961) further proposed that motivation consists of five components (i.e., personality factors, situational factors, resultant tendencies, emotional reactions, and achievement-related behaviors). According to this view, known as "Need Achievement Theory," it is through the interaction of these variables that the motivational level within the individual is determined. However, because of concerns about the appropriateness of general theories of motivation in the context of athletics as well as findings that suggest that the putative mechanisms of motivation may differ from athlete to athlete, researchers have developed theories of motivation specific to the context of sport and physical activity.

Sport and exercise-based theories of motivation

Harter (1981) attempted to explain motivation in terms of an individual's perceptions of self-worth, and her work was among the earliest to describe motivation in terms of physical appearance and competence. According to Harter's Competence Motivation Theory, humans are motivated to feel "worthy" and "competent" and to seek out environments in which these feelings can be attained, while avoiding situations that make one feel incompetent. Among general theories of motivation, Weiner's Attribution Theory has been widely applied to the context of sport (Weiner 1986). It purports that the multifaceted variables that influence motivation can be categorized in one of three domains: stability, locus of causality, and locus of control. According to this view a factor is considered stable if it is attributed to such permanent states as talent, while unstable if attributed to a temporary factor such as "good luck." Locus of causality can be either an external or an internal motivational influence, while locus of control refers to whether or not the factor is something over which the individual can exert control.

Recently, Duda and Hall (2001) have proposed that three interrelated factors act to determine individual levels of motivation. The Achievement Goal Theory contends that achievement goals, the perceived ability to attain these goals, and achievement

behavior (e.g., effort, persistence) interact to determine what success and failure mean to an individual, and thus the level of motivation. In some cases athletes are motivated to succeed through being rewarded for their efforts. Extrinsic motivation is typified by the desire for approval from others, or receiving awards and recognitions for success. However, Foster and Walker (2005) have contended that an athlete that becomes over-reliant on extrinsic motivation may experience several negative outcomes, including the loss of self-worth, in part because athletic prowess has become their primary source of self-esteem. In efforts to gain approval from their coach, the athlete may become injured or burned-out through excessive training. On the other hand, intrinsic motivation is typified by an athlete that performs an action for the pure enjoyment of it, without the primary urge to obtain external rewards (Foster & Walker 2005). While both extrinsic and intrinsic motivation may exert a salient influence, it is believed that the enduring positive impact of intrinsic motivation on sport performance holds the greatest benefit for athletes.

Motivational differences have been found in relation to levels of athletic performance. For example, LeUnes and Nation (2001) reported that athletes with greater ability appear to have more internalized motivational traits than those with average abilities. Similarly, Butt and Cox (1992) conducted an investigation that examined motivational patterns in tennis players of differing ability levels. The participants in the study were categorized into three groups based on ability: elite players of Davis Cup calibre, a university competitive tennis team, and recreational tennis players. Results revealed significantly different levels of ambition, aggression, competence, and competition between the groups, with the elite athletes exhibiting the highest scores with all variables. Similarly, Sloan and Wiggins (2001) reported that professional American football players exhibited significantly higher levels of both intrinsic and extrinsic motivation than collegiate American football players. Experience can also exert a significant role in motivational patterns. In a study of elite young soccer players, Stewart (2004) examined the roles of playing position and age on motivation. While no significant findings were reported for position, the older players were more motivated to avoid failure and were less prone to place their locus of control on external sources. The younger players had a greater external locus of control and appeared to be less afraid of failure situations.

Unfortunately, some athletes develop what is termed "amotivation," a state experienced by people who feel powerless to produce a desired result through their own efforts. Ryan and Decci (2000) suggested that amotivated athletes exhibit signs of distraction and appear uninvolved or disengaged from their sport, and that they feel no sense of control and believe it is impossible to positively alter their situation. Amotivated athletes typically can no longer find a good reason to continue participating in sport and will soon abandon their attempts (Foster & Walker 2005). Sport psychologists have advocated a variety of behavioral techniques to prevent amotivation as well as enhance motivation, but simpler approaches can often be very effective. The legendary Indiana University swim coach James "Doc" Counsilman once wrote: "Only if a swimmer is motivated properly will he be able to achieve physical conditioning" (Counsilman 1977). He also stressed the importance of structuring a practice environment that made the swimmer look forward to daily practice sessions rather than dreading each day's workout. Counsilman indicated that he motivated swimmers through enthusiasm, interest, and personal attention to their performances. One of the most successful motivational techniques employed was his annual "jellybean day," where swimmers could win small bags of candy by successfully completing a particularly grueling workout. The event soon became so popular that these training sessions drew an audience of several hundred enthusiastic students and faculty. Through these personal and environmental strategies, Counsilman believed that he was able to maintain high motivational levels in his swimmers, while also coaxing them to exert their utmost effort.

Psychological responses to the stress of athletic training: mood state, overload training, and the staleness syndrome

In some of the early mental health model studies it was found that differences in mood state profiles between successful and unsuccessful endurance athletes were most pronounced during or immediately following intensive training (Raglin 2001). This suggests that athletes with similar personality profiles may exhibit very different psychological responses to the stress of training, which in turn may have consequences for performance. The implications of these findings have taken on greater significance as it has now become the norm for endurance and non-endurance sports alike to incorporate periods of intense overload training with the goal of optimizing athletic condition. Most athletes are able to tolerate the stress of overload training and, following an appropriate reduction in training or taper, will exhibit modest (e.g., 2–4%) improvements in performance. But some athletes show little benefit and ominously, between 10 and 20% respond adversely and experience decrements in performance. This condition, labeled "overtraining syndrome" or "staleness" (Kuipers & Keizer 1988; Raglin & Wilson 2000), occurs when an athlete experiences a chronic drop in the capacity to train and compete at customary levels as a direct result of overload training. Staleness is commonly accompanied by infectious disorders, clinical depression, and other mood disturbances, as well as a host of less frequent symptoms (Kuipers & Keizer 1988; Raglin & Wilson 2000).

There is no single accepted treatment for staleness but affected athletes are generally advised to stop training for a period of weeks if not longer. Medical and psychological treatment is often required, yet even following successful recovery there is evidence that these individuals will be at an increased risk of relapse. Among college varsity swimmers it has been found that 91% who developed staleness their first season of collegiate competition became stale in one or more of the following three competition seasons, whereas the rate was only 34% among swimmers who did not become stale during their first season (Raglin 1993). A study of Swedish junior elite skiers found that 35% who developed staleness during their first competitive high school season became stale at least once the following two years of training, a rate higher than chance (Raglin & Kenttä 2005).

The efficacy of various putative markers of staleness has been reviewed extensively, and psychological changes have often been found to be more sensitive than physiological indicators of stress, such as cortisol (O'Connor 1997). Most of the psychological research on overload training has utilized the POMS (McNair *et al.* 1993). The standard instructions of the POMS yield somewhat stable (0.45–0.74) measures of mood that can fluctuate in response to significant stressors, making it appropriate for assessing the psychological responses to intensive physical training. Findings from POMS research indicate that mood state is consistently altered as a consequence of training load (Raglin & Wilson 2000): as training loads are raised there is a proportional increase in scores for global mood disturbance and negative mood states (and a decrease in the positive factor of vigor) with disturbances reaching their greatest intensity at the peak of training. Conversely, as training is reduced, mood disturbances decrease in magnitude, and by the end of the training season mood state scores typically do not differ from the desirable pre-season values. This dose-response relationship between training load and mood disturbance has been observed both in endurance and non-endurance sports where training loads are periodized (Raglin & Wilson 2000), and mood responses rarely differ between male and female athletes who undergo similar training regimens (O'Connor 1997; Raglin & Wilson 2000). An example of typical POMS profiles at three discrete phases of training is presented in Fig. 17.2.

Not all training cycles are implemented gradually, and so the psychological responses to rapid increases in training load imposed over a period of days have also been studied. In this case the administration of the POMS is modified so that athletes complete the questionnaire according to how they are feeling "today" or "right now." The result is a more transient or "state" measure of mood that is responsive to acute stressors experienced within the course of a single day. The findings of this work indicate that significant mood disturbances can occur following as few as two days of increased training (Raglin & Wilson 2000).

During periods of intensive training total it has been found that mood disturbance scores are consistently highest in those athletes with performance decrements indicative of staleness. Stale athletes also exhibit a unique pattern of mood disturbances. Data comparing the mood state responses in healthy and stale collegiate swimmers indicate that the most pronounced changes in mood state factors following overload training occur in the traits of vigor and fatigue for healthy athletes who do not develop staleness, with the smallest change occurring in depression. In contrast, swimmers who develop staleness exhibit larger shifts in each of the POMS variables factors but, most notably, depression exhibits the greatest increase of any specific mood state (Raglin & Wilson 2000).

The previous findings have led some researcher to propose that mood state monitoring might provide a practical means of reducing the risk of staleness for athletes who must undergo intensive overload training, and some research had been conducted to examine the efficacy of the POMS in this capacity. Berglund and Säfstrom (1994) administered the POMS repeatedly to a sample of elite race canoeists during the training season before an Olympic competition. Training loads were decreased in cases when an athlete's total mood state score was excessive high compared to a baseline established off-season. It was also assumed that a comparatively low levels of mood disturbance indicated that training was insufficient and so the load was increased in such an event. The majority of the sample (64%) needed to have their training loads altered on the basis of mood scores, but unexpectedly over half

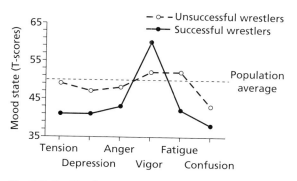

Fig. 17.2 Profile of mood states (POMS) T-scores for successful and unsuccessful candidates of the 1976 US Men's Olympic freestyle wrestling team. (Adapted with permission from Morgan 1985.)

(57%) also had training increased at some point because of positive mood. None of the athletes developed staleness and the authors attributed this directly to the intervention paradigm.

Additional research of this type incorporating appropriate control conditions as well as relevant physiological information will be needed before psychological assessments can be used routinely in efforts to avoid staleness. However, the findings of mood monitoring studies of overload training support the efficacy of applying evidence-based psychological applications to address complex issues in sport.

Psychological responses to the stress of athletic competition: pre-competition anxiety

Psychologists define anxiety as an emotional reaction to a situation or stimulus perceived to be threatening or dangerous (Spielberger 1972), and it is not surprising that the stress of sport competition often results in large increases in anxiety and other negative emotions. In the field of sport psychology it has been a long-standing belief that performance will invariably suffer as anxiety begins to reach high intensities (Oxendine 1970), but some sport psychologists regard even minor elevations to be harmful. These assumptions are largely derived from the inverted-U hypothesis (Yerkes & Dodson 1908), a theoretical paradigm that has exerted more influence on the field of sport psychology than any other. Based on applications of this hypothesis to sport, optimal performance should be most likely to occur when anxiety is within a moderate range of intensity. As anxiety begins to exceed or fall below the moderate range, performance will progressively worsen. It is further predicted that athletes competing in events involving gross motor activities requiring strength and speed (e.g., shot put, football) will perform better at a higher but still moderate levels of anxiety compared to athletic tasks that require fine muscle movements, steadiness, coordination, and general concentration (e.g., golf, archery; Oxendine 1970). It is also assumed that as athletes develop in both motor skill expertise and experience, the optimal level of anxiety will increase in parallel, with highly skilled individuals benefiting from anxiety intensities that would debilitate those with less ability.

Despite the intuitive appeal and widespread acceptance of the inverted-U hypothesis and its sport modifications, there has been an absence of compelling empirical support (Fazey & Hardy 1988). Instead it has been found that the role of anxiety is far more complex and individualized, with many athletes performing optimally at high anxiety intensities (Raglin 1992). Such findings have spurred the development of sport-specific and individualized theories that conceptualize anxiety as having harmful or beneficial consequences depending on the athlete and the competitive situation. Among them, one of the most intuitively appealing and empirically grounded is the Individual Zones of Optimal Functioning (IZOF) model developed by the Russian psychologist, Juri Hanin (1986, 1997). According to the IZOF model the optimal intensity of anxiety is highly variable across athletes, and may range from very low to extremely high. Another distinction of the IZOF model from the inverted-U hypothesis and other traditional perspectives, is that it contends that the level of optimal anxiety is not reliably influenced by either the sport task or skill level of the athlete (Raglin & Hanin 2000). As a consequence, it predicts that among similarly skilled athletes competing in the same event, a substantial percentage will perform best when anxiety is actually high. In fact there is substantial support for this prediction. IZOF research involving athletes in a number of different sports and skill levels has demonstrated that between 30 and 45% perform best when anxiety is high, a finding that has been observed in athletes as young as nine years old (Wilson & Raglin 1997; Raglin & Hanin 2000).

Determining the optimal anxiety zone

In early IZOF research the optimal zone of athletes was determined by assessing state anxiety approximately one-hour prior to the actual competitions using validated anxiety questionnaires such as the State-Trait Anxiety Inventory (Spielberger et al. 1983) until an outstanding or best performance occurred. According to procedures described by Hanin (1986), the optimal zone was established by adding and subtracting four anxiety units (approximately half a standard deviation) to the anxiety score obtained for the outstanding performance. However, the logistical challenges of following an athlete throughout a competitive season can make this method impractical, and repeatedly completing questionnaires prior to competitions can become intrusive and distracting (Raglin & Hanin 2000). In response to these problems Hanin (1986) developed a retrospective method for assessing the IZOF where athletes fill out anxiety questionnaires in non-competition settings according to how they remember feeling immediately before their best past performance. The derived scores are treated as optimal and again four anxiety units are added and subtracted to yield the optimal zone. Research using the retrospective method to establish optimal anxiety zones indicates that athletes are quite accurate in recalling anxiety levels of past performances. More importantly, it has been found that sport performance was significantly better in cases where pre-competition anxiety was within the optimal zone obtained with the recall technique than when anxiety either exceeded or fell below the optimal zone (Raglin & Hanin 2000).

Hanin (2000) has more recently extended the IZOF model to include other emotions beyond anxiety and has also developed questionnaires that allow athletes to identify how their own optimal emotional state can change during a performance. The findings of this and other related work support the use of ideographic models in the consequences of competition-related stressors whereby the influence of emotions experienced before and during competition on sport performance is determined on an individual basis. They also indicate that the common practice by many sport psychologists of routinely reducing anxiety prior to a competition in the effort of enhancing performance is likely to be counterproductive for a significant proportion of athletes. However, before implementing any anxiety regulation technique with the goal of enhancing performance it is crucial to determine the root cause of the athlete's anxiety. In some cases elevations in anxiety assumed to be associated with the stress of competition are in fact be a symptom of an underlying psychological or medical condition.

Cognitive strategies during the stress of endurance events: association and dissociation

The stress and discomfort of athletic competition is rarely as intense as during competitive endurance events such as distance running or cycling, and psychological research on endurance sports indicates that athletes employ very different psychological strategies to deal with this discomfort in practice and competition. Elite male and female distance runners have been found to utilize a cognitive strategy during competition in which they deliberately focus their attention on physiological sensations of exertion including pain, muscular fatigue, thirst, body temperature, and respiration (Morgan & Pollock 1977). Athletes using this strategy, known as "association," report using it to gauge their current state of performance and to make decisions whether to increase or decrease their pace. In other words, these individuals are actively and continuously engaging their sense of perception of effort to optimize efficiency and pace throughout the sporting event (Morgan 1981).

In contrast, it has been found that non-elite athletes typically adopt a very different cognitive strategy during competition known as "dissociation" (Morgan & Pollock 1977). Rather than closely monitoring internal feedback, these athletes use a variety of means to purposefully distract themselves from the discomfort of intense physical exertion. Morgan (1997) has found individuals to report using such exotic examples of dissociation as performing complicated mathematical calculations, reliving past experiences, or mentally designing and building a house, all done to distract themselves from or diminish the painful sensations of vigorous physical effort. Another form of dissociation is to utilize a pre-race strategy, such as following the pace of another runner, irrespective of one's own sense of perceived exertion. In this case an athlete utilizing this form of dissociation would stay with a predetermined pace or strategy despite the sensation that the work is either too hard or easy to maintain.

Although there is evidence that dissociation can actually prolong the time to exhaustion in steady-state treadmill running (Morgan 1997), in actual sporting events it more commonly results in sub-par performance. For example, Stevinson and Biddle (1998) found that recreational marathoners who used a dissociative strategy during a race were more likely to "hit the wall" as a result of ignoring intrinsic information related to pace and hydration. Elite athletes, however, do not exclusively use association strategies in all situations. Research with Olympic distance runners has found that approximately 50% report using some form of dissociation during training, whereas none relied on this strategy during competition (Morgan 1997). Morgan and Pollock (1977) further noted that athletes differ in the degree to which they accurately monitor bodily feedback during physical activity. They found that non-elite distance runners tended to underrate physical exertion during treadmill running compared to World Class distance runners who underwent the same protocol. Similarly, in a study of wrestlers competing for positions on the US Olympic freestyle team, Nagle *et al.* (1975) reported that unsuccessful competitors exhibited higher exercise heart rates during standardized exercise tests compared with wrestlers who successfully made the team. Despite this indication that the unsuccessful wrestlers were less physically fit, the perceived exertion ratings did not differ between the successful and unsuccessful groups. Based on these findings, Morgan (1997) has theorized that elite athletes are more likely to use association on a routine basis, and not simply during competition. O'Connor (1992) has proposed that such differences may be attributed to the fact that elite athletes associate because they can afford to monitor bodily signals, partly as a result of their higher level of pain tolerance. There is evidence that pain tolerance is greater for athletes than non-athletes, and in elite than in non-elite competitors (O'Connor 1992). Hence, it may be that repeated exposure to pain during intense training may influence individual perceptions of discomfort.

Summary

There has been considerable interest in identifying personality traits and other psychological factors associated with athleticism. Carefully conducted personality research has shown that several traits are consistently associated with success in a variety of sports at the group (i.e., nomothetic) level. Although the level of accuracy yielded by this research is insufficient for the purpose of selecting athletes for competition, the findings underscore the fundamental influence of mental health on sport performance. Research on the psychological responses to sport training indicates that athletes who initially possess positive psychological profiles will routinely experience mood disturbances when exposed to intense overload training. Not all athletes successfully tolerate this stress and 10% or more will develop the staleness syndrome, a condition that results in chronically worsened performance and clinical depression.

Other stresses associated with sport influence have psychological consequences for athletes, but these changes are even more individualized (i.e., ideographic). Athletes can be motivated by both internal and external factors, and for some individuals the stress of training and competition can lead to amotivation. The stress of competition also affects athletes differently, with some exhibiting very high anxiety levels, whereas it appears to have little emotional impact on others. More importantly, the effect of anxiety on sport performance is quite variable. The results of research based on the IZOF model reveals that between 30 and 45% of athletes actually benefit from high anxiety, independent of their sport, age, or skill level. These and other findings raise concerns with the common practice in sport psychology of administering a single psychological technique (e.g., relaxation) to an entire team or group of athletes in an attempt to enhance performance. Instead they indicate that the influence of psychology on sport performance must be considered at both team and individual level. Moreover, in the quest to optimize an athlete's performance it is simplistic and inappropriate to focus exclusively on the mental as it is the physical, a perspective expressed many years ago by the pioneering American sport psychologist, Coleman Roberts Griffith, who said: "The athlete, at work and at play constitutes a fine laboratory for the study of vexing physiological and psychological problems, many of which are distorted by the attempt to reduce them to simpler terms" (Griffith 1929). The complex interplay of the mind and body found in athletics truly requires an inclusive psychobiologic inquiry that unites psychologists and physiologists.

References

Berglund, B. & Säfström, H. (1994) Psychological monitoring and modulation of training load of world-class canoeists. *Medicine and Science in Exercise and Sport* **26**, 1036–1040.

Butt, D.S. & Cox, D.N. (1992) Motivational patterns in Davis Cup, university and recreational tennis players. *International Journal of Sport Psychology* **23**, 1–13.

Cooper, L. (1969) Athletics, activity and personality: a review of the literature. *Research Quarterly* **40**, 17–22.

Counsilman, J.E. (1977) *Competitive Swimming Manual for Coaches and Swimmers* Counsilman Co., Inc. Bloomington, Indiana: 266–273.

Duda, J.L. & Hall, H. (2001) Achievement goal theory in sport: Recent extensions and future directions. In: *Handbook of sport psychology*, 2nd edn. (Singer, R., Hausenblas, H. & Janelle, C., eds.) Wiley, New York: 417–443.

Dudley, A.T. (1888) The mental qualities of an athlete. *Harvard Alumni Magazine* **6**, 43–51.

Eysenck, H.J., Nias, K.B.D. & Cox, D.N. (1982) Personality and Sport. *Advances in Behavioral Research and Therapy* **1**, 1–56.

Fazey, J. & Hardy, L. (1988) *The inverted-U hypothesis: A catastrophe for sport psychology?* (BASS Monograph 1) White Line Press, Leeds, UK.

Foster, S. & Walker, B. (2005) Motivation. In: *Applying Sport Psychology; Four Perspectives* (Taylor, J. & Wilson, G.S., eds.) Human Kinetics, Champaign: 3–19.

Griffith, C.R. (1929) *The Psychology of Coaching* Charles Scribner's Sons, New York.

Hanin, Y.L. (1986) State-trait anxiety research in the USSR. In: *Cross Cultural Anxiety*, vol. 3 (Spielberger, C.D. & Diaz-Guerrero, R., eds.) Hemisphere, Washington D.C.: 45–54.

Hanin, Y.L. (1997) Emotions and athletic performance. Individual zones of optimal functioning model. In: *European Yearbook on Sport Psychology*, vol. 1 (Seiler, R., ed.) FEBSAC, Sank Augustin, Germany: 30–70.

Hanin, Y.L. (2000) *Emotions in Sport* Human Kinetics, Champaign.

Harter, S. (1981) A model of intrinsic mastery motivation in children: Individual differences and developmental change. In: *Minnesota Symposium on Child Psychology*, vol. 14 (Collins, W.A., ed.) Erlbaum, Hillsdale, New Jersey: 215–255.

Kuipers, H. & Keizer, H.A. (1988) Overtraining in elite athletes: review and directions for the future. *Sports Medicine* **6**, 79–92.

LeUnes, A. & Nation, J.R. (2002) *Sport Psychology*, 3rd edn Pacific Wadsworth, Grove, CA.

Mahoney, M.J. (1989) Psychological predictors of elite and non-elite performance in Olympic weight lifting. *International Journal of Sport Psychology* **20**, 1–12.

Martens, R. (1975) The paradigmatic crisis in American sport personology. *Sportwissenschaft* **5**, 9–24.

McClelland, D.C. (1961) *The Achieving Society* Free Press, New York.

McClelland, D.C., Atkinson, J.W., Clark, R.W. & Lowell, E.L. (1953) *The Achievement Motive* Appleton-Century-Crofts, New York.

McNair, D.M., Lorr, M. & Dropplemann, L.F. (1992) *Profile of Mood States Manual* Educational and Testing Service, San Diego, California.

Morgan, W.P. (1978) The credulous-skeptical argument in perspective. In: *An Analysis of Athlete Behavior* (Straub, W.F., ed.) Movement Publications, Ithaca, New York: 218–227.

Morgan, W.P. (1980) The trait psychology controversy. *Research Quarterly for Exercise and Sport* **51**, 50–76.

Morgan, W.P. (1981) Psychophysiology of self-awareness during vigorous physical activity. *Research Quarterly for Exercise and Sport* **52**, 385–427.

Morgan, W.P. (1985) Selected psychological factors limiting performance: a mental health model. In: *Limits of Human Performance* (Clarke, D.H. & Eckert, H.M., eds.) Human Kinetics, Champaign: 70–80.

Morgan, W.P. (1997) Mind games: The psychology of sport. In: *Optimizing Sport Performance: Perspectives in Exercise and Sports Medicine*, vol. 10 (Lamb, D.R. & Murray, R., eds.) Cooper Publications, Carmel, Indiana: 1–54.

Morgan, W.P. & Costill, D.L. (1996) Selected psychological characteristics and health behaviors of aging marathon runners: a longitudinal study. *International Journal of Sports Medicine* **17**, 305–313.

Morgan, W.P. & Pollock, M.L. (1977) Psychological characterization of the elite distance runner. *Annals of the New York Academy of Sciences* **301**, 382–403.

Nagle, F.J., Morgan, W.P., Hellickson, R.O., Serfas, R.C. & Alexander, J.C. (1975) Spotting success traits in Olympic contenders. *The Physician and Sports Medicine* **3**, 3–34.

Newcombe, P.A. & Boyle, G.A. (1995) High school students' sports personalities: variations across participation level, gender, type of sport, and success. *International Journal of Sport Psychology* **26**, 277–294.

O'Connor, P.J. (1992) Psychological aspects of endurance performance. In: *Endurance in Sport* (Shephard, R. & Åstrand, P.O., eds.) Blackwell Scientific Publications, Oxford: 139–145.

O'Connor, P.J. (1997) Overtraining and staleness. In: *Physical Activity and Mental Health* (Morgan, W.P. ed.) Hemisphere, New York: 145–160.

Oxendine, J.B. (1970) Emotional arousal and motor performance. *Quest* **13**, 23–30.

Raglin, J.S. (1992) Anxiety and sport performance. In: *Exercise and Sports Sciences Reviews*, vol. 20 (Holloszy, J.O., ed.) Williams & Wilkins, New York: 243–274.

Raglin, J.S. (1993) Overtraining and staleness: psychometric monitoring of endurance athletes. In: *Handbook of Research in Sport Psychology* (Singer, R.N., Murphey, M. & Tennet, L.K., eds.) Macmillan, New York: 840–850.

Raglin, J.S. (2001) Psychological factors in sport performance: the mental health model revisited. *Sports Medicine* **31**, 875–890.

Raglin, J.S. & Hanin, Y.L. (2000) Competitive anxiety. In: *Emotions in Sport* (Hanin, Y.L., ed.) Human Kinetics, Champaign: 93–111.

Raglin, J.S. & Kenttä, G. (2005) Incidence of the staleness syndrome across a three year period in elite age-group skiers. *Medicine and Science in Sports and Exercise* **37**, S40.

Raglin, J.S. & Wilson, G.S. (2000) Overtraining and staleness in athletes. In: *Emotions and Sport* (Hanin, Y.L., ed.) Human Kinetics, Champaign: 191–207.

Rushall, B.S. (1970) An evaluation of the relationship between personality and physical performance categories. In: *Contemporary Psychology of Sport* (Kenyon, G.S., ed.) Athletic Institute, Chicago: 157–165.

Ryan, R.M. & Deci, E.L. (2000) Self-determination theory and the facilitation of intrinsic motivation, social development, and subjective well-being. *American Psychologist* **55**, 68–78.

Sage, G. (1977) *Introduction to Motor Behavior: A Neuropsychological Approach*, 2nd edn. Addison-Wesley, Reading, Massachusetts.

Sloan, R.G. & Wiggins, M.S. (2001) Motivational differences between American collegiate and professional football players. *International Sports Journal* **5**, 17–24.

Spielberger, C.D. (1972) Anxiety as an emotional state. In: *Anxiety: Current trends in theory and research*, vol. 1 (Spielberger, C.D., ed.) Academic Press, New York: 23–49.

Spielberger, C.D., Gorsuch, R.L., Lushene, P.E., Vagg, P.R. & Jacobs, G.A. (1983) *Manual for the State-Trait Anxiety Inventory (Form Y)* Consulting Psychologist Press, Palo Alto, California.

Stevinson, C.D. & Biddle, S.J.H. (1998) Cognitive orientations in marathon running and 'hitting the wall'. *British Journal of Sports Medicine* **32**, 229–235.

Stewart, C. (2004) Motivational traits of elite young soccer players. *Physical Education* **61**, 213–218.

Thorndike, E.L. (1935) *The Psychology of Wants, Interest, and Attitudes* Appleton-Century-Crofts, New York.

Vanden Auweele, Y., DeCuyper, B., VanMele, V. & Rzenicki, R. (1993) Elite performance and personality: From description and prediction to diagnosis and intervention. In: *Handbook of Research on Sport Psychology* (Singer, R.N., Murphey, M. & Tennant, L.K., eds.) Macillian, New York: 257–289.

Warburton, R.W. & Kane, J.E. (1966) Personality related to sport and physical activity. In: *Readings in Physical Education* (Kane, J.E., ed.) P.E. Association, London: 61–89.

Weiner, B. (1986) *An Attribution Theory of Achievement Motivation and Emotion* Springer-Verlag, New York.

Wilson, G.S. & Raglin, J.S. (1997) Sport anxiety variability in 9–12 year old track and field athletes. *Scandinavian Journal of Medicine and Science in Sports* **7**, 253–258.

Yerkes, R.M. & Dodson, J.D. (1908) The relation of strength of stimulus to rapidity of habit-formation. *Journal of Comparative Neurology and Psychology* **18**, 459–482.

Part 8

Pharmacology

Chapter 18

Performance-Enhancing Drugs

MARIO THEVIS AND WILHELM SCHÄNZER

The temptation for athletes to enhance their physical performance by means of legal as well as illegal drugs has become a serious issue in professional and amateur sport. The progressively developing markets in pharmaceutical products for the treatment of serious diseases, as well as the contemporary search for effective anti-ageing medications, provides a continuously growing pool for drug abuse, in particular in elite sports. Besides "traditional" performance-enhancing drugs such as stimulants and anabolic androgenic steroids (AAS), novel and recently-introduced therapeutics, some of which have not yet passed clinical trials or obtained regulatory body approval, are considered relevant for restriction and monitoring. Peptide hormones synthesized by recombinant biotechnology with structures that are identical to or modifications of natural analogues, and new low-molecular weight drugs have extended the portfolio of compounds possessing great potential for misuse in sports. Moreover, gene doping has become an issue of great concern as gene therapy has demonstrated tremendous progress during recent years. Performance enhancement based on genetic manipulation is not detectable using conventional drug testing approaches; hence, current opinions on how to cope with genetic manipulation primarily include non- or minimally-invasive sampling of blood and/or other bodily samples followed by comprehensive protein profiling.

In the following chapter an overview will be given of the general and analytical aspects of the most frequently observed performance-enhancing drugs in doping controls, and therapeutics that are likely to enter the pharmaceutical market in the future.

Anabolic agents

Anabolic androgenic steroids (AAS)

GENERAL ASPECTS

The chemical structure of testosterone (Fig. 18.1a), the principal AAS, was identified in 1935 (Butenandt & Hanisch 1935; David et al. 1935; Ruzicka & Wettstein 1935), and since then its beneficial effects have been observed and substantiated in many clinical studies (reviewed in Nieschlag & Behre 2004). Endogenous AAS are of the utmost importance for male development and for changes in, for example, muscle and bone mass, and body composition. Numerous synthetic anabolic androgenic analogues such as nandrolone, metandienone, and stanozolol (Fig. 18.1a–d) have been developed for the treatment of anemia and other debilitating diseases. More recently, their suitability for the treatment of hypogonadal conditions or delayed puberty as well as the regulation of male fertility has been investigated (Kamischke & Nieschlag 2004; Kamischke & Nieschlag 2005).

Anabolic steroids are derived from testosterone, and there are virtually unlimited options for chemical modification of the parent compound. Between 1940 and 1960 thousands of analogues were prepared

The Olympic Textbook of Science in Sport, 1st edition. Edited by R.J. Maughan. Published 2009 by Blackwell Publishing. ISBN: 978-1-4051-5638-7.

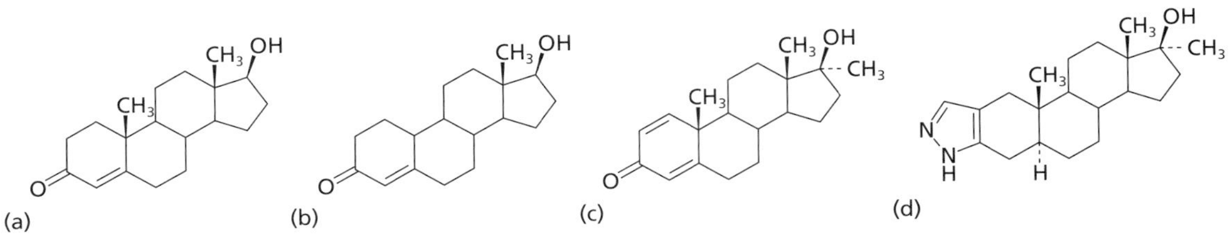

Fig. 18.1 Structural formulae of selected steroids: (a) testosterone (mw 288), (b) nandrolone (mw 274), (c) metandienone (mw 300), and (d) stanozolol (mw 328).

to dissociate the anabolic and androgenic properties, as the latter were found undesirable in most clinical applications (Maisel 1965; Kochakian 1976). Preclinical tests revealed numerous side-effects associated with chronic steroid replacement therapies, and only a few drug candidates have advanced to clinical trials and subsequently onto the pharmaceutical market. However, the evaluation of consequences attributed to the misuse of these drugs is considerably more complex due to the lack of prospective studies and assumed supra-physiological doses. Case reports, retrospective (post-mortem) analyses, and animal models revealed serious side-effects including cardiovascular, endocrine, hepatic, psychiatric, and musculoskeletal health issues. Most frequently, elevated risks of atherosclerosis have been reported that correlate with decreased serum levels of high-density lipoprotein and concomitantly increased values for low-density lipoprotein (Hall 2005). In addition, hepatotoxicity, especially resulting from 17-alkylated steroids such as metandienone and stanozolol, has been reported (Ishak & Zimmerman 1987; Hickson *et al.* 1989), and endocrine consequences such as a reduction in the levels of gonadotrophins luteinizing hormone (LH) and follicle-stimulating hormone (FSH) were observed. Consequently, azoospermia and (reversible) infertility occurred. Moreover, the conversion of steroidal hormones to estrogens, a reaction catalyzed by aromatases, caused feminization of men in terms of voice pitch and, more seriously, irreversible gynecomastia (Kerr & Congeni 2007).

Nevertheless, the anabolic properties of therapeutic agents based on AAS have presented enormous potential for abuse in sports and as lifestyle drugs. As far back as the early 1950s the first suspicions of testosterone misuse by Soviet weightlifters were mentioned along with equivocal attitudes of American athletes towards anabolic steroid misuse (Todd 1987). As officially known now, the former German Democratic Republic maintained a comprehensive and top-secret doping program with AAS (Franke & Berendonk 1997). Anabolic steroids have therefore represented one of the most frequently observed classes of drugs in doping controls and their misuse, as well as the willingness of some athletes to try to obtain the cutting edge advantage in competition through AAS abuse, has been substantiated with the recent discovery of "designer steroids" such as tetrahydrogestrinone (THG) and desoxymethyltestosterone (DMT, madol; Catlin *et al.* 2004; Sekera *et al.* 2005).

The therapeutic use of AAS requires medical indication and prescription; hence, supplement companies introduced so-called pro-hormones as legal alternatives in 1998. the anabolic properties of these compounds were advertised on the basis of an assumed conversion of pro-hormones to AAS *in vivo* and, being "protected" by The Dietary Supplement Health and Education Act (DSHEA), pro-hormones as well as new modified steroidal derivatives were available as nutritional supplements for over-the-counter (OTC) sales in the US until the implementation of the Anabolic Steroid Control Act in 2004. However, production and/or packaging of non-hormonal and steroidal nutritional supplements by companies has led to numerous cases of contamination. In a recent study, approximately 15% of more than 400 analyzed dietary supplements contained trace amounts of steroids, which would not exert an anabolic effect but could cause an adverse finding in doping controls (Geyer 2004).

A considerable tendency to AAS misuse in sports is evident, including the application of xenobiotic steroidal drugs (e.g., nandrolone, metandienone, stanozolol), pro-hormones (e.g., norandrostenedione, norandrostenediol), and designer steroids (e.g., THG, DMT) as well as synthetically-derived testosterone. Thus, sports drug-testing laboratories and regulatory authorities have been forced to update their list of target analytes continuously, and new strategies to cope with the possible abuse of new or unknown compounds, regardless of whether these compounds have received clinical approval or not, have been established during recent years.

DOPING CONTROLS

In 1974, the International Olympic Committee (IOC) Medical Commission included AAS in their list of prohibited substances, and ever since then detection assays have been improved in terms of sensitivity and specificity, and also extended to cover the broad range of possible misused drugs (Thevis & Schänzer 2005a). In particular, the application of chromatographic separation techniques interfaced to mass spectrometry (MS) analyzers has significantly enhanced the traceability of AAS misuse, and numerous studies have demonstrated the extensive metabolic conversion of the administered drugs (Schänzer 1996). Metabolites, as well as applied therapeutics have been characterized and employed as target candidates in doping control screening procedures. Gas chromatography (GC) coupled to MS has been the preferred technique for qualitatively and quantitatively determining AAS and their metabolic products in urine specimens, which has required chemical derivatization of these compounds in order to accomplish adequate GC-MS properties. In this respect, the generation of trimethylsilyl ethers from hydroxyl functions and trimethylsilyl enol ethers from keto residues has been the most frequently employed strategy. However, steroidal structures such as estra-4,9,11-trien-3-one or numerous corticosteroids have demonstrated poor GC-MS qualities using the commonly applied screening approaches; hence, these compounds have tended to be analyzed using liquid chromatography (LC) combined with (tandem) MS when soft ionization

techniques such as electrospray ionization (ESI) and atmospheric pressure chemical ionization (APCI) became commercially available (Thevis & Schänzer 2005a, 2007).

These detection methods require knowledge of the target analytes, i.e., administered drugs and/or their metabolites. The main advantages of analytical approaches that are optimized for particular compounds are their sensitivity and specificity, but a major shortcoming is the fact that unknown substances are provided with the "cloak of invisibility" due to the lack of consideration. For example, the designer drug THG remained undetected for several years, and was only discovered when residues of an empty syringe were investigated. Since then, more comprehensive screening assays have been suggested and established, which are based on three principal strategies: (i) precursor ion scan MS (Thevis et al. 2005a); (ii) bioassays in concert with high-resolution MS (Nielen et al. 2006); and (iii) steroid profiling (Donike et al. 1983; Geyer et al. 1996, 1997).

The first-mentioned approach utilizes knowledge of the gas-phase dissociation behavior of known steroids with particular nuclei. Product ions with diagnostic character are obtained from known steroid molecules, protonated by ESI, and fragmented by collision-induced dissociation (CID). These product ions are used as targets in precursor ion-scan experiments with triple-quadrupole mass spectrometers; i.e., ions obtained by ESI are scanned over a selected m/z range and each individual precursor ion is subjected to CID. Those yielding the selected product ion(s) are recorded and displayed in terms of a precursor ion scan in the respective chromatogram. Typical product ions representing the principle nuclei of steroids are m/z 109 (e.g., testosterone and nandrolone), 187 (e.g., 1-testosterone), 227 (e.g., trenbolone), and 241 (e.g., gestrinone).

The second approach to determine unknown AAS in biological matrices is based on LC of urine extracts with effluent splitting into two well plates, yielding two copies of each fraction collected. One copy is used for androgen bioactivity detection employing a yeast reporter gene assay and, in case of a "positive" result, the corresponding second copy is subjected to high-resolution LC interfaced to high-resolution/high-accuracy MS. Accurate mass measurements enable the calculation of elemental compositions of detected compounds, which allow for automated substance database searches and concretize possible steroid structures and constitutions in suspicious doping control samples.

Another important indicator for the abuse of synthetic and endogenous steroids (e.g., testosterone, dihydrotestosterone (DHT), dehydroepiandrosterone, and androstenedione) is the so-called "steroid profile." The administration of steroids, regardless of their natural or synthetic origin, causes a significant change in endogenous steroid biosynthesis, and thus in respective urinary concentrations. As endogenous steroids belong to the biosynthetic pathway of testosterone, the detection of their surreptitious application is more challenging and complicated than the identification of xenobiotic substances. Consequently, the use of hormone ratios, as determined by gas chromatography and MS, was suggested to identify artificially elevated steroid concentrations in athletes' urine samples. Numerous endocrinological studies have identified a urinary steroid profile (Donike *et al.* 1983; Geyer *et al.* 1996, 1997) that provides a detailed insight into natural and unnatural variations in steroid concentrations and ratios. This makes it possible to identify the administration of endogenous steroids, e.g., by the comparison of concentrations of testosterone and epitestosterone or metabolites such as androsterone and etiocholanolone, which requires the quantitative and qualitative determination of these analytes.

Clenbuterol

GENERAL ASPECTS

Clenbuterol (4-amino-α-[(*tert*-butylamino)methyl]-3,5-dichlorbenzyl alcohol (Fig. 18.2) belongs to the class of β2-agonists, which are considered as non-steroidal anabolic agents according to the World Anti-Doping Agency (WADA). It is one of the most frequently mentioned anabolic agents, along with AAS, in underground literature. As a representative of the class of sympathomimetic agents, clenbuterol has demonstrated a distinguished medical versatility in the past. It was developed for the treatment of pulmonary diseases such as asthma bronchiale or bronchial hyper-reactivity (e.g., as observed with exercise-induced asthma) owing to its bronchodilator activity. Its anabolic properties have led to numerous additional therapeutic applications, such as the prevention of skeletal muscle atrophy caused by injury or denervation (Zeman *et al.* 1987; Reeds *et al.* 1988; von Deutsch *et al.* 2000, 2002). There is evidence that it may counteract microgravity-induced atrophy in astronauts, and the beneficial effects of clenbuterol in the treatment of heart failure have been discussed, in particular in combination with ventricular assist devices (Prezelj *et al.* 2003).

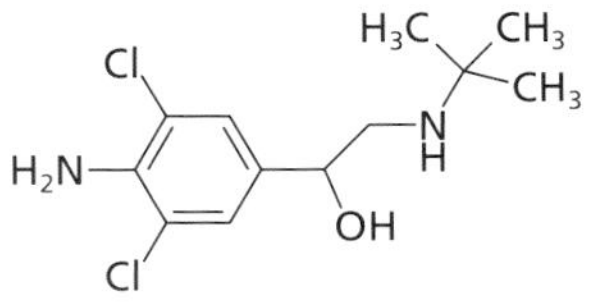

Clenbuterol exerts numerous effects, the most recognized being growth-promotion, which has led to several cases of misuse in animal production. The considerable increase seen in muscle size and general changes in body composition (reduction of body fat, increased nitrogen retention) have been the subject of various studies, but the detailed mechanisms underlying these effects have not yet been established. The increase in skeletal muscle mass has been attributed to several complementary actions of on muscle tissue. On the one hand, mass gain may result from improved nitrogen retention associated with protein biosynthesis. Additionally, a clenbuterol-induced transient activation of the insulin-like growth factor (IGF)-2 gene transcript in muscle has been suggested, and an increased diameter of fast twitch type 2 muscle fibers has been reported (Sneddon *et al.* 2001; Downie *et al.* 2008). On the other hand, clenbuterol is considered to inhibit protein breakdown as it demonstrably reduces the protein-degrading enzymes calpain 1 and 2 while concomitantly up-regulating calpastatin (Prezelj *et al.* 2003). In particular the calpains have been shown to trigger the catabolism of myofibrils.

In addition to an increased muscle size, fat tissue is also influenced by clenbuterol administration.

Fig. 18.2 Chemical structure of clenbuterol (monoisotopic mass 277).

A reduction of body fat has been reported, which is explained by concerted effects including the stimulation of lipolysis, inhibition of lipogenesis, enhancement of fatty acid turnover and oxidation, and reduction in adipocyte volume (Kearns *et al.* 2001, 2006).

These "positive" aspects must be balanced against the considerable side-effects that occur when clenbuterol is administered in doses that are significantly greater than those recommended therapeutically. These are characterized by, for example, tachycardia, palpitations, tremors, headaches, fever and hypo-kalemia, and acute poisoning can lead to interruption of breathing. However, the temptation to abuse clenbuterol is apparent and has led to numerous adverse findings in elite athletes' urine specimens during the last decade. A comprehensive review on clenbuterol and its clinical profile was published by Prezelj *et al.* in 2003.

DOPING CONTROLS

In 1992, sympathomimetics were added to the list of prohibited substances and methods of doping compiled by the IOC, and the IOC and WADA have classified β_2-agonists as stimulants as well as anabolic agents, with specific regulations in terms of competition and out-of-competition testing. While all β_2-agonists are considered as stimulants in competition (except for salbutamol, salmeterol, terbutaline, and formoterol when used via inhalation), only clenbuterol and salbutamol are referred to as anabolic agents, and for the latter a threshold of $1 \ \mu g \cdot mL^{-1}$ in urine has been established. Misuse of clenbuterol has been reported many times in professional as well as amateur sport, and because clenbuterol is effective at relatively low doses, a minimum required performance limit (MRPL) was established at $2 \ ng \cdot mL^{-1}$ for urine samples. Numerous assays allowing its unambiguous identification have been developed for sports drug testing, and these are based on different strategies including GC-MS, LC-MS, LC combined with tandem MS (LC-MS/MS), and immunological assays (Politi *et al.* 2005; Thevis *et al.* 2005b). In general, β_2-agonists possess poor gas chromatographic properties. Hence, sophisticated derivatization procedures have been developed including

trimethylsilylation, acylation, combined trimethylsilylation and acylation, and the formation of cyclic methylboronates or tetrahydrochinoline derivatives that allow adequate GC-MS screening and confirmation analyses (Damasceno *et al.* 2000; Henze *et al.* 2001). In addition, the mass spectrometric part contributed considerable improvements regarding detection limits for β_2-agonists in doping controls as GC combined with high-resolution MS, MS/MS, or multiple MS (MS/MS/MS) enabled the detection of trace amounts of clenbuterol (i.e., $< 0.2 \ ng \cdot mL^{-1}$) in human urine (Amendola *et al.* 2002). The use of LC-MS(/MS) has enabled faster screening and confirmation analyses for β_2-agonists as no derivatization of the analytes is required. Owing to excellent proton affinities and efficient gas-phase dissociation behaviors, comprehensive procedures and sensitive confirmation methods have been developed (Thevis *et al.* 2003, 2005b), which cover up to 19 different β_2-agonists and allow the qualitative and quantitative determination of clenbuterol in plasma and urine at $0.1–0.2 \ ng \cdot mL^{-1}$. In Fig. 18.3, the extracted ion chromatogram of a urine sample that tested positive for clenbuterol is illustrated to demonstrate the sensitivity and selectivity of modern LC-MS(/MS) analytical tools.

Selective androgen receptor modulators (SARMs)

GENERAL ASPECTS

As mentioned above, endogenous androgens are of the utmost importance for male development in general and the acquirement of secondary characteristics. Numerous AAS have been developed to mimic these properties for the treatment of various symptoms of serious diseases, but the limitations of anabolic-androgenic steroid therapies, such as decreased levels of high-density lipoprotein (HDL)-cholesterol and negative influences on prostate and cardiovascular systems, have led to the development of a novel class of anabolic agents – selective androgen receptor modulators (SARMs). SARMs act as full agonists in anabolic target tissues such as muscle and bone, but demonstrate only partial agonist activity in androgenic tissues such as prostate and seminal vesicles. Their main advantage over steroids in testosterone replacement therapies is

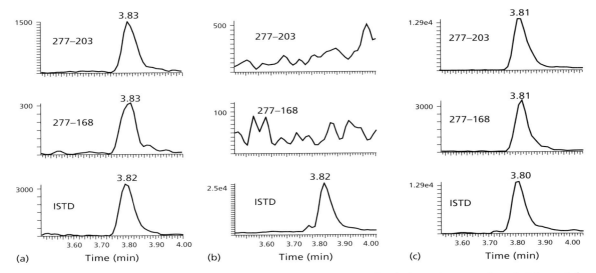

Fig. 18.3 Extracted ion chromatograms of (a) a urine specimen tested positive for clenbuterol at approximately 0.1 ng·mL^{-1}, (b) a blank urine sample, and (c) a reference urine specimen containing 0.2 ng·mL^{-1} of clenbuterol. Clenbuterol and the internal standard (d$_6$-clenbuterol) are determined using the ion transitions 277–203 and 283–204, respectively.

the fact that they do not represent substrates for 5α-reductases, one main route of metabolism for steroids related to testosterone. The resulting metabolic product of testosterone, DHT, is considered a more potent androgenic steroid than testosterone. In addition, due to the significant amount of DHT produced locally in organs such as the prostate, it is believed to amplify the androgenic activity of testosterone considerably. This effect is not seen with synthetic SARMs, which are not metabolized by this pathway, making them a promising class of anabolic agents that have no, or significantly reduced androgenic side-effects (Chen *et al.* 2005). Numerous SARMs are currently being evaluated for their anabolic and androgenic efficiency and their oral bioavailability. Drug candidates can be categorized by their chemical structures into four classes (Fig. 18.4): aryl-propionamide, bicyclic hydantoin, quinoline, and tetrahydroquinoline analogues. As early as 1998 the first report on a successful preparation of an aryl-propionamide-based SARM was published. It was derived from a closely-related androgen receptor antagonist, bicalutamide, and numerous structurally-related compounds have been tested for anabolic and/or androgenic potency since. Two products (Ostarine and Andarine, GTx Inc.,

Memphis, Tennessee) have recently entered clinical trials, demonstrating the fast progress of this class of therapeutics (Mohler *et al.* 2005).

Only a few pharmacokinetic studies have been published that deal with the metabolic fate of SARMs, with the exception of several aryl-propionamide-derived compounds. These drugs demonstrate a high degree of bioavailability after oral administration, and their rate of metabolic conversion is strongly dependent on the substituent "R" within the phenol residue (Fig. 18.4). Drugs bearing an acetamido function were found to be extensively metabolized by deacetylation, a fact that led to the development of structural analogues containing different halogen atoms instead of an acetamido residue. Most aryl-propionamide SARMs resulting from this alteration demonstrated a considerably increased metabolic stability, which initiated a new series of SARM drug candidates.

DOPING CONTROLS

Due to the promising results with synthetic SARMs, in particular with regard to anabolic effects on muscle strength, body composition, and bone density, and

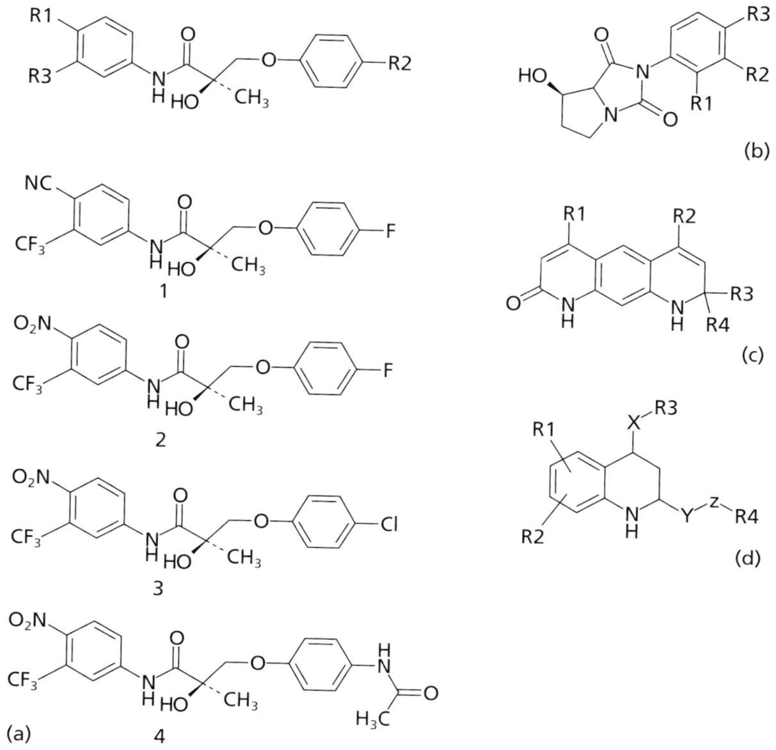

Fig. 18.4 Chemical structures for four categories of selective androgen receptor modulators SARMs: (a) aryl-propionamide-derived compounds (1–4), (b) bicyclic hydantoines, (c) quinolines, and (d) tetrahydroquinolines.

the reduced side-effects compared to conventional AAS, the potential for misuse in sports is extremely high. SARMs are currently not officially available, but doping-control laboratories must be prepared to measure this class of compounds as incidences in the past have demonstrated that misused therapeutics are not necessarily clinically approved, and WADA has prohibited these compounds since January 2008. As a consequence, traditional doping-control strategies have been complemented by preventive anti-doping research, an approach that includes the incorporation of new drugs or drug candidates into analytical screening protocols. The determination of SARMs in sports drug testing has required a novel assay (Thevis *et al.* 2006a), the analytical principle of which is comparable to that established for the detection of designer steroids, as described above. Due to the fact that SARMs are still under development and clinical trials are not yet complete, numerous derivatives must be considered in doping controls that are not available as reference material.

Hence, traditional target analysis, as commonly used for most drugs prohibited by WADA, is difficult to apply to SARMs because defined structures are only available for two candidates. Hence, precursor-ion scanning is once more the method of choice for this comprehensive group of therapeutics. One analytical approach has recently been published focusing on aryl-propionamide-derived SARMs (Fig. 18.4a–d). These compounds comprise a common bisubstituted phenyl residue generating abundant and characteristic product ions in negative ESI-MS/MS analyses at either 241 or 261 m/z, depending on the nature of substituents. In Fig. 18.5, ESI-MS/MS spectra obtained from deprotonated molecules of four aryl-propionamide-derived SARMs are shown, with base peaks at 241 (a) or 261 (b–d) m/z. These product ions have been structurally elucidated, and their elemental compositions were determined as $C_{11}H_8F_3N_2O$ and $C_{10}H_8F_3N_2O_3$, respectively. By means of concerted target analysis and precursor-ion scanning, numerous aryl-propionamide-derived drug candidates as

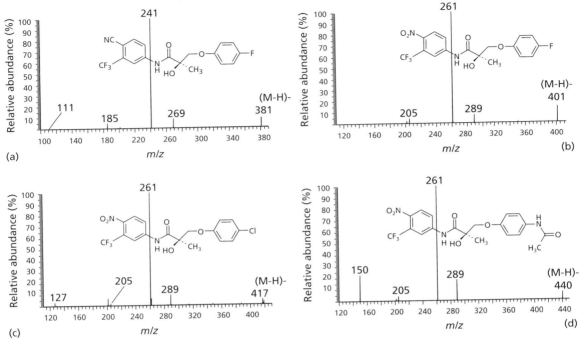

Fig. 18.5 Electrospray ionization (ESI) product ion spectra for the deprotonated molecules of four aryl-propionamide-derived SARMs (a–d). All spectra were recorded on a Thermo LTQ Orbitrap instrument using normalized collision energies of 27.

well as putative metabolites are detectable, and an expansion of this assay to cover additional SARM structures is expected in the near future.

Stimulants

Amphetamine and ephedrine derivatives

GENERAL ASPECTS

Psychostimulating agents have a long history of use and abuse. Drugs belonging to this class of thera-peutics have been consumed in different cultures and continents in different eras. The Incas, for instance, were known to chew coca leaves (from *Erythroxylon coca*) as a source of cocaine; African and Arabian cultures have used Khat leaves (from *Catha edulis*) owing to its high content of cathinone, which was converted to cathine *in vivo*. Effects such as increased alertness and feelings of mood elevation have been reported, and with the availability of chemically-synthesized stimulating principles and potent derivat-ives, controlled research but also considerable misuse was initiated around 1930 (Wadler & Hainline 1989). A general definition of psychostimulation using respective drugs was composed by Coper *et al.* in 1987, which attempted to distinguish between ana-leptics, nootropics, and stimulants. The latter were defined as "drugs which induce an overall, i.e., peripheral and central, but unphysiological, activa-tion of the organism combined with a short-lasting elevation in mood and performance" (Palm 1987).

Amphetamine and ephedrine (Fig. 18.6a & b, respectively), as well as numerous chemical derivat-ives, are psychostimulants that indirectly act as sympathomimetic agents. Both are powerful central nervous system (CNS) effectors and also act on peripheral α- and β-adrenergic receptors. Different modes of action resulting in organ-specific responses have been proposed to originate from: (i) the dis-placement and direct release of catecholamines (i.e., epinephrine, norepinephrine, and dopamine) into

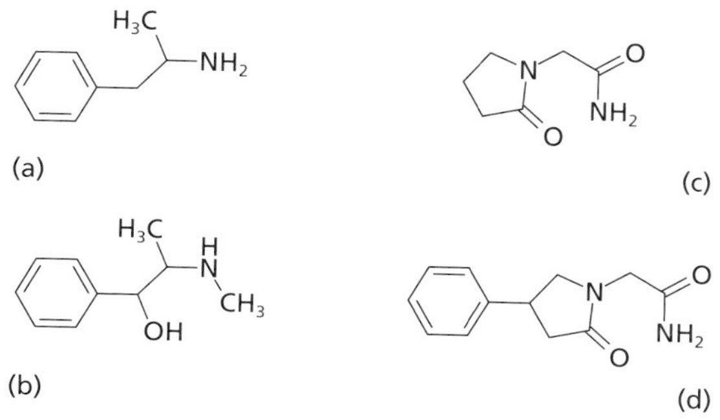

Fig. 18.6 Chemical structures of (a) amphetamine (mw 135), (b) ephedrine (mw 165), (c) piracetam (mw 142), and (d) carphedone (mw 218). The latter is considered a hybrid composed by amphetamine (left part) and piracetam (right part), initially designed for the Russian military.

synaptic clefts; (ii) a partial agonist activity, thus mimicking the presence of endogenously-produced catecholamines; (iii) inhibition of the reuptake of synaptic catecholamines, which causes an increased availability; and (iv) inhibition of monoamine oxidase activity, which is responsible for the metabolic elimination of endogenous catecholamines (Wadler & Hainline 1989). Numerous physiological effects of drugs related to amphetamine have been studied and elucidated in detail, including primarily an increased heart rate and contractile force of the myocardium, elevated glycogenolysis and gluconeogenesis in skeletal muscle and liver, increased plasma levels of free fatty acids, and bronchial dilatation. Also considerable psychic effects have been described, including wakefulness, a decreased sense of fatigue, decreased appetite, increased initiative and self-confidence as well as an elevation in motor and speech activity (Palm 1987).

All these facts have led to an enormous interest in drugs based on amphetamine, which was initiated with its chemical synthesis in 1887. Besides therapeutic application, including for instance the treatment of narcolepsy, obesity, hyperkinetic syndrome, and hypotensive states, particular interest arose from the military who intended to delay the onset of fatigue in troops. In addition, studies demonstrating the effects of amphetamines on athletic performance were conducted as early as 1959. Highly-trained runners, swimmers, and weight-throwers conducted

exercise tests after administration of either amphetamine or placebo proving a positive influence of the stimulating agent by increasing the performance of 75% of participating athletes by 0.6–4.0% (Beecher & Smith 1965). Considering the corresponding gain in seconds, participating swimmers for instance finished races of 100 and 200 yards 0.60–1.65 s faster, respectively (Smith & Beecher 1959). These and other subsequent investigations (Wadler & Hainline 1989) suggest that athletic performance may be significantly increased using stimulants such as amphetamine and related drugs. Components of sporting performance such as endurance (i.e., time to exhaustion), speed, power, and fine motor coordination have been the subject of numerous studies and provide an indication of improvements caused by therapeutics possessing psychostimulating properties.

These facts may have led to the considerable abuse of stimulating drugs in sports, which has been reported since they were prohibited by the IOC and WADA. One of the most recently detected stimulants is carphedone (see Fig. 18.4d), which is theoretically a hybrid composed of an amphetamine-like (Fig. 18.6a) and a piracetam-like (Fig. 18.6c) element. The drug originates from Russia, where it was developed for soldiers and astronauts to improve physical performance and resistance to low temperatures, and is a structural combination of a stimulating and a nootropic agent, first recognized in doping controls in 1997. For several years, it has been available as "Phenotropil" in Russian pharmacies.

DOPING CONTROLS

Stimulants were one of the first groups of compounds to be included on the prohibited list of the IOC, and were determined in terms of doping controls for the first time in horse saliva at the beginning of the 20th century. The first scientific procedures were developed by Russian and Austrian scientists, and in 1910 and 1911 about 220 samples were investigated for administration of alkaloids (Thevis & Schänzer 2005d). Between 1938 and 1954 the principal procedures for the detection of stimulants such as amphetamines were established. These had limited sensitivity and were susceptible to interferences by biological matrices, but in 1956 a commonly-accepted assay based on liquid extraction, paper chromatography, and visualization was introduced (Vidic 1956). Analytical results were further improved with the introduction of GC coupled to nitrogen-phosphor specific detectors (NPD) as well as MS for the qualitative and quantitative determination of stimulants in human urine, and the first comprehensive screenings for the use of stimulating agents were conducted during the 1972 Olympic Games in Munich (Donike *et al.* 1970; Donike & Derenbach 1976).

The principal sample preparation procedure for stimulants related to amphetamine and ephedrine is based on a liquid-liquid extraction of urine at pH 14 using ether as the organic solvent. This strategy has remained unchanged since it was first established more than 30 years ago, but the subsequent handling of organic extracts has been adjusted to employ more modern analytical tools. Ether extracts have commonly been measured for stimulants using GC-NPD/MS instruments, providing detailed information on the presence or absence of prohibited drugs using comprehensive mass spectra libraries. Typical mass spectra of amphetamine and ephedrine after electron ionization (EI) are shown in Fig. 18.7, which contain characteristic fragment ions that indicate the general structure of respective stimulants. The amines are likely ionized by EI at the nitrogen atom, which induces a typical α-cleavage (also referred to as β-bond cleavage) yielding dominant fragment ions upon electron bombardment. Fission of carbon-carbon bonds adjacent to the nitrogen results in base peaks at either m/z 44 for amphetamines bearing a primary amino function, or m/z 58 for those carrying

an additional methyl residue. These general fragment ions, in addition to many other factors, enable a broad screening for drugs related to amphetamine and ephedrine.

For ephedrine and phenylpropanolamine, as well as their stereoisomers pseudoephedrine and cathine, the WADA prohibited list provides different regulations. The detection of these drugs represents a doping offence whenever they exceed a specific threshold, except for pseudoephedrine, which has not been considered relevant for sports drug testing since January 2004. Hence, suspicious urine samples require a quantitative analysis of detected compounds, which includes the chromatographic separation of stereoisomers, but the separation of isomers of ephedrine by gas chromatography has proved to be a challenging task. Without chemical treatment of the analytes, a differentiation of ephedrine and pseudoephedrine has barely been accomplished, but by means of selective derivatization of hydroxyl and amine functions with *N*-methyl-*N*-trimethylsilyltrifluoroacetamide (MSTFA) and *N*-methyl-*N*-bistrifluoroacetamide (MBTFA), a gas chromatographic isolation of the derivatives was achieved enabling the unambiguous qualitative and quantitative detection of ephedrine and related compounds (Donike 1973; Donike & Derenbach 1976). A comprehensive review of the development of screening and confirmation strategies for stimulants, narcotics, and β-blockers was published by Hemmersbach and de la Torre in 1996.

Complementary approaches for the determination of stimulants have recently been reported, which

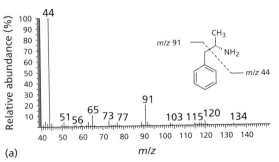

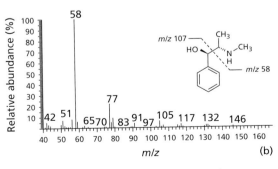

(a) m/z (b)

Fig. 18.7 Electron ionization (EI) mass spectra of (a) amphetamine and (b) ephedrine containing characteristic fragment ions at m/z 44 and 58, respectively, which result from typical α-cleavages upon electron impact ionization.

are based on comparable sample preparation procedures, but MS analyses have been conducted by employing modern LC-MS(/MS) instruments (Thevis & Schänzer 2005b; Deventer *et al.* 2006). The first-mentioned assay utilizes isotope-dilution MS (IDMS) to allow accurate quantification plus qualitative determination of ephedrine in urine specimens. Here, no sample extraction is performed, but specimens are fortified with three-fold deuterated ephedrine, and 2 µL aliquots are directly injected into LC-MS/MS systems for analysis. The second procedure qualitatively covers 27 amphetamine-related drugs in terms of a screening procedure complementing existing strategies. Its advantage over the traditional GC-NPD/MS assay is an increase in sensitivity for most drugs, but this is accomplished on the expense of the comprehensiveness of GC-NPD/MS approaches due to its focus on particular therapeutics.

Peptide hormones

Erythropoietin and mimetic agents

GENERAL ASPECTS

In 1977, Miyake *et al.* purified milligram amounts of erythropoietin (EPO) from 2550 L of urine that was collected from patients suffering from aplastic anemia. This incredible effort was the starting point for all subsequent studies that led to the characterization of EPO (Miyake *et al.* 1977), a glycoprotein of mainly renal origin with an approximate molecular weight of 34 kDa. It comprises 165 amino acid residues, three tetra-antennary *N*-linked (Asn 24, 38, and 83) carbohydrate side-chain and one *O*-linked (Ser 126) side-chain, as well as two disulphide bonds (Cys 7-Cys 161 and Cys 29-Cys 33). EPO inhibits the apoptosis of erythrocyte progenitors in the bone marrow and is thus an essential factor for the growth of red blood cells. The peptide core of EPO is crucial for receptor-binding while the carbohydrate structure, which accounts for approximately 40% of the molecular weight, allows *in vivo* survival of the hormone. A comprehensive review on the molecular biology of EPO was published by Jelkmann in 2004. A variety of clinically approved recombinant human EPO preparations has been commercialized since

EPO became available via biotechnological production in 1989. Moreover, chemically modified EPO, referred to as continuous erythropoiesis receptor activator (CERA), which bears a spacious methoxy-polyethylene glycol residue and possesses a significantly prolonged plasma half-life, has recently been launched. An erythropoietin derivative produced entirely by chemical synthesis has recently also been described, which was named synthetic erythropoiesis protein (SEP) (Kochendoerfer *et al.* 2003). SEP was assembled by sequential chemo-selective ligation reactions from individual peptide segments, yielding a protein core composed of 166 amino acid residues. The primary amino acid structure differs from human EPO at seven positions. Three asparagines (residues 24, 38, and 83) as well as one serine (residue 126) that are usually connected to carbohydrate moieties of EPO were replaced by lysine residues, two of which (24 and 126) are linked to precision polymers that terminate in negative charge-control units. Glutamate residues (89 and 117) were exchanged for cysteines by ligation reactions during synthesis, and sulfhydryl functions were adequately derivatized to mimic missing glutamates. Finally, a C-terminal arginine was attached that is removed from circulating and urinary EPO.

Primary and secondary structures of human urinary EPO and synthetic/recombinant analogues epoetin alpha, beta, delta, and omega are identical, whilst darbepoietin alpha comprises five different amino acid residues (Ala30Asn, His32Thr, Pro87Val, Trp88Asn, and Pro90Thr). These substitutions allow for additional oligosaccharide attachment at asparagines resulting in prolonged biological activity. Minor differences in glycan structures including different sialyation levels and modifications such as sulfonation have also been detected between human and recombinant EPO with identical peptide backbones. Numerous studies have reported the possibility of characterizing recombinant as well as natural EPO by means of capillary electrophoresis, isoelectric focusing (IEF), two-dimensional gel electrophoresis, MALDI-MS(/MS) and ESI-MS(/MS), and fundamental principles have been applied to allow the determination of recombinant EPO abuse in sports.

In addition to modified proteins closely related to EPO, mimetic agents have been clinically investigated, and these are based either on peptide- or non-peptide structures. Both types of compounds are designed to dimerize the EPO receptor and thus imitate an EPO presence. The reason for the search for agents mimicking the action of EPO is the option of an alternative route of administration, i.e., to avoid subcutaneous injection and, preferably, to allow for oral applications. Small peptides have been demonstrated to possess considerable *in vitro* and *in vivo* potencies, in particular after covalent dimerization (e.g., the EPO mimetic peptide 1, EMP1) as described by Wrighton *et al.* in 1997. Owing to limitations caused by a short half-life, a fusion protein generated from EMP1 was prepared resulting in increased *in vivo* activity, but the protein structure of the new product precluded oral administration (Sytkowski 2004). The determination of non-peptide EPO mimetics has also been reported recently. These compounds, which exhibited *in vitro* activity as a minimum, were based on either *N,N*-disubstituted amino acids or dimeric iminodiacetic diamides, both of which provided a proof of principle for the possibility of developing orally-active erythropoietic drugs. Until now, no EPO mimetic therapeutic agent has entered the pharmaceutical market.

Novel alternatives to EPO and its mimetic agents are the so-called hypoxia-inducible factor (HIF) stabilizers, which are currently in clinical trials for the treatment of anemia. Progress in understanding the adaptation of the human organism to hypoxia at the molecular level has led to the development of a new class of small molecules which up-regulate endogenous EPO production via factor HIF-1 and its degrading enzymes. Hypoxia is the physiological trigger that activates HIF, the 1α-subunit of which responds to changes in oxygen tension. HIF-1 in particular is a transcription factor that, under hypoxic conditions, binds specifically to hypoxia-responsive elements in the promoter or enhancer of inducible genes such as the EPO gene. Under normoxia, the half-life of HIF-1α is less than 5 min as hydroxylases modify the protein at different positions and "mark" it for degradation by von Hippel-Lindau (VHL) conjugation and ubiquitin conjugation, followed by proteasomal degradation. This process requires a certain oxygen level; hence, HIF production is not increased upon hypoxia but its destruction is slowed, which allows increased EPO production (Huang & Bunn 2003). As a consequence, the artificial stabilization of HIF-1 by orally-bioavailable therapeutics enables the treatment of anemia by stimulating erythropoiesis, thus increasing the red blood cell mass and hemoglobin concentration.

DOPING CONTROLS

Since 1990, EPO has been prohibited by the IOC and WADA. A study published by Videman *et al.* in 2000 stressed the rationale; it being that a considerable increase in total hemoglobin mass in elite cross country skiers has been measured since recombinant EPO has become commercially available. Hence, the search for an adequate assay to determine the misuse of EPO in sports has been an important item of anti-doping research, and has shown promising results from the beginning of the 21st century. In 2000, Lasne and de Ceaurriz reported the possibility of differentiating human urinary EPO profiles from those obtained from recombinant analogues by means of IEF (Lasne & de Ceaurriz 2000). Subsequently, a strategy to determine the presence of recombinant EPO in athletes' urine samples was presented in 2002, based on the concentration in 20 mL of urine and using ultrafiltration to give a final retentate volume of 20–80 μL (Lasne *et al.* 2002). This concentrate was then subjected to IEF utilizing a pH 3–5 polyacrylamide gel along with recombinant EPO controls and, after focusing of analytes, the gel was subjected to semidry blotting. The membrane was incubated with anti-EPO antibodies, and these were subsequently transferred to a second membrane and incubated in a solution containing biotinylated anti-mouse IgG antibodies. The addition of a streptavidin-biotinylated peroxidase complex allowed visualization of EPO profiles via chemiluminescence detection. A typical image obtained by the above described procedure is depicted in Fig. 18.8. Differences in the acidity of human and recombinant EPO cause distinct glycoform patterns, which appear in defined pH ranges and allow for a differentiation between endogenously-produced and biotechnologically-derived EPO in urine specimens. Due to the hyperglycosylation of darbepoietin alpha (NESP, novel erythropoiesis stimulating

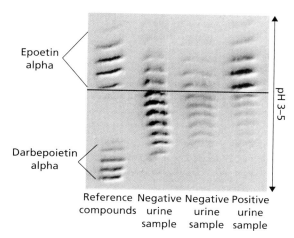

Epoetin alpha

Darbepoietin alpha

pH 3–5

Reference compounds | Negative urine sample | Negative urine sample | Positive urine sample

Fig. 18.8 Image obtained from an analysis of erythropoietin (EPO) using isoelectric focusing (IEF). Reference compounds (epoetin alpha and darbepoietin alpha) and both negative and positive urine samples have been applied, and respective bands are obtained within the typical pH ranges.

protein) a considerably increased acidity is obtained, which results in a glycoform pattern observed at pH 3–4, while the main isoforms of endogenous EPO occur in the range pH 4–4.5 and recombinant epoetins appear at a more alkaline of pH 4.5–5. This assay, in combination with models based on indirect blood parameters, was employed for EPO testing at the summer Olympic Games in Sydney (2000) and Athens (2004) as well as the winter Olympics in Salt Lake City (2002; Kazlauskas *et al.* 2002).

The double-blotting technique is a commonly accepted method for the determination of EPO misuse in sports and has a detection limit of approximately 50 pg per 20 mL of urine (0.3 IU/L). Since the procedure was first established, a few important modifications/additions have been made, such as a test for urinary bacterial activity that could simulate EPO misuse by shifting endogenously-produced EPO bands from "normal" pH values to those frequently observed with recombinant EPO preparations. In addition, a so-called stress-induced shift of EPO bands has also been observed in the past, which resulted in more specific guidelines for data interpretation to prevent false positives occurring.

The prospect of increasing endogenous EPO production by means of HIF stabilizers will require drug testing strategies that are comparable to approaches developed for small molecule therapeutics. One product (FG-2216; FibroGen Inc., South San Francisco, California) has recently passed phase 1 clinical trials and demonstrated a significant increase in erythrocyte and hemoglobin mass in healthy volunteers. In addition, an activation of enzymes involved in iron processing, transport, and utilization, as well as the activation of enzymes involved in the conversion of heme for the synthesis of hemoglobin, has been observed. Hence, the class of HIF stabilizers should definitely be considered relevant for sports drug testing in the near future.

Insulin and synthetic derivatives

GENERAL ASPECTS

Insulin is a small protein with a molecular weight of 5807 Da, consisting of two peptide chains cross-linked by two disulfide bonds. It is generated in the β-cells of the pancreas from proinsulin, a single-chain protein with a molecular weight of 9388 Da, by enzymes such as proconvertases and carboxypeptidase H, yielding insulin and C-peptide (Fig. 18.9). Insulin counteracts post-prandial hyperglycemia by inhibiting hepatic glucose production, facilitating glucose-uptake into target tissues such as hepatocytes and myocytes, and stimulating glycogen formation (Sönksen 2001). Disorders of this sensitively balanced endocrine system have become a serious issue during the last century. They are commonly referred to as (type 1) insulin-dependent diabetes mellitus (IDDM) and (type 2) non-insulin-dependent diabetes mellitus, depending on whether the main pathogenic factors are impaired insulin release owing to a lack of pancreatic β-cells or peripheral insulin resistance. IDDM has usually been treated by insulin substitution using recombinant preparations, but the inconvenience of so-called "lag phases," describing the period from subcutaneous administration of the drug to the appearance of its bioavailabile form, has led to the development of synthetic insulin derivatives with improved time-to-onset profiles. Human insulin tends to aggregate to form non-covalent hexamers, which is the major reason for the above-mentioned lag phase, and these require a dilution of

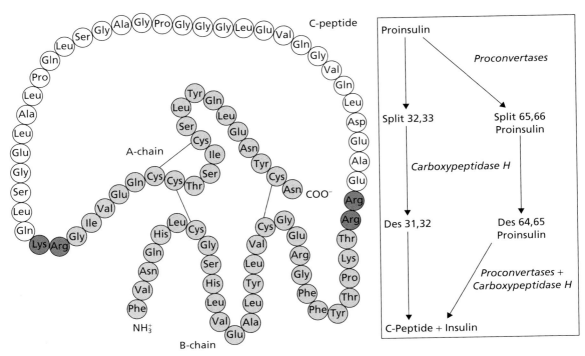

Fig. 18.9 Generation of insulin from proinsulin, a single-chain protein with two intramolecular disulfide bonds. Enzymes such as proconvertases and carboxypeptidase H cleave proinsulin at distinct positions yielding insulin (darker gray amino acid residues) and C-peptide (plain amino acid residues).

concentration by a factor of approximately 1000 to dissociate them into corresponding bioactive monomers (Polonsky & O'Meara 2001). Modifications of the primary structure of human insulin, preferably at the C-terminus of the B-chain, has yielded several insulin derivatives with full receptor-binding activity, but considerably reduced self-association, which results in rapidly bioavailable insulin monomers. This new class of insulin derivatives are referred to as rapid-acting insulins, and three products are now commercially available (Humalog LisPro, Novolog Aspart, and Glulisine Apidra).

In 1998, the question of whether insulin was a performance-enhancing drug arose, and the IOC added insulin to the list of prohibited compounds for athletes that were not suffering from IDDM. Sönksen summarized the physiological effects of insulin in 2001, and concluded that indications justifying its ban are several-fold. First, insulin facilitates glucose uptake into muscle cells via an increased

translocation of GLUT4 glucose transporters from the cytoplasm to the cell membrane. This causes increased glycogen formation due to the uptake of glucose in amounts greater than those required for cellular respiration. Second, hyperinsulinemic clamps during training and also after competition may improve stamina and recovery. Third, insulin exerts a chalonic action on proteolysis; i.e., (muscle) protein degradation is inhibited and the net anabolic effect of insulin is mainly indirect, via a reduction in the rate of protein degradation. However, other research groups also reported a stimulation of protein biosynthesis by insulin in the presence of sufficient amounts of particular amino acids (Wolfe 2005).

DOPING CONTROLS

Owing to the fact that insulin may have a significant effect on athletic performance, strategies for the detection of insulin misuse have been developed, which have been focused so far on rapid-acting synthetic insulins (Thevis *et al.* 2005c, 2006b). As the primary specimen for sports drug testing has been urine, and urinary levels of intact insulins are very low (approximately 50 fmol·mL^{-1}), approaches using immunoaffinity purification followed by sensitive LC-MS/MS have been established. Rapid-acting insulins comprise at least one modification site compared to endogenously-produced human insulin. This fact allows an unambiguous determination of these drugs as MS/MS considers the molecular weight of target analytes (which is different from human insulin in two out of three drugs), as well as characteristic product ions derived from cleavage of the peptide backbone. The molecular weight of human insulin (5807 Da) is reduced by 19 and 16 Da compared to Novolog Aspart (5826 Da) and Glulisine Apidra (5823 Da), respectively, while Humalog LisPro is composed of the same set of amino acids as human insulin but differs in its primary structure by two switched amino acid residue positions. Hence, diagnostic product ions obtained by MS/MS experiments are of the utmost importance when differentiating between these two compounds.

The principal identification of synthetic insulins is based on their affinity to immobilized anti-insulin antibodies, which allowed their isolation from 10–20 mL human urine. Extracts are concentrated using solid-phase extraction and vacuum centrifuges, and resulting residues are subjected to chromatographic separation and LC-MS/MS analysis. Additionally, isolated insulins are optionally cleaved into A- and B-chains using reducing agents that separate the intra-molecular disulfide bonds. Product ion mass spectra of human (endogenous) insulin, Humalog, Novolog, and Apidra are obtained by CID of five-fold protonated precursor ions, and diagnostic product ions for human insulin and Humalog are found at *m/z* 226 (y_3–y_1) and 217 (y_2), respectively. The proline-directed dissociation of the charged analytes allows an MS distinction despite identical precursor ions and closely-related chromatographic properties. The differentiation of Novolog and Apidra from human insulin is accomplished by considerably different masses and product ion spectra due to the exchange of the proline residue (B_{28}) of human insulin by aspartic acid (Novolog) or the substitution of the asparagine (B_3) and lysine (B_{29}) residues by lysine and glutamic acid (Apidra), respectively. Levels of synthetic insulins as low as 9 fmol·mL^{-1} have been determined using this novel approach in doping control.

Growth hormone

GENERAL ASPECTS

Growth hormone (GH) is produced by the human pituitary gland and is characterized owing to considerable structural heterogeneity (Baumann 1991). Detailed investigations allowed the determination of reasons for the appearance of numerous GH variants, which were found to originate from an alternative splice site at the mRNA level, from post-translational modifications such as N-terminal acylation or deamidation, as well as from oligomerization (Baumann 1999). All cells of the human body bear GH receptors, and GH appears to be active on almost all of them. Its primary action is the stimulation of metabolic processes, the most important one of which is the production of IGF-1 and its binding proteins. In most tissues IGF-1 exerts autocrine and paracrine effects. However, hepatocytes secrete IGF-1 into the circulation and thus are responsible for recordable blood levels. Interestingly, recent studies have demonstrated that hepatic IGF-1 production in particular is primarily dependent on nutrition and thyroid status rather than GH *per se* (Sönksen 2001). IGF-1 is an important mediator of GH activity and has similar biological effects to GH, one of which is the stimulation of protein biosynthesis. GH has the additional effect of fat mobilization by mediating direct lipolysis, and the concerted and synergistic actions of GH, IGF-1, and insulin – i.e., increased protein synthesis and reduced protein degradation, respectively – may suggest certain benefits for athletes when abusing GH. Hence, for doping control analysis, GH has become a serious issue. However, numerous studies have been conducted in order to verify or falsify the hypothesis of a performance-enhancing effect of GH, but the outcome is unclear (e.g., see Jenkins 1999). GH administration reverses symptoms of deficiency disorders such as increased body fat, decreased bone density, and impaired muscle strength. Administration of GH to normal subjects, however, did not provide evidence for improved exercise tolerance or endurance (Berggren *et al.* 2005; Ehrnborg *et al.* 2005).

DOPING CONTROLS

The heterogeneous GH family of is of great interest for doping control analysis. Several assays enabling the determination of GH levels as well as the potential misuse of recombinant preparations have been published, primarily utilizing sophisticated immunoassays (Baumann 1999; Bidlingmaier *et al.* 2001; Wallace *et al.* 2001). The optimization of these assays in terms of cross-reactivity as well as specificity has required the detailed investigation of target antigens and their natural and artificial variants. Extensive research has been conducted in the past, which yielded details on natural monomers (e.g., 22 kDa and 20 kDa variants), covalent, and non-covalent oligomers, and chemical, proteolytic, or metabolic GH degradation products (Singh *et al.* 1974; Baumann 1991; Thevis & Schänzer 2005c).

Two principal approaches have been evaluated to enable doping control analysis to identify GH misuse. The first was established by the GH2000 consortium and elucidated changes in the GH/IGF-1 axis as well as the regulation of collagen and bone turnover (Ehrnborg *et al.* 2003; Powrie *et al.* 2007). In particular, the parameters procollagen type III N-terminal extension peptide (PIIIP) and osteocalcin have been considered as potential markers as their concentrations were significantly increased for to 84 days following GH administration (Wallace *et al.* 2000; Healy *et al.* 2005). The second approach is based on changes in molecular isoforms of GH after administration of recombinant GH (Wu *et al.* 1999; Bidlingmaier *et al.* 2000). The so-called "differential immunoassay approach" includes two analyses of each serum sample employing two monoclonal antibodies with distinct affinities to either the predominant 22 kDa variant (assay 1), or preferably to the other endogenously-produced isoforms (assay 2). The ratio between the quantities derived from assays 1 and 2 is then calculated, as recombinant GH consists of the 22 kDa isoform only. In cases of recombinant GH administration, values greater than 1.0 were obtained (owing also to the suppressive effects of exogenous application on endogenous production and secretion of GH), while "normal" ratios have been determined at values below 1.0 (Bidlingmaier *et al.* 2000).

Conclusion

An enormous variety of drugs that presumably or demonstrably enhance athletic performance is available through legitimate pharmaceutical sources and also on the "black market." Some have been investigated in detail in order to establish their influence on parameters such as endurance and strength, and also their negative side-effects on health. However, for the majority of therapeutic agents, no scientifically sound data is available to suggest that athletes may gain a competitive edge by (mis)using these drugs. Nevertheless, doping-control laboratories have been screening for known as well as unknown compounds for decades, and the emerging markets of new therapeutics, which definitely include drugs with a great potential for being misused in sports, will force them to extend their assays day after day to reveal cheating in sports and to protect athletes from unjustified accusation. Hence, "preventive doping research" approaches have also been introduced that are based on various cornerstones, which include the development of detection methods for new drugs that may enter the pharmaceutical market in the near future, for the comprehensive education of professionals coaching elite athletes regarding the risks of dietary supplements, as well as for drug (mis)use.

References

Amendola, L., Colamonici, C., Rossi, F. & Botre, F. (2002) Determination of clenbuterol in human urine by GC-MS-MS-MS: confirmation analysis in antidoping control. *Journal of Chromatography B* **773**, 7–16.

Baumann, G. (1991) Growth hormone heterogeneity: genes, isohormones, variants, and binding proteins. *Endocrine Reviews* **12**, 424–449.

Baumann, G. (1999) Growth hormone heterogeneity in human pituitary and plasma. *Hormone Research* **51**, 2–6.

Beecher, H.K. & Smith, G.M. (1965) Drugs and athletic performance. In: *Doping* (de Schaependryver, A. & Hebbelinck, M., eds.) Pergamon Press, Oxford: 133–144.

Berggren, A., Ehrnborg, C., Rosen, T., Ellegard, L., Bengtsson, B. & Caidahl, K. (2005) Short-term administration of supraphysiologic rhGH does not increase maximum endurance exercise capacity in healthy, active young men and women with normal GH-IGF-1 axes. *Journal of Clinical Endocrinology and Metabolism* **90**, 3268–3273.

Bidlingmaier, M., Wu, Z. & Strasburger, C.J. (2000) Test method: GH. *Baillière's Best Practice and Research Clinical Endocrinology and Metabolism* **14**, 99–109.

Bidlingmaier, M., Wu, Z. & Strasburger, C.J. (2001) Doping with growth hormone. *Journal of Pediatric Endocrinology and Metabolism* **14**, 1077–1084.

Butenandt, A. & Hanisch, G. (1935) Über testosteron. Umwandlung des dehydroandrosterons in androstendiol und testosteron, ein weg zur darstellung des testosterons aus cholesterin. *Hoppe-Seyler's Zeitschrift für Physiologische Chemie* **237**, 89–97.

Catlin, D.H., Sekera, M.H., Ahrens, B.D., Starcevic, B., Chang, Y.-C. & Hatton, C.K. (2004) Tetrahydrogestrinone: discovery, synthesis, and detection in urine. *Rapid Communications in Mass Spectrometry* **18**, 1245–1249.

Chen, J., Kim, J. & Dalton, J.T. (2005) Discovery and therapeutic promise of selective androgen receptor modulators. *Molecular Interventions* **5**, 173–188.

Coper, H., Herrmann, W.M. & Woite, A. (1987) Psychostimulantien, analeptika, nootropika. versuch einer differenzierung von arzneimitteln zur behandlung von hirnleistungsstörungen. *Deutsches Ärzteblatt* **84**, C248–C252.

Damasceno, L., Ventura, R., Ortuno, J. & Segura, J. (2000) Derivatization procedures for the detection of beta(2)-agonists by gas chromatographic/mass spectrometric analysis. *Journal of Mass Spectrometry* **35**, 1285–1294.

David, K., Dingemanse, E., Freud, J. & Laquer, E. (1935) Über kristallines männliches Hormon aus Hoden (Testosteron), wirksamer als aus harn oder Cholesterin bereitetes Androsteron. *Hoppe-Seyler's Zeitschrift für Physiologische Chemie* **233**, 281–282.

Deventer, K., Van Eenoo, P. & Delbeke, F.T. (2006) Screening for amphetamine and amphetamine-type drugs in doping analysis by liquid chromatography/mass spectrometry. *Rapid Communications in Mass Spectrometry* **20**, 877–882.

Donike, M. (1973) Acylierung mit bis(acylamiden); N-methyl-bis(trifluoracetamid) und bis(trifluoracetamid), zwei neue reagenzien zur trifluoracetylierung. *Journal of Chromatography* **78**, 273–279.

Donike, M. & Derenbach, J. (1976) Die selektive derivatisierung unter kontrollierten bedingungen: ein weg zum spurennachweis von aminen. *Zeitschrift Analytische Chemie* **279**, 128–129.

Donike, M., Jaenicke, L., Stratmann, D. & Hollmann, W. (1970) Gas chromatographic detection of nitrogen-containing drugs in aqueous solutions by means of the nitrogen detector. *Journal of Chromatography* **52**, 237–250.

Donike, M., Bärwald, K.R., Klostermann, K., Schänzer, W. & Zimmermann, J. (1983) Detection of endogenous testosterone. In: *Leistung und Gesundheit, Kongressbd. Dtsch. Sportärztekongress* (Heck, H., Hollmann, W. & Liesen, H., eds.) Deutscher Ärtze-Verlag, Köln: 293–298.

Downie, D., Delday, M.I., Maltin, C.A. & Sneddon, A.A. (2008) Clenbuterol increases muscle fiber size and GATA-2 protein in rat skeletal muscle *in utero*. *Molecular Reproduction and Development* **75**(5): 785–794.

Ehrnborg, C., Lange, K.H., Dall, R., Christiansen, J.S., Lundberg, P.A., Baxter, R.C., et al. (GH-2000 Study Group) (2003) The growth hormone/insulin-like growth factor-I axis hormones and bone markers in elite athletes in response to a maximum exercise test. *Journal of Clinical Endocrinology and Metabolism* **88**, 394–401.

Ehrnborg, C., Ellegard, L., Bosaeus, I., Bengtsson, B.A. & Rosen, T. (2005) Supraphysiological growth hormone: less fat, more extracellular fluid but uncertain effects on muscles in healthy, active young adults. *Clinical Endocrinology* **62**, 449–457.

Franke, W.W. & Berendonk, B. (1997) Hormonal doping and androgenization of athletes: a secret program of the German Democratic Republic government. *Clinical Chemistry* **43**, 1262–1279.

Geyer, H., Schänzer, W., Mareck, U. & Donike, M. (1996) Factors influencing the steroid profile. In: *Recent Advances in Doping Analysis*, vol. 3 (Donike, M., Geyer, H., Gotzmann, A. & Mareck, U., eds.) Sport und Buch Strauss, Cologne: 95–114.

Geyer, H., Mareck, U., Schänzer, W. & Donike, M. (1997) The Cologne protocol to follow up high testosterone/epitestosterone ratios. In: *Recent Advances in Doping Analysis*, vol. 4 (Schänzer, W., Geyer, H., Gotzmann, A. and Mareck, U., eds.) Sport und Buch Strauss, Cologne: 107–126.

Geyer, H., Parr, M.K., Mareck, U., Reinhart, U., Schrader, Y. & Schänzer, W. (2004) Analysis of non-hormonal nutritional supplements for anabolic-androgenic steroids – results of an international study. *International Journal of Sports Medicine* **25**, 124–129.

Hall, R.C. (2005) Abuse of supraphysiologic doses of anabolic steroids. *Southern Medical Journal* **98**, 550–555.

Healy, M.L., Dall, R., Gibney, J., Bassett, E., Ehrnborg, C., Pentecost, C., et al. (2005) Toward the development of a test for growth hormone (GH) abuse: a study of extreme physiological ranges of GH-dependent markers in 813 elite athletes in the postcompetition setting. *Journal of Clinical Endocrinology and Metabolism* **90**, 641–649.

Hemmersbach, P. & de la Torre, R. (1996) Stimulants, narcotics and β-blockers: 25 years of development in analytical techniques for doping control. *Journal of Chromatography B* **687**, 221–238.

Henze, M.K., Opfermann, G., Spahn-Langguth, H. & Schänzer, W. (2001) Screening of beta-2 agonists and confirmation of fenoterol, orciprenaline, reproterol and terbutaline with gas chromatography-mass spectrometry as tetrahydroisoquinoline derivatives. *Journal of Chromatography B* **751**, 93–105.

Hickson, R.C., Ball, K.L. & Falduto, M.T. (1989) Adverse effects of anabolic steroids. *Medical Toxicology and Adverse Drug Experience* **4**, 254–271.

Huang, L.E. & Bunn, H.F. (2003) Hypoxia-inducible factor and its biomedical relevance. *Journal of Biological Chemistry* **278**, 19575–19578.

Ishak, K.G. & Zimmerman, H.J. (1987) Hepatotoxic effects of the anabolic/androgenic steroids. *Seminars in Liver Disease* **7**, 230–236.

Jelkmann, W. (2004) Molecular biology of erythropoietin. *Internal Medicine* **43**, 649–659.

Jenkins, P. (1999) Growth hormone and exercise. *Clinical Endocrinology* **50**, 683–689.

Kamischke, A. & Nieschlag, E. (2004) Progress towards hormonal male contraception. *Trends in Pharmacological Sciences* **25**, 49–57.

Kamischke, A. & Nieschlag, E. (2005) Hormonal contraception for males – an option for adolescents? *Gynäkologisch-Geburtshilfliche Rundschau* **45**, 241–246.

Kazlauskas, R., Howe, C. & Trout, G. (2002) Strategies for rhEPO detection in sport. *Clinical Journal of Sport Medicine* **12**, 229–235.

Kearns, C.F., McKeever, K.H., Malinowski, K., Struck, M.B. & Abe, T. (2001) Chronic administration of therapeutic levels of clenbuterol acts as a repartitioning agent. *Journal of Applied Physiology* **91**, 2064–2070.

Kearns, C.F., McKeever, K.H. & Malinowski, K. (2006) Changes in adipopnectin, leptin, and fat mass after clenbuterol treatment in horses. *Medicine and science in sports and exercise* **38**, 262–267.

Kerr, J.M. & Congeni, J.A. (2007) Anabolic-androgenic steroids: use and abuse in pediatric patients. *Pediatric Clinics of North-America* **54**(4), 771–785, xii.

Kochakian, C.D. (1976). Metabolic effects of anabolic-androgenic steroids in experimental animals. In: *Anabolic-Androgenic Steroids* (Kochakian, C.D., ed.) Springer, New York: 5–44.

Kochendoerfer, G.G., Chen, S.-Y., Mao, F., Cressman, S., Traviglia, S., Shao, H., *et al.* (2003) Design and chemical synthesis of a homogeneous polymer-modified erythropoiesis protein. *Science* **299**, 884–887.

Lasne, F. & de Ceaurriz, J. (2000) Recombinant erythropoietin in urine. *Nature* **405**, 635.

Maisel, A.Q. (1965). *The Hormone Quest* Random House, New York.

Lasne, F., Martin, L., Crepin, N. & de Ceaurriz, J. (2002) Detection of isoelectric profiles of erythropoietin in urine: differentiation of natural and administered recombinant hormones. *Analytical Biochemistry* **311**, 119–126.

Miyake, T., Kung, C.K. & Goldwasser, E. (1977) Purification of human erythropoietin. *Journal of Biological Chemistry* **252**, 5558–5564.

Mohler, M.L., Nair, V.A., Hwang, D.J., Rakov, I.M., Patil, R. & Miller, D.D. (2005) Nonsteroidal tissue selective androgen receptor modulators: a promising class of clinical candidates. *Expert Opinion on Therapeutic Patents* **15**, 1565–1585.

Nielen, M.W.F., Bovee, T.F.H., van Engelen, M.C., Rutgers, P., Hamers, A.R.M., van Rhijn, J.A. *et al.* (2006) Urine testing for designer steroids by liquid chromatography with androgen bioassay detection and electrospray quadrupole time-of-flight mass spectrometry identification. *Analytical Chemistry* **78**, 424–431.

Nieschlag, E. & Behre, H.M. (2004) *Testosterone – Action, Deficiency, Substitution* Cambridge University Press, Cambridge.

Palm, D. (1987) Effects and side effects of doping with psychostimulants and beta-adrenoceptor blocking drugs. In: *Official Proceedings of the International Athletic Foundation World Symposium on Doping in Sport* (Bellotti, P., Benzi, G. & Ljungqvist, A., eds.) Arti Grafiche Danesi, Florence: 111–133.

Politi, L., Groppi, A. & Polettini, A. (2005) Applications of liquid chromatography-mass spectrometry in doping control. *Journal of Analytical Toxicology* **29**, 1–14.

Polonsky, K.S. & O'Meara, N.M. (2001) Secretion and metabolism of insulin, proinsulin and C-peptide. In: *Endocrinology* (DeGroot, L.J. & Jameson, J.L., eds.) Elsevier, Philadelphia: 697–727.

Powrie, J.K., Bassett, E.E., Rosen, T., Jørgensen, J.O., Napoli, R., Sacca, L., *et al.* (GH-2000 Project Study Group) (2007) Detection of growth hormone abuse in sport. *Growth Hormone and IGF Research* **17**, 220–226.

Prezelj, A., Obreza, A. & Pecar, S. (2003) Abuse of clenbuterol and its detection.

Current Medicinal Chemistry **10**, 281–290.

Reeds, P.J., Hay, S.M., Dorward, P.M. & Palmer, R.M. (1988) The effect of beta-agonists and antagonists on muscle growth and body composition of young rats (Rattus sp.). *Comparative Biochemistry and Physiology C* **89**, 337–341.

Ruzicka, L. & Wettstein, A. (1935) Sexualhormone VII. Über die künstliche herstellung des testikelhormons testosteron (androsten-3-on-17-ol). *Helvetica Chimica Acta* **18**, 1264–1275.

Schänzer, W. (1996) Metabolism of anabolic androgenic steroids. *Clinical Chemistry* **42**, 1001–1020.

Sekera, M.H., Ahrens, B.D., Chang, Y.C., Starcevic, B., Georgakopoulos, C. & Catlin, D.H. (2005) Another designer steroid: discovery, synthesis, and detection of "madol" in urine. *Rapid Communications in Mass Spectrometry* **19**, 781–784.

Singh, R.N.P., Seavey, B.K. & Lewis, U.J. (1974) Heterogeneity of human growth hormone. *Endocrine Research Communications* **1**, 449–464.

Smith, G.M. & Beecher, H.K. (1959) Amphetamine sulphate and athletic performance. *Journal of the American Medical Association* **170**, 542–557.

Sneddon, A.A., Delday, M.I., Steven, J. & Maltin, C.A. (2001) Elevated IGF-II mRNA and phosphorylation of 4E-BP1 and p70(S6k) in muscle showing clenbuterol-induced anabolism. *American Journal of Physiology and Endocrinology and Metabolism* **281**, E676–E682.

Sönksen, P.H. (2001) Hormones and sport (insulin, growth hormone and sport). *Journal of Endocrinology* **170**, 13–25.

Sytkowski, A.J. (2004) *Erythropoietin – Blood, Brain and Beyond* Wiley-VCH, Weinheim.

Thevis, M. & Schänzer, W. (2005a) Mass Spectrometry in Doping Control Analysis. *Current Organic Chemistry* **9**, 825–848.

Thevis, M. & Schänzer, W. (2005b) Examples of doping control analysis by liquid chromatography-tandem mass spectrometry: ephedrines, beta-receptor blocking agents, diuretics, sympathomimetics, and cross-linked hemoglobins. *Journal of Chromatographic Science* **43**, 22–31.

Thevis, M. & Schänzer, W. (2005c) Identification and characterization of peptides and proteins in doping control analysis. *Current Proteomics* **2**, 191–208.

Thevis, M. & Schänzer, W. (2005d) Analysis of low molecular weight substances in doping control. In: *The Endocrine System in Sports and Exercise* (Kraemer, W.J. & Rogol, A.D., eds.) Blackwell Publishing, Oxford: 47–68.

Thevis, M. & Schänzer, W. (2007) Mass spectrometry in sports drug testing: structure characterization and analytical assays. *Mass Spectrometry Reviews* **26**, 79–107.

Thevis, M., Opfermann, G. & Schänzer, W. (2003) Liquid chromatography/ electrospray ionization tandem mass spectrometric screening and confirmation methods for β_2-agonists in human or equine urine. *Journal of Mass Spectrometry* **38**, 1197–1206.

Thevis, M., Geyer, H., Mareck, U. & Schänzer, W. (2005a) Screening for unknown synthetic steroids in human urine by liquid chromatography-tandem mass spectrometry. *Journal of Mass Spectrometry* **40**, 955–962.

Thevis, M., Schebalkin, T., Thomas, A. & Schänzer, W. (2005b) Quantification of clenbuterol in human plasma and urine by liquid chromatography-tandem mass spectrometry. *Chromatographia* **62**, 435–439.

Thevis, M., Thomas, A., Delahaut, P., Bosseloir, A. & Schänzer, W. (2005c) Qualitative determination of synthetic analogues of insulin in human plasma by immunoaffinity purification and liquid chromatography-tandem mass spectrometry for doping control purposes. *Analytical Chemistry* **77**, 3579–3585.

Thevis, M., Kamber, M. & Schänzer, W. (2006a) Screening for metabolically stable aryl-propionamide-derived selective androgen receptor modulators for doping control purposes. *Rapid Communications in Mass Spectrometry* **20**, 870–876.

Thevis, M., Thomas, A., Delahaut, P., Bosseloir, A. & Schänzer, W. (2006b) Doping control analysis of intact rapid-acting insulin analogues in human urine by liquid chromatography-tandem mass spectrometry. *Analytical Chemistry* **78**, 1897–1903.

Todd, T. (1987) Anabolic steroids: the gremlins of sport. *Journal of Sport History* **14**, 87–107.

Videman, T., Lereim, I., Hemmingsson, P., Turner, M.S., Rousseau-Bianchi, M.P., Jenoure, P., *et al.* (2000) Changes in hemoglobin values in elite cross-country skiers from 1987 to 1999. *Scandinavian Journal of Medicine and Science in Sports* **10**, 98–102.

Vidic, E. (1956) Eine methode zur identifizierung papierchromatographisch isolierter arzneistoffe. *Archiv für Toxikologie* **16**, 63–73.

von Deutsch, D.A., Abukhalaf, I.K., Wineski, L.E., Aboul-Enein, H.Y., Pitts, S.A., Parks, B.A., *et al.* (2000) Beta-agonist-induced alterations in organ weights and protein content: comparison of racemic clenbuterol and its enantiomers. *Chirality* **12**, 637–648.

von Deutsch, D.A., Abukhalaf, I.K., Wineski, L.E., Roper, R.R., Aboul-Enein, H.Y., Paulsen, D.F., *et al.* (2002) Distribution and muscle-sparing effects of clenbuterol in hindlimb-suspended rats. *Pharmacology* **65**, 38–48.

Wadler, G.I. & Hainline, B. (1989) *Drug and the Athlete* F.A. Davis Company, Philadelphia.

Wallace, J.D., Cuneo, R.C., Lundberg, P.A., Rosen, T., Jorgensen, J.O., Longobardi, S. *et al.* (2000) Responses of markers of bone and collagen turnover to exercise, growth hormone (GH) administration, and GH withdrawal in trained adult males. *Journal of Clinical Endocrinology and Metabolism* **85**, 124–133.

Wallace, J.D., Cuneo, R.C., Bidlingmaier, M., Lundberg, P.A., Carlsson, L., Boguszewski, C.L., *et al.* (2001) The response of molecular isoforms of growth hormone to acute exercise in trained adult males. *Journal of Clinical Endocrinology and Metabolism* **86**, 200–206.

Wolfe, R.R. (2005) Regulation of skeletal muscle protein metabolism in catabolic states. *Current Opinion in Clinical Nutrition and Metabolic Care* **8**, 61–65.

Wrighton, N.C., Balasubramanian, P., Barbone, F.P., Kashyap, A.K., Farrell, F.X., Jolliffe, L.K., *et al.* (1997) Increased potency of an erythropoietin peptide mimetic through covalent dimerization. *Nature Biotechnology* **15**, 1261–1265.

Wu, Z., Bidlingmaier, M., Dall, R. & Strasburger, C.J. (1999) Detection of doping with human growth hormone. *Lancet* **353**, 895.

Zeman, R.J., Ludemann, R. & Etlinger, J.D. (1987) Clenbuterol, a beta 2-agonist, retards atrophy in denervated muscles. *American Journal of Physiology* **252**, E152–E155.

Part 9

Limitations to Performance

Chapter 19

Cardiorespiratory Limitations to Performance

NIELS H. SECHER

The cardiorespiratory system provides oxygen and substrates to tissues, transports metabolic waste products to the liver and kidneys, and eliminates carbon dioxide and heat via exhalation and evaporation of water from the lungs and skin, respectively. Even though limitations to exercise performance vary depending on the duration of exercise, the involved muscle mass, and the ambient temperature, oxygen transport from the atmosphere to the working muscles remains critical. During whole-body exercise no single factor limits the oxygen transport cascade, expressed as the sum of the resistances presented by each step. Yet, in order to preserve arterial pressure, blood flow to working muscles (Secher & Volianitis 2006) and internal organs, including the brain (Ide & Secher 2000), is restrained with adverse outcomes for metabolism and fatigue (Nybo & Secher 2004; Dalsgaard 2006). Resistance to oxygen transport is adjusted to daily life activities, while endurance training affects most steps along the transport chain, primarily by decreasing total peripheral vascular resistance (Clausen 1976).

Animals have developed to enable them to overcome specific critical situations, and training adaptations can only moderate the pre-set evolutionary characteristics of the organism. Some reptiles depend on anaerobic metabolism for increased activity because their lungs encompass a sparse number of alveoli and their vasculature is not separated into pulmonary and systemic circulations, as is the case

in mammals (Wang & Hicks 2002). Conversely, the hearts of certain mammals may be large and their skeletal muscles encompass red fibers that are designed for sustained activity while others, like the cat family, possess relatively small hearts and their skeletal muscles are dominated by fibers that are geared for a fast short hunt.

The human heart weighs ~300 g while 380 g is expected when compared to animals of similar size (Brody 1945). Human skeletal muscles with ~50% slow-twitch (ST) fibers (Saltin & Gollnick 1983) are equally not well-prepared for enduring high-intensity activity. Exceptionally, the expiratory internal intercostal muscles demonstrate extreme adaptation to continued activity, where all fast-twitch (FT) fibers appear to be trained (specifically FTa fibers), perhaps to facilitate the important human function of talking. Internal intercostal muscles are also provided with a denser capillarization than other skeletal muscles (Fig. 19.1). For a given muscle large inter-individual variations (a standard deviation of 17% exists for the distribution of ST vs. FT fibers) form a structural background that explains why some athletes possess talent for endurance activities while others are inclined to sprinting.

In many sporting activities body size and, more specifically, the relative weight of different body segments plays a role (Larsen 2003) as most Olympic events favor tall individuals (Khosla 1983). Body size is a determinant of maximal oxygen uptake ($\dot{V}o_{2max}$) with a 0.73 power association with body weight (Jensen et al. 2001). This illustrates an advantage for light people when body weight is lifted, such as during running, in contrast to when the body weight is

The Olympic Textbook of Science in Sport, 1st edition. Edited by R.J. Maughan. Published 2009 by Blackwell Publishing. ISBN: 978-1-4051-5638-7.

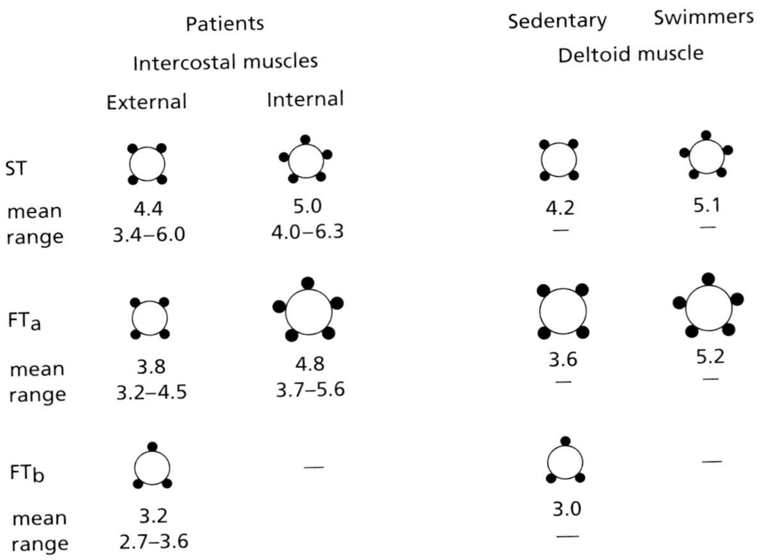

	Patients Intercostal muscles		Sedentary Swimmers Deltoid muscle	
	External	Internal		
ST				
mean	4.4	5.0	4.2	5.1
range	3.4–6.0	4.0–6.3	—	—
FT$_a$				
mean	3.8	4.8	3.6	5.2
range	3.2–4.5	3.7–5.6	—	—
FT$_b$				
mean	3.2	—	3.0	—
range	2.7–3.6		—	

Fig. 19.1 Capillarization of external and internal intercostal muscles obtained from patients during thoractomy and of the deltoid muscle of sedentary subjects and swimmers. FT$_a$, trained fast twitch muscle fibers; FT$_b$, untrained fast twitch muscle fibers; ST, slow twitch muscle fibers. (Reproduced with permission from Secher *et al.* 1984.)

supported, such as during rowing, which favors large, heavy individuals. In a dimensionally-neutral comparison of small and large individuals, $\dot{V}o_{2max}$ for distance runners and cyclists reaches 234 mL·kg$^{-0.73}$·min^{-1} and the largest reported absolute value of 7.46 L·min^{-1} is for a cross country skier (Saltin 1996).

It is probable that structural adaptations are more responsive during childhood and early adolescence rather than when fully-grown, but people of all ages maintain work capacity related to their daily activity, including during training (Yoshiga *et al.* 2002). Talent is further based upon genetically-determined cardiovascular responses to a given intervention (Snyder *et al.* 2006), and genetic influences on cardiovascular control can in turn affect athletic performance (Gayagay *et al.* 1998). Even though it is likely, it remains to be established whether the inherent cardiovascular adaptations to exercise are coupled to developments of the heart and skeletal muscles in humans. In this review, oxygen transport in the body is followed with little consideration to interindividual differences in oxygen-carrying capacity.

Ventilation

Oxygen enters the body through the lungs, which have an enormous gas diffusion capacity with an alveolar area of 50–100 m^2. Increased ventilation is coupled intimately to exercise, but the contribution of the lungs to oxygen transport during submaximal and maximal exercise remains unknown for two reasons. First, lung function is described as a capacity rather than as the actual contribution to the transport of oxygen during a given intervention, including exercise. Second, evaluation of the lungs is combined with the capacity of hemoglobin in pulmonary capillaries to take up oxygen, expressed as the pulmonary carbon monoxide diffusion capacity (DLCO; Krogh 1915). The more relevant value for the diffusion capacity of oxygen is 23% larger than the DLCO, and the value for carbon dioxide is 24.6-times the DLCO value (Dittmer & Grebe 1958).

DLCO is a non-invasive measure of lung function because the affinity of carbon monoxide (CO) to hemoglobin is 200-times that of oxygen. When ~1% CO is added to inspired air, CO binds with hemoglobin over the entire length of the pulmonary capillary (Fig. 19.2) and DLCO therefore represents the gas transport capacity. Conversely, DLCO is dominated by acute changes in the pulmonary capillary blood volume. For example, DLCO decreases by 15% from the supine to the seated position at rest (Hanel *et al.* 1997) because pulmonary capillary blood volume is reduced while the pulmonary membrane diffusion is enhanced by 30% (Fig. 19.3). During exercise, there is a doubling of DLCO

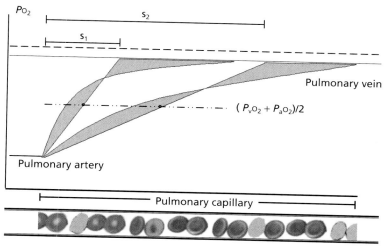

Fig. 19.2 A diagram showing the oxygen tension of blood (P_{O_2}) during its course through a pulmonary capillary at two flow rates. Also shown is a cartoon of red cells passing through a pulmonary capillary with carbon monoxide (CO) binding to hemoglobin. The apparent pulmonary diffusion for oxygen (Dm_{O_2}) describes the effective area for diffusion rather than the diffusion capacity established when the whole capillary is engaged in oxygen transfer. Because there is little or no transport of oxygen in the venous end of the capillary, the effective capillary diffusion area (s_1 or s_2) is approximated by the insertion of a line integrating the considered increase in P_{O_2}. When it takes longer for the alveolar to capillary oxygen equilibrium to be established because of doubled flow during exercise or because of low inspired oxygen tension, the venous end of the capillary becomes increasingly important and an enhanced effective diffusion area is expressed as an elevated Dm_{O_2}. Discrepancy between a doubling of the diffusion capacity for CO and an eightfold increase in Dm_{O_2} during exercise indicates that at rest, in normoxia, an equilibrium is established between PA_{O_2} and Pc_{O_2} within one-quarter of the length of the pulmonary capillary. During hypoxemia, however, an equilibrium is not reached and the entire capillary contributes to diffusion, which is expressed as a maximal Dm_{O_2}. Any venous admixture to arterial blood is reported as a change in Dm_{O_2}, representing an integrated measure of pulmonary function rather than of diffusion *per se*. To validate the absolute value, pulmonary venous oxygen tension needs to replace Pa_{O_2} in the calculation of Dm_{O_2}.

Fig. 19.3 Pulmonary function in supine and upright positions at rest and during progressive exercise on a cycle ergometer. The apparent pulmonary membrane diffusion for oxygen (Dm_{O_2}) reached a maximal value (i.e., its capacity) during ergometer cycling exercise but not during one-legged exercise. $\dot{V}E$, ventilation; $\dot{V}_{O_2}$, pulmonary oxygen uptake; (PA_{O_2}), alveolar tension for oxygen; PA_{O_2}-Pc_{O_2}, alveolar to pulmonary capillary oxygen tension difference. Values are presented as mean ± SE for 16 and 8 subjects for the cycle ergometer and one-legged exercise, respectively. (Reproduced with permission from Mortensen *et al.* 2005.)

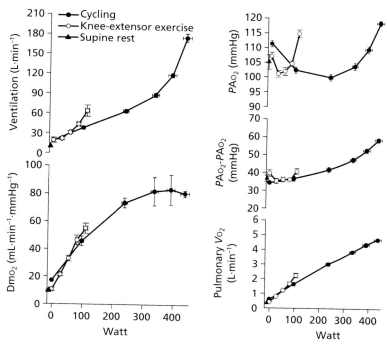

(25–50 mL·mmHg^{-1}·min^{-1}; Dittmer & Grebe 1958) reflecting the support of the muscle pump to the pulmonary blood volume, with recruitment of capillaries in the apical parts of the lungs.

Transport of oxygen

In contrast to CO, which is taken up over the entire length of the capillary, in normoxia equilibrium between alveolar and capillary oxygen tensions is established within a fraction of the capillary blood transit time (Fig. 19.2). During exercise, as the velocity of red cells in pulmonary capillaries increases, equilibrium takes longer to be established and, ultimately, the entire capillary partakes in diffusion of oxygen and hence the capacity is utilized. As the length of the capillary involved in diffusion increases during exercise, it becomes difficult to maintain alveolar oxygen tension (PAo_2) and an increase in ventilation is required to compensate for oxygen taken up by capillary blood (Fig. 19.3). Ventilation during exercise follows two distinct patterns. Low-intensity exercise is associated with little drive to ventilation from the central nervous system (termed "central command;" Galbo et al. 1987). Relative hypoventilation is expressed as a 0.5 kPa elevation in the arterial CO$_2$ tension ($Paco_2$; Jørgensen et al. 1992), which is the dominant stimulus for ventilation. As exercise intensity increases then ventilation increases exponentially, an effect that is influenced by the decreased blood pH. The important effect of blood pH on driving ventilation is demonstrated by the ~15 L·min^{-1} reduced ventilation following normalization of pH with bicarbonate administration, despite the 1 kPa increase in $Paco_2$ (Nielsen et al. 2002a). With marked hyperventilation during intense exercise PAo_2 increases to high levels (17 kPa) but $Paco_2$ decreases to below the resting value.

Even though the lungs facilitate oxygen transport during light to moderate exercise by recruiting alveoli and enhancing the within capillary diffusion area (Fig. 19.2), a diffusion capacity of ~80 mL·mmHg^{-1}·min^{-1} (an eight-fold increase from rest; Fig. 19.3) is insufficient to account for the often more than 15-fold increase in $\dot{V}o_2$ during maximal exercise. Further, during intense exercise $\dot{V}o_2$ depends on a widening of the alveolar-capillary oxygen tension difference because gas diffusion is impeded by high pulmonary arterial pressure that provokes the accumulation of fluid in the alveolar-capillary space (Hanel et al. 2003). Thus, arterial oxygen tension (Pao_2) – expressed as a "physiologic shunt" or "exercise-induced hypoxemia" (Dempsey & Wagner 1999) – decreases, (e.g., from 12 to 10 kPa; Nielsen et al. 1999) although PAo_2 increases during intense exercise.

During intense exercise the elevated ventilation, as demonstrated by the extraordinarily large ventilatory rates observed in endurance-trained athletes (up to 314 L·min^{-1}; Saltin 1996), increases PAo_2, and Pao_2 is maintained at the highest possible level. Such a mechanism may explain the enhanced exercise performance following specific respiratory muscle training that supports large ventilation and Pao_2, as indicated by the elevated end-tidal oxygen tension during exercise (Volianitis et al. 2001).

In contrast, the pulmonary diffusion capacity does not seem to respond to training and the large reported values for DLCO represent a selection of gifted individuals with exceptionally large vital capacities, as is the case for competitive rowers with ~7 L being the average lung capacity and the highest recorded value being 9.1 L (Secher 1983). DLCO varies from 15 to 45 mL·mmHg^{-1}·min^{-1} (Dittmer & Grebe 1958) and this range reflects differences in body size and the amount of hemoglobin within the central blood volume (termed the "pulmonary capillary blood volume"), in addition to variations in pulmonary membrane diffusion capacity. Pulmonary membrane diffusion capacity is larger than DLCO because it does not include the resistance to diffusion of oxygen in plasma or the binding of CO to hemoglobin; however, values for athletes versus control subjects or for a potential training effect have yet to be established.

Hemoglobin

The transport of oxygen in blood by hemoglobin is described by the oxyhemoglobin dissociation curve (Fig. 19.4), reserving ~2% of the transport to oxygen dissolved in plasma during maximal exercise (Mortensen et al. 2005). At rest and during moderate exercise, when the Pao_2 value is ~13 kPa, pH has little influence on the amount of oxygen

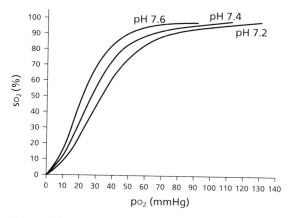

Fig. 19.4 The oxyhemoglobin dissociation curve for three pH values of blood, illustrating the Bohr effect. (Modified with permission from Dittmer & Grebe, 1958.)

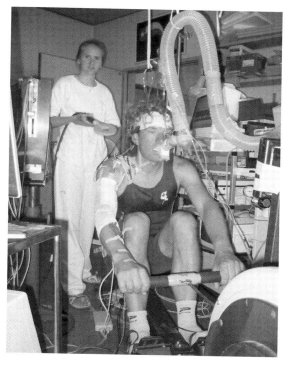

Fig. 19.5 Evaluation of metabolism, circulation, and brain function during ergometer rowing.

transported. During maximal exercise, when Pao_2 is reduced, a right-shift ("Bohr effect") of the oxyhemoglobin dissociation curve demonstrates that any deviation in pH affects the ability of hemoglobin to transport oxygen; $\dot{V}o_{2max}$ decreases in proportion to the reduction in hemoglobin saturation. During maximal ergometer rowing the Bohr effect reduces arterial oxygen saturation to ~90% and imposes a 5–10% restraint on $\dot{V}o_{2max}$. When arterial oxygen saturation is restored, both in response to hyperoxic breathing (Dempsey & Wagner 1999) and to pH normalization following bicarbonate administration (Nielsen *et al.* 2002a), $\dot{V}o_{2max}$ increases (Fig. 19.5). On the other hand, oxygen delivery to tissues is enhanced both by the effect of exercise-induced body temperature elevation and the Bohr effect, and augmented by the lower pH of venous compared to arterial blood (e.g., 7.0 vs. 7.2) as carbon dioxide is exhaled ($Paco_2$ reduced from 12 to 5 kPa, venous vs. arterial; Mortensen *et al.* 2005). The record low pH value of 6.74, corresponding to a blood lactate level of 32 mM, was measured following a ergometer rowing championship (Nielsen 1999).

Blood lactate during exercise

The Bohr effect on the oxyhemoglobin dissociation curve illustrates the delicate balance between aerobic and anaerobic metabolism during maximal exercise,

but little is known about that balance during actual sporting competitions (Fig. 19.6). Appreciating the various tactics that athletes apply during a race, it is likely that the degree to which oxygen transport is affected by acidity varies between individuals depending on Pao_2, which in turn is influenced by the balance between hyperventilation and pulmonary membrane diffusion capacity. Competitions start at high speed to accelerate the increase in $\dot{V}o_2$ (Secher 1983) because the total aerobic metabolism is represented by the accumulated $\dot{V}o_2$ during the race rather than the highest level that $\dot{V}o_2$ reaches. For unknown reasons, early in exercise a "stitch," corresponding to the attachment of the diaphragm to the ribs, may be experienced, especially by untrained individuals. Also, there may be a partial recovery as the load becomes easier after a minute or so, described as a "second wind".

More is known about exercise at high altitude. When the inspired oxygen tension is low it is

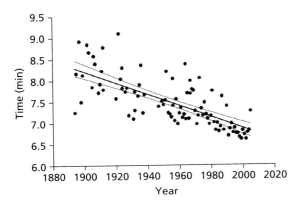

Fig. 19.6 Results obtained during the Federation International Societes d'Aviron (FISA) Single Sculling Championships, 1893–2006, with a 95% confidence interval for the regression line. (Updated by T. Vogelsang with permission from Secher 1973.)

disadvantageous to work at an intensity that provokes lactate acidosis, because any anaerobic contribution to metabolism attenuates the more important oxygen-carrying capacity of blood. While it is possible to work at an intensity that provokes lactate acidosis, endurance activity in hypoxic environments is usually associated with a small deviation in pH, a condition that has been defined as the high altitude "lactate paradox" (Ward *et al.* 1989). Following high altitude acclimatization, when ventilation and Pao_2 increase, plasma lactate during maximal exercise is comparable with sea-level values (Lundby *et al.* 2000). The unproven but likely beneficial effect of moderate altitude training (~2000 m) for sea-level performance (Jensen *et al.* 1993) may be explained by the adaptation of the respiratory muscles to the large exercise ventilation in hypoxia. Upon return to sea level it feels easier to maintain a large ventilation during competition, to increase Pao_2, and hence, to enhance the anaerobic contribution to exercise without affecting the oxygen-transport capacity of hemoglobin.

Lactate threshold

The Bohr effect on the oxyhemoglobin dissociation curve explains why the work-rate at a given blood lactate level is a sensitive predictor of performance

(Coen *et al.* 2002). Blood lactate increases exponentially with workload but their relationship is right-shifted following training, i.e., blood lactate increases with relative workload. The workload that elicits a given lactate level (often set at 4 mM) is, therefore, an indirect measure of $\dot{V}o_{2max}$, which is in itself a predictor of performance (Secher 1983). Blood lactate is a more precise performance predictor than $\dot{V}o_{2max}$ because blood lactate reflects not only $\dot{V}o_{2max}$ but also the ability to work without affecting the oxy-hemoglobin dissociation curve.

For a given workload less lactate is produced during the recruitment of ST compared to FT muscle fibers, as illustrated when ST fibers are prevented from contracting with curare-induced (South American arrow poison) partial neuromuscular blockade (Gallagher *et al.* 2001a). The workload that elicits a given blood lactate level reflects the work capacity of ST muscle fibers. The composition of muscles depends not only on the percent of ST vs. FT fibers but also on their relative size. For example, weight-lifters develop large FT fibers in adaptation to rapid lifts, while rowers' muscles are characterized by large ST fibers (Larsson and Forsberg 1980) reflecting the relatively slow movements involved in rowing. Furthermore, considering that "central fatigue" inhibits ST muscle fiber recruitment (Secher 1992), during exercise that requires increased central command a smaller contribution from ST muscle fibers necessitates that work has to be carried out with a larger contribution from FT muscle fibers, and hence lactate production increases. In other words, evaluation of blood lactate during submaximal exercise reflects the mental preparation and automatization that determines the central command requirements for a given activity.

It should also be noted that although it is lactate that is measured in blood, it is the deviation in pH that influences oxygen transport. Lactate is a substrate for tissues including muscle, liver, kidney, and brain (Dalsgaard 2006), but its exponential accumulation in the blood as the work-rate increases is a manifestation of attenuated elimination by the liver and kidneys (Nielsen *et al.* 2002b). Blood lactate is, therefore, also an indicator of how well organ blood flow is preserved during various levels of exercise.

Blood volume and cardiac preload

The heart delivers oxygen to the tissues. The heart of quadruped animals is at a level with the main portion of blood within the body, but upright humans face a circulatory challenge as the indifference point for volume is at the level of the pelvis (Perko *et al.* 1995) and about 80% of the blood volume is positioned below the heart. Thus, in response to reduced central blood volume, cardiovascular reflexes including sympathetic activation (Pedersen *et al.* 1995) and the veno-arterial reflex (Henriksen & Skagen 1986) are important for maintaining the upright position. Yet, it is not possible to remain upright without the muscle pump preventing the accumulation of blood in dependent parts of the body (van Lieshout *et al.* 2001). If humans stand still for prolonged periods of time, as known from soldiers standing in-line, they become prone to fainting with a concomitant decrease in heart rate and blood pressure recorded. This reflex, defined as "vasovagal syncope," is elicited when the central blood volume is reduced by 30% due to hemorrhage or gravitational pooling in the upright posture, and the associated reduction in blood pressure is attributed to a "Bezold-Jarish-like reflex" that induces vasodilatation in skeletal muscles at the expense of flow to the brain (Secher & van Lieshout 2005).

Starling's law of the heart

The influence of central blood volume, or "cardiac preload," on the function of the heart is described by Starling's law of the heart (Fig. 19.7). In this context, "normovolaemia," defined by the absence of a further increase in stroke volume or cardiac output when central blood volume increases, is achieved in the supine posture. During a head-down tilt that increases diastolic filling of the heart, there is no further stroke volume increase indicating that the upper flat part of the Starling curve is reached (Harms *et al.* 2003; van Lieshout *et al.* 2005). Conversely when upright, central blood volume is reduced and the heart operates on the ascending part of the Starling curve with cardiac output depending on preload.

During exercise central blood volume and the ~10% increase in the blood volume of working

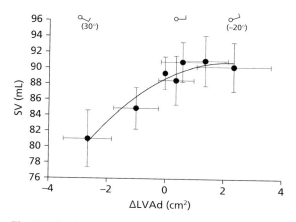

Fig. 19.7 Starling curve for the human heart as evaluated during a head-up and head-down tilt. During supine rest the upper flat part of the curve is reached. SV, stroke volume; ΔLVAd, change in left ventricular end-diastolic area. (Reproduced with permission from Jans *et al.* 2008.)

muscles (Pawelczyk *et al.* 1992) are supported by the muscle pump promoting venous return and the redistribution of blood volume by differentiated vasoconstriction in the splanchnic area (Perko *et al.* 1998). However, with increasing blood flow requirements in working muscles and the skin as body temperature increases (Cai *et al.* 2000), splanchnic vasoconstriction does not recruit enough blood to enable the central blood volume to reach the level established in the seated or supine position at rest. During exercise central blood volume contributes to the level of sympathoexcitation established, as illustrated by changes in heart rate. For example, when in the supine position resting heart rate may be 60 bpm; this increases to 80 bpm when standing, but decreases to 70 bpm during contraction of the leg muscles. Muscle contractions increase sympathetic activity but the concomitant enhancement of central blood volume and central venous pressure by the muscle pump elicits a "paradoxical" reduction in sympathetic activity (Ray *et al.* 1993; van Lieshout *et al.* 2001). Similarly, during running a smaller central blood volume manifests as a lower central venous pressure and distension of the atria, as reflected by the plasma level of atrial natriuretic peptide (ANP), and heart rate is higher than during rowing at a given exercise $\dot{V}O_2$. Furthermore, the lowest heart rate response to exercise is observed in the supine posture (Stenberg *et al.* 1967). This gravitational influence on heart rate is sustained during maximal exercise, as indicated by the lower value during rowing than during running, despite the higher $\dot{V}_{O_{2max}}$ value established by the larger active muscle mass during rowing (Yoshiga & Higuchi 2001).

The heart rate response to exercise is of particular interest because an almost linear relationship between heart rate and workload (or $\dot{V}_{O_2}$) is widely applied for the evaluation of $\dot{V}_{O_{2max}}$ in population studies (Åstrand 1960). Following endurance training that enhances central blood volume – as detected by electrical impedance of the thoracic region (Ogoh *et al.* 2003b) – heart rate at a given workload, including maximal effort, decreases. Nevertheless, it should be noted that the heart rate response to training is more complicated than this implies, and some observations remain unexplained. For example, following one-legged training, training-induced bradycardia does not manifest during two-legged cycling even though both legs are trained (Davies & Sargeant 1975; Klausen *et al.* 1982).

Blood volume

The cardiac output depends on the volume of blood that the heart receives or its preload. As the total capacitance of the vasculature is larger than the total blood volume, distribution of the blood volume is critical for maintenance of blood pressure and regional flow. Blood volume encompasses the volumes of both red cells and plasma, the latter of which changes rapidly in response to physical activity. For example, plasma volume is elevated by 20% following short-term training and it decreases during bed rest (Saltin *et al.* 1968) or during space flight. The enlargement of plasma volume following training and the reduction in plasma volume when the central blood volume remains elevated, demonstrate that central blood volume rather than total blood volume is the regulated variable.

During exercise humans lose weight by sweating, but even after body weight is restored by drinking the central blood volume remains reduced for many hours and plasma volume is expanded by further drinking as thirst is maintained. Central blood volume is reduced following exercise due to muscle edema provoked by the combined effects of elevated perfusion pressure and muscle vasodilatation. In addition, cutaneous vasodilatation induced by the elevated body temperature contributes to the attenuation of central blood volume (Cai *et al.* 2000). Even though body temperature normalizes and muscle edema is cleared rapidly after exercise (Clausen *et al.* 1973; Rasmussen *et al.* 1992), muscle blood volume recruited from the central circulation, as detected by DLCO and thoracic electrical impedance, remains elevated for almost 24 h (Hanel *et al.* 1997).

The reduced central blood volume following exercise is reflected in the levels of hormones that regulate fluid balance, including plasma vasopressin (alternatively named antidiuretic hormone, ADH) and plasma ANP (Hanel *et al.* 1997). Plasma vasopressin remains elevated while plasma ANP is low following exercise and both these hormonal changes reduce urine production, resulting in positive fluid balance. Conversely, during bed rest or space flight, central blood volume remains elevated and plasma volume is down-regulated by a reverse hormonal profile to that established following exercise.

It is less clear why the red cell volume increases in response to training. Bone marrow is stimulated to produce hemoglobin by erythropoietin (EPO), which is released mainly from the kidneys. Exposure to high-altitude hypoxia increases hemoglobin production, but the acute increase in hematocrit is caused by loss of plasma volume. Conversely, kidney diseases are associated with anemia attributed to low EPO production, and the administration of EPO is integrated into the treatment of these patients. Thus, whole-body exercise, in addition to the exercise-induced hypoxemia stimulus for EPO production, may stimulate hemoglobin production via a sympathetically-induced reduction in kidney blood flow.

The increase in total hemoglobin is an important adaptation to training because $\dot{V}_{O_{2max}}$ is related to red cell volume or to hemoglobin (Åstrand 1952; Heinicke *et al.* 2001). In an apparent paradox, athletes often present somewhat low hemoglobin concentrations (or hematocrit: 44% vs. 46% in untrained individuals) because of their enlarged plasma volume. For athletes, plasma and red cell volumes may be 61 and 46 mL·kg^{-1}, respectively, compared to reference values of 46 and 33 mL·kg^{-1}, respectively, for men (Heinicke *et al.* 2001); training-induced increases in both plasma and red cell volumes support preload to the heart.

The heart

As known from the study of cardiac diseases, the heart adapts to the load it is exposed to and this adaptation also applies to training (Secher 1921). With endurance training especially, the internal diameters of the heart increase. The highest values recorded were observed in professional cyclists, with an internal diameter of 55 mm and a wall thickness of 10 mm, compared to values of 50 and 8.7 mm, respectively, for divers (Pelliccia *et al.* 1991). The heart of weightlifters is different because they develop high blood pressure during each maximal effort by concomitantly performing a Valsalva-like maneuver (Pott *et al.* 2003) that stabilizes the spine. To overcome the high blood pressure, the wall thickness of the heart is 10 mm, with the same internal diameter as cyclists despite a larger body mass.

In rowing and kayaking, as in many other activities, there is a combined demand for a large $\dot{V}o_{2max}$, cardiac output, and stroke volume, in addition to overcoming the high blood pressure (e.g., at the beginning of each rowing stroke; Clifford *et al.* 1994). It follows that both the internal dimensions and wall thickness of the heart increase and these athletes possess the largest "sports heart," with a left ventricular mass of 330 g compared to 142 g for divers. Correspondingly, the internal diameter may be 56–59 mm and wall thickness 11–14 mm (Pelliccia *et al.* 1991). In these athletes the heart is so enlarged that myocardial perfusion becomes inhomogeneous (Bartram *et al.* 1998). This, combined with a high vagal tone and low "intrinsic heart rate" (after combined vagal and sympathetic blockade; Katona *et al.* 1982), creates a complicated electrocardiographic presentation. As in skeletal muscles, training increases capillarization of the heart (Brown 2003) and, following detraining, the size of the heart returns to its control values (Secher 1923).

While maintaining an adequate preload to the heart during upright exercise is a problem, it is not difficult for the heart to pump the blood it is provided with. In contrast to the pain experienced in skeletal muscles during sustained exercise, healthy people do not complain of chest pain upon exertion, indicating that myocardial oxygen demand does not limit cardiac output. Furthermore, it is energy-efficient for the heart to provide a large cardiac output. The energy requirements of the heart depend on its rate and (systolic) pressure expressed as the "rate-pressure product," and in cardiac patients "angina pectoris" is provoked at the same rate-pressure product before and after training (Clausen & Trap-Jensen 1976). In fact, vascular impedance or "cardiac afterload" decreases to 3–4 Hz with increasing heart rate.

Following endurance training the enlarged blood volume ensures filling of the heart and reduces sympathetic activity, which attenuates heart rate by the same mechanism observed during supine and seated exercise. Furthermore, the enhanced central blood volume attenuates the pressure that arterial baroreceptors control during exercise, as exemplified by the blood pressure reduction when leg exercise is added to arm cranking (Fig. 19.8; Volianitis *et al.*

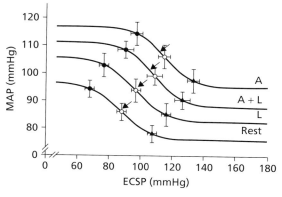

Fig. 19.8 The carotid baroreflex at rest and during arm (A), leg (L), and combined arm and leg exercise (A + L). At rest the actual pressure (arrow) corresponds to the maximum gain of the reflex (o), while during exercise it may be positioned at a slightly lower estimated carotid sinus pressure (ECSP), suggesting that the baroreflex detects hypotension even though blood pressure is elevated. HR, heart rate; MAP, mean arterial pressure. (Reproduced with permission from Volianitis *et al.* 2004a.)

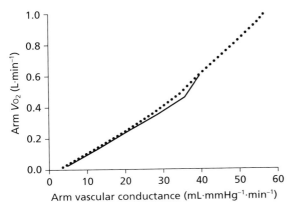

Fig. 19.9 Arm vascular conductance at rest and during exercise for untrained (full line) and trained rowers (broken line). (Modified with permission from Secher & Volianitis 2006.)

2004a). Cardiac output is elevated following endurance training with no additional strain on the heart (i.e., same rate–pressure product during maximal exercise), indicating that the enhanced blood flow to active muscles is provided by means of increased vascular conductance (Fig. 19.9; Clausen 1976; Secher & Volianitis 2006). Yet, the muscle pump cannot provide enough blood to the heart and sometimes, at exhaustion, a constraint on cardiac preload is illustrated by decreasing central venous pressure (Mortensen et al. 2005).

Stroke volume

The stroke volume of endurance-trained athletes is impressive – 195 vs. 110 mL for control subjects (Ekblom & Hermansen 1968) and 227 mL for a $\dot{V}o_{2max}$ of 7.46 (Saltin 1996). However, it is not limited by the capacity of the heart to encompass a large volume of blood. The problem upright humans face in increasing cardiac output during exercise is different from that experienced by quadruped animals (Stray-Gundersen et al. 1986). In puppies, work capacity increases following pericardiectomy, which allows the heart to expand. In upright humans there is no similar restraint on stoke volume, as illustrated by the filling of the heart during supine exercise and

by the ability of the heart to increase stroke volume in response to a volume overload. With the administration of the plasma expander Macrodex® heart rate during maximal exercise decreases (183 vs. 188 bpm), while stroke volume is enhanced by 10% (from 155 to 144 mL; Kanstrup & Ekblom 1982).

Despite the fact that following volume expansion the enhanced stroke volume confirms that the heart operates at the ascending part of the Starling curve when humans are upright, stroke volume during exercise does not increase via enhanced filling. On the contrary, the size of the heart remains unchanged and it may decrease somewhat when heart rate exceeds 150 bpm (Holmgren 1956), indicating that the heart propels the blood it is provided with. During exercise stroke volume increases due to enhanced contractility and the systolic duration shortens to about one-half while the diastolic duration is further limited to one-third of the resting value. Exercise tachycardia develops although plasma potassium increases, e.g., to 6–7 mM (Nielsen et al. 1998; Volianitis et al. 2004b), signifying that sympathetic activation (Kjær et al. 1987) is needed not only to maintain function of the heart but also to clear plasma potassium during and after exercise (Schmidt et al. 1995).

A short diastolic interval during exercise may present a problem for the filling of the heart, as illustrated in patients with atrial fibrillation where cardiac output is compromised when the heart rate exceeds 120 bpm. However, during exercise venous return is enhanced and contractility of the heart is increased. The influence of sympathetic activation on the heart is supported by a small increase in free plasma calcium released from albumin as pH decreases (Nielsen et al. 2002a; Volianitis et al. 2004b). In addition, relaxation of the left ventricle may draw blood into the heart and this action is enhanced when the end-systolic volume is attenuated during vigorous exercise. Yet the attenuated heart rate response to exercise following training is an advantageous adaptation for the filling of the heart. Conversely, following cardiac transplantation, where the heart is denervated, stroke volume is determined by diastolic volume (a Starling mechanism; Kjær et al. 1999).

Extreme exercise

The ability of the heart to cope is less impressive during extreme exercise. Reports on horses running to death are not uncommon. It is also well-known that Pheidippides died after running the original Marathon course to report to Athens the Greek victory over the Persians (battle of Marathon, 490 BC). (It may be noted that previously he had been fighting in the battle after running 2×250 km in a round trip from Athens to Sparta to request support!) While running to exhaustion, the heart of rats is dilated and the blood volume encompassed within the cavities is elevated by 50% and takes days to normalize (Secher 1921). That degree of exhaustion is further characterized by a state simulating thyroid insufficiency, as illustrated by reduced spontaneous activity, increased food consumption, and increased body weight in rats that were forced to swim to exhaustion (Richter 1958).

The extent that the post-exercise stress syndrome in rats relates to overtraining in humans is only a speculation, but long-distance events such as the triathlon or the Ironman provoke cardiac fatigue (Dawson et al. 2003). This presents primarily as reduced diastolic and systolic functions. Both chronotropic and inotropic functions are affected by competitions lasting for hours, as illustrated by attenuated responses to sympathomimetic drugs (e.g., by beta-receptor downregulation or desensitization; Welsh et al. 2005).

Cardiac output

Cardiac output provides blood flow to tissues including working skeletal muscles and there is, on average, a 7.3 : 1 coupling between cardiac output and $\dot{V}o_2$ (Mitchell et al. 1958), or 6.5 : 1 in athletes (Ekblom & Hermansen 1968). The largest reported $\dot{V}o_{2max}$ of 7.46 L·min^{-1} was associated with a maximal cardiac output of 42.5 L·min^{-1} (Saltin 1996), and values of 40 L·min^{-1} are regularly reported for athletes (Ekblom & Hermansen 1968). There are, however, large inter-individual variations in cardiac output both at rest and during exercise. At rest some of this variation relates to body size and cardiac output

is expressed as the "cardiac index" ($\sim$3.1 m^{-2}) in cardiology, with body surface area based on height and weight ($\sim$1.7 m^{-2}). More important, cardiac output varies according to polymorphisms in the β_2-adrenergic receptor (Snyder et al. 2006) and with hematocrit (Krantz et al. 2005).

During exercise pulmonary $\dot{V}o_2$ increases in relation to metabolism in exercising muscles with the oxygen uptake of non-exercising tissues being 0.7 L·min^{-1} during leg exercise (Secher et al. 1977). Such observations underscore a tight coupling between cardiac output, regional blood flow, and metabolism, with some attenuation of blood flow seen at the highest workloads (Åstrand et al. 1964; Mortensen et al. 2005). However, it is not blood flow per se that is regulated but rather oxygen-carrying capacity, defined as venous oxygen saturation. Such regulation is demonstrated in patients with anemia who present a large cardiac output (may be 15 L·min^{-1}) and regional blood flows, while their venous hemoglobin saturation is close to that of healthy people (75%). Equally, with manipulation of hematocrit, there is an inverse relationship between cardiac output and regional blood flow, including working muscles, and hematocrit (Gonzàlez-Alonso et al. 2006). Oxyhemoglobin liberates vasodilatatory substances such as nitric oxide (NO) and adensine triphosphate (ATP) when it is deoxygenated and creates its own flow (Gonzàlez-Alonso et al. 2002). At a low hematocrit, a given oxygen consumption is provided by deoxygenation of the red cells passing through the tissue and flow is enlarged until the normal venous saturation is re-established. Conversely, when hematocrit is high, as in some patients with pulmonary disease or following chronic exposure to high altitude, little oxygen is liberated from hemoglobin and blood flow is maintained at a low level. Cardiac output compensates for a low hematocrit until it is reduced to $\sim$50% during isovolaemic hemodilution (Krantz et al. 2005).

The postulate of an oxygen-dependent regulation of cardiac output and regional blood flow assumes that the heart can meet the demand for cardiac output, but that is not always the case. When the circulating blood volume is reduced, as exemplified by blood letting or dehydration, cardiac output may become limiting. Where cardiac function may be compromised, the influence of posture and other situations associated with a reduced circulating blood volume, such as sweating and fasting, become important; thus, cardiac output evaluation is recognized as an important element of preoperative assessment of patients (Ejlersen *et al.* 1995). In addition, the heart may be unable to generate an adequate cardiac output in patients with cardiac insufficiency (Schmidt *et al.* 1995; Ide & Secher 2000) and in normal individuals after the administration of a beta-adrenergic receptor antagonist (Pawelczyk *et al.* 1992).

Blood pressure

Arterial pressure has two roles in the regulation of blood flow to tissues. First, it is the primary regulated circulatory variable controlled beat by beat from the arterial baroreceptors, which modulate peripheral resistance (Ogoh *et al.* 2003a), including that of skeletal muscles (Collins *et al.* 2001). Second, it serves to regulate perfusion pressure to the tissues, and notably to the brain. There are two theories for the control of regional blood flow and specifically of flow to the brain. It is considered that flow to the brain is supported by a "siphon" in the sense that potential energy required to raise blood from the level of the heart to the brain could be regained when flow leaves the brain through the veins. Such a mechanism would require that venous pressure is negative in the internal jugular vein that drains the brain (vertical distance to the heart 35 cm; negative pressure 25 mmHg). However, in the upright posture the internal jugular veins collapse and their pressure is close to zero (Dawson *et al.* 2004). In neck veins, as with other veins raised above the level of the heart, blood flows like water piling down a window (termed a "Starling resistor"). Cerebral blood flow is dependent on mean arterial pressure and venous pressure influences perfusion pressure to the brain only in supine humans (Pott *et al.* 2000). Similarly, perfusion of the arms is limited when they are held over the head, as demonstrated by the pain experienced while painting the roof and, conversely, leg blood flow is supported by the hydrostatic distance from the heart (Folkow *et al.* 1971).

During exercise, regulation of arterial pressure by the arterial baroreceptors implies that their operating range is right-shifted and elevated by neural influence from central command and by the "muscle pressor reflex," as illustrated in Fig. 19.8 (Gallanger *et al.* 2001a,b). Two strategies may be applied in establishing the pressure that the baroreceptors are reset to control. Ideally, the set pressure can be established by an increase in cardiac output to compensate for the marked decrease in total peripheral resistance induced by exercise. However, if that is not possible because of strain on cardiac output either by a restricted preload or by an inability of the heart to produce the required cardiac output, then the mean arterial pressure is maintained by vasoconstriction, not only to internal organs (Perko *et al.* 1995) but also to working muscles (Secher & Volianitis 2006) and the brain (Ide & Secher 2000).

Regional blood flow

Skeletal muscle blood flow is modulated by deoxygenation of hemoglobin adjusting flow to metabolism and that takes place despite the enhanced sympathetic activity during exercise. Such "sympatholysis" (Remensnyder *et al.* 1962) also depends on other factors such as elevated muscle temperature, potassium, nitric oxide and, significantly, by mechanical distortion of the feed-arteries to the muscles (Clifford *et al.* 2006). It is likely that flow is coupled to tissue metabolism through the arterial pyruvate/lactate ratio (Mintun *et al.* 2004). However, muscle blood flow is not allowed to increase at the expense of blood pressure. Priority for blood pressure regulation over regulation of flow is demonstrated when comparison is made between flow to a muscle working in isolation and to one working with other muscles. As an example, flow to working legs ($\sim$10 L·min^{-1}) is reduced when the arms are working intensely at the same time (Fig. 19.10; Secher *et al.* 1977). Equally, arm blood flow (4.6 L·min^{-1} in untrained vs. 6.4 l L·min^{-1} in rowers) and oxygenation are larger during arm cranking alone than when arm cranking is performed together with high-intensity cycling exercise; similar observations are available for roller skiing (Calbert *et al.* 2004).

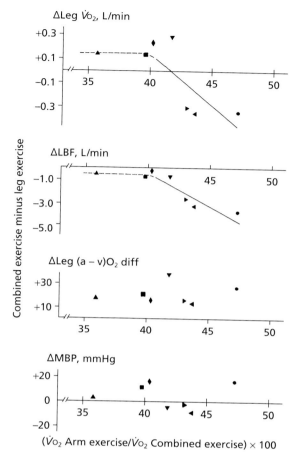

Fig. 19.10 The effect of adding arm exercise to leg exercise on leg oxygen uptake ($\dot{V}o_2$), leg blood flow (LBF), the leg arterial to venous oxygen difference [(a-v̄)O_2 diff], and mean arterial pressure (MBP). (Reproduced with permission from Secher *et al.* 1977.)

Skeletal muscles seldom receives the blood flow that their vasculature can handle as only a few exercise modalities involve a single muscle group. Even during normal cycling single-leg blood flow may be lower than when that leg is working alone (Klausen *et al.* 1982). During whole-body exercise in particular, flow to the working muscles is reduced by ~20–40% compared to the flow they receive during exercise involving small muscle mass, and this reduction is manifested primarily via sympathetically-mediated enhanced vascular resistance (Pawelczyk *et al.* 1992; Saito *et al.* 1992). However, when leg exercise is added

to arm cranking, blood pressure decreases and perfusion pressure to the arm accounts for ~50% of the reduction in arm blood flow (Volianitis *et al.* 2004b).

Muscles

The final step in the oxygen transport chain to muscle is by diffusion. Krogh (1929) found that capillaries are recruited when muscles are activated, suggesting that the capillary network is designed to provide the muscle with oxygen during exercise rather than at rest. In fact, arteries are not gas-impermeable and a considerable amount of gas exchange (oxygen uptake and elimination of CO_2) takes place in vessels larger than the capillaries (Shibata *et al.* 2006). However, during exercise muscle cells are provided with oxygen through diffusion from the capillaries. There is a coupling between $\dot{V}o_{2max}$ and capillary density and more capillaries surround ST than FT muscle fibers (Fig. 19.1). Typical values for the vastus lateralis muscle are 1.8 capillaries per fiber for untrained and 2.6 capillaries per fiber for trained subjects. The highest capillarization is observed in the internal intercostal muscles with 6.0 capillaries per fiber.

As with the lungs, the oxygen diffusion capacity of the muscles can be calculated (Wagner *et al.* 1977). The available oxygen diffusion capacity of the muscles is not always used: during moderate exercise capillary recruitment enhances the gas diffusion capacity, but during maximal whole-body exercise blood flow is limited and, thus, gas diffusion is restricted. During arm exercise gas diffusion values for the arm may be 20 mL·min^{-1}·mmHg^{-1} in untrained subjects and 50 mL·min^{-1}·mmHg^{-1} in trained subjects, but it decreases to 32 mL·min^{-1}·mmHg^{-1} in trained subjects when leg exercise is added to arm cranking (Volianitis *et al.* 2004b).

Brain

Ultimately, it is the brain that limits performance. During maximal exercise the ratio between oxygen and glucose and lactate uptake by the brain (cerebral metabolic ratio: molecular uptake of oxygen/uptake of glucose + 1/2 lactate) decreases from a resting value of 6.0 to nearly 3.0 at exhaustion; i.e., the brain behaves as if it has a substantial capacity for anaerobic metabolism and its glycogen deposits decrease upon activation (Dalsgaard 2006). Several factors may challenge brain oxygenation during maximal exercise. Brain blood flow depends on Pa_{CO_2} which decreases with hyperventilation during maximal exercise. Furthermore, maximal whole-body exercise may be associated with exercise-induced hypoxemia, and together these two factors may reduce brain oxygenation by ~10% (Nielsen et al. 1999). The brain is much more sensitive to a reduction in its oxygenation than skeletal muscles (Gonzàlez-Alonso et al. 2004) because the cerebral capillaries are surrounded by the astrocytes. These cells represent the "blood-brain barrier" but at the same time make the diffusion distance for oxygen from the capillaries to the neurons longer than the diffusion distance to the myocytes. It is therefore likely that central fatigue relates to an energy crisis faced by the neurons and/or the inability of the brain to maintain a given level of central command when its temperature reaches 40–41°C (Nybo & Secher 2004). Conversely, proper hydration allows for evaporation of water and control of temperature while training may be interpreted as the preparation of the cardiorespiratory system to provide oxygen and substrates to working muscles so that work can be carried out without the brain being aware of the effort (Secher 1992).

Taken together, the cardiorespiratory system has the capacity to increase $\dot{V}_{O_{2max}}$ by modulating each of the different steps in the transport system with the exception of the pulmonary system, which is the only organ for which adaptation to endurance training has not been demonstrated. Endurance-type activity is limited primarily by the ability to provide the muscle with oxygen, as originally suggested by A.V. Hill who defined $\dot{V}_{O_{2max}}$. However, the ultimate decision to stop exercise is made by the central nervous system and this may be linked to when glycogen stores in associated astrocytes are depleted and the relevant neurons do not receive lactate for accelerated activity.

References

Åstrand, I. (1960) Aerobic working capacity in men and women with special reference to age. *Acta Physiologica Scandinavica* **49**(Suppl 169), 83.

Åstrand, P.-O. (1952) *Experimental Studies of Physical Working Capacity in Relation to Sex and Age.* Munksgaard, Copenhagen.

Åstrand, P.-O., Cuddy, T.E., Saltin, B. & Stenberg, J. (1964) Cardiac output during submaximal and maximal exercise. *Journal of Applied Physiology* **19**, 268–274.

Bartram, P., Toft, J., Hanel, B., Ali, S., Gustafsson, F., Mortensen, J. et al. (1998) False-positive defects in technetium-99m sestamibi myocardial single-photon emission tomography in healthy athletes with left ventricular hypertrophy. *European Journal of Nuclear Medicine* **25**, 1308–1312.

Brody, S. (1945) *Biogenetics and Growth.* Reinhold, New York.

Brown, M.D. (2003) Exercise and coronary vascular remodeling in the healthy heart. *Experimental Physiology* **88**, 645–658.

Cai, Y, Jenstrup, M., Ide, K., Perko, M. & Secher, N.H. (2000) Influence of temperature on blood volume distribution as assessed by electrical impedance. *European Journal of Applied Physiology* **81**, 443–448.

Calbert, J. Jensen-Urstad, M., van Hall, G., Holmberg, H.-C., Rosdahl, H. & Saltin, B. (2004) Maximal vascular conductance during whole body upright exercise in humans. *Journal of Physiology* **558**, 319–331.

Clausen, J.P. (1976) Circulatory adjustments to dynamic exercise and effect of physical training in normal subjects and in patients with coronary artery disease. *Progress in Cardiovascular Diseases* **18**, 459–495.

Clausen, J.P., Klausen, K., Rasmussen, B. & Trap-Jensen, J. (1973) Central and peripheral circulatory changes after training of the arms or legs. *American Journal of Physiology* **255**, 675–682.

Clausen, J.P. & Trap-Jensen, J. (1976) Heart rate and arterial blood pressure during exercise in patients with angina pectoris. Effect of training and nitroglycerin. *Circulation* **53**, 436–442.

Clifford, P.S., Hanel, B. & Secher, N.H. (1994) Arterial blood pressure response to rowing. *Medicine and Science in Sports and Exercise* **26**, 715–719.

Clifford, P.S., Kluess, H.A., Hamann, J.J., Buckwalter, J.B. & Lesperse, J.L. (2006) Mechanical compression elicits vasodilatation in rat skeletal muscle feed arteries. *Journal of Physiology* **572**, 561–567.

Coen, B., Urhausen, A. & Kinderman, W. (2002) Sports specific performance diagnostics in rowing: an incremental graded exercise test in coxless pairs. *International Journal of Sports Medicine* **24**, 428–432.

Collins, H.L., Augusttyniak, R.A. & O'Lery, D.S. (2001) Carotid baroreflex pressor responses at rest and during exercise: cardiac output vs. regional vasoconstriction. *American Journal of Physiology* **280**, H642–H648.

Dalsgaard, M.K. (2006) Fuelling cerebral activity in exercising man. *Journal of Cerebral Blood Flow and Metabolism* **26**, 731–750.

Davies, C.M.T. & Sargeant, A.J. (1975) Effects of training on the physiologic response to one- and two-leg work. *Journal of Applied Physiology* **38**, 377–381.

Dawson, E.E., George, K., Shave, R., Whyte, G. & Ball, D. (2003) Does the human heart fatigue subsequently to prolonged exercise? *Sports Medicine* **33**, 365–380.

Dawson, E.A., Secher, N.H., Dalsgaard, M.K., Ogoh, S., Yoshiga, C.C., Gonzàlez-Alonso, J., et al. (2004) Standing up to the challenge of standing: a siphon does not support cerebral blood flow in humans. *American Journal of Physiology* **287**, R911–R914.

Dempsey, J.A. & Wagner, P.D. (1999) Exercise-induced arterial hypoxemia. *Journal of Applied Physiology* **87**, 1997–2006.

Dittmer, D.S. & Grebe, R.M., eds. (1958) *Handbook of Respiration* Saunders, Philadelphia: 52, 77.

Ejlersen, E., Skak, C., Møller, K., Pott, F. & Secher, N.H. (1995) Central cardiovascular variables at a maximal mixed venous saturation in severe hepatic failure. *Transplantation Proceedings* **27**, 3506–3507.

Ekblom, B. & Hermansen, L. (1968) Cardiac output in athletes. *Journal of Applied Physiology* **25**, 619–625.

Folkow, B., Haglund, M., Jodal, M. & Lundgren, O. (1971) Blood flow in the calf muscle of man during rhythmic exercise. *Acta Physiologica Scandinavica* **81**, 157–161.

Galbo, H., Kjær, M. & Secher, N.H. (1987) Cardiovascular, ventilatory and catecholamine responses to maximal dynamic exercise in partially curarized man. *Journal of Physiology* **389**, 557–568.

Gallagher, K.M., Fadel, P.J., Strømstad, M., Ide, K., Smith, S.A., Querry, R.G., et al. (2001a) Effects of partial neuromuscular blockade on carotid baroreflex function during exercise in humans. *Journal of Physiology* **533**, 861–870.

Gallagher, K.M., Fadel, P.J., Strømstad, M., Ide, K., Smith, S.A., Querry, R.G., et al. (2001b) Effects of exercise pressor reflex activation on carotid baroreflex function during exercise in humans. *Journal of Physiology* **533**, 871–880.

Gayagay, G., Yu, B., Hambly, B., Boston, T., Hahn, A., Celermajer, D.S. et al. (1998) Elite endurance athletes and the ACE I allele-role of genes in athletic performance. *Human Genetics* **103**, 48–50.

Gonzàlez-Alonso, J., Olsen, D.B. & Saltin, B. (2002) Erythrocyte and the regulation of human skeletal muscle blood flow and oxygen delivery: role of circulating ATP. *Circulation Research* **91**, 1046–1055.

Gonzàlez-Alonso, J., Dalsgaard, M.K., Osada, T., Volianitis, S., Dawson, E.A., Yoshiga, C.C. et al. (2004) Brain and central haemodynamics and oxygenation during maximal exercise in humans. *Journal of Physiology* **557**, 331–142.

Gonzàlez-Alonso, J., Mortensen, S., Dawson, E.A., Secher, N.H. & Damsgaard, R. (2006) Erythrocyte and the regulation of human skeletal muscle blood flow and oxygen delivery: Role of erythrocyte count and oxygenation state of haemoglobin. *Journal of Physiology* **572**, 295–305.

Hanel, B., Teunissen, I., Rabøl, A., Warberg, J. & Secher, N.H. (1997) Restricted postexercise pulmonary diffusion capacity and central blood volume depletion. *Journal of Applied Physiology* **83**, 11–17.

Hanel, B., Law, I. & Mortensen, J. (2003) Maximal rowing has an acute effect on the blood-gas barrier in elite athletes. *Journal of Applied Physiology* **95**, 1076–1082.

Harms, M.P., van Lieshout, J.J., Jenstrup, M., Pott, F. & Secher, N.H. (2003). Postural effects on cardiac output and mixed venous saturation in humans. *Experimental Physiology* **88**, 611–616.

Heinicke, K., Wolfarth, B., Winchenbach, P., Biermann, B., Schmid, A. Huber, G., et al. (2001) Blood volume and hemoglobin mass in elite athletes of different disciplines. *International Journal of Sports Medicine* **22**, 504–512.

Henriksen, O. & Skagen, K. (1986) Local and central sympathetic vasoconstrictor reflexes in human limbs during orthostatic stress. In: *The Sympathoadrenal System. Physiology and Pathophysiology* (Christensen, N.J., Henriksen, O. & Lassen, N.A., eds.) Munksgaard, Copenhagen: 83–94.

Holmgren, A. (1956) Circulatory changes during muscular work in man. *Scandinavian Journal of Clinical and Laboratory Investigations* **8**(Suppl. 24), 1–97.

Ide, K. & Secher, N.H. (2000) Cerebral blood flow and metabolism during exercise. *Progress in Neurobiology* **61**, 397–414.

Jans, Ø., Tollund, C., Bundgaard-Nielsen, M., Selmer, C., Warberg, J. & Secher, N.H. (2008) Goal-directed fluid therapy: stroke volume optimisation and cardiac dimensions in healthy humans. *Acta Anaesthesiologica Scandinavica* **52**, 536–540.

Jensen, K., Nielsen, T., Fiskestrand, Å., Lund, J.O., Christensen, N.J. & Secher, N.H. (1993) High altitude training does not increase maximal oxygen uptake or work capacity at sea level in rowers. *Scandinavian Journal of Medicine and Science in Sports and Exercise* **3**, 256–262.

Jensen, K., Johansen, L. & Secher, N.H. (2001) Influence of body mass on maximal oxygen uptake: importance of sample size. *European Journal of Applied Physiology* **84**, 201–205.

Jørgensen, L.G., Perko, M., Hanel, B., Schroeder, T.V. & Secher, N.H. (1992) Middle cerebral artery flow velocity and blood flow during exercise and muscle ischemia in humans. *Journal of Applied Physiology* **72**, 1123–1132.

Kanstrup, I.-L. & Ekblom, B. (1982) Acute hypervolemia, cardiac performance and aerobic power during exercise. *Journal of Applied Physiology* **52**, 1186–1191.

Katona, P.G., McLean, M., Dighton, D.H. & Guz, A. (1982) Sympathetic and parasympathetic cardiac control in athletes and nonathletes at rest. *Journal of Applied Physiology* **52**, 1652–1657.

Khosla, T. (1983) Sports for tall. *British Medical Journal* **287**, 736–738.

Kjær, M., Secher, N.H. & Galbo, H. (1987) Physical stress and catecholamine release. *Balliere's Clinical Endocrinology and Metabolism* **1**, 279–298.

Kjær, M., Beyer, N. & Secher, N.H. (1999) Exercise and organ transplantation. *Scandinavian Journal of Medicine and Science in Sports* **9**, 1–14.

Klausen, K., Secher, N.H., Clausen, J.C., Hartling, O. & Trap-Jensen, J. (1982) Central and regional circulatory adaptations to one-leg training. *Journal of Applied Physiology* **52**, 976–983.

Krantz, T., Warberg, J. & Secher, N.H. (2005) Venous oxygen saturation during normovolaemic haemodilution in the pig. *Acta Anaesthesiologica Scandinavica* **49**, 1149–1156.

Krogh, A. (1929) *The Anatomy and Physiology of Capillaries*. Yale University Press, New Haven.

Krogh, M. (1915) The diffusion of gases through the lung of man. *Journal of Physiology* **49**, 271–296.

Larsen, H. (2003) Kenyan dominance in distance running. *Comparative Biochemistry and Physiology* **136**, 161–170.

Larsson, L. & Forsberg, A. (1980) Morphological muscle characteristics in rowers. *Canadian Journal of Applied Sports Sciences* **5**, 239–244.

Lundby, C., Saltin, B. & van Hall, G. (2000) The "lactate paradox", evidence for a transient change in the course of acclimatization to severe hypoxia in lowlanders. *Acta Physiologica Scandinavica* **170**, 265–269.

Mitchell, J.H., Sproule, B.J. & Chapman, C.B. (1958) The physiologic meaning of the maximal oxygen intake test. *Journal of Clinical Investigation* **37**, 538–547.

Mintun, M.A., Vlassenko, A.G., Rundle, M.M. & Raichle, M.E. (2004) Increased lactate/pyruvate ratio arguments blood flow in physiologically activated human brain. *Proceeding of Natural Academy of Science* **101**, 659–664.

Mortensen, S.P., Dawson, E.A., Yoshiga, C.C., Dalsgaard, M.K., Damsgaard, R., Secher, N.H. *et al.* (2005) Limitations to systemic and locomotor limb muscle oxygenation delivery and uptake during maximal exercise in humans. *Journal of Physiology* **566**, 273–285.

Nielsen, H.B. (1999) pH after competitive rowing: the lower physiologic range? *Acta Physiologica Scandinavica* **165**, 113–114.

Nielsen, H.B., Madsen, P., Svenden, L.B., Roach, R.C. & Secher, N.H. (1998) The influence of Pao$_2$, pH and SaO$_2$ on maximal oxygen uptake. *Acta Physiologica Scandinavica* **164**, 89–97.

Nielsen, H.B., Boushel, R., Madsen, P. & Secher, N.H. (1999) Cerebral desaturation during exercise reversed by O$_2$ supplementation. *American Journal of Physiology* **277**, H1045–H1052.

Nielsen, H.B., Bredmose, P., Strømstad, M., Volianitis, S., Quistorff, B. & Secher N.H. (2002a) Bicarbonate attenuates arterial desaturation during exercise in humans. *Journal of Applied Physiology* **93**, 724–731.

Nielsen, H.B., Clemmesen, J.O., Skak, C., Ott, P. & Secher, N.H. (2002b) Attenuated hepatic elimination of lactate during intense exercise in humans. *Journal of Applied Physiology* **92**, 1677–1683.

Nybo, L. & Secher, N.H. (2004) Cerebral perturbations provoked by prolonged exercise. *Progress in Neurobiology* **72**, 223–261.

Ogoh, S., Fadel, P.J., Nissen, P., Jans, Ø., Selmer, C., Secher, N.H. *et al.* (2003a) Carotid baroreflex-mediated changes in cardiac output and total peripheral conductance during exercise in humans. *Journal of Physiology* **550**, 317–324.

Ogoh, S., Volianitis, S., Nissen, P., Wray, D.W., Secher, N.H. & Raven, P.B. (2003b) Carotid baroreflex responsiveness to head-up tilt-induced central hypovolaemia: effect of aerobic fitness. *Journal of Physiology* **551**, 601–608.

Pawelczyk, J.A., Hanel, B., Pawelczyk, R.A., Warberg, J. & Secher, N.H. (1992)

Leg vasoconstriction during dynamic exercise with reduced cardiac output. *Journal of Applied Physiology* **73**, 1838–1846.

Pedersen, M., Madsen, P., Klokker, M., Olesen, H.L. & Secher, N.H. (1995) Sympathetic influence on cardiovascular responses to sustained head-up tilt in humans. *Acta Physiologica Scandinavica* **155**, 435–444.

Pelliccia, A., Maron, B.J., Spataro, A., Proschan, M.A. & Spirito, P. (1991) The upper limit of physiologic cardiac hyperthrophy in highly trained elite athletes. *New England Journal of Medicine* **324**, 295–301.

Perko, G., Tilgren, R. & Secher, N.H. (1995) Venous pump does not affect the indifference point for electrical impedance in man. *European Journal of Applied Physiology* **72**, 179–195.

Perko, M.J., Nielsen, H.B., Skak, C., Clemmensen, J.O., Schroeder, T.V. & Secher, N.H. (1998) Mesenteric, coeliac and splanchnic blood flow during exercise. *Journal of Physiology* **513**, 907–913.

Pott, F., van Lieshout, J.J., Ide, K., Madsen, P. & Secher, N.H. (2000) Middle cerebral artery flow velocity during a Valsalva maneuver the standing position. *Journal of Applied Physiology* **88**, 1545–1550.

Pott, F., van Lieshout, J.J., Ide, K., Madsen, P. & Secher, N.H. (2003) Middle cerebral artery blood velocity during intense static exercise is dominated by a Valsalva maneuver. *Journal of Applied Physiology* **94**, 1335–1344.

Rasmussen, J., Hanel, B., Saunamaki, K. & Secher, N.H. (1992) Recovery of pulmonary diffusion capacity after maximal exercise. *Journal of Sports Sciences* **10**, 525–531.

Ray, C.A., Rea, R.F., Clary, M.P. & Mark, A.L. (1993) Muscle sympathetic nerve responses to dynamic one-legged exercise: effect of body posture. *American Journal of Physiology* **264**, H1–H7.

Remensnyder, J.P., Mitchell, J.H. & Sarnoff, S.J. (1962) Functional sympatholysis during muscular activity; observations on influence of carotid sinus oxygen uptake. *Circulation Research* **11**, 370–380.

Richter, C.P. (1958) Neurological basis for responses to stress. In: *Neurological Basis of Behaviour.* Ciba Foundation Symposium (Wolstenholme, G.E.W., ed.) Churchill, London: 204–221.

Saito, M., Kagaya, A., Ogta, F. & Shinohara, M. (1992) Changes in muscle sympathetic nerve activity and calf blood flow during combined leg and forearm exercise. *Acta Physiologica Scandinavica* **146**, 449–456.

Saltin B (1996) The physiology of competitive c.c. skiing across a four decade perspective; with a note on training induced adaptations and role of training at medium altitude. In: *Science and Skiing* (Müller, E., Schwameder, H., Kornexl, E. & Rascher C., eds.) E & FN Spon, London: 435–469.

Saltin, B. & Gollnick, P.O. (1983) Skeletal muscle adaptability: significance for metabolism and performance. In: *Handbook of Physiology, Skeletal Muscle* (Peachy, L.D., Hadrian, R. & Geiger, S.R., eds.) American Physiololgcal Society. William & Wilkins, Washington: 555–631.

Saltin, B., Blomqvist, G., Mitchell, J.H., Johnson, R.L., Wildenthal, K. & Chapman, C.B. (1968) Response to submaximal and maximal exercise after bed rest and training. *Circulation* **38**(Suppl. 7), 1–78.

Schmidt, T.A., Bundgaard, H., Olesen, H.L., Secher, N.H. & Kjeldsen, K. (1995) Digoxin affects potassium homeostasis during exercise in patients with heart failure. *Cardiovascular Research* **29**, 506–511.

Secher, K. (1921) Experimentelle untersuchungen ueber den einfluss der anstrengungen auf die grösse des herzens. *Zeitscrift für die gesamte experimentelle Medizin* **14**, 113–129.

Secher, K. (1923) Experimentelle untersuchungen ueber die grösse des herzens nach einem aufhören des trainierens. *Zeitscrift für die gesamte experimentelle Medizin* **32**, 290–295.

Secher, N.H. (1973) Development of results in international rowing championships 1893–1971. *Medicine and Science in Sports* **5**, 195–199.

Secher, N.H. (1983) The physiology of rowing. *Journal of Sports Science* **1**, 23–53.

Secher, N.H. (1992) Central nervous influence on fatigue. In: *The Olympic Book of Endurance Sports* (Shepherd, R.J. & Åstrand, P.-O., eds.) Blackwell, London: 96–107.

Secher, N.H. & van Lieshout, J.J. (2005) Normovolaemia defined by central blood volume and venous oxygen saturation. *Clinical and Experimental Pharmacology and Physiology* **32**, 901–910.

Secher, N.H. & Volianitis, S. (2006) Are the arms and legs in competition for cardiac output? *Medicine and Science in Sports and Exercise* **38**, 1797–1803.

Secher, N.H., Clausen, J.P., Klausen, K., Noer, I. & Trap-Jensen, J. (1977) Central and regional circulatory effects of adding arm exercise to leg exercise. *Acta Physiologica Scandinavica* **100**, 288–297.

Secher, N.H., Mizuno, M. & Saltin, B. (1984) Adaptation of skeletal muscles to training. *Bulltin European Physiopathologie et Respiratori* **20**, 453–457.

Shibata, M., Ichioka, S., Togawa, T. & Kamiya, A. (2006) Arterioles contribution to oxygen supply to skeletal muscles at rest. *European Journal of Applied Physiology* **97**, 327–331.

Snyder, E.M., Beck, H.C., Diez, N.M., Eisenach, J.H., Joyner, M.J., Turner, S.T. *et al.* (2006) Arg16Gly polymorphism of the β$_2$-adrenergic receptor is associated with differences in cardiovascular function at rest and during exercise in humans. *Journal of Physiology* **571**, 121–130.

Stenberg, J., Åstrand, P.-O., Ekblom, B., Royce, J. & Saltin, B. (1967).

Hemodynamic response to work with different muscle groups in sitting and supine position. *Journal of Applied Physiology* **22**, 61–70.

Stray-Gundersen, J., Musch, T.I., Haidet, G.C., Ordway, G.A. & Mitchell, J.H. (1986) The effect of pericardiectomy on maximum oxygen consumption and maximal cardiac output in untrained dogs. *Circulation Research* **58**, 523–530.

van Lieshout, J.J., Pott, F., Madsen, P.L., van Goudoever, J. & Secher, N.H. (2001) Muscle tensing during standing. Effects on cerebral tissue oxygenation and cerebral artery blood velocity. *Stroke* **32**, 1546–1551.

Volianitis, S., McConnell, A.K., Koutedakis, Y., McNaughton, L., Backx, K. & Jones, D.A. (2001) Inspiratory muscle training improves rowing performance. *Medicine and Science in Sports and Exercise* **33**, 803–809.

Volianitis, S., Yoshiga, C.C., Vogelsang, T. & Secher, N.H. (2004a) Arterial blood pressure and carotid baroreflex function during arm and combined arm and leg exercise. *Acta Physiologica Scandinavica* **181**, 289–295.

Volianitis, S., Yoshiga, C.C., Nissen, P. & Secher, N.H. (2004b) Effect of fitness on arm vascular and metabolic responses to

upper body exercise. *American Journal of Physiology* **286**, H1736–H1174.

Wagner, P.D., Hoppler, H. & Saltin, B. (1977) Determinants of maximal oxygen uptake. In: *The Lung* (Crystal, R.G. & West, J.B., eds.) Lippencott-Raven, Philadelphia: 2033–2041.

Wang, T. & Hicks, J.W. (2002) An integrative model to predict maximum O$_2$ uptake in animals with central vascular shunts. *Zoology* **105**, 45–53.

Ward, M.P., Milledge, J.S. & West, J.B., eds. (1989) *High Altitude Medicine and Physiology* Chapman and Hall, London: 220–221.

Welsh, R.C., Warburton, D.E.R., Humen, D.P., Taylor, D.A., McGavock, J. & Haykowsky, M.J. (2005) Prolonged strenuous exercise alters the cardiovascular response to dobutamine stimulation in male athletes. *Journal of Physiology* **569**, 325–330.

Yoshiga, C.C. & Higuchi, M. (2001) Heart rate is lower during ergometer rowing than during treadmill running. *European Journal of Applied Physiology* **87**, 97–100.

Yoshiga, C.C., Yadhiro, K., Higuchi, M. & Oka, J. (2002) Rowing prevents muscle wasting in older men. *European Journal of Applied Physiology* **88**, 1–4.

Chapter 20

Metabolic Limitations to Performance

FRANCIS B. STEPHENS AND PAUL L. GREENHAFF

Adenosine triphosphate (ATP) is the sole substrate that can be used directly by skeletal muscle to fuel contraction. However, the store of ATP in human skeletal muscle is relatively small (approximately 24 mmol·kg dry muscle^{-1}) and, therefore, must be continually resynthesized from its breakdown products adenosine diphosphate (ADP), adenosine monophosphate (AMP), and inorganic phosphate (P_i). Resynthesis of ATP during exercise is provided by anaerobic (non-oxygen using) and aerobic (oxygen using) processes (Fig. 20.1), with the contribution from each depending principally on the relative exercise intensity and duration.

During prolonged submaximal exercise, ATP resynthesis can be adequately achieved by the oxidative combustion of fat and carbohydrate stores within the mitochondria (protein breakdown contributes less than 5% of the energy provision for muscle activity). The fat and carbohydrate (glycogen) stores within the body are large enough to maintain the required rate of ATP resynthesis during submaximal exercise for a number of hours (Table 20.1a). However, during high intensity to maximal exercise, the relatively slow activation and relatively low rate of energy delivery of oxidative ATP resynthesis cannot meet the energy requirements of contraction and therefore anaerobic ATP resynthesis from phosphocreatine (PCr) hydrolysis and glycolysis is essential if the energy demand of contraction is to be met. However, PCr hydrolysis and glycolysis can sustain the high ATP demand of

maximal exercise for only a few seconds (Table 20.1a). Once the rate of ATP demand outstrips the rate of ATP resynthesis at any given exercise intensity, then fatigue (defined as the inability to maintain a given or expected power or work output) is inevitable and exercise performance declines. However, it is important to remember that other metabolic factors, occurring as a consequence of achieving high rates of ATP turnover rate, are also involved in bringing about the onset of fatigue.

It is beyond the scope of this chapter to consider all potential metabolic limitations to performance in detail. Therefore, we focus on the premise that metabolic-based fatigue development in contracting skeletal muscle occurs as a direct consequence of the inability of muscle to maintain the required ATP demand of contraction as a result of fuel substrate depletion limiting ATP provision, or as a consequence of product inhibition limiting ATP utilization processes. By way of example, mechanisms thought to be responsible for fatigue development during both prolonged submaximal exercise and high intensity to maximal exercise are described.

Prolonged submaximal exercise

Prolonged "submaximal" exercise is typically defined as the intensity of exercise that can be sustained for durations of 30–180 min. In practice, this is usually an exercise intensity of 60–85% of maximal oxygen consumption ($\dot{V}o_{2max}$). Continuous exercise of any longer duration (i.e., at an exercise intensity of less than 60% [$\dot{V}o_{2max}$]) is probably not limited by muscle substrate availability and, providing adequate

The Olympic Textbook of Science in Sport, 1st edition. Edited by R.J. Maughan. Published 2009 by Blackwell Publishing. ISBN: 978-1-4051-5638-7.

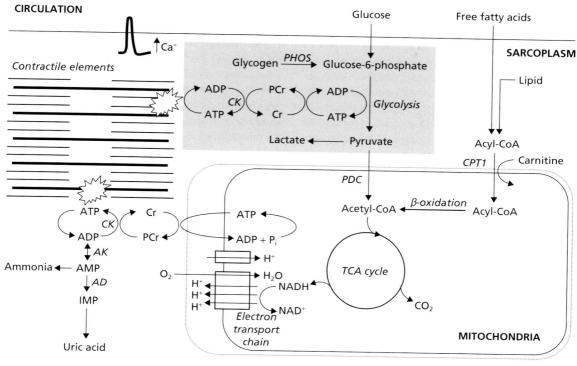

Fig. 20.1 Schematic diagram of the pathways involved in anaerobic (shaded) and aerobic ATP resynthesis. AD, adenosine monophosphate deaminase; ADP, adenosine diphosphate; AK, adenylate kinase; AMP; adenosine monophosphate; ATP, adenosine triphosphate; CK, creatine kinase; CPT1, carnitine palmitoyltransferase 1; IMP, inosine monophosphate; NAD$^+$, nicotinamide-adenine dinucleotide (oxidized form); NADH, nicotinamide-adenine dinucleotide (reduced form); PDC, pyruvate dehydrogenase complex; PHOS, glycogen phosphorylase; TCA, tricarboxylic acid.

Table 20.1 (a) Amounts of fuel substrate available in a 70-kg person, and maximal rates of adenosine triphosphate (ATP) resynthesis from these substrates. (b) Rates of ATP demand of different athletic events.

(a) Substrate	Amount available (mol)	Maximal rate (mol ATP·min^{-1})	(b) Event	ATP demand (mol·min^{-1})
ATP, PCr	0.67	4.40	100 m sprint	2.6
Muscle glycogen	1.6		400 m sprint	2.3
(glycolysis)	(theoretically 6.7)	2.35	800 m run	2.0
Muscle glycogen	84	0.85–1.14	1500 m run	1.7
(complete oxidation)			Marathon	1.0
Liver glycogen	19	0.37	Rest	0.07
Fatty acids	4000	0.40		

PCr, phosphocreatine.

hydration in maintained, can be sustained for several hours. Because the rate of muscle ATP resynthesis required during prolonged exercise is relatively low (Table 20.1), PCr, carbohydrate, and fat all contribute to ATP resynthesis.

Is fat limiting to prolonged submaximal exercise performance?

Fat (stored mainly as triacylglycerol) constitutes the largest energy reserve in the body (Table 20.1) and in terms of the amount available it is not limiting to prolonged exercise performance. For example, using only fat as an energy source, a marathon run would require only about 300 g body fat to be oxidized for a 70-kg runner. Unfortunately, fat exhibits a relatively low maximum rate of oxidation (0.4 mol ATP·min^{-1}; Table 20.1a) and cannot resynthesize ATP at a rate sufficient to maintain exercise at an intensity of more than around 60% $\dot{V}o_{2max}$.

By way of example, an experiment in human volunteers, which involved the intravenous infusion of trace amounts of stable isotopes in order to directly quantify fuel selection during exercise, demonstrated that as exercise intensity increases from rest to a moderate intensity (approximately 55% $\dot{V}o_{2max}$), the contribution from both fat and carbohydrate oxidation to total energy expenditure (i.e., ATP resynthesis) increased (Fig. 20.2; van Loon *et al.* 2001). However, whereas the contribution from carbohydrate sources to energy expenditure continued to increase further when exercise intensity was increased to approximately 75% $\dot{V}o_{2max}$, the contribution from fat oxidation (derived from plasma and intramuscular sources) declined.

This would suggest that during prolonged submaximal exercise at around 75% $\dot{V}o_{2max}$ the rate of

fat oxidation is limiting to ATP resynthesis and, if it were the sole substrate available, exercise performance. Consequently, in order to meet the ATP demand of muscle contraction, carbohydrate is also utilized, particularly at exercise intensities close to and above 75% $\dot{V}o_{2max}$. Looked at another way, it can be calculated that if an elite marathon runner depended solely on carbohydrate as an energy source he would be exhausted after about 90 min of running (Table 20.1b). As the world record for the marathon is around 125 min, this clearly exemplifies the importance of fuel integration during prolonged exercise. This also answers the question of the present section in that, because the carbohydrate stores within the body (i.e., muscle and liver glycogen) are relatively small, carbohydrate availability is the limiting factor to prolonged submaximal exercise performance rather than the rate of fat oxidation per se. Indeed, one of the main adaptations observed in endurance trained individuals is an increased rate of fat oxidation during exercise, perhaps primarily because of an increase in carnitine palmitoyltransferase 1 (CPT1) activity (the rate-limiting enzyme for fatty acid entry into the mitochondria; Fig. 20.1). A mechanism behind the increase in prolonged submaximal exercise performance with this increased capacity to oxidize fat is likely to be the sparing of the muscle glycogen store during exercise. This, in turn, would delay fatigue development and increase exercise performance, which is discussed in more detail in the following section. However, fat feeding before or during exercise does not appear to have a positive effect on prolonged submaximal exercise performance in humans. On the contrary, the literature currently suggests that physical and psychological performance is more likely to be impaired by attempting to increase fat availability.

Carbohydrate availability limits prolonged submaximal exercise performance

The concept that carbohydrate availability limits prolonged exercise performance is well established. As early as 1939, Christensen and Hansen demonstrated that prolonged exercise capacity can be markedly increased (two- to threefold) by feeding a carbohydrate-rich diet in the days before exercise

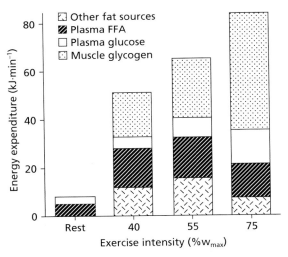

Fig. 20.2 Energy expenditure and fuel selection during 30 min of submaximal exercise at intensities of 40, 55, and 75% of maximal work load. FFA, free fatty acids. (Reproduced with permission from van Loon *et al.* 2001.)

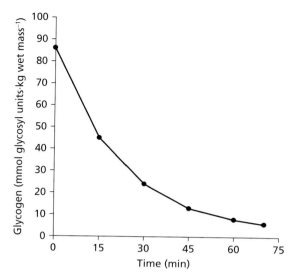

Fig. 20.3 Muscle glycogen content during bicycling exercise at 80% $\dot{V}_{O_{2max}}$ until voluntary exhaustion. (Reproduced with permission from Bergström & Hultman 1967.)

compared with a high-fat diet. Furthermore, in the 1960s, using the muscle biopsy technique, Bergstrom and Hultman demonstrated a clear relationship between pre-exercise muscle glycogen content and exercise performance. The muscle glycogen store in healthy humans is approximately 350 mmol·kg dry muscle^{-1}, or 80 mmol·kg^{-1} wet muscle (to convert muscle metabolite content from wet muscle to dry muscle [dm] we use a factor of 4.3), and is fairly resistant to change in non-exercised muscles. However, Bergstrom and Hultman (1967) demonstrated that the point of volitional exhaustion in 10 healthy human subjects bicycling at an exercise intensity of 80% $\dot{V}_{O_{2max}}$ (approximately 70 min) coincided with near-complete depletion of the muscle glycogen store (Fig. 20.3). In fact, it is likely that some muscle fibers were completely depleted of muscle glycogen (discussed below).

By taking muscle biopsy samples every 15 min during exercise it was observed that the rate of muscle glycogen depletion was greatest at the onset of exercise, with nearly half of the muscle glycogen store being utilized within the first 15 min. This could perhaps be because muscle glycogen content in itself can regulate the rate of glycogenolysis, but most probably because it takes time for mitochondrial ATP production from fat and carbohydrate oxidation to reach a steady state following the onset of exercise. Hence, there is a greater contribution from anaerobic glycolysis during this period, resulting in greater glycogen degradation, and a pronounced elevation of the blood lactate concentration, which then declines as exercise progresses.

It was noted in an experiment by Bergstrom and Hultman (1966) that if subjects consumed a high-carbohydrate diet following glycogen-depleting one-legged bicycling exercise, then muscle glycogen stores in the exercised muscles were increased to supranormal levels (approximately 900 mmol·kg dm^{-1}), with the most rapid period of glycogen resynthesis in the first few hours after exercise, whereas it was relatively unchanged in the non-exercised leg. The supracompensatory effect on glycogen storage was probably brought about by a residual effect of an exercise-induced increase in the muscle glucose transporter (GLUT4) and glycogen synthase activity.

In another of Bergström and Hultman's pioneering experiments (Bergstrom et al. 1967), muscle glycogen content was altered in six healthy male volunteers by feeding normal, low, or high carbohydrate isoenergetic diets for 3 days following glycogen depleting exercise. The subjects then performed prolonged cycling exercise to exhaustion and it was clearly demonstrated in all subjects that the greater the pre-exercise muscle glycogen content, the longer it took for the subjects to fatigue (Fig. 20.4). In the 40 years that have passed since publication, these findings have been confirmed on many occasions and clearly demonstrate that muscle glycogen availability is a limiting factor to prolonged exercise performance. Furthermore, based on these experiments, the practice of "carbohydrate loading" to improve prolonged exercise performance is now common amongst athletes worldwide.

Human skeletal muscle contains at least two major fiber types, which can be distinguished by differences in their myofibrillar ATPase activity and oxidative capacity. Contractile speed is closely related to ATPase activity and therefore fiber types with low or high ATPase activity are designated slow (type 1) and fast (type 2) twitch, respectively (although type 2 fibers can be further subclassified). These characteristics of muscle fibers result in different patterns of

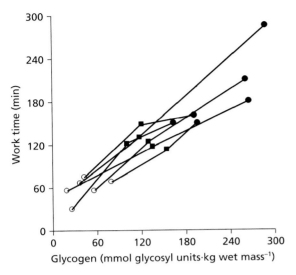

Fig. 20.4 The relationship between pre-exercise muscle glycogen content and exercise time to exhaustion at 75% $\dot{V}O_{2max}$ in six subjects following 3 days of normal (squares), low (open circles) or high (closed circles) dietary carbohydrate intake. (Reproduced with permission from Bergström *et al.* 1967.)

use (recruitment) depending on the exercise intensity. During prolonged submaximal exercise, type 1 (high oxidative capacity) muscle fibers are the first to become depleted of glycogen. (By contrast, high intensity exercise results in initial glycogen depletion in type 2 [high glycolytic capacity] muscle fibers, which are discussed later.) For example, it was observed in a study by Gollnick *et al.* (1974), where healthy human volunteers cycled at 31% $\dot{V}O_{2max}$ for 3 h, that muscle glycogen content (measured by histochemical staining) was almost completely depleted in approximately 33% of the type 1 fibers, but only slightly reduced in type 2 muscle fibers at the end of exercise. Furthermore, when the exercise intensity was increased to 64% and 83% $\dot{V}O_{2max}$, muscle glycogen content was depleted in a greater number of type 1 fibers at exhaustion in relation to the exercise intensity, whereas glycogen content was still elevated in type 2 fibers (albeit to a lesser degree). As would be expected, the rate of muscle glycogen depletion was positively correlated with the exercise intensity such that exhaustion occurred much sooner at the higher exercise intensity.

By measuring muscle glycogen content biochemically in pooled muscle fibers, it was later demonstrated in healthy human volunteers that the rate of muscle glycogen depletion during the first 15 min of one-legged cycling exercise at 61% $\dot{V}O_{2max}$ was around 2.5-fold greater in type 1 compared with type 2 muscle fibers, resulting a decrease in muscle glycogen content from approximately 340 to 170 and 280 mmol·kg dm^{-1}, respectively (Ball-Burnett *et al.* 1991). Thereafter, muscle glycogen depletion followed the same pattern in both fiber types for 2 h, albeit at a progressively reduced rate. These findings have also been confirmed during isometric exercise and prolonged running exercise. The most likely explanation for the selective fiber type depletion is that type 1 fibers are preferentially recruited (via the motor unit) at the onset of exercise because of their physiological characteristics (i.e., slow twitch, highly oxidative), and that with increasing exercise intensities more fibers (including type 2) become recruited.

Taken together, these findings confirm that during prolonged submaximal exercise, muscle glycogen availability is limiting to performance and fatigue will occur specifically as a result of glycogen depletion in the recruited muscle fibers, in this case type 1 fibers. It should be noted that in the studies discussed above the muscle samples were obtained from the vastus lateralis which has a mixed muscle fiber content of approximately 50% type 1 and 50% type 2 in healthy humans. Thus, when muscle glycogen content is measured in mixed muscle samples taken following exhaustive exercise a significant amount of whole muscle glycogen is still present, which could, perhaps misleadingly, be interpreted to suggest that muscle glycogen availability does not have an important role in prolonged exercise performance.

It should be acknowledged that liver glycogen stores also have an important role in providing carbohydrate during exercise, particularly as studies using animals and human volunteers have shown that liver glycogen depletion during exercise can limit performance either indirectly, by bringing about a more rapid depletion of muscle glycogen stores, or directly, by causing hypoglycemia, which will inhibit neurologic function. Liver biopsy studies in healthy human volunteers have clearly demonstrated that the liver is extremely sensitive to changes in dietary carbohydrate intake. For example, work by Nilsson and Hultman in the 1970s demonstrated that 1 day of carbohydrate restriction depleted liver glycogen stores from approximately 270 to 30 mmol·kg wet muscle^{-1}, and that further dietary carbohydrate restriction for several days maintained liver glycogen at this low content, which was then supercompensated following a high-carbohydrate diet. In the absence of exogenous carbohydrate (i.e., from carbohydrate feeding during exercise), hepatic glycogenolysis is the principal means of maintaining euglycemia during exercise, and the rate of glycogenolysis is directly related to the hepatic glycogen content. Thus, increasing the liver glycogen store prior to exercise via carbohydrate ingestion will increase the potential for glucose delivery to skeletal muscle during a subsequent bout of exercise. Indeed, research using magnetic resonance spectroscopy (MRS) has demonstrated that following exhaustive exercise in healthy volunteers, liver glycogen is depleted to a considerable degree and, if post-exercise carbohydrate feeding is inadequate, liver glycogen resynthesis may impair glucose release from the liver and subsequent exercise capacity (Casey et al. 2000).

The exact metabolic mechanism(s) by which fatigue is brought about in the carbohydrate depleted state are unclear. However, it is most likely caused by an inability to rephosphorylate ADP to ATP at the required rate. For example, towards the end of prolonged exercise the depletion of the muscle glycogen store results in a reduction in glycolytic intermediates and there is an accumulation of ADP, AMP, and inosine monophosphate (IMP; at the point of fatigue there is up to a 20-fold increase in muscle IMP content). It has been suggested that the decrease in glycolytic flux may reduce the rate of oxidative ATP resynthesis. A decrease in oxidative ATP resynthesis, in the face of high ATP demand, will result in an accumulation of ADP. The increase in ADP, coupled with a decreased capacity to rephosphorylate ADP (because of low PCr content and decreased glycolytic flux), will result in an increase in AMP via the adenylate kinase reaction (2 ADP $\leftrightarrow$ ATP + AMP). When its concentration becomes excessive, AMP is dephosphorylated to adenosine or deaminated to IMP, particularly under conditions that favor the AMP deaminase reaction (AMP + H_2O + H^+ $\rightarrow$ IMP + NH_4^+)

i.e., an increase in hydrogen ion concentration (see p. 333). Thus, the increase in IMP concentration reflects a decline in cellular phosphate potential, and it is possible that the decrease in phosphate potential is related to the impairment of the contractile process. It is also important to note that the energy yield of ATP hydrolysis decreases when the products of its hydrolysis (ADP and P_i) increase in concentration, which may also accelerate the development of fatigue by impairing ATP utilizing reactions. Support for this hypothesis is highlighted in patients who lack glycogen phosphorylase (McArdle's disease) and therefore are unable to utilize muscle glycogen during exercise, resulting in maximal exercise capacities that are around 50% of expected normal values. These patients also exhibit exaggerated adenine nucleotide (ATP, ADP, and AMP) degradation and IMP accumulation during exercise.

Carbohydrate feeding improves performance during prolonged submaximal exercise by maintaining muscle glucose delivery

It has been known since the 1930s that the ingestion of carbohydrate during exercise can increase endurance capacity during prolonged submaximal exercise. More recently, this has been attributed to carbohydrate ingestion maintaining a high rate of carbohydrate oxidation during exercise and preserving muscle glycogen stores, particularly in type 1 fibers. Indeed, it has been suggested that the ability to perform prolonged submaximal exercise becomes increasingly dependent on blood glucose availability as exercise progresses, particularly in well-trained subjects, and that as muscle glycogen stores are reduced, the oxidation of carbohydrate from alternative sources is increased to meet the energy demands of contraction.

For example, a study by Bjorkman et al. (1984) in healthy volunteers demonstrated that ingestion of glucose (250 mL of a 7% solution) every 20 min during bicycling exercise at approximately 70% $\dot{V}o_{2max}$ until exhaustion, increased exercise time by around 20% compared to the ingestion of water or fructose (250 mL, 7%). Furthermore, the increase in exercise performance with glucose ingestion corresponded with a lower rate of glycogen degradation compared to water or fructose ingestion (1.3 vs. 2.3 and 2.1 mmol/kg dm/min, respectively), suggesting that intermittent glucose ingestion during prolonged submaximal exercise increases exercise performance by delaying muscle glycogen depletion. In contrast, although fructose ingestion maintained blood glucose concentration to the same degree as glucose ingestion, it failed to influence glycogen depletion or exercise performance.

In recent years a wealth of studies have been published that demonstrate that carbohydrate ingestion during prolonged submaximal exercise can increase exercise performance, usually when the exercise duration is 45 min or more. Such studies have also addressed what are the most effective forms of carbohydrate, what is the most effective feeding schedule during exercise, and what is the optimal amount of carbohydrate to be ingested. However, this is beyond the scope of this chapter and so the reader is directed to other reviews on the subject (Jeukendrup & Jentjens 2000; Tsintzas & Williams 1998).

In agreement with the selective type 1 muscle fiber depletion of glycogen, it has been demonstrated that the sparing of muscle glycogen content during prolonged exercise with carbohydrate ingestion occurs predominantly in type 1 fibers. Tsintzas *et al.* (1996) demonstrated that the ingestion of a 5.5% carbohydrate-electrolyte solution during prolonged running to exhaustion at 70% $\dot{V}O_{2max}$ was associated with a 25% reduction in utilization of muscle glycogen in type 1 fibers, compared with placebo ingestion, and an increase in exercise performance. Indeed, 65 g carbohydrate was ingested during 105 min of the running exercise and 50 g glycogen was spared in the thigh muscles compared with controls. Furthermore, a very good correlation ($r = 0.95$) was observed between the amount of glycogen spared (70 mmol·kg dm^{-1}) and the amount of glycogen used (60 mmol·kg dm^{-1}) in type 1 fibers to sustain the exercise intensity for an additional 30 min. In agreement with the aforementioned cycling studies, type 1, but not type 2, muscle fibers were glycogen depleted at the point of exhaustion, suggesting that the impairment of the contractile process during running exercise is also restricted to slow twitch fibers and not to the muscle as a whole.

Indeed, it was later demonstrated in a study by Tsintzas *et al.* (2001) that carbohydrate ingestion during prolonged running exercise attenuated the decline in type 1 muscle fiber PCr concentration by 46%. The sparing of PCr in the absence of a decline in ATP concentration was likely to reflect a better maintained resynthesis of ATP by aerobic processes during exercise, and thus reduced accumulation of ADP, AMP, and P_i. In support of this theory, carbohydrate feeding has been demonstrated to improve performance during prolonged cycling exercise at 70% $\dot{V}O_{2max}$ by maintaining muscle glucose delivery and attenuating the decline in muscle glycolytic (hexomonophosphates) intermediates, and offset the accumulation of IMP (Spencer *et al.* 1991).

It is also important to remember that even if muscle glycogen utilization is unaffected by carbohydrate ingestion, it may still favorably affect exercise performance by postponing the rate of liver glycogen depletion, or by taking the place of liver glycogen stores when they become depleted, thereby delaying the onset of hypoglycemia. Indeed, an increase in exercise time to exhaustion has been associated with the improved maintenance of blood glucose levels on several occasions.

In one such study, performed by Coyle *et al.* (1983), it was demonstrated that (paradoxically) there was no difference in muscle glycogen utilization during 3 h of exercise when subjects were fed a flavored placebo or a glucose polymer solution every 20 min during exercise. When the subjects ingested the placebo solution they became exhausted after approximately 180 min of exercise and this was accompanied by a fall in blood glucose concentration to 2.5 mmol·L^{-1} and a decline in carbohydrate oxidation towards the end of exercise. When the glucose polymer solution was ingested, the subjects cycled for over 240 min and blood glucose concentration and carbohydrate oxidation were maintained throughout. However, it should be noted that this study was performed using highly trained endurance athletes and it is unclear whether such high rate of glucose oxidation (up to 2.2 g·min^{-1}) could be maintained from circulatory sources in untrained individuals, or whether the same degree of muscle glycogenolysis would be observed. Nevertheless, it would appear that blood glucose availability, whether supplied from exogenous carbohydrate or liver glycogenolysis, is important to endurance exercise performance.

Taken the above findings together, it is not surprising that carbohydrate ingestion during exercise, particularly in the form of carbohydrate beverages, has become a very popular practice among both recreational and endurance athletes. The rationale underpinning the ingestion of any carbohydrate solution during exercise is that, in preventing hypoglycemia and providing a fuel source that is immediately usable by the working muscles, muscle glycogen content will be spared, the onset of fatigue will be delayed, and prolonged submaximal exercise performance will be increased.

High intensity and maximal exercise

In contrast to prolonged exercise, during high intensity (greater than 85% $\dot{V}o_{2max}$) and maximal intensity exercise work output can be sustained for periods lasting minutes to seconds before performance declines. Because of the high energy demand of high intensity exercise (Table 20.1b), the majority of ATP resynthesis is derived from PCr hydrolysis, anaerobic glycolysis, and aerobic carbohydrate utilization (Fig. 20.1). PCr is broken down by the enzyme creatine kinase to produce creatine and P_i, which is then transferred to ADP in order to resynthesize ATP ($PCr + ADP + H^+ \rightarrow ATP + Cr$). In the process of anaerobic glycolysis, glucose-6-phosphate, derived from muscle glycogen or the irreversible phosphorylation of blood-borne glucose, is converted to lactate via a series of metabolic reactions, two of which (1,3-diphosphoglycerate → 3-phosphoglycerate and phosphoenolpyruvate → pyruvate) rephosphorylate ADP to form ATP. Pyruvate that is not reduced to lactate enters the mitochondria via the pyruvate dehydrogenase complex (PDC), where it provides acetyl-CoA for the tricarboxylic acid (TCA) cycle and oxidative ATP resynthesis, albeit at a much lower maximal rate of ATP resynthesis compared with PCr hydrolysis or glycolysis. Fatigue is an inevitable feature of high intensity to maximal intensity exercise, and it has been demonstrated that force production and power output during intermittent, electrically evoked maximal isometric contractions, and maximal treadmill sprinting in human

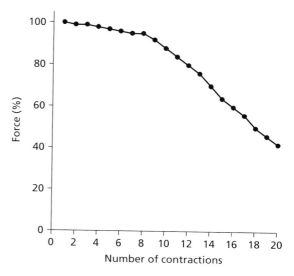

Fig. 20.5 Reduction in force development during 20 intermittent (1.6-s contraction at 50 Hz, 1.6 s rest) maximal electrically evoked isometric quadriceps femoris contractions in human volunteers. (Reproduced with permission from Soderlund *et al.* 1992.)

volunteers can decline by as much as 40% after only 30 s (Fig. 20.5). The onset of fatigue during maximal exercise is likely to be a multifactorial process.

Is muscle acidosis limiting to high intensity/maximal exercise performance?

A high rate of glycolytic flux is a prerequisite for a high muscle power output and, in order to achieve this, muscle lactic acid production must increase (Fig. 20.1). Classically, the accumulation of lactic acid has been suggested as being responsible for fatigue development during high intensity exercise. At physiological pH values, lactic acid almost completely dissociates into its constituent lactate and hydrogen ions (H^+), and the accumulation of hydrogen ions causes the pH of the muscle to fall (acidosis). The normal resting pH of the muscle cell is approximately 7.1. However, during high intensity exercise muscle pH can fall to about 6.5, and studies using animals have demonstrated that this causes the contractile mechanism to begin to fail, resulting in a reduction in force production, and also inhibits key enzymes such as glycogen phosphorylase (PHOS) and phosphofructokinase (PFK; the rate-limiting step in glycolysis). [It is generally accepted that a pH-mediated decrease in the activity of PHOS and PFK during maximal exercise can be overcome by the accumulation of their activators (e.g., AMP).]

A low pH also stimulates free nerve endings in the muscle, resulting in the perception of pain. It would also appear that lactate and hydrogen ion accumulation can result in muscle fatigue independent of one another, but the latter is the more commonly cited mechanism, and there is a vast literature in which a decline in muscle force generation is correlated with muscle acidosis. In support of this, it can be seen in examples in nature that animals that experience severe hypoxia (such as deep diving mammals) or can develop high muscle power outputs (such as animals that hunt or escape by running) have a high glycolytic capacity and a high muscle buffering capacity. In the context of the latter, their muscles, particularly type 2 fibers, contain high concentrations of histidine dipeptides, such as carnosine, which sequester hydrogen ions and maintain muscle pH better (Table 20.2). β-alanine (a non-proteogenic amino acid) is a precursor for muscle carnosine synthesis, and it has recently been demonstrated that 4 weeks of β-alanine feeding at a dose of 3.2–6.4 g·day^{-1} (as multiple doses of 400 or 800 mg) increased muscle carnosine content by approximately 40–65% in healthy human subjects (Harris et al. 2006). Moreover, the same group also demonstrated that this feeding regimen was associated with a 13% increase in high intensity bicycling exercise capacity (Hill et al. 2007). The authors attributed the increase in exercise performance to a calculated 10% increase (at least) in

muscle hydrogen ion buffering capacity as a result of the observed increase in muscle carnosine content. In support of this hypothesis, sprint athletes have a higher muscle buffering capacity than endurance athletes, and it has been demonstrated that high intensity exercise training can increase muscle buffering capacity and thereby offset the deleterious effects of muscle acidosis during exercise. Similarly, sodium bicarbonate ingestion, which buffers hydrogen ions, has also been used in an attempt to reduce hydrogen ion accumulation and/or accelerate muscle hydrogen ion efflux during high intensity exercise in order to improve performance. It has been demonstrated in one such animal experiment that intravenous sodium bicarbonate infusion increased isometric force by 20% during 5 min of ischemic maximal contraction. Taken together, these results demonstrate that an improvement in high intensity exercise capacity is linked to an increase in intracellular hydrogen ion buffering capacity in muscle, suggesting that muscle acidosis could indeed exert a limiting effect on exercise performance.

At the onset of high intensity exercise there is a lag in oxidative ATP resynthesis, resulting in the rapid hydrolysis of PCr and lactic acid generation. It is now established that this is, at least in part, brought about by an inertia in mitochondrial ATP resynthesis (acetyl group deficit) at the onset of exercise, and in particular at the level of the PDC. This was demonstrated in a series of experiments in ischemic (blood flow occluded) muscle by Timmons et al. (1997) and Roberts et al. (2002) in which the PDC was activated pharmacologically at rest (via intravenous dichloroacetate infusion), resulting in the accumulation of mitochondrial acetyl-CoA and acetylcarnitine (carnitine is a buffer of acetyl groups) in mitochondria prior to contraction. This provided a readily available substrate (acetyl groups) pool for the TCA cycle and oxidative ATP resynthesis at the onset of exercise, thereby overcoming the inertia in mitochondrial ATP production at the level of the PDC. The removal of this metabolic inertia resulted in a 30% greater contribution from oxidative ATP resynthesis and a 35% reduction in PCr hydrolysis and lactate accumulation during the first minute of high intensity exercise, and brought about 30% less fatigue after 6 min of contraction. These experiments also suggest that the

Table 20.2 Histidine dipeptide contents and H$^+$ ion buffering capacity in muscles from various animals (from Harris et al. 1990).

Buffering capacity	Animal	Histidine dipeptide content (mmol·kg dry muscle^{-1})
High	Little piked whale	400
Medium	Horses and deer	110
	Greyhound dog	90
Low	Man	17–5

lactic acid production at the onset of high-intensity exercise may be one of the factors determining the onset of fatigue as exercise progresses. Indeed, in the study of Timmons *et al.* (1997) muscle lactic acid production was almost abolished over 6 min of contraction. It is worthy of note that acetyl groups can also accumulate within muscle during a period of warm-up exercise, which may partly explain the reported metabolic and performance benefits of warm-up before exercise prior to competition.

Although clearly likely to be related to the fatigue process, is it unlikely that both lactate and hydrogen ion accumulation can be wholly responsible for the development of muscle fatigue during high intensity maximal exercise. For example, studies involving human volunteers have demonstrated that muscle force generation following fatiguing exercise can recover rapidly, despite still having a very low muscle pH value. Thus, it has been suggested that the maintenance of force production during high intensity exercise is pH dependent, but the initial force generation is more related to PCr availability. Also, several studies have suggested that muscle acidosis is merely coincidental and may have little causal effect on contraction in skeletal muscle, particularly at physiological temperatures (Westerblad *et al.* 2002). For example, studies in isolated and skinned (cell surface removed) muscle fibers have noted that, whereas muscle acidosis (around pH 6.5) impairs force production at 15°C, it has little effect at 30°C (although a more recent study demonstrated that acidosis impairs peak power to a greater extent at 30°C than 15°C).

However, some caution should be exhibited when interpreting *in vitro* findings (particularly in skinned fibers where there is no cytosol) in the context of the *in vivo* setting. There are also reports that muscle acidosis does not reduce glycogenolysis and/or glycolysis during high intensity exercise in healthy human volunteers (Gladden 2004). Nevertheless, following over 150 years of research on the topic, it would be premature to dismiss muscle acidosis as an important factor in high intensity exercise performance, particularly as buffering or inhibiting hydrogen ion accumulation (i.e., protecting against acidosis) improves contractile function and exercise performance *in vivo*. It is also important to remember that although the negative effects of acidosis resulting from lactic acid production are often stressed, the energy made available by anaerobic glycolysis and the production of lactate allows the performance of high intensity exercise that would otherwise be impossible. Also, metabolic acidosis is important in optimizing flux in several regulatory pathways in intermediary metabolism (e.g., the AMP deaminase reaction).

Inability to maintain extremely high rates of ATP turnover during maximal exercise also limits performance

A decline in muscle anaerobic ATP production and/or the parallel increase in ADP accumulation, caused by a depletion of PCr and/or a fall in the rate of glycogenolysis, have also been implicated in fatigue development during maximal exercise, particularly in type 2 muscle fibers.

The PCr concentration in mixed fiber skeletal muscle is three- to fourfold greater than the ATP reservoir, amounting to around 80 mmol·kg dm^{-1} at rest, although this value is higher in type 2 muscle fibers than type 1 (85 vs. 75 mmol·kg dm^{-1}). At the immediate onset of contraction there is a momentary rise in muscle ADP concentration, which triggers PCr hydrolysis, via the creatine kinase reaction (Fig. 20.1), in order to rapidly rephosphorylate ADP and thus resynthesize ATP. For each mole of PCr degraded, one mole of ATP is resynthesized via creatine kinase, with the rate of PCr hydrolysis being greater in type 2 muscle fibers. The importance of this immediate onset of PCr hydrolysis lies in the extremely rapid rates at which it can resynthesize ATP, especially during maximal short duration exercise. However, the muscle PCr store is finite, and can only maintain ATP resynthesis during maximal exercise for a few seconds. For example, Fig. 20.6 shows the results of an experiment in human volunteers by Hultman *et al.* (1991), which demonstrated the rate of ATP resynthesis from PCr hydrolysis during 30 s of fatiguing maximal isometric contraction in mixed fiber muscle was at its greatest within 1.3 s of the onset of contraction, at around 9 mmol·kg dm^{-1}·s^{-1} (approximately 4 mol·min^{-1}). However, after only 2.6 s of contraction the rate of ATP resynthesis from PCr had declined by about 15% and in the final 10 s of a 30-s bout of

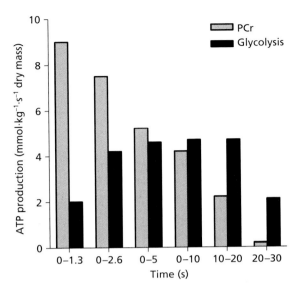

Fig. 20.6 Rates of anaerobic adenosine triphosphate (ATP) resynthesis from phosphocreatine (PCr) and glycolysis during 30 s of near-maximal intensity isometric contraction in humans. (Reproduced with permission from Hultman *et al.* 1991.)

muscle contraction was relatively small, amounting to just 2% of the initial yield.

If we then allow for a further level of complexity by considering PCr degradation in different muscle fiber types during this type of exercise, it can be seen that during the first 10 s of maximal muscle contraction, the rate of PCr utilization in type 1 and 2 fibers is around 3.3 and 5.3 mmol·kg dm^{-1}·s^{-1}, respectively (around 4.2 mmol·kg dm^{-1}·s^{-1} in mixed fiber muscle; Fig. 20.6). However, as contraction continues from 10 to 20 s, the rate of PCr utilization in type 2 fibers declines by about 60% to 2.1 mmol·kg dm^{-1}·s^{-1}, such that by the end of contraction PCr stores are nearly depleted. The corresponding rate of PCr degradation in type 1 fibers remains relatively unchanged, perhaps because of the oxidative nature of type 1 fibers (Soderlund *et al.* 1992). The mechanisms responsible for the almost instantaneous decline in the rate of PCr utilization during maximal exercise are unknown, but it could be related to a local myofibrillar decline in its availability coupled with the inability of mitochondrial (oxidative) ATP resynthesis to match this extremely rapid rate of PCr hydrolysis. Thus, if

maximal exercise is to be continued beyond only a few seconds there must be a marked increase in the contribution from glycogenolysis and glycolysis to ATP resynthesis (note, the ATP demand could never be matched by ATP generation because of inertia in this system at the onset of exercise and relatively low maximal rate of mitochondrial ATP generation).

Anaerobic glycolysis involves several more steps than PCr hydrolysis, resulting in a lower maximum rates of ATP resynthesis, but compared with oxidative phosphorylation, glycolysis is still very rapid. It was thought for many years that PCr was the sole fuel utilized at the initiation of contraction with glycogen utilization occurring at the onset of PCr depletion but this now known not to be the case and, as Fig. 20.6 shows, ATP resynthesis from glycolysis during maximal contraction begins to occur almost immediately at the onset of exercise. Indeed, the activation of muscle contraction by calcium and the accumulation of the products of ATP and PCr hydrolysis (ADP, AMP, IMP, and P_i) act as stimulators of glycogenolysis. Furthermore, unlike PCr hydrolysis, ATP resynthesis from glycolysis does not reach its maximal rate until after 5 s of exercise (suggesting that PCr may act as a buffer of ATP resynthesis until glycolysis is fully activated) and is maintained at this high rate for several seconds, such that over 30 s of maximal exercise, the contribution from anaerobic glycolysis to ATP resynthesis is nearly double that from PCr hydrolysis. This is reflected by the very high muscle lactate concentrations (more than 100 mmol·kg dm^{-1}) that are achieved during maximal exercise lasting 30 s or more.

In keeping with the higher glycogen content in type 2 muscle fibers, the rate of glycolysis is very close to maximal in type 2 fibers (6.3 mmol·kg dm^{-1}·s^{-1}) during the initial 20 s of maximal contraction, and is far in excess of the relatively low rate observed in type 1 fibers (0.6 mmol·kg dm^{-1}·s^{-1}). Indeed, it is in excess of both the measured and calculated maximal rates of glycolysis for mixed fiber muscle (Fig. 20.6). However, glycolysis in muscles with mixed fiber types begins to decline after 20–30 s (Fig. 20.6), and this parallels the 45% decline in glycolytic rate observed in type 2 fibers (to around 3.5 mmol·kg dm^{-1}·s^{-1}). The mechanisms responsible for the decline in glycolysis during maximal exercise are unclear, but are unlikely to be related to a depletion of muscle glycogen stores as levels are still high at the end of maximal exercise (providing that the pre-exercise glycogen store is not depleted to below 100 mmol·kg dm^{-1}). However, the decline could be a result of a reduction in glycogen phosphorylase activity. For example, it has been suggested that once the rate of glycogen utilization has reached its peak during maximal exercise, a decrease in the concentration of muscle free AMP (as a result of a decrease in the rate of ADP formation and/or a pH-induced increase in the activity of AMP deaminase) will result in a decrease in glycogen phosphorylase activity and thus a decline in the rate of glycogenolysis and glycolysis during exercise (Greenhaff *et al.* 1993).

It would appear that in parallel with the loss of force production during 30 s of maximal exercise (Fig. 20.5), there is also a marked decline in the rates of muscle PCr and glycogen utilization, predominantly in type 2 muscle fibers. Indeed, after 20 s of maximal contraction, the type 2 fiber PCr store is almost totally depleted and the rate of glycogen utilization begins to decline. At this point, it would appear that there is no means whereby type 2 fibers can overcome or compensate for the declining rate of anaerobic ATP resynthesis and/or ADP rephosphorylation in order to maintain force production, and fatigue is inevitable. In support of this suggestion, studies involving repeated bouts of maximal exercise have shown that a significant relationship exists between the extent of PCr resynthesis in type 2 fibers during recovery between exercise bouts and subsequent exercise performance. With this in mind, research over the past 15 years has provided a growing body of evidence to indicate that dietary creatine (Cr) supplementation is a useful tool by which individuals can increase their ability to perform high intensity exercise.

In human skeletal muscle, Cr is present at a concentration of about 125 mmol·kg dm^{-1}, approximately 60% of which is in the form of PCr in resting muscle. Ingesting 20 g·day^{-1} Cr (in 4 × 5 g doses) for 5 days can lead to an increase of more than 20% in muscle total Cr concentration, 20% of which is in the form of PCr. The performance benefits in certain types of exercise of increasing muscle total Cr content have been well documented, and it is generally accepted that performance during short single or multiple bouts of high intensity exercise can be improved by Cr supplementation. For example, ingesting Cr for 5 days (20 g·day^{-1}) has been shown to significantly increase the amount of work that can be performed by healthy volunteers during repeated bouts of maximal concentric and isokinetic cycling exercise (e.g., three bouts of maximal cycling exercise interspersed with 4 min recovery) by about 5–7%. The exact mechanisms by which performance is improved by Cr feeding are unclear. However, considering that PCr availability is thought to be limiting to maximal exercise performance (as discussed above), an increase in muscle PCr content, via Cr feeding, and/or an increase in the capacity for PCr resynthesis during and immediately following exercise would increase muscle performance capability by maintaining anaerobic ATP resynthesis during exercise. In support of this stance, Cr feeding has been shown to reduce plasma ammonia and hypoxanthine accumulation (markers of IMP degradation) and the magnitude of ATP depletion during maximal exercise, while at the same time increasing work output. Furthermore, individuals who demonstrate more than a 25% increase in muscle Cr content as a result of Cr feeding, show an accelerated rate of PCr resynthesis during recovery. To date, however, there is no evidence to suggest Cr supplementation can benefit prolonged submaximal exercise, nor is there any reason to expect that it would given the metabolic demands of this type of exercise.

The breakdown of PCr, via the creatine kinase (CK) reaction, during intense muscle contraction results in an increase in muscle P$_i$ concentration, and it has been suggested that an increase in intracellular P$_i$ is also a major factor in the development of muscular fatigue. It has been demonstrated in a number of studies in isolated skinned muscle fibers that increasing P$_i$ concentration can inhibit contractile force. Furthermore, maintaining a resting muscle P$_i$ concentration during contraction in intact muscle from a CK knockout mouse model delays fatigue development by up to 30% (although this could be a result of a compensatory effect, a phenomenon routinely observed in knockout models). The mechanisms involved in this reduction in contractile force are believed to be P$_i$-mediated reductions in calcium

(Ca^{2+}) sensitivity, calcium release, and calcium availability, as well as a direct impairment of cross-bridge cycling (an increase in muscle P_i may impair P_i release from the myosin head during the power stroke; Westerblad *et al.* 2002). For example, increasing P_i from 3 to 20 $mmol \cdot L^{-1}$ in rabbit muscle skinned fibers at pH 7, decreased ATPase activity by 15–20% and isometric tension by approximately 20%, although it did not affect the maximum shortening velocity (Cooke *et al.*, 1988). However, we should again exhibit some caution when interpreting these *in vitro* findings in the context of the *in vivo* setting. For example, during maximal exercise *in vivo* muscle PCr hydrolysis (and thus muscle P_i accumulation) is at its greatest within the first few seconds of muscle contraction, and this does not appear to coincide with the period of greatest fatigue development.

Thus, taking the above findings together, it is clear that an inability to maintain extremely high rates of ATP turnover during maximal exercise also limits performance. It should be noted, however, that the decline in the rate of glycolysis, at least during maximal short-duration exercise, may be of an insufficient magnitude to account for the decline in muscle force generation observed under these conditions, implying that other factors must be involved in the fatigue process.

Calcium handling is disrupted during high intensity exercise

Calcium (Ca^{2+}) is essential for the activation of muscle excitation–contraction coupling. Upon muscle depolarization, calcium is released by the sarcoplasmic reticulum (SR) within the muscle cell, which leads to muscle contraction. Subsequently, calcium is removed from the contractile proteins and pumped back into the SR by an active (ATP-dependent) process, which results in relaxation of the muscle. This cyclic process creates a calcium transient. The ability of the SR to regulate calcium movement within the muscle declines during fatiguing contractions and calcium transients become progressively smaller: this effect has been attributed to a reduction in calcium reuptake by the SR and/or increased calcium binding to contractile proteins. These alterations in calcium release and reuptake may therefore disturb

normal skeletal muscle contractile characteristics. Strong evidence that a disruption of calcium handling is responsible for fatigue comes from studies in isolated muscle showing that stimulation of SR calcium release by the administration of caffeine can improve force production, even in the face of a low muscle pH (hence one use of caffeine supplementation as an ergogenic aid).

Interestingly, PCr concentration appears to affect caffeine-induced SR calcium release and reuptake. Duke and Steele (2001) demonstrated that acute PCr depletion in skinned rat skeletal muscle fibers results in a loss of calcium from the SR and a reduced rate of SR calcium reuptake. Thus, it would appear that the depletion of the muscle PCr store that occurs during maximal exercise may also bring about fatigue by disrupting SR calcium handling and thus excitation–contraction coupling. The mechanism whereby PCr depletion disrupts calcium handling is unclear, but it could be because of a local reduction in ATP resynthesis by PCr and therefore a reduced capacity of the SR to actively reuptake calcium.

Extracellular potassium accumulation may impair performance during high intensity exercise

In order for a skeletal muscle fiber to contract, calcium must be released by the SR. The trigger for this release is a nerve impulse sent from the motor nerve to the muscle fiber that it innervates, which results in the opening of sodium ion (Na^+) channels on the muscle fiber membrane, the influx of sodium down its concentration gradient into the muscle fiber, and depolarization of the membrane potential. Repolarization of the muscle fiber membrane potential occurs via the opening of potassium ion (K^+) channels and the efflux of potassium down its concentration gradient from the muscle fiber into the extracellular space. Sodium and potassium are actively (by hydrolyzing ATP) pumped against their respective concentration gradients by the Na^+, K^+-ATPase pump and the cycle (action potential) is repeated. However, during high intensity exercise potassium ions are gradually released from skeletal muscle into the extracellular space, and the accumulation of potassium in the muscle interstitium has been suggested to cause fatigue as a result of impaired membrane excitability. Several studies in isolated muscles have shown that extracellular potassium concentrations above 8 mmol·L^{-1} reduce contractility.

In a study by Nielsen *et al.* (2004), healthy male volunteers performed a one-legged incremental exercise test to exhaustion, using both of their legs, following 7 weeks of intense knee-extensor training of one leg only. The rate of release of potassium from the muscle into the interstitium (determined by microdialysis) was greater in the untrained leg than in the trained leg. However, the venous and interstitial potassium concentrations were identical in both legs at the point of fatigue, despite the trained leg taking around 30% longer to fatigue than the untrained leg. Furthermore, there was a calculated 30% decrease in membrane potential at the point of fatigue in both legs. These findings support the hypothesis that interstitial potassium accumulation is involved in the development of fatigue, and suggest that intense training reduces the accumulation of potassium in human skeletal muscle interstitium during exercise, probably through a larger reuptake of potassium because of greater skeletal muscle Na$^+$,K$^+$-ATPase pump activity (there was also an increase in muscle Na$^+$,K$^+$-ATPase pump protein content with training). Interestingly, it has been suggested that skeletal muscle potassium release during contraction is increased at a lower muscle pH, perhaps because of an increase in potassium conductance.

Conclusions

ATP is the sole fuel that can be used directly for skeletal muscle force generation. However, the ATP store of skeletal muscle is small and therefore muscle must be constantly resynthesized during exercise by aerobic (i.e., carbohydrate and fat oxidation) and anaerobic (i.e., PCr hydrolysis and glycolysis) processes depending upon the duration and intensity of exercise.

Prolonged submaximal exercise is typically is defined as the intensity of exercise that can be sustained for durations of 30–180 min. In practice, this is usually an exercise intensity of 60–85% of maximal oxygen consumption ($\dot{V}o_{2max}$). Because the rate of muscle ATP resynthesis required during prolonged exercise is relatively low, oxidation of fat and carbohydrate is the main contributor to ATP resynthesis.

The availability of fat within the body is not limiting to prolonged exercise performance, but fat exhibits a relatively low maximum rate of oxidation, and cannot resynthesize ATP at a rate sufficient to maintain exercise at an intensity of more than about 60% $\dot{V}o_{2max}$. Thus, for higher submaximal exercise intensities to be achieved, carbohydrate must also be utilized and it appears that, because the carbohydrate stores within the body (i.e., muscle and liver glycogen) are relatively small, carbohydrate availability is the limiting factor to prolonged submaximal exercise performance rather than the rate of fat oxidation per se. Endurance training can increase the rate of fat oxidation during prolonged exercise, and as a result spare muscle glycogen usage and increase exercise performance.

Carbohydrate availability, in the form of muscle and liver glycogen stores, is limiting to prolonged submaximal exercise performance. Carbohydrate stores are depleted at the point of fatigue, particularly in type 1 muscle fibers, and pre-exercise carbohydrate availability is strongly correlated with exercise performance. The mechanisms responsible for fatigue during prolonged submaximal exercise with carbohydrate depletion are probably directly related to an inability to rephosphorylate ADP at the required rate and hypoglycemia. Carbohydrate feeding during exercise delays muscle glycogen and PCr depletion in type 1 fibers and maintains euglycemia, resulting in an increase in exercise performance.

In contrast to prolonged exercise, during high intensity (greater than 85% $\dot{V}o_{2max}$) and maximal intensity exercise, work output can be sustained for periods lasting only minutes to seconds before there is a loss of force production and performance declines. Because of the very high energy demand of high intensity exercise, the majority of ATP resynthesis is derived from PCr hydrolysis, anaerobic glycolysis, and aerobic carbohydrate metabolism. The onset of fatigue is likely to be a multifactorial process.

The accumulation of hydrogen ions (H$^+$) within the muscle during high intensity exercise results in a fall in muscle pH (acidosis), which has long been thought to be limiting to high intensity exercise performance. Indeed, examples from nature and experiments in humans and animals have demonstrated that buffering hydrogen ion accumulation increases glycolytic capacity and improves high intensity exercise performance. However, to date the mechanism whereby muscle acidosis brings about fatigue and a decline in exercise performance remains unclear but it is likely to be multifactorial.

In parallel with the loss of force production during maximal exercise, there is a marked decline in the rate of muscle PCr and glycogen utilization, predominantly in type 2 muscle fibers. Under these conditions it would appear that there is no means whereby type 2 fibers can overcome or compensate for the declining rate of anaerobic ATP resynthesis in order to maintain force production, and fatigue is inevitable. The accumulation of P_i from the breakdown of PCr may also impair force production during maximal exercise. Research over the past 15 years has indicated that dietary creatine supplementation is a useful tool by which individuals can increase their ability to perform high intensity exer-

cise, perhaps because of an increase in muscle PCr content and an increase in the capacity for PCr resynthesis during exercise.

Calcium (Ca^{2+}) release and reuptake by the SR is essential for the activation of muscle excitation–contraction coupling, and SR calcium handling is impaired during maximal exercise. Stimulation of SR calcium release by caffeine can improve muscle force production *in vitro*, even when muscle pH is low. The impairment of SR calcium handling may be a result of local PCr depletion reducing ATP resynthesis and therefore the capacity of the SR to actively reuptake calcium.

During high intensity exercise, potassium ions (K^+) are gradually released from skeletal muscle into the extracellular space, and the accumulation of potassium in the muscle interstitium may cause fatigue as a result of impaired membrane excitability. Intense training reduces the accumulation of potassium in human skeletal muscle interstitium during exercise, probably through a larger reuptake of potassium because of greater skeletal muscle Na^+,K^+-ATPase pump activity.

References

Ball-Burnett, M., Green, H.J. & Houston, M.E. (1991) Energy metabolism in slow and fast twitch fibres during prolonged cycle exercise. *Journal of Physiology* **437**, 257–267.

Bergstrom, J. & Hultman, E. (1966) Muscle glycogen synthesis after exercise: an enhancing factor localized to the muscle cells in man. *Nature* **210**, 309–310.

Bergstrom, J. & Hultman, E. (1967) A study of the glycogen metabolism during exercise in man. *Scandinavian Journal of Clinical and Laboratory Investigation* **19**, 218–228.

Bergstrom, J., Hermansen, L., Hultman, E. & Saltin, B. (1967) Diet, muscle glycogen and physical performance. *Acta Physiologica Scandinavica* **71**, 140–150.

Bjorkman, O., Sahlin, K., Hagenfeldt, L. & Wahren, J. (1984) Influence of glucose and fructose ingestion on the capacity for long-term exercise in well-trained men. *Clinical Physiology* **4**, 483–494.

Casey, A., Mann, R., Banister, K., Fox, J., Morris, P.G., Macdonald, I.A., *et al.* (2000) Effect of carbohydrate ingestion

on glycogen resynthesis in human liver and skeletal muscle, measured by (13)C MRS. *American Journal of Physiology. Endocrinology and Metabolism* **278**, E65–E75.

Christensen, E.H. & Hansen, O. (1939) Arbeitsfähigkeit und Ernährung. *Skandinavisches Archiv für Physiologie* **81**, 160–175.

Coyle, E.F., Hagberg, J.M., Hurley, B.F., Martin, W.H., Ehsani, A.A. & Holloszy, J.O. (1983) Carbohydrate feeding during prolonged strenuous exercise can delay fatigue. *Journal of Applied Physiology* **55**, 230–235.

Cooke, R., Franks, K., Luciani, G.B. & Pate, E. (1988) The inhibition of rabbit skeletal muscle contraction by hydrogen ions and phosphate. *Journal of Physiology* **395**, 77–97.

Duke, A.M. & Steele, D.S. (2001) Interdependent effects of inorganic phosphate and creatine phosphate on sarcoplasmic reticulum Ca^{2+} regulation in mechanically skinned rat skeletal muscle. *Journal of Physiology* **531**, 729–742.

Gladden, L.B. (2004) Lactate metabolism: a new paradigm for the third millennium. *Journal of Physiology* **558**, 5–30.

Greenhaff, P.L., Soderlund, K., Ren, J.M. & Hultman, E. (1993) Energy metabolism in single human muscle fibres during intermittent contraction with occluded circulation. *Journal of Physiology* **460**, 443–453.

Gollnick, P.D., Piehl, K. & Saltin, B. (1974) Selective glycogen depletion pattern in human muscle fibres after exercise of varying intensity and at varying pedal rates. *Journal of Physiology* **241**, 45–57.

Harris, R.C., Marlin, D.J., Dunnett, M., Snow, D.H. & Hultman, E. (1990) Muscle buffering capacity and dipeptide content in the thoroughbred horse, greyhound dog and man. *Comparative Biochemistry and Physiology A* **97**, 249–251.

Harris, R.C., Tallon, M.J., Dunnett, M., Boobis, L., Coakley, J., Kim, H.J., *et al.* (2006) The absorption of orally supplied beta-alanine and its effect on muscle carnosine synthesis in human vastus lateralis. *Amino Acids* **30**, 279–289.

Hill, C.A., Harris, R.C., Kim, H.J., Harris, B.D., Sale, C., Boobis, L.H., *et al.* (2007) Influence of beta-alanine supplementation on skeletal muscle carnosine concentrations and high intensity cycling capacity. *Amino Acids* **32**, 225–233.

Hultman, E., Greenhaff, P.L., Ren, J.M. & Soderlund, K. (1991) Energy metabolism and fatigue during intense contraction. *Biochemical Society Transactions* **19**, 347–353.

Jeukendrup, A.J. & Jentjens, R. (2000) Oxidation of carbohydrate feedings during prolonged exercise: current thoughts, guidelines and directions for future research. *Sports Medicine* **29**, 407–424.

Nielsen, J.J., Mohr, M., Klarskov, C., Kristensen, M., Krustrup, P., Juel, C., *et al.* (2004) Effects of high-intensity intermittent training on potassium kinetics and performance in human skeletal muscle. *Journal of Physiology* **554**, 857–870.

Nilsson, L.H. & Hultman, E. (1973) Liver glycogen in man: the effect of total starvation or a carbohydrate-poor diet followed by carbohydrate refeedings.

Scandinavian Journal of Clinical and Laboratory Investigation **32**, 325–330.

Roberts, P.A., Loxham, S.J., Poucher, S.M., Constantin-Teodosiu D. & Greenhaff P.L. (2002) Bicarbonate-induced alkalosis augments cellular acetyl group availability and isometric force during the rest-to-work transition in canine skeletal muscle. *Experimental Physiology* **87**, 489–498.

Soderlund, K., Greenhaff, P.L. & Hultman, E. (1992) Energy metabolism in type I and type II human muscle fibres during short term electrical stimulation at different frequencies. *Acta Physiologica Scandinavica* **144**, 15–22.

Spencer, M.K., Yan, Z. & Katz, A. (1991) Effect of low glycogen on carbohydrate and energy metabolism in human muscle during exercise. *American Journal of Physiology* **262**, C975–C979.

Timmons, J.A., Poucher, S.M., Constantin-Teodosiu, D., Macdonald, I.A. & Greenhaff, P.L. (1997) The metabolic responses from rest to steady-state determine contractile function in ischemic canine skeletal muscle. *American Journal of Physiology* **273**, E233–E238.

Tsintzas, K. & Williams, C. (1998) Human muscle glycogen metabolism during exercise: effect of carbohydrate supplementation. *Sports Medicine* **25**, 7–23.

Tsintzas, O.K., Williams, C., Boobis, L. & Greenhaff, P. (1996) Carbohydrate ingestion and single muscle fiber glycogen metabolism during prolonged running in men. *Journal of Applied Physiology* **81**, 801–809.

Tsintzas, K., Williams, C., Constantin-Teodosiu, D., Hultman, E., Boobis, L., Clarys, P., *et al.* (2001) Phosphocreatine degradation in type I and type II muscle fibres during submaximal exercise in man: effect of carbohydrate ingestion. *Journal of Physiology* **537**, 305–311.

van Loon, L.J., Greenhaff, P.L., Constantin-Teodosiu, D., Saris, W.H. & Wagenmakers, A.J. (2001) The effects of increasing exercise intensity on muscle fuel utilisation in humans. *Journal of Physiology* **536**, 295–304.

Westerblad, H., Allen, D.G. & Lannergren, J. (2002) Muscle fatigue: lactic acid or inorganic phosphate the major cause? *News in Physiological Sciences* **17**, 17–21.

Further reading

Gladden, L.B. (2004) Lactate metabolism: a new paradigm for the third millennium. *Journal of Physiology* **558**, 5–30.

Greenhaff, P.L., Campbell-O'Sullivan, S.P., Constantin-Teodosiu, D., Poucher, S.M., Roberts, P.A. & Timmons, J.A. (2002) An acetyl group deficit limits mitochondrial ATP production at the onset of exercise. *Biochemical Society Transactions* **30**, 275–280.

Greenhaff, P.L., Hultman, E. & Harris, R.C. (2004) Carbohydrate metabolism. In *Principles of Exercise Biochemistry*, 3rd edn. (Poortmans J.R., ed.) Karger, Basel: 108–151.

Greenhaff, P.L., Nevill, M.E., Soderlund, K., Bodin, K., Boobis, L.H., Williams, C.,

et al. (1994) The metabolic responses of human type I and II muscle fibres during maximal treadmill sprinting. *Journal of Physiology* **478**, 149–155.

Hultman, E., Greenhaff, P.L., Ren, J.M. & Soderlund, K. (1991) Energy metabolism and fatigue during intense contraction. *Biochemical Society Transactions* **19**, 347–353.

Jeukendrup, A.J. & Jentjens, R. (2000) Oxidation of carbohydrate feedings during prolonged exercise: current thoughts, guidelines and directions for future research. *Sports Medicine* **29**, 407–424.

Maughan, R., Gleeson, M. & Greenhaff, P.L. (1997) Metabolic responses to high

intensity exercise. In *Biochemistry of Exercise*. Oxford University Press, Oxford: 138–157.

Maughan, R., Gleeson, M. & Greenhaff, P.L. (1997) Metabolic responses to prolonged exercise. In *Biochemistry of Exercise*. Oxford University Press, Oxford: 158–176.

Tsintzas, K. & Williams, C. (1998) Human muscle glycogen metabolism during exercise: effect of carbohydrate supplementation. *Sports Medicine* **25**, 7–23.

Westerblad, H., Allen, D.G. & Lannergren, J. (2002) Muscle fatigue: lactic acid or inorganic phosphate the major cause? *News in Physiological Sciences* **17**, 17–21.

Chapter 21

The Brain and Fatigue

TIMOTHY D. NOAKES, HELEN CREWE AND ROSS TUCKER

"Now if you are going to win any battle you have to do one thing. You have to make the mind run the body. Never let the body tell the mind what to do. The body will always give up. It is always tired morning, noon and night. But the body is never tired if the mind is not tired. When you were younger the mind could make you dance all night, and the body was never tired ... You've always got to make the mind take over and keep going". George S. Patton, US Army General, 1912 Olympian.

Currently there are two popular models of exertional fatigue – the peripheral and central models. Both are examples of linear, catastrophic systems (Noakes & St. Clair Gibson 2004; St. Clair Gibson & Noakes 2004), in which a failure of homeostasis must first occur before fatigue develops. Both models reflect a fundamental shift from the historic understanding that the human, like all known creatures, has evolved a complex biology, with one purpose: "All the vital mechanisms, varied as they are, have only one object, that of preserving constant the conditions of life in the internal environment" (Bernard 1974). Neither model allows the human brain the freedom to anticipate what will occur in the future and hence to take preventive action in order to protect the body's internal environment.

More recently we have proposed a novel model in which the brain regulates exercise performance "in anticipation," specifically to ensure protection of the "milieu intérieur" (Bernard 1974). We have called this the central governor model (Noakes 1998, 2000; Noakes *et al.* 2001, 2005). Here, we briefly review the evidence for this model and, in particular, why this model is better able to explain many fundamental observations in sport and exercise.

The peripheral fatigue model

Currently the most popular model of exercise fatigue posits that fatigue results from metabolite-induced skeletal muscle contractile failure – so-called peripheral fatigue (Noakes & St. Clair Gibson 2004). This model originates in a series of classical studies performed in the early 1900s by Fletcher and Hopkins (1907) and by Nobel Laureate A.V. Hill and colleagues (Hill & Lupton 1923; Hill *et al.* 1924a,b,c; Hill 1924). On the basis of some quite scanty evidence abetted with a heavy dose of interpretation, these authors postulated that fatigue develops during exercise when the oxygen demands of both the heart and the active skeletal muscles exceed the heart's capacity to provide an adequate oxygen supply to those organs.

Thus, as first formulated by A.V. Hill and his colleagues, this model (Fig. 21.1) proposes that exercise of a high intensity and short duration is limited by an inadequate oxygen supply to the exercising muscles as the output of the heart (cardiac output) reaches its maximum, leading first to an inadequate blood supply to the heart muscle itself, inducing myocardial ischemia. This ischemia causes a fall in cardiac output, reducing blood flow to muscle and hence leading to skeletal muscle anaerobiosis

The Olympic Textbook of Science in Sport, 1st edition. Edited by R.J. Maughan. Published 2009 by Blackwell Publishing. ISBN: 978-1-4051-5638-7.

Fig. 21.1 The Hill model of exercise physiology. A.V. Hill believed that maximal exercise performance was limited by a "catastrophic" failure of myocardial function resulting from a developing myocardial ischemia when maximum cardiac output was achieved. The failure of cardiac output caused the development of skeletal muscle anaerobiosis, which in turn prevented oxidation of the lactic acid that Hill believed initiated skeletal muscle contraction. To ensure that the heart was not damaged whilst it was ischemic, Hill postulated the existence of a "governor" in either the brain or the heart. The function of the governor was to reduce cardiac contractile function, thereby protecting the ischemic heart by reducing cardiac work.

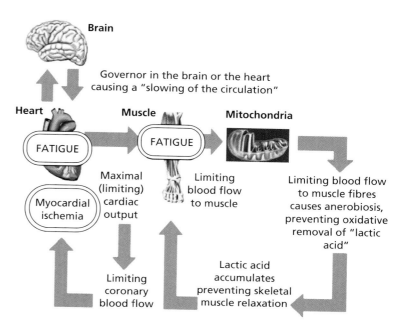

which, according to Fletcher and Hopkins' original theory that lactic acid is "associated with" fatigue (1907), would then cause a lactic acid-induced failure of skeletal muscle contraction. Hill (1924) understood that contraction resulted from muscle recruitment by the brain (central command) but he believed that lactic acid was the chemical messenger that induced muscle contraction. We now know that calcium release from the sarcoplasmic reticulum plays this role. He also believed that the oxidative removal of lactic acid produced muscle relaxation. Therefore, his model actually predicted that exercise must terminate with the development of a lactic acid-induced skeletal muscle rigor, resulting from skeletal muscle anaerobiosis.

Hill *et al.* (1924c) also acknowledged that uncontrolled ischemia would cause irreversible damage to the heart, which was of greater relevance. As a result of this observation they suggested that a "governor" must exist, either in the heart or the brain, which would protect the heart from damage during exercise (Fig. 21.1). Whilst there is currently debate as to whether cardiac output ever reaches a limiting value during maximum exercise (Gonzalez-Alonso *et al.* 2007), with two notable exceptions from the same laboratory (Gonzalez-Alonso & Calbert 2003;

Mortensen *et al.* 2005), few others find evidence that cardiac output reaches a maximum ("plateau") during exercise (Vella & Roberts 2005). Certainly none show that cardiac output fails precipitously at maximum exercise as a result of myocardial ischemia, as predicted by Hill's model. Indeed one of the more fervent supporters of this model, P.O. Astrand, noted as early as 1952 that "there was no sign of a decrease in stroke volume when work became maximum, at least not in the older subjects. This would have been the case if the central circulation had failed"; so that, "during maximal running and cycling, the heart probably works submaximally" (Astrand 1952). Yet Astrand nevertheless concluded that: "The working capacity of the heart should determine that of the muscles". It is unclear from this logic how a heart working submaximally can "determine" the performance of the muscles, unless the heart is itself subject to some external regulation.

Taylor and colleagues (1955) contributed significantly to the legitimization and global acceptance of Hill's interpretation by proposing that a "plateau" in oxygen consumption occurs during maximal exercise testing in the laboratory. They attributed this plateau to the attainment of the maximal capacity of the cardiovascular system to deliver oxygen to the

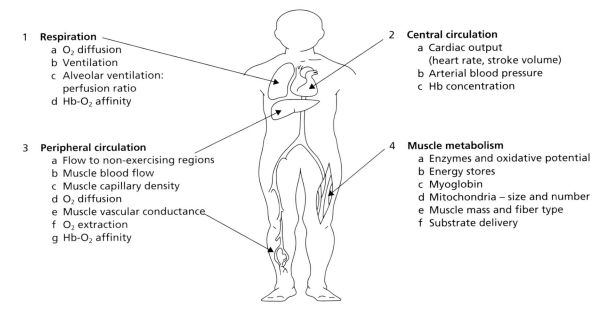

1 **Respiration**
   a O_2 diffusion
   b Ventilation
   c Alveolar ventilation:
      perfusion ratio
   d Hb-O_2 affinity

2 **Central circulation**
   a Cardiac output
      (heart rate, stroke volume)
   b Arterial blood pressure
   c Hb concentration

3 **Peripheral circulation**
   a Flow to non-exercising regions
   b Muscle blood flow
   c Muscle capillary density
   d O_2 diffusion
   e Muscle vascular conductance
   f O_2 extraction
   g Hb-O_2 affinity

4 **Muscle metabolism**
   a Enzymes and oxidative potential
   b Energy stores
   c Myoglobin
   d Mitochondria – size and number
   e Muscle mass and fiber type
   f Substrate delivery

Fig. 21.2 The classic diagram depicting the physiological factors that are believed to limit the $\dot{V}O_{2max}$. However, the (missing) factor in this diagram that clearly does "limit the ability to increase oxygen uptake" is the absence of the CNS because, in its absence, no muscle work is possible. This model is the natural extension of the belief, implicit in A.V. Hill's original model (Fig. 21.1), that it is the rate of provision of oxygen and hence of adenosine triphosphate (ATP) to the exercising muscles that determines exercise performance. However, this diagram is valid only if all the motor units in the active limbs are active during maximum exercise. If this is not the case, then the recruitment of additional motor units might further increase $\dot{V}O_{2max}$, showing that skeletal muscle recruitment regulates the rate of ATP use and hence $\dot{V}O_2$ during maximal exercise in humans. In which case, the true regulator of skeletal muscle function during maximum exercise is not the rate of ATP production but rather the number of actin and myosin cross-bridges that are formed in response to calcium release into the myoplasm, consequent to neural recruitment by the CNS (Noakes *et al.* 2004b). (Reproduced with permission from Rowell 1993.)

working muscles and suggested that "there is a linear relationship between oxygen intake and work-load until the maximum oxygen intake is reached. Further increases in work load beyond this point merely result in an increase in oxygen debt and a shortening of the time in which the work can be performed." However, they also observed that increasing the working muscle mass, by adding arm work while running, caused an increase in oxygen consumption. Therefore, they might equally have concluded that the plateau in oxygen consumption does not guarantee that the individual's true maximum $\dot{V}O_2$ had been achieved. The factors that are typically considered to limit $\dot{V}O_{2max}$ according to this model are presented in Fig. 21.2.

Further refinements to this theory were added by Wassermann and colleagues (1964, 1967) and

Hollmann *et al.* (1985) who identified a (submaximal) work-rate corresponding to an "anaerobic threshold" (AT). Continued exercise at work-rates above the AT caused blood lactate concentrations to rise sharply. Thus, according to the original logic of Fletcher and Hopkins (1907), lactic acid accumulation occurs in "anaerobic" working muscles receiving an inadequate oxygen supply. Since this lactic acid accumulation would lead ultimately to fatigue (as the result of a direct metabolic effect in the exercising muscles according to the original interpretation of A.V. Hill), testing for AT would be a useful method to predict athletic ability and future athletic performances.

One perhaps unrecognized consequence of the widespread acceptance of Hill's model of fatigue during maximal exercise has been its effect on how exercise physiologists explain all forms of fatigue.

Thus, since this model requires that the body must first fail (catastrophically) before fatigue occurs and exercise terminates, then this explanation must also apply to all other forms of exercise. Accordingly, fatigue in any form of exercise must always occur after there has been a failure of homeostasis, i.e., a failure to protect the "milieu intérieur." In retrospect this is a surprising proposal since death is the only known condition in which there is a complete loss of homeostasis.

As a consequence of this subconscious mindset, the original studies to determine a metabolic basis for fatigue during prolonged exercise concluded that such fatigue must occur as the result of a catastrophe, specifically complete depletion of energy substrates, i.e., muscle and occasionally liver glycogen stores. For example, in a review published to mark the 20th anniversary of these original studies, Conlee (1987) wrote: "When glycogen runs out . . . the muscle fails from lack of aerobic adenosine triphosphate (ATP) production. However plausible and attractive this theory, it is unproven . . . what is clear is that, in glycogen-depleted muscle, ATP is being used up faster than it can be manufactured, and so force output is diminished." However, there is no evidence that muscle glycogen ever "runs-out" completely in the exercising muscle. Nor are ATP concentrations abnormally reduced at exhaustion during prolonged exercise (Noakes & St. Clair Gibson 2004). Thus, Baldwin *et al.* (2003) concluded that "our data do not support the concept that a decrease in muscle tricarboxylic acid cycle intermediates (TCAI) during prolonged exercise in humans compromises aerobic energy provision or is the cause of fatigue;" and hence, "our results refute the hypothesis that links attenuated glycogen availability with fatigue via impaired aerobic energy provision, impaired adenine nucleotide metabolism, or TCAI pool size."

Indeed, what is clearly true is that the explanation proposed by Conlee (1987), in the absence of any other influence, cannot be true. If the rate of ATP production during prolonged exercise falls below the rate of ATP use, then the muscle ATP concentrations must fall progressively, terminating ultimately not in fatigue but in muscle rigor. In a detailed review Noakes and St. Clair Gibson (2004) argue that for the Hill model of the mechanisms causing fatigue

during maximal exercise to be correct, six conditions must be met:

1 If the development of oxygen deficiency in the active muscles is the exclusive factor limiting maximum exercise performance, and if the "plateau phenomenon" is the external marker of this skeletal muscle anaerobiosis, then the plateau phenomenon must occur in 100% of subjects at exhaustion during progressive exercise;

2 Skeletal muscle anaerobiosis must develop at exhaustion during maximum exercise;

3 To maximize skeletal muscle blood flow and hence oxygen delivery, cardiac output must always be maximum at fatigue because, according to the Hill model, the heart is merely the slave to the oxygen demand of the exercising muscles;

4 Models of peripheral fatigue predict that, at the point of fatigue in all exercise regardless of its intensity or duration, there must always be complete recruitment of all motor units in the active limbs;

5 Fatigue must always develop when a similar level of peripheral (inhibiting) metabolites has been reached; and

6 Fatigue must always be absolute, requiring a period of recovery during which the inhibitory metabolites are removed from the previously active muscles so that their function can recover and the exercise can again begin.

Perhaps the fourth condition is the most important test of the generalized model that fatigue always results from catastrophic homeostatic failure according to Hill's original concept. This is because if fatigue is truly due either to the metabolite-induced "poisoning" of skeletal muscle function or to a complete energy depletion, neither of which can be prevented by the action of the brain, then every single muscle cell (fiber) in the exercising limbs must be activated (recruited) at exhaustion. Furthermore, if some cells are inactive because they have yet to be recruited, the logical question becomes: why does the brain not simply recruit those inactive and yet-to-be "poisoned" or yet-to-be energy-depleted fibers, in order to allow the exercise to continue until every single muscle cell is either "poisoned" or completely depleted of energy?

In fact a multiplicity of evidence shows that humans essentially never recruit all cells in their exercising muscles either during maximal effort or at the point of fatigue during prolonged exercise (St. Clair Gibson *et al.* 2001; St. Clair Gibson & Noakes 2004; Place *et al.* 2006; Noakes 2007a). Accordingly we have concluded that the peripheral model cannot fully explain the fatigue that occurs during exercise. Rather if even some muscle cells have yet to be recruited at the point of fatigue during exercise, then the brain must be in control and must be "choosing" how many muscle cells it wishes to recruit in the active muscles. This choice must be made on the basis of calculations, the nature of which we are only now beginning to appreciate (St. Clair Gibson & Noakes 2004; Lambert *et al.* 2005; Rauch *et al.* 2005; Tucker *et al.* 2006c).

The central fatigue model

According to this model, it is argued that changes occur within the brain as a direct (but passive) consequence of exercise. These changes typically involve alterations in the concentrations of key neurotransmitters, especially those that are believed to have an inhibitory action on brain function. As a result of these changes, the athlete develops the sensations of fatigue, which ultimately cause the termination of exercise by mechanisms not yet fully described.

As is the case with the traditional peripheral model of fatigue, this central model is also a linear/catastrophic model in which the brain is an innocent victim of what is happening elsewhere in the body. Thus, changes in neurotransmitter balance produced perhaps as a result of metabolic changes in the active muscles or elsewhere, somehow impair brain functioning causing the termination of exercise. However, like the peripheral model, the central fatigue model is also "brainless" because it predicts that there can be no anticipation of future events. Rather, humans, driven by the "will" of their muscles, will continue to exercise until such time as the catastrophe occurs in the brain, causing the termination of exercise.

Similar to the linear peripheral fatigue model, this model also predicts that exercise performance cannot increase near to the end of exercise – the "end-spurt phenomenon" (Catalano 1974) – since the progressive accumulation of poisonous metabolites in either the muscles or brain not only limits the

athlete's pace during exercise but also ensures that he or she can go no faster, not just at the finish but throughout the race. Furthermore, this model also requires a period of time for the restoration of the "poisonous" brain metabolites before exercise can again begin.

In addition, as is the case with the peripheral model, if this model is correct it must also be able to explain why fatigue is partial and not absolute; why even the most exhausted marathon runner or Ironman triathlete can still walk. Or conversely, why after hours or days of unusual exertion there can be an almost complete collapse, the moment the subject believes that no further exertion is necessary. Consider for example the case of Joe Simpson, the British mountaineer who, despite a shattered leg dragged himself for four days to return to his base-camp after an epic climbing accident. Only when he reached the safety of his companions did he suddenly believe that "I was nearer to death than when I had been alone. The minute I knew help was at hand something had collapsed inside me. Whatever had been holding me together had gone. Now I could not think for myself, let alone crawl. There was nothing to fight for, no patterns to follow, no *voice*, and it frightened me to think that, without these, I might run out of life" (Simpson 1997). Or, conversely, the experience of Reinhold Messner and Peter Habeler, the first humans to climb Mount Everest without oxygen. Despite reaching the summit of Everest in a state of complete exhaustion, they were able to descend within minutes of reaching the summit: "Now . . . at a height of 8,800 metres, we can no longer keep on our feet while we rest. We crumple to our knees, clutching our axes . . . Every ten or fifteen steps we collapse into the snow to rest, then crawl on again" (Messner 1979). Yet both subsequently descended more than 800 m in less than 2 h successfully, but only after considerable effort, as described by Messner: "I have now to summon every last ounce of resolve, and make myself stand up and leave this place" (Messner 1979).

The central governor model

It is our argument that for many reasons, not least the absence of any evidence showing the catastrophic failure of any biological system during exercise, even when performed to "maximum" capacity, there must be another mechanism controlling exercise performance, and that the symptoms of fatigue contribute in some way to this control process (Noakes & St. Clair Gibson 2004; Noakes *et al.* 2005).

The central governor model proposes that the brain regulates the mass of skeletal muscle that is recruited during exercise specifically to ensure that bodily homeostasis is never threatened (Noakes *et al.* 2001, 2005). Accordingly, the key prediction of this model is that the brain acts "in anticipation" to ensure that exercise is always at an intensity and of a (safe) duration that does not threaten a catastrophic failure of homeostasis. According to Hill's original model (Fig. 21.1), the central governor would prevent myocardial ischemia, not be slowing the work-rate of the (ischaemic) heart by some direct action (presumably the withdrawal of sympathetic activation and its replacement with powerful vagal stimulation), but by reducing the extent of skeletal muscle recruitment. The immediate consequence of a reduced skeletal muscle recruitment would be reduced muscle work, reduced skeletal muscle blood flow and, as a consequence, a reduced cardiac output. This model therefore predicts that whilst the heart may indeed be the slave to the working muscles (Noakes *et al.* (2004a), at least it has the brain on its side to ensure that the muscles never make excessive demands on the pumping capacity of the heart.

Clear examples of fatigue without catastrophic failure or disruption of whole-body homeostasis have been demonstrated during exercise in extreme hypoxia at real or simulated high altitudes (Green *et al.* 1989; Kayser *et al.* 1994; Calbet *et al.* 2003a,b; Amann *et al.* 2006, 2007), and in severely hot conditions (Gonzalez-Alonso *et al.* 1999; Nybo & Nielsen 2001a). In both conditions exercise terminates without any evidence of a failure of homeostasis. Furthermore, even exercise of high intensity terminates without any evidence that profoundly reduced pH levels are reached or that all available sources of energy production are maximally utilized (Calbet *et al.* 2003c).

Therefore, during maximal exercise at extreme altitude, cardiac output and heart rate are lower than during maximal exercise at sea level (Kayser 2003); hence exercise terminates at submaximal rates of heart work (Noakes 2007c). There is also no evidence for disturbed metabolic homeostasis at exhaustion during exercise at extreme altitude (Kayser 2003). Rather, blood and muscle lactate concentrations are low and blood pH is only modestly acidotic (Green *et al.* 1989), situations that are termed the "lactate and cardiac output paradoxes" of fatigue at extreme altitude (Noakes & St. Clair Gibson 2004). In contrast, the traditional Hill model predicts that exercise in the most profoundly hypoxic conditions known to man should occur at the highest possible cardiac outputs (Noakes *et al.* 2004a; Noakes 2007c) and with high blood lactate concentrations, including a severe acidosis. Yet the opposite holds true. This suggests that the traditional model can simply not be correct.

Kayser and colleagues (1994) have suggested that the exercise limitation at high altitude is the result of a reduced central neural drive, as first proposed by Bigland-Ritchie and Vollestad (1988). In their studies, Kayser *et al.* showed that whereas the performance of upper-limb exercise was not altered by hypoxia, peak power output during cycling was 24% lower in hypoxia than in normoxia. When subjects switched suddenly to 100% O_2 at the point of exhaustion in hypoxia, they were able to continue cycling, indicating that peripheral fatigue caused by "anaerobic muscle poisoning" could not explain the fatigue at exhaustion. This is because reversal of fatigue occurred too rapidly, disproving condition six of Hill's model (see the list above).

The authors concluded that performance during high-intensity exercise involving small muscle groups is not impaired at altitude, whereas the performance of exercise using large muscles groups is reduced. More importantly, they showed that muscle electromyographic (EMG) activity was reduced during maximal exercise in hypoxia but increased when fatigue was reversed, allowing exercise to continue when 100% O_2 was inhaled. This could be explained if the central governor limited exercise in hypoxia by responding to sensory feedback from some variable that alters rapidly when the oxygen content of the inspired air is changed suddenly from a hypoxic to hyperoxic mixture. One such obvious factor would be the arterial partial pressure of oxygen (Pa_{O_2}).

More recent studies by Calbet *et al.* (2003a,b) and Amann *et al.* (2006, 2007) confirm some of the findings of Kayser *et al.* (1994) and also provide further evidence for the central governor hypothesis, although other groups have tended to dismiss this possibility (Noakes *et al.* 2004a) or to interpret the evidence somewhat differently (Noakes & Marino 2007). All of these studies have also shown that exercise performance, which was impaired in hypoxia, improved the instant a hyperoxic gas mixture was substituted for the hypoxic mixture. Furthermore, subjects in the studies by Calbet and colleagues (2003a,b) reached lower peak cardiac outputs and rates of oxygen consumption in hypoxia, but terminated exercise at blood lactate concentrations and metabolic acidosis levels that were lower than those recorded at higher work-rates in hyperoxia. Accordingly, the authors concluded that: "The reduction in cardiac output experienced with severe acute hypoxia could be envisaged as a regulatory mechanism aimed at protecting either the heart itself or, more importantly, the central nervous system (CNS) from hypoxic damage due to the risk of increased desaturation at very high cardiac output . . . The down-regulation of maximal cardiac output was likely mediated by Pa_{O_2} and presumably Ca_{O_2}- and Sa_{O_2}-sensing mechanisms that adjust the output drive from cardiovascular nuclei in the CNS." This explanation is essentially the same as Hill's original concept of a governor that protects the heart from damage by reducing its pumping capacity. But a more effective method of protecting the heart would be to control the demands for blood flow by regulating the amount of work the exercising muscles are able to do (Noakes *et al.* 2004a).

Indeed, one of the crucial weaknesses of most studies purporting to "prove" that a failure of oxygen delivery secondary to a failure to increase the cardiac output can explain the limitations of maximal exercise performance in both hypoxia and normoxia, is that the study design is cross-sectional. In these studies, multiple biological variables are measured as they change, for example, during a maximal exercise test (Noakes *et al.* 2004a). Associations are then sought between these variables in an attempt to determine which biological variable "limits" exercise performance. But this research model is unable to prove causation since the determination of causation is dependant on the model used to make that interpretation. The sole method for establishing causation is to evaluate the results of an intervention, the outcome of which will differentiate between the predictions of two different models. Thus, the best experiments are those designed to produce results which differentiate precisely between two competing theories (or models).

In a second study Calbet *et al.* (2003b) studied the exercise performance of subjects before and after a period of living at high altitude, which greatly increased their blood hemoglobin concentrations, thereby increasing the potential for oxygen delivery to exercising skeletal muscles by 40%. The aim of the investigation was to determine whether or not oxygen delivery to muscle limits maximal exercise performance (as is predicted by the Hill model). By substantially increasing the potential for oxygen delivery to muscle their experimental design allowed the distinction between the two opposing exercise models – the original Hill model and the central governor model. If oxygen consumption increased as a result of the increase in oxygen delivery, then the former would be supported; if not, then some other model would be favored. However, neither maximum oxygen consumption nor peak work-rate increased significantly after altitude exposure, which should have increased oxygen delivery to the muscles by 40%. Hence, the traditional Hill model was unable to explain why, in the face of a substantial potential increase in oxygen delivery to skeletal muscle, neither oxygen consumption nor exercise performance increased significantly. On the other hand, the introduction of hyperoxia improves exercise performance (Bannister & Cunningham 1954) probably by increasing skeletal muscle recruitment (Amann *et al.* 2006, 2007; Tucker *et al.* 2006c), perhaps secondary to improved cerebral oxygenation (Noakes & Marino 2007).

We have therefore used these findings as evidence that the factors regulating maximal exercise performance cannot reside in oxygen delivery to muscle (Noakes *et al.* 2004a; Noakes & Marino 2007). But oxygen is clearly important since exercise performance in hypoxia is instantly improved by increasing the fraction of oxygen in the inspired air

(Kayser *et al.* 1994; Calbet *et al.* 2003a; Amann *et al.* 2007). The more logical explanation is that Pao_2, the determinant of cerebral oxygenation, may play a crucial role. Thus, a falling Pao_2 must be prevented if cerebral function is to be sustained and the brain protected. The logical way in which a fall in Pao_2 can be prevented is to control the function of the organ that consumes the largest volume of oxygen during exercise – i.e., active skeletal muscles (Noakes *et al.* 2001). This is logically regulated by a brain controller sensitive to an index of arterial oxygenation that reduces skeletal muscle recruitment during hypoxia, as has already been shown to occur (Kayser *et al.* 1994; Kayser 2003; Noakes 2007c).

Similarly, during exercise in the heat, effort normally terminates before a dangerous core temperature is reached, that is, before there is a catastrophic failure of thermal regulation (Tucker *et al.* 2004, 2006c). Numerous studies have established that the voluntary termination of prolonged exercise in the heat at a fixed work-rate occurs at a similar core temperature, regardless of the pre-exercise body temperature (Gonzalez-Alonso *et al.* 1999; Walters *et al.* 2000), the ambient temperature (Gonzalez-Alonso *et al.* 1999), state of heat acclimatization (Nielsen *et al.* 1993), and the rate of rise of core temperature (Gonzalez-Alonso *et al.* 1999). These findings have supported the hypothesis that fatigue during exercise in the heat always occurs when a critical core body temperature of approximately 40°C is reached (Nielsen *et al.* 1993; Nybo & Nielsen 2001a). The presumption according to the model of central fatigue is that this effect is due to the effects of heat on cerebral function, thus inducing a catastrophic failure of brain function. There are, however, also numerous studies to show that higher core temperatures are achieved at the point of fatigue during exercise in the heat than when the same exercise is performed in cool or temperate conditions (e.g., Febbraio *et al.* 1994; Galloway & Maughan 1997).

However, all these studies were performed at a fixed work-rate, either a constant running or cycling speed in the laboratory, so that each exerciser's brain was unable to modify the work-rate – that is, to adopt a personal pacing strategy. Yet the singular feature of human exercise, especially during competition, is the use of different pacing strategies to complete exercises of different durations and intensities in different environmental conditions. Thus, when subjects are allowed to pace themselves during laboratory exercise it is found that they respond as if the body anticipates what will happen in the future, so it acts pro-actively to ensure that harm does not occur (Tucker *et al.* 2004, 2006c). This concept of "teleoanticipation" was first proposed by Ulmer (1996), although athletes have been warned for more than 100 years of the dangers of starting competitive races too rapidly (Downer 1901; Noakes 2003).

The central governor model (Noakes *et al.* 2004b; St. Clair Gibson *et al.* 2004; Lambert *et al.* 2005) therefore proposes that the initial pace during exercise is based on prior experience of the average pace that can be sustained for the expected duration of the exercise bout. As a result, an appropriate number of motor units are recruited by the brain (central command) in the exercising limbs at the start of exercise; more for higher-intensity exercise of short duration, less for more prolonged exercise of a lower intensity. Afferent feedback is sent continually from multiple systems in the body to the brain during exercise and this produces a continuous modification of the pace that typifies all forms of competitive exercise (Tucker *et al.* 2006a,b). Calculations are made and efferent commands are relayed in order to complete the required task within the body's metabolic and biomechanical limits (Fig. 21.3). An important point is that this control can only be observed during "self-paced" exercise in which the subject is free to vary his or her work-rate, and not when the exercise intensity is fixed and imposed by the researcher – the more usual form of laboratory exercise.

Once the importance of studying self-paced exercise instead of exercise at a constant, externally imposed workload was grasped, it became rather easier to show that exercise regulation "in anticipation" is a normal, indeed defining, feature of human physiology. Of course, an anticipatory response cannot be explained by a system that is regulated solely in the periphery (Noakes & Marino 2007), and which is activated only after a catastrophic failure of homeostasis has occurred in either the exercising muscles (peripheral fatigue model) or in the brain (central fatigue model).

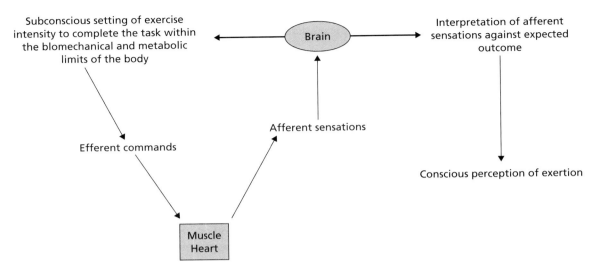

Fig. 21.3 Teleoanticipation and perceived exertion. A precise regulation of exercise performance may be achieved through a process of teleoanticipation. According to this model, the subconscious brain sets the exercise intensity prior to the onset of exercise, on the basis of prior experience. This feed-forward system sends efferent commands to many organs in the body, including the active skeletal muscles and the heart. Sensory (afferent) feedback produces a continual update, which is then used by the subconscious brain to modify the original pacing strategy. This information is also used to establish the conscious rating of perceived exertion (RPE) on the basis largely of the anticipated duration of the exercise bout that remains (Noakes 2004). The perception of exertion results from the interpretation of afferent sensations against an expected outcome (Hampson *et al.* 2001).

For example, Marino *et al.* (2004) compared the running performance of African and Caucasian athletes in both cool (15°C) and hot environmental conditions (35°C). After a 30 min run at 70% of the peak treadmill speed achieved during $\dot{V}o_{2max}$ testing, both groups of athletes reached rectal temperatures of ~38.4°C. They then performed a self-paced 8 km time-trial run on the treadmill in either hot or cold conditions. Whereas the performance of both groups was the same in cold conditions, the African runners who were significantly smaller and therefore had lower rates of heat production and heat storage at any given running speed (Dennis & Noakes 1999) maintained higher running speeds throughout the time-trial. More importantly, the difference in running speed in the time-trial in the heat was observed essentially from the start of exercise (Fig. 21.4a). Furthermore, despite different running speeds in the time-trial in the heat, the two groups' rectal temperatures increased similarly during the time-trial (Fig. 21.4b).

It therefore appeared that, in this study the rate of heat storage was the variable that regulated running speed in the heat. Since the Caucasian runners were heavier and therefore produced more heat when running at the same speed as the lighter African runners, to achieve the same rate of heat production they were forced to reduce their running speed almost from the start of the time-trial, well before hyperthermic body temperatures were reached. Indeed at the moment they chose the slower running speeds, the core temperatures of the Caucasian runners were the same as those of the African runners. Thus, the slower speeds of the Caucasian runners were selected "in anticipation" and could only have been produced by voluntarily-chosen, reduced skeletal muscle recruitment and not by a temperature-induced failure of either skeletal muscle or cerebral function (since core temperatures in African and Caucasian runners were the same). The most probable conclusion must be that both groups regulated their running speeds in the heat on the basis of rates of heat

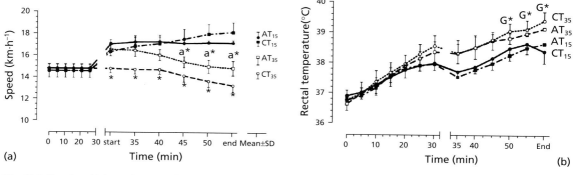

Fig. 21.4 Results of (a) running speeds and (b) rectal temperatures in black African and Caucasian runners of different body weights during an 8-km laboratory time-trial at 15°C and 35°C. Results showed that in cool conditions African runners (15°C; ■-AT_{15}) maintained the same speeds (start to end) as Caucasian runners (●-CT_{15}). But, in hot conditions, heavier Caucasians (○-CT_{35}) ran slower from the onset than smaller and lighter black Africans (□-AT_{35}). Despite different running speeds, rectal temperatures rose similarly in black African and Caucasian runners (G-right panel) when running in the heat. A reasonable conclusion might be that heavier Caucasian runners ran slower in the heat on the basis of an anticipatory decision by the subconscious brain (teleoanticipation), the function of which is to ensure that safe body temperatures are maintained during exercise (Tucker *et al.* 2004, 2006c). (a): *$P < 0.001$, Caucasians in warm conditions compared to Africans and Caucasians in cool conditions (a*); *$P < 0.01$, Africans in warm conditions compared to Caucasians in warm conditions. (b) (G*) *$P < 0.001$, Caucasians in warm compared to Caucasians in cool conditions. (Reproduced with permission from Marino *et al.* 2004.)

storage, which were chosen specifically to ensure that an excessive rate of storage leading to catastrophic hyperthermia did not occur.

Tucker *et al.* (2004) extended this finding and studied cyclists that performed two 20-km time-trials, one in hot (35°C) and one in cool conditions (15°C). As shown in Fig. 21.5a, although power output was the same in both hot and cool conditions for the first 20% of the trial, thereafter power output fell in the hotter environment, as did skeletal muscle activation measured via EMG activity. However, at that moment and for the remainder of the trials, the rectal temperatures (Fig. 21.5b) were the same in both conditions, indicating that the reduction in power output in the heat was not caused by excessive heat accumulation. Interestingly, the highest EMG activities occurred at the end of both trials, when core temperatures were at their highest. This proves that the impaired performance in the heat was not due directly to higher core temperatures acting (catastrophically) on motor control regions of the brain, as is required by the central fatigue model (Nybo & Nielsen 2001a). Rather, this study provides clear evidence that this was an anticipatory control mechanism that enabled the body to regulate its

power output and, hence, the rate of heat storage, thus maintaining thermal homeostasis. Another key finding of this study was that ratings of perceived exertion (RPE) increased linearly over time during both trials, despite the differences in power output (Fig. 21.5c).

Perhaps the most obvious evidence that the peripheral fatigue model cannot be a singular, absolute truth comes from two clear observations of how athletes pace themselves during competition. First, it is an obvious truth that athletes do not begin races of 100 m and 1000 km at the same pace; rather they begin the shorter-distance race at a much higher intensity. But this cannot be explained by the peripheral fatigue model that argues that the pacing strategy is determined exclusively by the action of poisonous metabolites that accumulate in the exercising muscles, thus impairing their function (Fig. 21.1). Running at 100-m speed will rapidly produce much higher levels of "poisonous" metabolites than will exercise at the pace required to complete 1000 km. Thus a race of 100 m should be run at a slower pace than a race of 1000 km. Clearly this is the opposite of what actually occurs. Second, as argued in detail elsewhere (Noakes & St. Clair Gibson 2004;

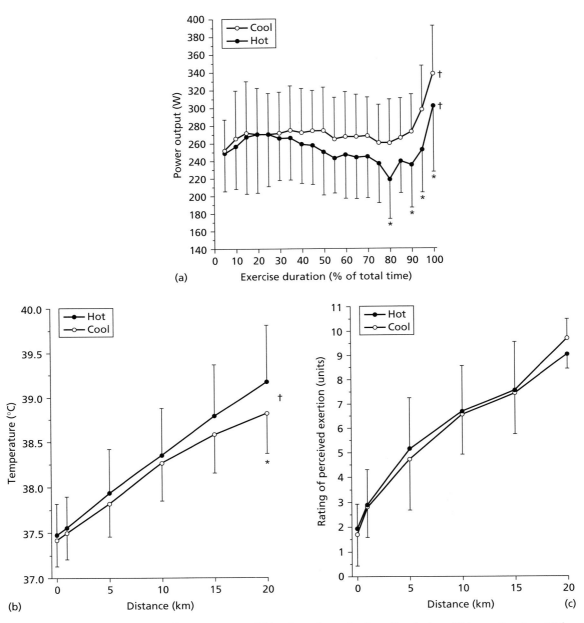

Fig. 21.5 (a) Power output, (b) rectal temperature, and (c) ratings of perceived exertion during a 20-km cycling time-trial at 35°C (filled symbols) and 15°C (open symbols). Note that power output in the heat begins to fall below that in the cool after about 20% of the exercise bout has been completed, and that rectal temperatures and ratings of perceived exertion rise similarly in both hot and cool conditions despite differences in power output. $^†P < 0.05$, power output and temperature in hot compared to cool conditions. (Reproduced with permission from Tucker *et al.* 2004.)

Tucker *et al.* 2006b; Noakes 2007b), athletes consistently increase their pace during the final 5–10% of races lasting more than about 20 min when, according to the peripheral model, fatigue should be at its greatest because the concentrations of "poisonous" intramuscular metabolites should be at their highest. Thus, this model is quite unable to explain how athletes can run their fastest when they are most fatigued.

These observations are more easily explained by the central governor model. Thus, the different paces observed at the start of races of different durations could be explained by varying levels of recruitment (activation) of the fibers in the active muscles: much less in a race of 1000 km, much more in a race of 100 m. The fact that the extent of EMG activity – an indirect measure of the extent of skeletal muscle activation – rises as a linear (Bigland-Ritchie & Woods 1974; Henriksson & Bonde-Petersen 1974) or curvilinear function (Gamet *et al.* 1993; Hug *et al.* 2004; Laplaud *et al.* 2006) of increasing power output, is an established finding; thus this theory is not purely hypothetical. Furthermore, magnetic resonance imaging also shows that muscle activation increases as a function of power output (Akima *et al.* 2005). Similarly, the increase in power output that can be achieved at the end of an exercise bout – the so-called end-spurt (Catalano 1974) – is associated with an increase in EMG activity, suggesting increased skeletal muscle activation (Ansley *et al.* 2004b; Tucker *et al.* 2004).

Further evidence for brain-regulated anticipatory pacing strategies comes from two recently-published studies. Ansley *et al.* (2004a,b) examined the adoption of pacing strategies during supramaximal exercise lasting approximately 30 s, the so-called Wingate Anaerobic Test (WAnT), and during successive 4-km cycling time-trials. A deception protocol was adopted during the WAnT so that some trials were slightly longer than the subject expected. The study found that power output over the last 3 s and the mean power index were lower, and the fatigue index was higher, during the trial in which subjects expected to perform trials of 30 s, but which actually lasted 36 s. This fall in power output did not occur when subjects exercised for 36 s after they had been truthfully informed that the exercise would last for 36 s. The authors concluded that athletes use previous

experience and knowledge of a pre-programmed "end-point" in order to pace themselves so that they can complete the exercise bout successfully (Ansley *et al.* 2004a).

In the second study (Ansley *et al.* 2004b), subjects performed three successive 4-km time-trials, with 17 min rest in between each. The only feedback given to the subjects during the trials was the distance they had traveled. The results showed that mean power output was similar in each trial but the performance time, although similar in the first and third trials, was slightly but not significantly longer in the second trial. In each trial, subjects increased their power output over the last 60 s (Fig. 21.6) and this was associated with an increase in EMG activity in the exercising limbs. EMG activity did not increase in successive time-trials, and only about 25% of the available motor units were recruited at any moment during exercise. Since less than 100% of the available motor units had been recruited, it could be concluded that the regulation of the exercise performance must have occurred centrally. Thus, the authors suggested that the pacing strategy was executed by central regulation of muscle recruitment and de-recruitment during the exercise bout (Ansley *et al.* 2004b), as predicted by the central governor model.

More recently, Nummela and colleagues (2006) have shown that performance during a 5-km time-trial is related to the sum of EMG activity (AEMG) in five lower limb muscles during the ground contact phase of the running stride. Furthermore, AEMG activity increased significantly as the athletes increased their pace in the final sprint. Since there was neuromuscular recruitment reserve during the first 4 km, it must be that the CNS determined performance in the time-trials by setting the number of motor units that were recruited throughout the exercise bout. This conforms to the predictions of the central governor model (Noakes & Marino 2007). Thus, there is clear evidence for an anticipatory regulation by the CNS of the exercise intensity even as the exercise begins. This probably occurs at both conscious and subconscious levels; the probable teleological purpose is to protect the body from harm (Noakes 1997; Kayser 2003; Noakes *et al.* 2005).

Finally, further evidence that this is a generalizable response and does not occur only, for example,

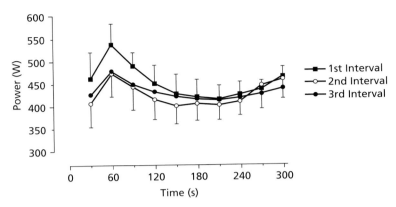

Fig. 21.6 Power output during three successive 4-km time-trials separated by rest periods of 17 min. Note that power outputs are remarkably similar from 120 to 300 s in all three trials despite the expected increase in fatigue. This suggests that the pacing strategy for all three bouts may have been decided in anticipation of the first interval. Note also the end-spurt in all three intervals, which occurred with an increase in EMG activity (not shown). However, maximal EMG activity in the lower limb muscles was not achieved at any time during exercise. This suggests that the regulation of the pacing strategy occurs centrally in the brain rather than in the peripheral muscles, since the peripheral fatigue model predicts that all motor units must always be active at exhaustion (Noakes *et al.* 2004b). (Reproduced with permission from Ansley *et al.* 2004b.)

because the body temperature is elevated by exercise (Tucker *et al.* 2004, 2006c), comes from the study of Morrison *et al.* (2004). They examined the effect of changes in core and skin temperature on maximal voluntary contraction (MVC) and voluntary activation (VA) of muscle during isometric knee-extension exercise. Subjects were passively heated from a core temperature of 37.5–39.5°C and then gradually cooled again to the starting temperature in order to separate the effects of hyperthermia from any cardiovascular or metabolic strain caused by exercise. A 10 s MVC was performed at every 0.5°C change in core temperature, with two muscle stimulations performed during each MVC to determine the magnitude of VA of the muscle. Their results showed a gradual decrease in MVC and VA during passive heating and a subsequent return to baseline with cooling (Fig. 21.7).

These results do not, therefore, support the hypothesis of the catastrophe model, which predicts that a reduction in skeletal muscle recruitment occurs only once a critically high core temperature has been reached. Rather, the findings of Morrison *et al.* (2004) and Tucker *et al.* (2004, 2006c) suggest that, during exercise in which force output is selected by the individual, motor command and VA are reduced well before a critical core temperature is reached. Indeed, the goal of the reduced muscle activation is specifically to prevent the development of a catastrophe.

All of these data contribute to the growing body of evidence for anticipatory regulation of exercise by an intelligent central governor that does not wait for the catastrophe to occur before it takes action. This is the opposite to the outcome predicted by both the peripheral and central fatigue models. An unsolicited letter received from a former professional cyclist indicates that these ideas resonate with the experiences of professional athletes:

"If I go and inject myself with 250 mg of speed amphetamine the drug will have a rapid effect on this 'governor' and I can guarantee that I was there all along but I was never able to access as my 'governor' is a tight b******! The only limiter will be when I drop dead or run out of fuel. Unfortunately for me I've seen both sides of the effects of drugs in sport. My wife's previous boyfriend died from racing in hot conditions whilst under the influence. Super natural rides used to be common here until drug testing came and they all had to switch to more subtle expensive products."

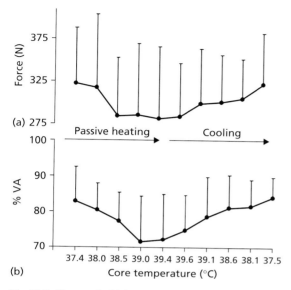

Fig. 21.7 Changes in (a) force produced during maximum voluntary contractions (MVC) of the knee extensor muscles and (b) voluntary activation (VA) with changes in core body temperature produced passively by exposure to external heating. Note that peak force during the MVC falls with increasing core temperature as does the extent of voluntary activation, but that both recover as core temperature returns to the normal range. (Reproduced with permission from Morrison *et al.* 2004.)

Of course, the traditional peripheral model of fatigue is quite unable to explain how amphetamines act in this way to improve performance.

Brain activity and fatigue

According to the central fatigue model, fatigue during prolonged exercise in the heat results from the effects of the elevated core temperature on brain function. Thus, the relationship between core temperature and electroencephalographic (EEG) activity has been investigated in an attempt to understand this concept of "central fatigue". Nielsen *et al.* (2001) reported a linear relationship between changes in EEG activity and core temperature during exercise in the heat. Specifically, they found that the high-frequency β-band on the EEG trace decreases gradually as core temperature rises. They used the α/β index (which is the ratio of slower-wave α-bands to high-frequency β-bands) as an indicator of fatigue, since arousal levels are reduced as the α/β index increases. This index was closely associated with changes in core temperature, increasing as temperature increased during the hot trial, and leveling off when core temperature reached a plateau during the cool trial. Accordingly, they concluded that these alterations in the electrical activity of the frontal area of the brain show the development of hyperthermia-associated cerebral "fatigue".

Nybo and Nielsen (2001b) then performed a similar study by measuring EMG activity, RPE, core temperature, and EEG activity during cycling. They again showed a close association between the α/β index and core temperature changes (Fig. 21.8c). Interestingly, they also found relationships between RPE and the α/β index, as well as between RPE and core temperature (Fig. 21.8a,b). Since EMG activity was unchanged during the trials, the authors concluded that hyperthermia of the extent measured in their study does not influence the extent of skeletal muscle recruitment during dynamic exercise (Nybo & Nielsen 2001b).

However, because this trial was at a fixed work-rate and subjects were unable to alter their power outputs during exercise, this result should have been expected. Instead, the authors might have concluded that, since their subjects were unable to alter their work-rates during exercise in the heat, their body temperatures rose more rapidly. As a result, the duration of exercise they could sustain until fatigue was reduced, as predicted by the findings of the studies of Tucker *et al.* (2004, 2006c).

Rasmussen *et al.* (2004) also reported a close relationship between the α/β index and core temperature changes during exercise, as well as between the α/β index and RPE. The authors suggested that changes in core temperature and the α/β index are the best predictors of an increase in RPE.

These results concur with the anticipatory model of exercise, as opposed to the catastrophic model, as reduced arousal (or fatigue) is already evident in electrical measurements of brain function well before the core body temperature reaches hyperthermic values. The gradual decrease in arousal coincides with the gradual increase in RPE. Thus, it may be that the α/β index is an electrical equivalent

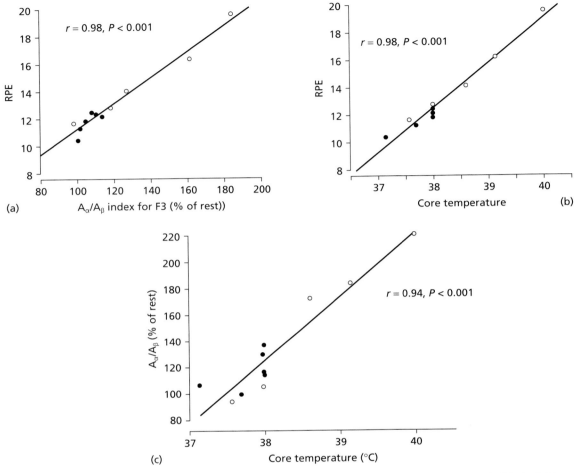

Fig. 21.8 (a) Rating of perceived exertion (RPE) plotted against electroencephalographic (EEG) activity (α/β index). (b) RPE plotted against core temperature. (c) α/β Index plotted against core temperature. Note that all variables are related to each other suggesting that the A_α/A_β index may be a brain determinant of the RPE. (Reproduced with permission from Nybo & Nielsen 2001b.)

of the RPE – one acting at the subconscious, and the other at the conscious level.

The conscious perception of fatigue

The central governor model posits that the conscious sensation of fatigue is protective since it influences behavior in order to ensure that no exerciser overrides the subconscious reductions in skeletal muscle recruitment and power output and so places the body at risk by continuing to generate too much power

(and heat) for too long (Morrison *et al.* 2004; Noakes 2004; Tucker *et al.* 2004, 2006; Albertus *et al.* 2005). Or, in the words of Lehmann *et al.* (1939), exercise may terminate "when the sum of all negative factors, such as fatigue and muscle pain, are felt more strongly than the positive factors of motivation and will power".

The perception of effort, measured as the RPE, is derived from the integration of a number of afferent signals (St. Clair Gibson *et al.* 2003; Morrison *et al.* 2004). Thus, cardiopulmonary factors such as respiratory rate, minute ventilation, heart rate, and oxygen uptake, as well as peripheral factors such as blood lactate concentration, mechanical strain, skin temperature, and core temperature, are all believed to play a role in the construction of effort perception (Hampson et al. 2001; St. Clair Gibson et al. 2003). However, many different studies have associated and then disassociated each of these variables from RPE. The extent to which each of these variables contributes to the perception of effort and fatigue is therefore unclear (Nybo & Nielsen 2001a). The central governor model is rather more inclusive and proposes that all these biological variables are monitored by the brain during exercise and, depending on the specific circumstances, exercise is regulated to prevent any one variable from deviating beyond its homeostatic range and so causing bodily harm.

The precise regions of the brain that are responsible for the production of these conscious sensations have yet to be conclusively identified (St. Clair Gibson et al. 2003). The extent to which changes in neurotransmitter concentrations in the brain contribute to these sensations has also been discussed (Nybo et al. 2003; St. Clair Gibson et al. 2003). Changes in brain serotonin, dopamine, and norepinephrine concentrations lead to alterations in both arousal and in behavioral responses to external stimuli. Acetylcholine is involved in synchronization and the generation of electrical activity in the brain. Therefore, changes in neurotransmitter concentrations may produce the conscious sensation of fatigue, and may play a role in the cognitive response to that sensation (St. Clair Gibson et al. 2003).

It has also recently been proposed that the RPE is set at the beginning of the exercise bout and that it will rise linearly to maximum levels at exercise completion (Noakes 2004). During open-ended exercise testing protocols, in which the exercise intensity is fixed so that subjects must maintain a constant power output until volitional exhaustion, it is proposed that the duration of exercise depends on the rate of increase in RPE so that, at any moment, RPE is a measure of the duration of exercise that can still be maintained at that exercise intensity (Noakes 2004).

This proposal comes from an analysis of the data from Baldwin et al. (2003), derived from a study of the effect of starting with different muscle glycogen concentrations on subjects exercising at a constant $\dot{V}o_2$ until fatigue. The subjects cycled significantly longer when starting with "high" glycogen than with "low" glycogen concentrations, but the RPE values were the same at the start and finish for both trials (Fig. 21.9). When the RPE data were plotted against the absolute duration of exercise (Fig. 21.9a), and against the percentage of time that had been completed (Fig. 21.9; right panel), they showed that the rate of rise of RPE was faster in the shorter duration (low-glycogen) trial (Fig. 21.9a); but when presented relative to the percentage of exercise duration, RPE increased at the same rate in both trials (Fig. 21.9b).

The author concluded that, at the start of exercise, the brain subconsciously calculates the anticipated duration of exercise that can be safely sustained at the required intensity without causing a disruption of whole body homeostasis (in this case, energy depletion). The RPE is then generated by the brain during the exercise bout, increasing as a function of the percentage of the total exercise time that has been completed (and that still remains). The maximum RPE is therefore reached before catastrophic failure of any bodily system. Thus, it is suggested that the rate at which RPE increases will determine the total duration of exercise (Noakes 2004).

That muscle glycogen content may indeed have a signaling role (Lambert et al. 2005) is suggested by the study of Rauch et al. (2005). These authors showed that, when subjects performed self-paced exercise, they began the exercise at a lower power output in the glycogen-depleted state. Yet they terminated exercise at essentially identical muscle glycogen concentrations. This suggests that the initial exercise intensity during self-paced exercise was chosen on the basis of the muscle glycogen concentrations sensed by the brain at the onset of exercise. This ensured that exercise terminated when the lowest safe muscle glycogen concentrations, also already established by the brain perhaps on the basis of prior experience, were reached.

Recent studies focusing on the anticipatory regulation of exercise performance in the heat lend further support for the role of the RPE in this regulation. For example, the study of Tucker et al. (2004) also showed a linear and identical rise in RPE during

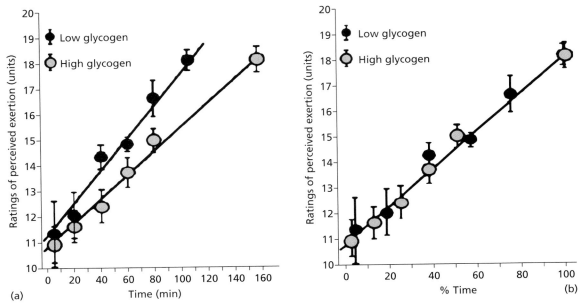

Fig. 21.9 Ratings of perceived exertion (RPE) plotted against absolute exercise duration (a) and against the percentage of total exercise time completed (b). Note that the RPE rises as a linear function of both absolute and relative exercise duration and that subjects terminate exercise at the same maximal RPE, regardless of the environmental conditions. This suggests that the rate at which the RPE rises is set at the onset of exercise in order to determine the duration of exercise before the maximal tolerable RPE is reached. If true, this suggests that the RPE provides a measure of the duration of exercise that remains (at that exercise intensity). (Reproduced with permission from Noakes 2004.)

two 20-km cycling time-trials (Fig. 21.5c), although (i) one was performed in hot and the other in cool conditions, and (ii) the subjects selected a lower power output in the heat. It was suggested that under the conditions of that study, the rate of heat storage was the regulated variable as core temperature increased linearly and identically in both trials despite differences in power output and rates of heat production. Thus, it may be that adjustments in power output were made in order to maintain a preset linear rise of RPE and, in so doing, to maintain thermal homeostasis.

To further examine the relationship between RPE and core temperature, Tucker *et al.* (2006c) performed an "RPE-clamp" study, in which cyclists rode in hot (35°C), normal (25°C), and cool (15°C) conditions while maintaining their RPE at sixteen on the Borg 15-point (6–20) scale. This allowed the cyclists to continuously adjust their power output so that RPE remained constant throughout the exercise. The trial was terminated when the subject's power output

declined to 70% of the initial power output, measured at the beginning of the trial.

The study found that the work-rate decreased during all trials but that the absolute rate of decline was faster in the hot than in the other two trials. However, when expressed as a percentage of total duration, all three trials showed similar rates of decrease in power output. Also, although rectal temperatures rose similarly throughout each trial, the rate of heat storage only differed during the first 4 min of exercise, after which the values for all trials were similar despite the different environmental conditions. This outcome can only have been achieved through the integration of afferent feedback regarding body temperature changes causing an altered efferent commands to the muscle, with the result that the work-rate is changed in an anticipatory manner in order to reduce the rate of heat storage. The authors concluded that this study proves that "exercise is regulated in anticipation by a complex intelligent system". This is, of course, the opposite of the brainless, catastrophic peripheral fatigue model which seeks to destroy, not to maintain homeostasis.

In a subsequent study, Crewe *et al.* (2008) examined changes in RPE and thermoregulatory variables during exercise in which the work-rate was fixed and not free to vary for the duration of the exercise bout. Subjects were required to exercise to exhaustion at a range of exercise intensities in either hot or cool conditions. It was found that RPE increased linearly in all exercise trials, irrespective of the exercise intensity and the environmental temperature (Fig. 21.10a). The linear increase occurred from the onset, suggesting that the subconscious brain must be able to forecast the duration of exercise and then set the rate of increase in RPE so that, in this case, volitional fatigue occurs before catastrophic hyperthermia can develop. The rate of increase in RPE then determines the time to volitional fatigue (Fig. 21.10a). Thus, in the trials at a higher exercise intensity of 65% and 70% of each subject's peak power output (PPO), the RPE rose more rapidly and fatigue occurred significantly sooner than in the trials at 55% of PPO. The duration of exercise to fatigue was thus a function of the absolute rate of increase in RPE.

The study also showed that, when expressed as a percentage of the completed exercise duration, the RPE increased at the same rate in all conditions, regardless of temperature or exercise intensity (Fig. 21.10b). This finding is similar to that described by Noakes (2004) in his analysis of the data of Baldwin *et al.* (2003) and further suggests that, at the onset of exercise, the subconscious brain calculates the exercise duration that can be maintained without disrupting whole-body homeostasis. The brain then generates a conscious sensation of exertion in a forecasted (feed-forward) manner, and effectively ensures that the maximal tolerable RPE occurs at the same moment that the full exercise duration (100% of completed duration) is achieved.

Finally, Albertus *et al.* (2005) have provided further evidence to support this theory of feed-forward, anticipatory control. Using a self-paced cycling protocol, they had subjects perform four 20-km time-trials, during which they were given feedback regarding the completed distance that was either accurate or inaccurate, depending on the requirements of each trial. The time taken to complete each time-trial did not differ. Power output decreased progressively

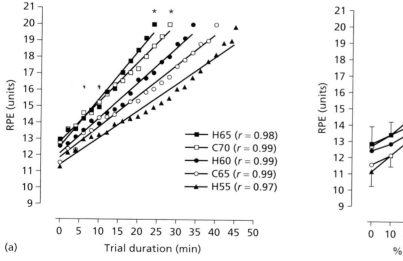

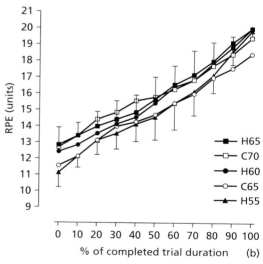

(a)   Trial duration (min)

% of completed trial duration   (b)

Fig. 21.10 Rating of perceived exertion (RPE) plotted against (a) mean exercise duration and (b) relative (% completed) trial duration in five trials at different exercise intensities (55, 60, 65, and 70% $\dot{V}o_{2max}$) at 15°C (C) or 35°C (H). Note that RPE rises as a linear function of absolute trial duration (a). Furthermore when expressed relative to % completed trial duration, RPE rose at the same rate in all conditions, regardless of the environmental temperature or the exercise intensity. (Reproduced with permission from Crewe *et al.* 2008)

from the start of each trial and then increased near the end, to levels that were similar to those measured at the start. But RPE increased linearly from start to finish and was similar across all trials, even though the subjects had received feedback which was sometimes inaccurate. The authors suggested that the rate of increase in RPE is set at the onset of exercise and that changes in power output are effected in order to ensure that the actual rate of increase in RPE does not exceed that preset rate. Thus, it appears that a pacing strategy is set in place according to the RPE and that this serves to ensure that the trial is completed without disruption of homeostasis.

The crucial point is that, presently, only the central governor model can explain these findings. It is also the sole model that explains all the currently reported findings of how the pace is set during exercise and why and when the decision to terminate exercise is taken.

Conclusion

The original theory for the "limitation" of maximal exercise performance proposed by A.V. Hill and his colleagues in 1923 had three important consequences for the global understanding of exercise physiology. Those consequences are essentially still acting more than 80 years later, as this article is written.

First, the idea was developed that exercise physiology is a special branch of physiology in which the risk is always present that whole-body homeostasis will fail. In contrast, the basic understanding of all other branches of physiology is that the integration of all bodily systems occurs specifically so that homeostasis is maintained, for when homeostasis fails the only outcome must be death.

Second, by extension, it was presumed that whenever fatigue develops and exercise terminates, regardless of the intensity or duration of the activity, the mechanism must be the same; specifically a failure of homeostasis in the organ system most taxed by that activity. But it is our contention that there is no evidence for a failure of homeostasis in healthy athletes during exercise (with the possible exception of heatstroke which, it may yet be proven, occurs only in those who are genetically predisposed (Noakes 2005) and hence are not entirely "healthy").

Third, the Hill model focused on the factors that cause "fatigue" and the termination of (maximal) exercise. Thus, it became popular to study fatigue and the factors that determine exercise termination in the wide variety of physical activities in which humans participate. However, we would argue that the much more interesting phenomenon is that of pacing (Noakes et al. 2005), which occurs from the onset of exercise and so has to be set "in anticipation" by the brain. In the context of pacing, the decision of when to terminate exercise is simply another component of the pacing strategy and may even be set before, or shortly after, the onset of exercise (Noakes et al. 2004). Once it is understood that pacing is the most important feature of how humans exercise, and it is appreciated that only the brain can determine the pacing strategy in response to prior experience and on the basis of sensory feedback by acting as an intelligent, complex system (Tucker et al. 2006c), the understanding of how a central governor might act becomes rather more obvious.

As Sir Roger Bannister, the first human to run the mile in less than 4 min, wrote in 1955: "The human body is centuries in advance of the physiologist, and can perform an integration of heart, lungs and muscles which is too complex for the scientist to analyse" (see Bannister 2004). More recently he has written that: "It is the brain not the heart or lungs that is the critical organ, it's the brain" (see Entine 2000). Or as A.V. Hill himself wrote in 1933: "In the case of bodily movement the nervous system is the steersman, who has to compound all the messages – the nerve waves – he receives to form one general impression on which to act . . . The continual reaction between muscles, nerves, end-organs and CNS is the physiologic basis of muscular skill, and on its smooth and efficient working depend many of the things that mankind finds worthy of accomplishment" (Hill 1965).

But perhaps the final word goes to the American physiologist L.W. Eichna and his colleagues: ". . . physical fitness cannot be defined nor can differences be detected by means of a few simple physiologic measurements (heart rate, body temperature, blood pressure) obtained during limited tests (step test, pack test, long march). To do so results in focusing attention on some small segment of the whole process and this at times gives an entirely erroneous concept. Man is not a pulse rate, a rectal temperature, but a complex array of many phenomena . . . Into performance enters the baffling yet extremely important factor of motivation, the will-to-do. This cannot be measured and remains an uncontrollable, quickly fluctuating, disturbing variable which may at any time completely alter the performance regardless of physical or physiologic state" (Eichna *et al.* 1945).

Indeed the crucial weakness of the reductionist (A.V. Hill) peripheral model of exercise fatigue is that the model allows no role for the brain and hence for a host of factors such as motivation, "mental toughness", prior experience, and pharmacological manipulations, which so obviously have major effects on human performance. Continuing to ignore the obvious would not seem to be particularly wise.

References

Akima, H., Kinugasa, R. & Kuno, S. (2005) Recruitment of the thigh muscles during sprint cycling by muscle functional magnetic resonance imaging. *International Journal of Sports Medicine* **26**, 245–252.

Albertus, Y., Tucker, R., St. Clair, G.A., Lambert, E.V., Hampson, D.B. & Noakes, T.D. (2005) Effect of distance feedback on pacing strategy and perceived exertion during cycling. *Medicine and Science in Sports and Exercise* **37**, 461–468.

Amann, M., Eldridge, M.W., Lovering, A.T., Stickland, M.K., Pegelow, D.F. & Dempsey, J.A. (2006) Arterial oxygenation influences central motor output and exercise performance via effects on peripheral locomotor muscle fatigue in humans. *Journal of Physiology* **575**, 937–952.

Amann, M., Romer, L.M., Subudhi, A.W., Pegelow, D.F. & Dempsey, J.A. (2007) Severity of arterial hypoxaemia affects the relative contributions of peripheral muscle fatigue to exercise performance in healthy humans. *Journal of Physiology* **581**, 389–403.

Ansley, L., Robson, P.J., St. Clair, G.A. & Noakes, T.D. (2004a) Anticipatory pacing strategies during supramaximal exercise lasting longer than 30 s. *Medicine and Science in Sports and Exercise* **36**, 309–314.

Ansley, L., Schabort, E., St. Clair, G.A., Lambert, M.I. & Noakes, T.D. (2004b) Regulation of pacing strategies during successive 4-km time trials. *Medicine and Science in Sports and Exercise* **36**, 1819–1825.

Astrand, P.O. (1952) *Experimental Studies of Physical Work Capacity in Relation to Sex and Age*. Munksgaard, Copenhagen.

Baldwin, J., Snow, R.J., Gibala, M.J., Garnham, A., Howarth, K. & Febbraio, M.A. (2003) Glycogen availability does not affect the TCA cycle or TAN pools during prolonged, fatiguing exercise. *Journal of Applied Physiology* **94**, 2181–2187.

Bannister, R.G. (2004) *The First Four Minutes*. Sutton Publishing, Stroud: 1–244.

Bannister, R.G. & Cunningham, D.J. (1954) The effects on the respiration and performance during exercise of adding oxygen to the inspired air. *Journal of Physiology* **125**, 118–137.

Bernard, C. (1974) *Lectures on the Phenomena of Life Common to Animals and Plants*. Charles C. Thomas Pub. Ltd., Illinois.

Bigland-Ritchie, B. & Woods, J.J. (1974) Integrated EMG and oxygen uptake during dynamic contractions of human muscles. *Journal of Applied Physiology* **36**, 475–479.

Bigland-Ritchie, B. & Vollestadt, N. (1988) Hypoxia and fatigue: how are they related? In: *Hypoxia: The Tolerable Limits* (Sutton, J.R., Houston, C.S. & Coates, G., eds.) Benchmark, Indianapolis, Illinois: 315–325.

Calbet, J.A., Boushel, R., Radegran, G., Sondergaard, H., Wagner, P.D. and Saltin, B. (2003a) Determinants of maximal oxygen uptake in severe acute hypoxia. American Journal of Physiology. Regulatory, Integrative and Comparative Physiology **284**, R291–R303.

Calbet, J.A., Boushel, R., Radegran, G., Sondergaard, H., Wagner, P.D. & Saltin, B. (2003b) Why is $\dot{V}o_{2max}$ after altitude acclimatization still reduced despite normalization of arterial O_2 content? American Journal of Physiology. Regulatory, Integrative and Comparative Physiology **284**, R304–R316.

Calbet, J.A., De Paz, J.A., Garatachea, N., Cabeza de Vaca, S. & Chavarren, J. (2003c) Anaerobic energy provision does not limit Wingate exercise performance in endurance-trained cyclists. *Journal of Applied Physiology* **94**, 668–676.

Catalano, J.F. (1974) End-spurt following simple repetitive muscular movement. *Perceptual and Motor Skills* **39**, 763–766.

Conlee, R.K. (1987) Muscle glycogen and exercise endurance: a twenty-year perspective. *Exercise and Sport Science Reviews* **15**, 1–28.

Crewe, H., Tucker, R. & Noakes, T.D. (2008) The rate of increase in rating of perceived exertion predicts the duration of exercise to fatigue at a fixed power output in different environmental conditions. *European Journal of Applied Physiology* **103**(5), 569–577.

Dennis, S.C. & Noakes, T.D. (1999) Advantages of a smaller body mass in humans when distance-running in warm, humid conditions. *European Journal of Applied Physiology and Occupational Physiology* **79**, 280–284.

Downer, A.R. (1901) *Running Recollections and How to Train*. Gale & Polden Ltd, London: 3–150.

Eichna, L.W., Bean, W.B., Ashe, W.F. & Nelson, N. (1945) Performance in relation to environmental temperature. *Bulletin of the Johns Hopkins Hospital* **76**, 25–58.

Entine, J. (2000) Taboo: *Why Black Athletes Dominate Sports and Why We're Afraid to Talk About it*. Public Affairs, New York: 3–387.

Febbraio, M.A, Snow, R.J., Stathis, C.G., Hargreaves, M. & Carey M.F. (1994) Effect of heat stress on muscle energy metabolism during exercise. *Journal of Applied Physiology* **77**: 2827–2831.

Fletcher, W.M. & Hopkins, W.G. (1907) Lactic acid in amphibian muscle. *Journal of Physiology* **35**, 247–309.

Galloway, S.D. & Maughan, R.J. (1997) Effects of ambient temperature on the capacity to perform prolonged cycle exercise in man. *Medicine and Science in Sports and Exercise* **29**, 1240–1249.

Gamet, D., Duchene, J., Garapon-Bar, C. & Goubel, F. (1993) Surface electromyogram power spectrum in human quadriceps muscle during incremental exercise. *Journal of Applied Physiology* **74**, 2704–2710.

Gonzalez-Alonso, J. & Calbet, J.A. (2003) Reductions in systemic and skeletal muscle blood flow and oxygen delivery limit maximal aerobic capacity in humans. *Circulation* **107**, 824–830.

Gonzalez-Alonso, J., Teller, C., Andersen, S.L., Jensen, F.B., Hyldig, T. & Nielsen, B. (1999) Influence of body temperature on the development of fatigue during prolonged exercise in the heat. *Journal of Applied Physiology* **86**, 1032–1039.

Gonzalez-Alonso, J., Warburton, D.E. & Gledhill, N. (2007) Point: Counterpoint: Stroke volume does/does not decline during exercise at maximal effort in healthy individuals. *Journal of Applied Physiology* **104**, 275–276.

Green, H.J., Sutton, J.R., Young, P.M., Cymerman, A. & Houston, C.S. (1989) Operation Everest II: Muscle energetics during maximal exhaustive exercise. *Journal of Applied Physiology* **66**, 1032–1039.

Hampson, D.B., St. Clair, G.A., Lambert, M.I. & Noakes, T.D. (2001) The influence of sensory cues on the perception of exertion during exercise and central regulation of exercise performance. *Sports Medicine* **31**, 935–952.

Henriksson, J. & Bonde-Petersen, F. (1974) Integrated electromyography of quadriceps femoris muscle at different exercise intensities. *Journal of Applied Physiology* **36**, 218–220.

Hill, A.V. (1924) Muscular activity and carbohydrate metabolism. *Science* **60**, 505–514.

Hill, A.V. (1965) *Trails and Trials in Physiology*. Edward Arnold Publishers Ltd, London: 1–374.

Hill, A.V. & Lupton, H. (1923) Muscular exercise, lactic acid, and the supply and utilization of oxygen. *Quarterly Journal of Medicine* **16**, 135–171.

Hill, A.V., Long, C.H.N. & Lupton, H. (1924a) Muscular exercise, lactic acid, and the supply utilization of oxygen: parts IV–VI. *Proceedings of the Royal Society B* **97**, 84–138.

Hill, A.V., Long, C.H.N. & Lupton, H. (1924b) Muscular exercise, lactic acid and the supply and utilisation of oxygen: parts VII–VIII. *Proceedings of the Royal Society B* **97**, 155–176.

Hill, A.V., Long, C.H.N. & Lupton, H. (1924c) Muscular exercise, lactic acid, and the supply utilization of oxygen: parts I–III. *Proceedings of the Royal Society B* **96**, 438–475.

Hollman, W. (1985) Historical remarks on the development of the aerobic-anaerobic threshold up to 1966. *International Journal of Sports Medicine* **6**, 109–116.

Hug, F., Bendahan, D., Le Fur, Y., Cozzone, P.J. & Grelot, L. (2004) Heterogeneity of muscle recruitment pattern during pedaling in professional road cyclists: a magnetic resonance imaging and electromyography study. *European Journal of Applied Physiology* **92**, 334–342.

Kayser, B. (2003) Exercise starts and ends in the brain. *European Journal of Applied Physiology* **90**, 411–419.

Kayser, B., Narici, M., Binzoni, T., Grassi, B. & Cerretelli, P. (1994) Fatigue and exhaustion in chronic hypobaric hypoxia: influence of exercising muscle mass. *Journal of Applied Physiology* **76**, 634–640.

Lambert, E.V., St. Clair, G.A. & Noakes, T.D. (2005) Complex systems model of fatigue: integrative homoeostatic control of peripheral physiologic systems during exercise in humans. *British Journal of Sports Medicine* **39**, 52–62.

Laplaud, D., Hug, F. & Grelot, L. (2006) Reproducibility of eight lower limb muscles activity level in the course of an incremental pedaling exercise. *Journal of Electromyography and Kinesiology* **16**, 158–166.

Lehmann, G., Straub, H. & Szakall, A. (1939) Pervitin as an ergogenic aid during exercise. *Arbeitsphysiology* **10**, 680–691.

Marino, F.E., Lambert, M.I. & Noakes, T.D. (2004) Superior performance of African runners in warm humid but not in cool environmental conditions. *Journal of Applied Physiology* **96**, 124–130.

Messner, R. (1979) *Everest: Expedition to the Ultimate*. Kaye & Ward, London: 179.

Morrison, S., Sleivert, G.G. & Cheung, S.S. (2004) Passive hyperthermia reduces voluntary activation and isometric force production. *European Journal of Applied Physiology* **91**, 729–736.

Mortensen, S.P., Dawson, E.A., Yoshiga, C.C., Dalsgaard, M.K., Damsgaard, R., Secher, N.H. *et al.* (2005) Limitations to systemic and locomotor limb muscle oxygen delivery and uptake during maximal exercise in humans. *Journal of Physiology* **566**, 273–285.

Nielsen, B., Hales, J.R., Strange, S., Christensen, N.J., Warberg, J. & Saltin, B. (1993) Human circulatory and thermoregulatory adaptations with heat acclimation and exercise in a hot, dry environment. *Journal of Physiology* **460**, 467–485.

Nielsen, B., Hyldig, T., Bidstrup, F., Gonzalez-Alonso, J. & Christoffersen, G.R. (2001) Brain activity and fatigue during prolonged exercise in the heat. *Pflugers Archives* **442**, 41–48.

Noakes, T.D. (1997) 1996 J.B. Wolffe Memorial Lecture. Challenging beliefs: ex Africa semper aliquid novi. *Medicine and Science in Sports and Exercise* **29**, 571–590.

Noakes, T.D. (1998) Maximal oxygen uptake: "classical" versus "contemporary" viewpoints: a rebuttal. *Medicine and Science in Sports and Exercise* **30**, 1381–1398.

Noakes, T.D. (2000) Physiologic models to understand exercise fatigue and the adaptations that predict or enhance athletic performance. *Scandinavian Journal of Medicine and Science in Sports* **10**, 123–145.

Noakes, T.D. (2003) *Lore of Running*. Human Kinetics Publishers, Champaign, Illinois: 1–930.

Noakes, T.D. (2004) Linear relationship between the perception of effort and the duration of constant load exercise that remains. *Journal of Applied Physiology* **96**, 1571–1572.

Noakes, T.D. (2005) Mind over matter: Deducing heatstroke pathology. *The Physician and Sportsmedicine* **33**, 44–46.

Noakes, T.D. (2007a) Determining the extent of neural activation during maximal effort: comment. *Medicine and Science in Sports and Exercise* **39**, 2092.

Noakes, T.D. (2007b) The central governor model of exercise regulation applied to the marathon. *Sports Medicine* **37**, 374–377.

Noakes, T.D. (2007c) The limits of human endurance: What is the greatest endurance performance of all time? Which factors regulate performance at extreme altitude? In: *Hypoxia and the Circulation* (Roach, R.C., Wagner, P.D. & Hackett, P.H., eds.) Springer, New York: 259–280.

Noakes, T.D. & Marino, F.E. (2007) Arterial oxygenation, central motor output and exercise performance in humans. *Journal of Physiology* **585**(3), 919–921.

Noakes, T.D. & St. Clair Gibson, A. (2004) Logical limitations to the "catastrophe" models of fatigue during exercise in humans. *British Journal of Sports Medicine* **38**, 648–649.

Noakes, T.D., Peltonen, J.E. & Rusko, H.K. (2001) Evidence that a central governor regulates exercise performance during acute hypoxia and hyperoxia. *Journal of Experimental Biology* **204**, 3225–3234.

Noakes, T.D., Calbet, J.A., Boushel, R., Sondergaard, H., Radegran, G., Wagner, P.D. *et al.* (2004a) Central regulation of skeletal muscle recruitment explains the reduced maximal cardiac output during exercise in hypoxia. *American Journal of Physiology. Regulatory Integrative and Comparative Physiology* **287**, R996–R999.

Noakes, T.D., St. Clair Gibson, A. & Lambert, E.V. (2004b) From catastrophe to complexity: a novel model of integrative central neural regulation of effort and fatigue during exercise in humans. *British Journal of Sports Medicine* **38**, 511–514.

Noakes, T.D., St. Clair Gibson, A. & Lambert, E.V. (2005) From catastrophe to complexity: a novel model of integrative central neural regulation of effort and fatigue during exercise in humans: summary and conclusions. *British Journal of Sports Medicine* **39**, 120–124.

Nummela, A.T., Paavolainen, L.M., Sharwood, K.A., Lambert, M.I., Noakes, T.D. & Rusko, H.K. (2006) Neuromuscular factors determining 5-km running performance and running economy in well-trained athletes. *European Journal of Applied Physiology* **97**, 1–8.

Nybo, L. & Nielsen, B. (2001a) Hyperthermia and central fatigue during prolonged exercise in humans. *Journal of Applied Physiology* **91**, 1055–1060.

Nybo, L. & Nielsen, B. (2001b) Perceived exertion is associated with an altered brain activity during exercise with progressive hyperthermia. *Journal of Applied Physiology* **91**, 2017–2023.

Nybo, L., Nielsen, B., Blomstrand, E., Moller, K. & Secher, N. (2003) Neurohumoral responses during prolonged exercise in humans. *Journal of Applied Physiology* **95**, 1125–1131.

Place, N., Matkowski, B., Martin, A. & Lepers, R. (2006) Synergists activation pattern of the quadriceps muscle differs when performing sustained isometric contractions with different EMG biofeedback. *Experimental Brain Research* **174**, 595–603.

Rasmussen, P., Stie, H., Nybo, L. & Nielsen, B. (2004) Heat induced fatigue and changes of the EEG is not related to reduced perfusion of the brain during prolonged exercise in humans. *Journal of Applied Physiology* **29**, 731–737.

Rauch, H.G., St. Clair Gibson, A., Lambert, E.V. & Noakes, T.D. (2005) A signalling role for muscle glycogen in the regulation of pace during prolonged exercise. *British Journal of Sports Medicine* **39**, 34–38.

Rowell, L.B. (1993) *Human Cardiovascular Control*. Oxford University Press, New York: 1–500.

Simpson, J. (1997) *Touching the Void*. Vintage, London: 9–216.

St. Clair Gibson, A. & Noakes, T.D. (2004) Evidence for complex system integration and dynamic neural regulation of skeletal muscle recruitment during exercise in humans. *British Journal of Sports Medicine* **38**, 797–806.

St. Clair Gibson, A., Lambert, M.L. & Noakes, T.D. (2001) Neural control of force output during maximal and submaximal exercise. *Sports Medicine* **31**, 637–650.

St. Clair Gibson, A., Baden, D.A., Lambert, M.I., Lambert, E.V., Harley, Y.X., Hampson, D., *et al.* (2003) The conscious perception of the sensation of fatigue. *Sports Medicine* **33**, 167–176.

Taylor, H.L., Buskirk, E. & Henschel, A. (1955) Maximal oxygen uptake as an objective measure of cardio-respiratory performance. *Journal of Applied Physiology* **8**, 73–80.

Tucker, R., Rauch, L., Harley, Y.X. & Noakes, T.D. (2004) Impaired exercise performance in the heat is associated with an anticipatory reduction in skeletal muscle recruitment. *Pflugers Archives* **448**, 422–430.

Tucker, R., Bester, A., Lambert, E.V., Noakes, T.D., Vaughan, C.L. & St. Clair, G.A. (2006a) Non-random fluctuations in power output during self-paced exercise. *British Journal of Sports Medicine* **40**, 912–917.

Tucker, R., Lambert, M.I. & Noakes, T.D. (2006b) An analysis of pacing strategies during men's world record performances in track athletics. *International Journal of Sports Physiology and Performance* **1**, 233–245.

Tucker, R., Marle, T., Lambert, E.V. & Noakes, T.D. (2006c) The rate of heat storage mediates an anticipatory reduction in exercise intensity during cycling at a fixed rating of perceived exertion. *Journal of Physiology* **574**, 905–915.

Ulmer, H.V. (1996) Concept of an extracellular regulation of muscular metabolic rate during heavy exercise in humans by psychophysiologic feedback. *Experientia* **52**, 416–420.

Vella, C.A. & Robergs, R.A. (2005) A review of the stroke volume response to upright exercise in healthy subjects. *British Journal of Sports Medicine* **39**, 190–195.

Walters, T.J., Ryan, K.L., Tate, L.M. & Mason, P.A. (2000) Exercise in the heat is limited by a critical internal temperature. *Journal of Applied Physiology* **89**, 799–806.

Wasserman, K. & McIlroy, M.B. (1964) Detecting the threshold of anaerobic metabolism in cardiac patients during exercise. *American Journal of Cardiology* **14**, 844–852.

Wasserman, K., Whipp, B.J., Koyal, S.N. & Beaver, W.L. (1967) Anaerobic threshold and respiratory gas exchange during exercise. *Journal of Applied Physiology* **22**, 71–85.

Part 10

Special Populations

Chapter 22

The Young Athlete

LYLE J. MICHELI AND MARGO MOUNTJOY

Organized sports participation and training by children is a relatively new phenomenon. With its apparent beginnings in Little League Baseball in North America in 1947, systematic training for child athletes is now a worldwide phenomenon. Young athletes may begin training in sports as early as 4 years of age and commence competitive sports by age 7. In the USA alone, more than 25 million children regularly engage in organized sports (Gotch & Gilchrist 2002; Conn *et al*. 2003), and 10 times that number participate worldwide. This extraordinary growth in the numbers of children participating in sports has stimulated interest in the study of both the training specifics of children's sports and the potential for injury, and in particular, the unique patterns of injury that arise as a result of repetitive training (O'Neill & Micheli 1988).

In the past, a clear demarcation existed between sports science and sports medicine. Sports science is the study of training and the physiological response of the athlete to training. Sports medicine, on the other hand, is the clinical medical care of athletes who have sustained illness or injury from athletic participation or training. It is becoming increasingly clear, however, that there is interdependence between these two disciplines, as evidenced by shared areas of interest such as overtraining, hydration, doping, and injury prevention. A further stimulus to this

integration is the growing emphasis on the practice of evidence-based medicine, which incorporates a critical review of the medical and scientific basis of therapeutic interventions, with determination of levels of evidence as part of the process (Oxford Centre for Evidence-Based Medicine; Davidoff *et al*. 1995).

Our strong conviction is that modern sports medicine must integrate the scientific investigation of sports performance and the clinical care of the athlete, and that every member of the sports medicine team should be responsible for advancing the science of the sports training and participation. The evolution of the scientific method in Renaissance Europe was often likened by its early practitioners to a three-legged stool: the first leg of the stool was the observation of the workings of nature, the second was the development of hypotheses to explain these workings, and the third incorporated the testing of these hypotheses by systematic experiments or observations. Without any one of the three legs, the stool would fall. This metaphor demonstrates how important it is that sports medicine and sports science exist as interrelated disciplines. In the area of sports science and sports medicine, the evolution of a new scientific advance that improves our care of the athlete often begins with the clinical observation of an apparent association between two variables, which is then tested by the researcher. Everyone involved in the care or training of the athlete should be a part of the scientific process that promotes the health of children through sports training and competition, a process that is founded on sound scientific principles.

The Olympic Textbook of Science in Sport, 1st edition. Edited by R.J. Maughan. Published 2009 by Blackwell Publishing. ISBN: 978-1-4051-5638-7.

Uniqueness of the child athlete

The child is by definition a human being who has not yet completed the growth process and attained full maturation of the body's various organ systems. The physiological response to training and the susceptibility to overtraining injury have been noted to be different in the child when compared to the adult (Bar-Or 1989a; Mountjoy *et al.* 2008). A truism puts it succinctly: "The child is not just a small adult." Differences between the child and adult in the areas of thermal regulation and cardiovascular response are covered in detail later in this chapter. Another area of concern is the effect of intense training on a child's growth and maturation.

Sports scientists and clinicians vigorously debate the growth and maturation of the child athlete and the potential benefits or harm of regular sports training (Theintz *et al.* 1993; Borer 1995; Malina 1998). The consequence of systematic sports training on the growth and maturation of children remains an area of scientific controversy. Some studies suggest that regular physical activity, including sports training, can stimulate growth and health (Bailey *et al.* 1978; Borer 1995); others posit that excessive sports training can have a deleterious effect on growth and maturation (Theintz *et al.* 1993; Tofler *et al.* 1996). It is clear that the volume and intensity of training is a critical determinant of whether an outcome in children's sports is positive or negative. However, this is not always accurately quantified, particularly in observational studies of a young athlete's training. It has frequently been observed by clinicians that there appears to be a delay in onset of menarche and a delay in longitudinal growth in some young athletes engaged in intense training, particularly if combined with nutritional deprivation (Daly *et al.* 2005). This appears to be more prevalent in the individual sports such as gymnastics, dance, or figure skating where high volumes of training have become relatively routine, even for athletes as young as age 10 or 11 (Daly *et al.* 2005).

In a recent review on this topic, Baxter-Jones *et al.* (2003) concluded that "there is limited evidence to suggest that intensive training for sport has a negative effect on the growth and maturation of young athletes." Nonetheless, clinicians caring for child athletes engaged in intensive sports training such as gymnastics, dance, or figure skating have observed that there is a significant acceleration in growth and maturation when the child is unable to train for 3–6 months (e.g., due to injury). It has yet to be determined whether this apparent delay in growth and maturation due to intensive training compromises ultimate growth. The study of overtraining of child athletes has just begun, but decline in the rate of growth in the course of training should be given serious consideration as one of the markers for overtraining in this age group (Balyi *et al.* 2005; Daly *et al.* 2005).

Readiness for participation

Readiness for sport is defined by "the child's level of growth, maturity, and development that enables him/her to perform tasks and meet demands of training and competition. Readiness and critical periods of trainability during growth and development of young athletes are also referred to as the correct time for the programming of certain stimuli to achieve optimum adaptation with regard to motor skills, muscular and/or aerobic power" (Balyi *et al.* 2005).

Physical readiness

When considering athlete readiness, it is essential to be cognizant of the variations in rates of maturation. At any given age, there will be children of the same chronological age who are up to 2 years older or younger in terms of developmental age. Awareness of this discrepancy is important when considering readiness to learn and to perform new tasks. Although there is an optimal window of trainability for athletic skills, it is important to realize that all systems are always trainable at all ages (Tables 22.1 & 22.2).

AGES 6–11

The child in the early stages of this age range has a greater proportion of developed large muscle groups than small muscle groups. As a result, these children are best suited for developing general motor skills involving the large muscle groups such as running,

Table 22.1 Recommendations for children ages 6–11. (Reproduced with permission from Balyi *et al.* 2005.)

Recommendations
- The optimal window of trainability for flexibility is 6–10 years of age
- The first optimal window for speed training is 7–9 years in males and 6–8 years in girls
- The optimal window of trainability for skill acquisition is from 9–12 years in males and 8–11 years in girls

Table 22.2 Recommendations for children ages 12–16. (Reproduced with permission from Balyi *et al.* 2005.)

Recommendations
- The optimal window of trainability for endurance occurs at the onset of peak height velocity.
- Aerobic capacity training is recommended prior to peak height velocity.
- The optimal window of trainability for strength in boys is 12–18 months after peak height velocity and in girls it is at the onset of menarche.
- The second optimal window of trainability for speed occurs in boys between the ages of 13–16 and in girls between the ages of 11–13.

jumping, swimming, climbing, etc. More coordinated activities requiring smaller muscle groups can be developed towards the end of this stage. A focus on sport-specific skill acquisition and specialization in sport should also occur at the end of this age range. Physical literacy – or competency in the fundamental movement and sport skills – should be developed at this stage. This includes balance, throwing, kicking, catching, skipping, coordination, hopping, agility, speed, dribbling, etc. The child in this age group has a larger heart size in relation to the rest of the body, resulting in an increasing endurance capacity. However, the anaerobic system is not well developed, resulting in poor performance during anaerobic training. The child requires more oxygen and energy to work at the same rate as adults; they also have higher heart rates. As a result of these physiological characteristics, their metabolism is less efficient than adults. Daily physical activity is recommended, which should become more sport-specific as the child matures. Emphasis should be on fun and participation.

AGES 12–16

The early adolescent undergoes significant morphological changes. There is considerable variation in growth and maturation rates between individuals. Girls on average reach their peak height velocity at age 12 and boys around the age of 14. As the child grows, there are significant proportional changes occurring in bone, muscle, and fat tissue. Different parts of the body grow at different rates. Arm and leg length increases before the trunk, and decreasing flexibility is common as muscle growth lags behind bone growth. Further development of the anaerobic system occurs enabling the introduction of anaerobic training. The central nervous system is also developing, thus facilitating the refinement of skill development through agility, balance, and coordination. Abstract thinking and egocentric thought processes develop, which enables psychological training to be expanded.

Psychological readiness

The psychological readiness of the child athlete is dependent upon the developmental stage of the child. Further information relating to specific age ranges is given in Tables 22.3–22.5. Awareness and attention to the developmental stage of each individual is essential, as psychological readiness is as important for optimal athlete development as physical readiness. Good coaches are aware of their athlete's psychological stage of development and they adapt the training program accordingly.

Coaching principles

The coach plays a critical role in the development of a successful athlete. Coaches are also influential in the development of healthy adults from the appropriate training of the child athlete. Coaches must be aware of the physical and psychological readiness principles, and planning and coaching techniques must be adapted accordingly. The following coaching principles should be followed when designing a training program for the child athlete:

1 The most important factor to consider in the training of the child athlete is that sport should be fun;

Table 22.3 Psychological characteristics and training recommendations for children ages 2–6. (Reproduced with permission from Committee on Sports Medicine and Fitness and Committee on School Health 2001.)

Characteristic	Training recommendation
Highly developed imagination	Creative play and experimentation
Developing self concept	Positive reinforcement
Unable to understand concept of competition	Sport sessions to consist of development of sport fundamentals
Basis for the development of life habits	Teach children to have an active lifestyle

Table 22.4 Psychological characteristics and training recommendations for children ages 7–11. (Reproduced with permission from Committee on Sports Medicine and Fitness and Committee on School Health 2001.)

Characteristic	Training recommendation
Improved memory and decision-making skills	Able to conceptualize basic strategies
Improved attention span	Able to understand longer training sessions and instructions
Reasoning ability skills are still limited	Training should be fun and well-planned
Unable to understand the concept of competition	Encourage the learning of basic skills and rules of sport
Developing a sense of fairness	Consistent coaching is essential
Enjoy being the centre of attention	Emphasize success with positive reinforcement

Table 22.5 Psychological characteristics and training recommendations for children ages 12–18. (Reproduced with permission from Committee on Sports Medicine and Fitness and Committee on School Health 2001.)

Characteristic	Training recommendation
Physical and psychological maturity do not always coincide	Awareness and accommodation for incongruence in maturation
Rapid morphological change occurs subsequently resulting in altered performance	Psychological consequences to physical changes should be supported emotionally by coach
Abstract thought development	Variation in coaching techniques are now possible
Change in social behavior	Sport allows opportunity to engage in appropriate social expression
Development of autonomy	Support of independence and inclusion in decision-making
Motivational change to more progressive internalization; becoming more personal and intrinsic	Focus on personal goal setting

2 The focus of sport should be on skill development, not on winning (Committee on Sports for Medicine and Fitness and Committee on School Health 2001);

3 Children should train and compete in programs designed for children, not for adults;

4 Equipment, rules, and the playing field should be adapted for the child's size and capabilities;

5 Developmental age not chronological age should be used in training planning;

6 The fundamental skills of sport should be taught to children;

7 Critical periods of accelerated adaptation to training should be recognized and planned for in the training program;

8 Children should be matched for skill, size, and developmental stage, not solely by chronological age;

9 Gender-specific training should occur at appropriate development stages when discrepancies in physical abilities exist; and

10 Children have the right to enjoy sport without negative influence and pressures from the media, sports administrators, over-zealous parents, and coaches.

Training recommendations

Aerobic and anaerobic training

Aerobic and anaerobic training are important components of the training program for most sports. Indeed, successful performance in most sports relies on peak aerobic and anaerobic fitness. Much scientific evidence exists to support the recommendations for aerobic and anaerobic training in the mature athlete; however, this is not the case with training in children. There are few well-designed, prospective studies of exercise training in children and adolescents and of those that have been published, the majority have inherent flaws such as inadequate training program duration and/or small sample size. To further ensure the safety of training programs for the child athlete and to validate the efficacy of such programs, more scientific evidence is necessary. There is, however, good scientific evidence to make the following observations and training recommendations.

EFFECT OF GROWTH ON AEROBIC AND ANAEROBIC TRAINING

As children grow and mature, their aerobic and anaerobic fitness increases. However, the acquisition of aerobic and anaerobic fitness is not uniform. Children experience more marked improvements in anaerobic performance during adolescence. The optimal window of trainability for aerobic capacity training is prior to peak height velocity. The difference between aerobic and anaerobic fitness in girls vs. boys is not evident until late childhood when boys out-perform girls. This gender difference becomes more pronounced through adolescence. Despite these differences, all children at all ages do show benefit

and improvement in aerobic and anaerobic fitness through age-appropriate training.

MODE OF EXERCISE

Many different modes of exercise have been studied in children to ascertain their effect on $\dot{V}O_{2max}$, including:

1 Continuous, sustained exercise;
2 Interval training;
3 Combined continuous and interval training; and
4 Resistance exercise.

It can be concluded from the scientific literature that exercise using large muscle groups – regardless of the mode – has the potential to increase peak aerobic fitness. Studies that utilize a combination of both interval training and continuous exercise appear to be the most successful in producing the greatest improvement in aerobic fitness (Obert *et al*. 2003). However, this benefit may be attributed to the retention of the child's interest and attention for longer periods as a result in the variation in activity, resulting in training sessions of longer duration.

TRAINING PROGRAM

Most studies evaluating aerobic and anaerobic training use a frequency of three to four training sessions per week. Significant increases in $\dot{V}O_{2max}$ are also demonstrated following two and five training sessions per week. Many studies demonstrate that sessions of 40–60 min duration are the most successful in terms of an improvement in $\dot{V}O_{2max}$. The intensity that has been reported to produce the most significant increases is 85–90% of maximum heart rate (HR_{max}; Savage *et al*. 1986). Studies evaluating the optimum program length are inconclusive.

Strength training

Strength training has become one of the most popular and rapidly evolving methods of enhancing athletic performance. Although it is widely used by adult athletes, the role of strength training for children and adolescents was actively debated when first introduced in the context of children's sports training. Three primary questions asked at that time were whether strength training could actually increase muscular strength in young athletes, whether it was safe, and whether it would result in increased athletic performance (Guy & Micheli 2001). Current evidence indicates that both children and adolescents can increase muscular strength as a consequence of strength training and, when properly supervised and by following appropriate programs, this is indeed a safe activity for the young athlete.

However, the physiological mechanisms responsible for this observed increase in strength by children in response to a progressive resistive program remains controversial. Present evidence suggests that the major mechanisms responsible appear to be an increased neuromuscular activation and coordination (Faigenbaum 2000). Longer-term studies will be necessary to address whether there is also a component of muscle hypertrophy in this age group. It should be noted further that there is no evidence to support the misconception that children need androgens for strength gain, or that they lose flexibility with strength training. A well-designed training regimen that incorporates components of flexibility should result in no loss of flexibility in conjunction with the gains in strength training. As with any form of training for children, additional care should be taken that safe lifting techniques are used, and that proper supervision and progression of resistance are employed at all times. As with adults, continued training is required to maintain strength gains, which dissipate when training is discontinued.

Periodization

Periodization is a coaching tool that facilitates the planning of the training program for the athlete. In addition to providing a framework for training, it is also a valuable tool to assist in time management. Periodization helps with the organization of the complex array of training processes into a logical and scientifically-based schedule designed to bring about optimal improvements in performance (Balyi *et al.* 2005). This is achieved by organizing the different components of training into weeks, days, and even particular training sessions. Macro-cycles refer to large blocks of time within a training phase, usually from 8 to 16 weeks in duration. Meso-cycles are smaller periods of time, usually of 4 weeks duration.

Micro-cycles refer to a period of 7 days. Periodization must link the developmental stage of the athlete with the specific skill requirements of the sport. It must also focus on the particular priorities of the training within the time context of the competitive season. Flexibility is also crucial, and ongoing athlete monitoring and evaluation will dictate program periodization, as will changes in the athlete's developmental stage.

Current examples of periodization models in sport performance literature focus on the elite and sub-elite athletes. There is a paucity of scientific evaluation of periodization models designed for children. More research is therefore needed in this area in order to ascertain effective and safe periodization models for the child athlete.

Many factors must be taken into consideration when designing a periodization plan (Table 22.6). Ideal periodization extends beyond the realm of coaching to sport organizations such as Regional, National, and International Federations. Ideal periodization should include competition planning to complement the physical, psychological, and athletic stage of development of the child (Table 22.7).

Table 22.6 Factors to be taken into consideration when designing a periodization plan.

Periodization planning factors:
Modality
Volume
Intensity
Frequency of training
Competition schedule
Recovery
Growth
Maturation
Trainability principles

Table 22.7 The ideal training : competition ratio.

Age range	Training : competition ratio
Males 6–9 years Females 6–8 years	Age-appropriate sport activities based on the development of fundamentals of sport
Males 9–12 years Females 8–11 years	70% training & 30% competition
Males 12–16 years Females 11–15 years	60% training & 40% competition

A common problem for the child athlete is over-competition and under-training as a result of competitive schedules that do not take into account their developmental needs.

Psychological training

The psychological training of the child athlete is as important as the physical training. Healthy and effective psychological training is most effective when based on the following premises (Committee on Sports Medicine and Fitness and Committee on School Health 2001):

1 Children are still developing and should not be considered as miniature adults;

2 Healthy psychological development in childhood is essential to ensure healthy adults; and

3 Children should be encouraged to play and have fun with sport.

When planning for the psychological training of the child athlete it is important to consider and respect the individual psychological developmental stage of the child. As is the case with physical development in children, there is variation amongst children of the same chronological age in terms of their stage of psychological development. The developmental stage of the individual child is determined by a combination of both individual talent and environmental factors.

PSYCHOLOGICAL PRESCRIPTION

When designing the psychological training prescription for the child athlete, the goal is to include appropriate activities that encourage healthy psychological growth and that are relevant for the specific developmental stage. It is also important to design activities that encourage the child to develop a passion for sport. The specific psychological skills that should be developed in the child athlete include motivation, self-confidence, emotional control, and concentration, and sport-related tasks should be designed to encourage growth and skill in these areas. Consistent coaching techniques and positive feedback can reinforce and foster these psychological skills. The child athlete should also be encouraged to develop strategies in goal setting, and cognitive and behavioral control. Independence is another

Table 22.8 Nutritional principles for the child athlete.

1. The attention to healthy eating habits
2. The provision of adequate energy for growth
3. The provision of adequate energy for physical activity
4. The provision of essential nutrients for growth

psychological skill that should be part of the training program (Tofler & Butterbaugh 2005).

In addition to the individual personal psychological skills listed above, sport provides a forum for children to learn other important psychological skills such as codes of behavior or conduct, team work and cooperation, and fair play. At all times, sport should foster a positive self concept in a healthy motivational climate.

Nutritional requirements

Growing, active children require a healthy diet. Many factors affect the nutritional requirements of the child athlete, for example age, gender, pubertal status, event, and competitive season. The nutritional plan for the child athlete should mimic basic nutritional concepts with the focus being on nutrient-rich foods (Table 22.8). They should be taught healthy food choices and healthy eating habits should be encouraged. There are no short-cuts to healthy nutrition. Ensuring a balance of energy, protein, and nutrient intake is most effective and efficiently accomplished through healthy and balanced nutrition. Meal replacements, nutritional supplements, and vitamin supplements are not necessary, and should be avoided in the diet of the child athlete. Likewise, convenience foods or fast foods, which are often high in saturated fats and sugars, should be discouraged as these foods do not provide the nutrients required for a healthy balanced diet, and are partially responsible for the increasing incidence of obesity in many societies. Likewise, snacks such as sweets, cakes, cookies, and pop should be replaced with healthier snacks such as fruit, yogurt, or muesli.

Carbohydrates

Carbohydrates are the most important energy source to fuel physical activity (Burke *et al.* 2003). Carbohydrate ingestion should be within the range of 45–65% of the total daily energy intake. The child athlete should ingest sufficient carbohydrate to meet the energy demands of their sport and to optimize recovery of the muscle stores of glycogen. They also require sufficient carbohydrate intake to accommodate growth (Morantz 2006a). The recommended intakes are as follows:

1 Carbohydrate ingestion to facilitate immediate recovery after exercise (0–4 h): 1–1.2 g·kg body weight (bw)$^{-1}$·h^{-1}, consumed at frequent intervals;

2 Daily recovery during moderate duration/low intensity training: 5–7 g·kg bw^{-1}·day^{-1};

3 Daily recovery during moderate-heavy endurance training: 7–12 g·kg bw^{-1}·day^{-1}; and

4 Daily recovery during an extreme exercise program (4–6 h+ per day): 10–12+ g·kg bw^{-1}·day^{-1}.

Carbohydrate-restricted, fad diets that are popular in some societies are not recommended for the healthy growth and development of children, nor do they provide adequate energy for the active child athlete. These diets should be avoided. Examples of healthy carbohydrate food choices include whole-grain breads, cereals, rice, noodles, fruits, and vegetables.

Protein

Protein can also be utilized as a fuel source. Adequate carbohydrate ingestion will spare proteins for utilization in other areas such as growth, muscle, and tissue repair. Protein ingestion should be within the range of 10–15% of the total daily energy intake, or 1.2–1.7 g·kg bw^{-1}·day^{-1} (Tipton & Wolfe 2003), with the protein obtained from foods rather than supplements. A positive nitrogen balance is needed for growth, and the protein needs – expressed relative to body mass – in children are greater than in adults due to the increase in relative lean body mass of the child. More protein is required during periods of active growth (7–9 years) and puberty. Examples of healthy protein sources include meat, fish, eggs, and dairy products.

Fat

Fat intake is also important for the healthy growth and development of the child athlete, and a child uses proportionately more fat and less carbohydrate than adults during exercise. The recommended range is 25–35% of the total daily energy intake. This should include a good source of unsaturated fats to ensure an adequate intake of omega-3 fatty acids. Special attention should be given to limiting fast-food consumption as these foods are often high in unhealthy saturated fats, which are partially responsible for the rise in obesity in many societies. Healthy fats including those found in vegetables such as avocadoes, in nuts, and in fish such as salmon should be encouraged over foods that have been deep-fried (Morantz 2006b).

Fluids

The child athlete is vulnerable to develop heat injury and attention to hydration is therefore especially important. A child makes more metabolic heat per unit of body mass than an adult (American Academy of Pediatrics 2000). As a result, body temperature increases during dehydration in a child more quickly than in adults. Adequate water intake is critical in the exercising child to prevent heat injury. Hydration should occur before, during, and after exercise with water, sports drinks, or diluted fruit juice. The use of high-sugar soda pop should be avoided.

Micronutrients

Micronutrients are also important in the diet of the exercising child. Iron is lost through sweat, feces, and menstrual losses. The recommended daily intake of iron is 15 mg·day^{-1} for females and 11 mg·day^{-1} for males. Iron supplementation is necessary only in cases of iron deficiency (Zlotkin 2003). Another important micronutrient is calcium, with the daily recommended intake being 1300 mg·day^{-1} from the ages of 8–18 years of age. Calcium is especially important during adolescence to ensure adequate bone health as this time period is thought to be a "critical window" for bone deposition. A well-balanced diet should contain all of the necessary nutrients and vitamins, thereby making supplementation unnecessary (Nicklas & Johnson 2004; Pettifor 2005). However, vitamin D may be necessary as a supplement for those athletes who do not drink milk, especially if exposure to sunlight is limited by indoor activities or through wearing protective clothing.

Unique problems in child athletes

Growth and injury in young athletes

Musculoskeletal sports injury can occur as a result of two distinct mechanisms: acute trauma or repetitive microtrauma (and sometimes a combination of the two). Acute trauma is the application of a single episode of excessive force that overwhelms the structural integrity of bone, ligament, or tendon. Repetitive microtrauma is the repetition of low-intensity mechanical force that ultimately disrupts the structural integrity of bone, ligament, tendon, or fascia. In the literature such injuries are frequently referred to as "overuse" or "overtraining" injuries, and include stress fractures, tendonitis, aphophysitis, and fasciitis (O'Neill & Micheli 1988; Kocher et al. 2000).

THE GROWTH FACTOR

It is believed that longitudinal growth in the child is initiated in the bones with secondary elongation of all other spanning structures. The growth of a child's bones is due to the presence of growth or physeal cartilage in their bones. This growth cartilage is present at three sites: the growth plate, or physis; the joint surfaces; and the sites of major muscle tendon insertions, or apophyses. An injury at any of these sites, whether the result of acute or repetitive trauma, may result in the permanent loss of growth or deformity in the child's limb, particularly if the trauma occurs at the physeal growth plate (Mann & Rajmaira 1990). In the growing child, the stage of relative maturation may affect the location of tissue disruption and the pattern of injury. As an example, a significant fall on the outstretched hand in the prepubescent child (Tanner stage II), usually results in a fracture at the junction of the diaphysis and the metaphysis of the radius and ulna distally. Whereas, an adolescent child (Tanner stage III or IV) who experiences a similar fall – especially when the child is in the midst of a growth spurt – will sustain a fracture through the relatively more vulnerable growth plate, or physis, of the distal radius. In the young adult,

the usual result would be a fracture of the scaphoid bone.

THE GROWTH SPURT

We now know that children's growth in not an uninterrupted continuum but rather a series of stop and start processes throughout the stages of maturation (Wales 1998). However, there is one characteristic period of rapid growth known as the "adolescent growth spurt" that appears to occur in every child, although at different times throughout the maturation process depending on a multiplicity of additional factors. During adolescent growth spurts there appears to be a relative tightening of the muscle tendons spanning the growing physeal plates. In certain conditions, such as Osgood–Schlatter's disease, this tightening may be more extreme and can lead to an increased risk of both apophyseal avulsions and repetitive injury to the apophyses. The relative increase in tension on the muscle tendon units at these times of rapid growth results in a decreased level of flexibility that may exacerbate the risk of injury during this period. During periods of rapid growth, training intensity should be reduced and, in our opinion, specific, slow stretching exercises should be initiated to prevent injury (Micheli 1983).

The articular cartilage of a child also undergoes a growth process and thus differs in anatomy and most probably in biomechanical characteristics from the adult cartilage. One of the characteristic results of overload of articular cartilage in the adult is the development of chondromalacia. By contrast, a similar pattern of repetitive overload in the child may result in the development of osteochondritis dissecans of the articular surface. There is growing clinical evidence for a higher incidence of osteochondritis dissecans in children exposed to systematic sports training compared to the general population (Hefti et al. 1999). Acute traumatic injuries to the physes, particularly during the period of the adolescent growth spurt when it is relatively weak, can result in the serious disruption of linear growth or possibly angular deformity at the joint level. These physeal injuries are treated with great respect by clinicians because of these potential complications. Fortunately, only approximately 15% of all fractures in children involve the physes, and of these, only a small portion result in growth, arrest, or deformity, depending on the specific physes involved, the type of injury, and the age of the child at the time of the injury (Committee on Sports Medicine and Fitness and Committee on School Health 2001). Repetitive microtrauma or stress injury to the physes has only very recently been documented. It has, however, been hypothesized for some years that repetitive impact to the lower extremities in activities such as distance running, and in particular marathon running, might cause microscopic injuries to the physes or the joint surface, with a concomitant inhibition of subsequent growth in the child (Rowland *et al.* 2006). Reports of physeal injury of the distal radius and ulna in young gymnasts from apparent repetitive impact or shearing have now been reported in many different nations (Tolat *et al.* 1992; DiFiori *et al.* 1997). Once again, these injuries may well be an additional marker for overtraining in the child.

Heat

Exercising in the extreme heat and humidity poses a unique problem for the child athlete. As discussed earlier, the child is less effective than the adult at regulating body temperature and, as a result, may be more vulnerable to heat-related illnesses or hyperthermia. This is more pronounced in the child who is particularly obese or extremely thin.

CONTRIBUTING FACTORS

Although a child can regulate their body temperature during exercise in warm climates, they are at risk of heat injury in hot or humid climates. Several factors contribute to the child's inability to effectively regulate heat balance. Most importantly, the child has immature sweat glands that produce a smaller amount of sweat than mature glands in adults. The adult production of sweat is an efficient cooling mechanism to lower the body temperature through evaporation. Another important factor is that the child has a large skin surface area relative to their body mass. They are also more sensitive to changes in temperature and are slower to acclimatize to exercise in warmer conditions. During exercise,

the child produces more metabolic heat per unit of body mass than the adult, resulting in a more rapid increase in body temperature during dehydration. This is further exacerbated by the fact that children are less likely to instinctively drink water during exercise to balance their heat production (Bar-Or 1989b; American Academy of Pediatrics 2000).

PREVENTING HEAT INJURIES

Coaches, trainers, and parents should be educated regarding the risks of heat injury in the child. They should be educated in preventative strategies, be able to recognize the early signs and symptoms, and be aware of the initial treatment principles. Exercising in extreme climatic conditions such as temperatures above 20°C and humidity above 70% should be avoided. Planning outdoor activities in shaded areas is also recommended. In seasons of extreme heat, exercise should be planned for the early morning or evening to avoid exposure during the warmest hours of the day. Adequate hydration before, during, and after exercise is important.

CONSEQUENCES OF HEAT INJURY

Heat cramps can result from prolonged exercise in the heat. This condition is characterized by a sudden onset of painful cramps in large muscle groups, most commonly in the legs. It is thought to be caused by an electrolyte imbalance as a result of excessive sweating and inadequate hydration.

Heat exhaustion can also occur as a result of prolonged exposure to heat. It is characterized by increasing thirst, dizziness, rising temperature, hypotension, tachycardia, nausea, excess sweating, oliguria, and fatigue. Prompt recognition and medical treatment is necessary to prevent the development of heat stroke. Treatment consists of cooling and fluid replacement.

Heat stroke is a serious, life-threatening consequence of heat exposure. If heat exhaustion is not treated, it can progress to heat stroke. In contrast to heat exhaustion, heat stroke is characterized by dry, hot skin. The athlete may be disoriented and hallucinating, and may convulse. Emergency medical treatment is essential.

Concussion

Concussion is defined as "a complex pathophysiologic process affecting the brain, induced by traumatic biomechanical forces." There are five features that further define a concussive head injury (McCrory *et al.* 2005):

1 It may be caused either by a direct blow to the head, face, neck or elsewhere on the body with an "impulsive" force transmitted to the head;

2 It typically results in the rapid onset of short-lived impairment of neurological function that resolves spontaneously;

3 It may result in neuropathological changes but the acute clinical symptoms largely reflect a functional disturbance rather than a structural injury;

4 It results in a graded set of clinical syndromes that may or may not involve loss of consciousness. Resolution of the clinical and cognitive symptoms typically follows a sequential course; and

5 Neuroimaging studies are typically normal in athletes who suffer from concussion.

CLASSIFICATION

The Prague Concussion Conference held in November 2004 defined a new classification of concussion (McCrory *et al.* 2005). First, simple concussion is an injury that progressively resolves without complication over 7–10 days. Second, complex concussion is one where the athlete suffers persistent symptoms that recur with exertion and specific sequelae, which include concussive convulsions, prolonged loss of consciousness of greater than one minute, or prolonged cognitive impairment following the injury. This group may also include those athletes who suffer multiple concussions over time or where repeated concussions occur with progressively less impact force.

PEDIATRIC CONCUSSIVE INJURY

With respect to the child athlete, the Prague conference confirmed that the previously-defined treatment guidelines for adults are applicable to children. In particular, the child athlete should not return to play until completely symptom-free, and the decision on when to return to play must be made by an experienced sports physician. A conservative approach to return-to-play is recommended. In the recovery period "cognitive rest" is recommended in addition to physical rest. During this time period, while symptomatic, the child should limit exertion and activities of daily living as well as scholastic activities (McCrory *et al.* 2005). Formal cognitive assessment using existing neuropsychological assessment tools before the late teen years is problematic as the ongoing cognitive maturation that occurs during this time period makes comparison to the athlete's own baseline norms problematic. It was thus recognized that additional research is needed to better clarify the potential differences between adults and children with respect to recovery.

SPORT CONCUSSION ASSESSMENT TOOL (SCAT)

Coaches and trainers should have the SCAT card on-hand for all sports that have a high risk of concussion. This standardized tool was designed from many existing tools to provide patient education as well as to facilitate physician assessment (available at: http://multimedia.olympic.org/pdf/en_report_1005.pdf).

Sudden cardiac death in sport

Thankfully, sudden death in young competitive athletes is an extremely rare phenomenon, occurring at an incidence rate of 2/100 000 persons per year in the 12–35 year age range. Of these, approximately 40% are under the age of 18. Sudden cardiac death is, however, quite visible and tragic. It is defined as "death occurring within one hour of the onset of symptoms in a person without a previously recognized cardiovascular condition that would appear fatal; this excludes cerebrovascular, respiratory, trauma, and drug-related causes" (Oswald *et al.* 2004). The leading cause of non-traumatic sudden death in athletes is a pre-existing cardiac abnormality. These structural cardiovascular diseases may be clinically identifiable. The cardiac syndromes most commonly associated with cardiac sudden death are summarized in Table 22.9.

Table 22.9 Cardiac syndromes most commonly associated with sudden death.

Disease process	Examples
Cardiomyopathy	Hypertrophic cardiomyopathy Arrythmogenic right ventricle Dilated cardiomyopathy
Rhythm abnormalities	Long QT syndrome Short QT syndrome Wolff–Parkinson–White syndrome
Connective tissue abnormalities	Marfan's syndrome
Other	Coronary artery anomalies Atherosclerosis Trauma Myocarditis

Table 22.10 All children at the beginning of their competitive activities should have pre-participation cardiac specific history and physical examination.

Evaluation tool	Cardiac: specific details
Personal history	Symptomatology of cardiovascular disease
Family history	Sudden death Cardiac illness
Physical examination	Peripheral pulses Marfan's stigmata Heart rate and rhythm Blood pressure Presence of murmurs or clicks

The Lausanne Recommendations on Sudden Cardiovascular Death in Sport published in December 2004 provided clear guidelines on the pre-participation screening for these disorders in the child athlete (Table 22.10). All children at the beginning of their competitive activities should have a pre-participation cardiac-specific history questionnaire completed along with a physical examination.

Diagnostic testing to assess rhythm and conduction or repolarization abnormalities should include a 12-lead resting electrocardiogram beginning after the onset of puberty. It is recommended that this screening procedure be repeated every 2 years. If any of the screening tests reveals positive findings, further evaluation and investigations are recommended. Referral to an age-appropriate cardiac specialist is recommended for assessment prior to the granting of permission for participation in sport. Investigations may include 24-hour ambulatory electrocardiographic (ECG) monitoring, trans-thoracic echocardiography and maximal exercise stress testing. Care with respect to patient confidentiality and the financial implications of testing should be considered. Participation in sport should occur only after a complete and thorough evaluation under the guidance of a cardiologist.

Disease states

At one time, children with medical conditions were restricted from participating in sport as physical activity was thought to be dangerous and detrimental to the disease process. It is now well-established in the scientific literature that participation in physical activity can provide substantial benefit both physically and emotionally to the child with a chronic medical illness. Of course, physical activity may pose some risks in certain conditions, thus the exercise prescription for the child at risk must be designed, monitored, and modified by an appropriately qualified specialist. Necessary education regarding precautions should include the child, parents, coaches, and trainers.

OBESITY

Obesity in children is quickly becoming an epidemic in many societies due to poor nutritional intake with the ubiquitous availability of fast-food and from increased inactivity exacerbated by excessive television viewing, video game-playing, and internet surfing by children and adolescents. The obese child is more likely to become an obese adult than the average-weight child (Reilly *et al*. 2004; Smith 2004). The obese adult has an increased risk of many diseases, such as hypertension, cardiovascular disease, and diabetes. Overweight children should therefore be encouraged to exercise regularly in an enjoyable sport. Special attention should be paid to the avoid heat stress with activity in these individuals.

ASTHMA

Asthma is one of the most common diseases suffered by children. The incidence varies depending on geographical location and season; in some countries it is as high as 30%. It is characterized by a narrowing of the airways or bronchospasm, accompanied by swelling of the bronchial mucosa as well as an increase in bronchial mucous production. The child may complain of shortness of breath, wheezing, and/or difficulty with expiration. Bronchospasm is often triggered by cigarette smoke, environmental allergens, dust, animal dander, pollution, and even exercise. Severity ranges greatly from a minimal cough to life-threatening airway compromise. In most cases, asthma is well-controlled via appropriately prescribed steroid inhalation and bronchodilators (beta-2 agonists). With appropriate treatment, the asthmatic child can participate in a variety of sports successfully. Indeed, there are Olympic champions in a variety of sports who suffer from asthma.

INFECTIOUS MONONUCLEOSIS

Children suffering form acute infections with fever, myalgias, and arthralgias should not exercise until symptoms abate. Special attention should be paid to the child athlete with infectious mononucleosis. This viral illness presents with fatigue, fever, sore throat, headaches, and swelling of the lymph glands. As the spleen may become enlarged in this illness, avoidance of physical activity that could lead to splenic rupture is essential, and medical supervision must be obtained prior to return to play.

DIABETES

Diabetes in children most often presents as the type I or insulin-dependent form. Exercise programs in children with diabetes must be medically supervised to ensure that modifications to the insulin prescription can adequately accommodate any change in glucose metabolism caused by the energy expended in exercise. The diabetic child should eat a meal or snack prior to exercise and have snacks at regular intervals if the exercise session is prolonged. Physical activity should be avoided in the child with poorly-controlled diabetes and also before bedtime. Coaches and trainers should be aware of the signs and symptoms of hypoglycemia and should be experienced in the management of this serious complication of diabetes. Children with diabetes should participate in a regular exercise pattern, avoiding sessions of intermittent, prolonged, excessive exercise.

ARTHRITIS

Unlike adults, children rarely suffer from osteoarthritis from overuse and aged joints. Children may, however, be limited by juvenile rheumatoid arthritis (JRA), which presents with painful, swollen joints, and stiffness, and may lead to a loss of mobility in the affected joints. The joints most commonly involved are the hands, wrists, shoulders, ankles, and knees. Children with JRA benefit from exercise in non-weight bearing sports such as swimming and cycling. Prudent and informed medical supervision is essential.

EPILEPSY

Epilepsy is characterized by the brief and intermittent disturbance of the electrical activity of the brain. There are a variety of different types of epileptic seizures ranging from the petit mal or absence seizure to the more extreme grand mal seizure. Epilepsy does not interfere with a child's ability to perform physical activity; however, safety precautions and supervision are important. Close supervision while swimming is essential to avoid drowning during a seizure. Likewise, rock climbing, SCUBA diving, or undertaking other high-risk sports should be avoided for safety reasons. Exercise in the postictal state is not recommended due to fatigue.

CARDIOVASCULAR DISEASE

Cardiac abnormalities are relatively rare in children. Of those children born with congenital heart disease, only half will have a significant enough defect to compromise or limit their ability to participate in sport. Children with cardiac defects should undergo medical evaluation and supervision for all physical activity.

CYSTIC FIBROSIS

Cystic fibrosis is a rare genetic disorder which affects the lungs, pancreas, and liver. Children with cystic fibrosis often suffer from shortness of breath due to the excessive production of mucous in the airways. It was once believed that children with this disease should not exercise due to their respiratory compromise, but regular, monitored exercise programs are now considered beneficial. Ideal sports for the child with cystic fibrosis include swimming, cycling, and walking. Due to involvement of the sweat glands, the child with cystic fibrosis does not regulate heat efficiently so attention to appropriate fluid intake and heat regulation is recommended.

Rehabilitation of the child athlete: scientific elements

The young athlete often receives appropriate initial treatment for sports injury, but thereafter may receive inadequate rehabilitation on the mistaken assumption that children heal rapidly and recover quickly from musculoskeletal derangement. Many adolescents return to their sport or competition too quickly following an injury, which can cause a recurrence, or place the athlete at increased risk of developing a new injury. A comprehensive rehabilitation program that is sports-specific includes the young athlete's goals, and an emphasis on education and communication with the athlete, parents, and coaches is essential to ensure a safe and effective return to the sport.

The overall goals of a rehabilitation program include:
1 Eduction on inflammation and pain;
2 Promotion of healing;
3 Restoration of function;
4 Safe return to sports training and competition; and
5 Prevention of future injury.
The immediate objective of physical therapy after injury includes restoration of a full range of motion and strength to within 10% of the uninjured extremity. Full restoration of strength and flexibility is also important and appropriate exercises for both strength and flexibility are mandatory (Cassella *et al.* 2006). In addition to restoring the health and function of the injured extremity, specific steps should be taken to maintain the athlete's level of physical fitness dur-

ing healing. Finally, sports-specific skills and strategies should be incorporated into the final stages of rehabilitation to ensure that when the athlete returns to their sport, he or she is able to meet the particular demands of the activity and its skill requirements without hesitation.

Prevention of sports injury in young athletes

Injury prevention has been somewhat overlooked in the relatively new discipline of pediatric and adolescent sports medicine and science, although we are seeing an emergence of efforts in this area.

One of the keys to injury prevention in child athletes is research into injury epidemiology. Both acute and overuse injuries are amenable to epidemiological study as a first step toward reducing the incidence or severity of injury in this population. The primary obstacle to epidemiological study is availability of necessary data. For this reason, establishment of sports injury surveillance systems was one of the primary recommendations of the Consensus Statement on Organized Sports for Children prepared by International Federation of Sports Medicine (FIMS) and the World Health Organization (WHO). Nevertheless, sports injury surveillance systems and comprehensive epidemiologic studies of sports injuries in child athletes are still rare and often focus on particular population groups for short periods of participation. Ideally, such systems can determine the incidence of injury per season and per population. They can also help determine the relative risk for exposure with the ideal measure being injuries per hour of participation. Injury surveillance systems can also establish trends in injury patterns, and can also help determine the effects of safety interventions.

Though comprehensive injury surveillance systems for child sports are rare in most countries and thus systematic injury prevention remains difficult at this level of sport, a review of the few existing studies suggests that the rate of sports-related injuries in children is relatively high and appears to be increasing in the pediatric age group. It has been estimated that up to one-half of all injuries sustained by children and adolescents participating in organized sports are preventable (Smith *et al.* 1993; Micheli *et al.* 2000).

Epidemiology is our most important tool in injury prevention. It is also essential to determine risk factors for injury in every sport. The risk factors in a contact sport such as gridiron football or rugby will vary significantly to those in an equipment-based sport such as tennis. Risk factors may be divided into two general categories: "host" and "environmental." Host factors are specific to the individual athlete at risk, while environmental factors are common to all participants, though the response to these risk factors may vary from individual to individual.

"Host" or "intrinsic" risk factors for injury include the following:
1 Anatomic malalignment;
2 Muscle tendon imbalances;
3 Stage of the growth process; and
4 Associated disease states present at the time of injury.

Psychological factors and sociological factors may also increase the risk of injury at a given time for a child athlete, and finally, as noted previously, there are specific gender risk factors, particularly for the female athlete (O'Neill & Micheli 1988; Loud & Micheli 2001).

The "extrinsic," or "environmental," factors that can contribute to injury in the young athlete include the following:
1 Errors in training or technique;
2 Improper coaching;
3 Improper footwear or protective equipment;
4 Inadequate or excessive irregularity or hardness of playing surface;
5 Nutritional status; and
6 Cultural deconditioning from lack of general exercise participation.

Each young athlete has his or her own individual risk factors and each sport poses its own specific risks for injury.

In order for the impact of preventive measures to be measured effectively it is important to determine what type of injuries are most prevalent in a given sport, who sustains the injuries, and why and where they occur. This again reinforces the necessity of having surveillance systems in place in all organized youth sports. Prevention strategies that can effectively decrease the rate of injury in youth sports include attention to playing conditions, volume, and intensity of training, and the credentialing of youth sport coaches at this level. Coaches and teachers should emphasize that general fitness is the basis for all safe sports participation. Fitness exercises should be included in the youth sports training regimens. In addition, the volume and intensity of sports training by children should be carefully monitored, and careful correlation between volume and intensity of training and evidence of overtraining should be noted.

Conclusion

There are vast numbers of children participating in organized sports all over the world. Despite this, very few scientific investigations into training, overtraining, and injury prevention for the young athlete have been published. However, there have been important advances in recent years in our understanding of strength training responses in young athletes. The study of nutrition for the child and child athlete has been stimulated by the growing incidence of obesity in this age group and the occurrence of eating disorders in child athletes and dancers. As noted in our introduction, it is essential that sports clinicians and sports scientists coordinate their efforts with this age group, especially in relation to developing meaningful studies based on direct observation of child athletes. Of greatest concern is that we are, as yet, unable to give parents, coaches, and national governing bodies scientifically-grounded guidelines for training and determinants of overtraining for the child athlete. It is a regrettable state of affairs that when it comes to training the child athlete we still too often determine "how much is enough" by observing "how much was too much."

References

American Academy of Pediatrics (2000) Committee on Sports Medicine and Fitness. Climatic heat stress and the exercising child and adolescent. *Pediatrics* **106**(1), 158–159.

Bailey, D.A., Malina, R.B. & Rasmussen, R.L. (1978) The influence of exercise, physical activity, and athletic performance on the dynamics of human growth. In: *Human growth 2: Post-natal growth* (Faulkner, F., ed.) Plenum Press, New York: 475–505.

Balyi, I., Cardinal, C., Higgs, C., Norris, S. & Way, R. (2005) *Long Term Athlete Development. Resource Paper.* Canadian

Sport for Life, Canadian Sport Centres, Ottawa: 5, 26, 28.

Bar-Or, O. (1989a) Temperature regulation during exercise in children and adolescents. In: *Perspectives in Exercise Sciences and Sports Medicine, II. Youth, Exercise and Sport* (Gisolfi, C. & Lamb, D.R., eds.) Benchmark Press, Indianapolis: 335–367.

Bar-Or, O. (1989b) Trainability of the prepubescent child. *Physician and Sportsmedicine* 17, 228–236.

Baxter-Jones, A.D.G., Maffulli, N. & Mirwald, R.L. (2003) Does elite gymnastics competition inhibit growth and maturation? Probably not! *Pediatric Exercise Science* 15, 373–382.

Borer, K.T. (1995) The effects of exercise on growth. *Sports Medicine* 20(6), 375–397.

Burke, L.M., Kiens, B. & Ivy, J.L. (2003) Carbohydrates and fat for training and recovery. *Journal of Sports Sciences* 22(1), 15–30.

Cassella, M., Richards, K. & Gustafson, C. (2006) Physical therapy and rehabilitation. In: *The Pediatric and Adolescent Knee* (Michel, L.J. & Kohe, M., eds.). Saunders, Philadelphia: 131–145.

Committee on Sports Medicine and Fitness and Committee on School Health (2001) Organized Sports for Children and Preadolescents. *Pediatrics* 107, 1459–1462.

Conn, J.M., Annest, J.L. & Gilchrist, J. (2003) Sports and recreation related injury episodes in the US population, 1997–99. *Injury Prevention* 9(2), 117–123.

Daly, R., Caine, D., Bass, S., Pieter, W. & Broekhoff, J. (2005) Growth and anthropometric comparisons of highly versus moderately trained competitive female artistic gymnasts. *Medicine and Science in Sports and Exercise* 37(6), 1053–1060.

Davidoff, F., Haynes, B., Sackett, D. & Smith, R. (1995) Evidence based medicine. *British Medical Journal* 310, 1085–1086.

DiFiori, J.P., Puffer, J.C., Mandelbaum, B.R. & Dorey, F. (1997) Distal radial growth plate injury and positive ulnar variance in nonelite gymnasts. *American Journal of Sports Medicine* 25(6), 763–768.

Faigenbaum, A.D. (2000) Strength training for children and adolescents. *Clinics in Sports Medicine* 19(4), 593–619.

Gotch, K. & Gilchrist, J. (2002) Nonfatal sports and recreation-related injuries treated in emergency departments – United States, July 2000–June 2001.

Morbidity Mortality Weekly Report 51, 736–740.

Guy, J.A. & Micheli, L.J. (2001) Strength training for children and adolescents. *Journal of the Amercan Academy of Orthopedic Surgeons* 9(1), 29–36.

Hefti, F., Beguiristain, J., Krauspe, R., Moller-Madsen, B., Riccio, V., Tschauner, C., *et al.* (1999) Osteochondritis dissecans: a multicenter study of the European Pediatric Orthopedic Society. *Journal of Pediatric Orthopaedics B* 8(4), 231–245.

Kocher, M.S., Waters, P.M. & Micheli, L.J. (2000) Upper extremity injuries in the paediatric athlete. *Sports Medicine* 30(2), 117–135.

Loud, K.J. & Micheli, L.J. (2001) Common athletic injuries in adolescent girls. *Current Opinions in Pediatrics* 13(4), 317–322.

Malina, R.B. (1998) Growth and maturation of young athletes – is training a risk factor? In: *Sports and Children* (Chan, K.M. & Micheli, L.J., eds.) William and Wilkins, Hong Kong: 133–161.

Mann, D.C. & Rajmaira, S. (1990) Distribution of physeal and nonphyseal fractures in 2650 long-bone fractures in children aged 0–16 years. *Journal of Pediatric Orthopaedics* 10(6), 713–716.

McCrory, P., Johnston, K., Meeuwisse, W., Aubry, M., Cantu, R., Dvorak, J. *et al.* (2005) Summary and agreement statement of the 2nd International Conference on Concussion in Sport, Prague 2004. *Clinical Journal of Sports Medicine* 15(2), 48–57.

Micheli, L.J. (1983) Overuse injuries in children's sports: the growth factor. *Orthopedic Clinics of North America* 14(2), 337–360.

Micheli, L.J., Glassman, R., Klein, M. (2000) The prevention of sports injuries in children. *Clinics in Sports Medicine* 19(4), 821–834.

Morantz, C.A. (2006a) AHA releases dietary recommendations for children and adolescents. *American Family Physician* 73(3).

Morantz, C.A. (2006b) Dietetary Recommendations for children and adolescents. *American Family Physician* 73(3).

Mountjoy, M., Armstrong, N., Bizzini, L., Blimkie, C., Evans, J., Gerrard, D. *et al.* (2008) IOC consensus statement: "training the elite child athlete." *British Journal of Sports Medicine* 42, 163–164.

Nicklas, T. & Johnson, R. (2004) Position of the American Dietetic Association: Dietary guidance for healthy children ages 2 to 11 years. *Journal of the American Dietetic Association* 104(4), 660–677.

Obert, P., Mandigout, S., Nottin, S., Vinet, A., N'Guyen, L.D. & Lecoq, A.M. (2003) Cardiovascular responses to endurance training in children: effect of gender. *European Journal of Clinical Investigation* 33, 199–208.

O'Neill, D.B. & Micheli, L.J. (1988) Overuse injuries in the young athlete. *Clinics in Sports Medicine* 7(3), 591–610.

Oswald D., Dvorak J., Corrado D., Brenner, J.I., Hoogsteen, J., McKenna, W., *et al.* (2004) *Sudden Cardiovascular Death in Sport.* Lausanne recommendations: preparticipation cardiovascular screening. http://multimedia.olympic.org/pdf/en_report_886.pdf

Pettifor, J.M. (2005) Rickets and vitamin D deficiency in children and adolescents. *Endocrinology and Metabolism Clinics of North America* 34(3), 537–553.

Reilly, J.J., Jackson, D.M., Mongomery, C., Kelly, L.A., Slater, C., Grant, S., *et al.* (2004) Total energy expenditure and physical activity in young Scottish children: mixed longitudinal study. *Lancet* 363, 211–212.

Rowland, T., Micheli, L., Caine, D., Anderson, S., Small, E., Pate, R., *et al.* (2006) Should children be allowed to run marathon races? A virtual round table. *Pediatric Exercise Science* 18(1), 1–10.

Savage, M.P., Petratis, M.M., Thomson, W.H., Berg, K., Smith, J.L. & Sady, S.P. (1986) Exercise training effects on serum lipids of prepubescent boys and adult men. *Medicine and Science in Sports and Exercise* 18(2): 197–204.

Smith, A., Andrish, J. & Micheli, L. (1993) The prevention of sports injuries in children and adolescents. *Medicine and Science in Sports and Exercise* 25(Suppl.), 1–7.

Smith, C.J. (2004) The current epidemic of childhood obesity and its implications for future coronary heart disease. *Pediatric Clinics of North America* 51(6), 1679–1695.

Theintz, G.E., Howald, H., Weiss, U. & Sizonenko, P.C. (1993) Evidence for a reduction of growth potential in adolescent female gymnasts. *Journal of Pediatrics* 122(2), 306–313.

Tipton, K.D. & Wolfe, R.R. (2003) Protein and amino acids for athletes. *Journal of Sports Sciences* 22(1), 65–79.

Tofler, I.R. & Butterbaugh, G.J. (2005)
Developmental overview of child and
youth sports for the twenty-first century.
Clinics in Sports Medicine **24**(4), 783–804,
vii–viii.

Tofler, I.R., Stryer, B.K., Micheli, L.J. &
Herman, L.R. (1996) Physical and
emotional problems of elite female
gymnasts. *New England Journal of
Medicine* **335**(4), 281–283.

Tolat, A.R., Sanderson, P.L., De Smet, L.
& Stanley, J.K. (1992) The gymnast's
wrist: acquired positive ulnar
variance following chronic epiphyseal
injury. *Journal of Hand Surgery* **17**:
678–681.

Wales, J.K.H. (1998) A brief -history of
the study of human growth dynamics.
Annals of Human Biology **25**(2), 175–184.

Zlotkin, S. (2003) Clinical nutrition: 8. The
role of nutrition in the prevention of iron
deficiency anemia in infants, children
and adolescents. *Canadian Medical
Association Journal* **168**(1), 59–63.

Chapter 23

The Female Athlete

MYRA A. NIMMO

Since the first involvement of women in the Olympic Games in 1900, great progress has been made in increasing the participation rates of women in sport as in most other activities of human society. In 2000, women represented 44% of the competitors at the Sydney Summer Games, although this was not matched by coverage of women's sports in the major newspapers of Belgium, Denmark, France, and Italy. In these countries, women's sport at the Sydney Olympics represented only 29% of the articles and 38% of photographs (Capranica *et al.* 2005).

The number of published research studies on females to support the increased participation is reflected in the number of publications in the *Journal of Applied Physiology* in the first 6 months of 2006. These data suggest that there is still a shortfall in the proportions of female studies compared to those on males. Of those articles specifically referring to exercise in humans ($n = 42$), 60% were on males only, 5% were on females only, 12% were on males and females with the genders being studied separately, and 23% were on males and females with no acknowledgment of the mixed gender. Collating these facts, together with the observation that many of the early findings on females and exercise have been found to be invalid because of poorly controlled studies, it is clear that there is still much to be done. The aim is to ensure that training sessions are optimized for performance enhancement in the female population

and that training and competition are not detrimental to the long-term health of female participants.

There are a number of different models of investigation. Studies that try to compare genders have difficulties in matching subjects and minimizing the confounding variables inherent in cross-sectional studies. Tarnopolsky and Saris (2001) recommend that subjects be matched on both training history and maximum oxygen uptake ($\dot{V}o_{2max}$). This permits account to be taken of the largely genetic ($\dot{V}o_{2max}$) and the environmental (training state) factors contributing to $\dot{V}o_{2max}$. If, in addition, data are expressed relative to lean body mass, account can be taken of the differences in body fat between the genders. Although this has allowed a focus on those differences that are truly the effect of gender, there are still possible errors in expressing exercise intensity as a percentage of $\dot{V}o_{2max}$ particularly when the percentage used the classic endurance intensity of 70%. Recently, studies (including those on a single sex) have exercised subjects at an intensity that expresses the intensity as a percentage of lactate threshold (LT). Notwithstanding the debate about the presence or otherwise of a discrete point at which the blood lactate concentration begins to increase, a definite increase in the blood lactate concentration is observed when the power output exceeds around 80% $\dot{V}o_{2max}$ although this can vary from below 60% to above 90% $\dot{V}o_{2max}$. Therefore, even if subjects are matched for training history, $\dot{V}o_{2max}$, and corrected for body mass, but have not been matched for LT, the results can still falsely signify gender differences where none exist.

An alternative approach, avoiding the need for cross-sectional studies, is based on the assumption

The Olympic Textbook of Science in Sport, 1st edition. Edited by R.J. Maughan. Published 2009 by Blackwell Publishing. ISBN: 978-1-4051-5638-7.

that gender differences are the result of the actions of the sex steroids. In this way, it is possible to investigate exercise responses during the natural fluctuation of these hormones during the female menstrual cycle. However, even in studies where methodology is tightly controlled, the physiological variability of the sex steroids affords large inter- and intravariability, with estradiol concentrations during mid-luteal phase ranging 82–232 ng·L^{-1} and progesterone 8–40 µg·L^{-1}. This has led, from a mechanistic as well as a practical perspective, to the investigation of the influence of exogenous female steroids on physiology and performance. Administration of the oral contraceptive (OC) pill offers a model for the investigation of the female sex steroids and can be mapped over a longitudinal time period, with individuals acting as their own controls. Casazza et al. (2002) suggest that administration should be for longer than 1 month to ensure that any chronic or cumulative effects of the steroids are not missed. OCs suppress normal menstrual cycle levels of estradiol and progesterone by inhibiting the pituitary release of gonadotropins and replacing the sex steroids with consistent levels of estradiol and progesterone, thus limiting the variation in circulating levels. A multiphase OC pill contains a changing dose of both hormones throughout three phases of the cycle with 21 days of administration (typically ~35 µg estradiol with increasing doses of progestagen from 200 to 250 mg) and 7 days of non-administration, thus closely mimicking the "natural" cycle of sex hormones. The monophonic OC pill provides a constant level of estradiol and progestagen for 21 days of a relatively low dose (~30 µg estradiol and 150 µg progestagen).

The administration of testosterone to females is a possible experimental model, but ethical considerations would permit this only in cases of clinical need, so the validity of extrapolating the data to healthy young women would inevitably be limited. Finally, extrapolation of data from animal studies is difficult because of the significantly higher estrogen and progesterone levels of animals (Jacobs et al. 2005).

Although it is clear there are still difficulties in the analysis of human data on the effects of the sex steroids on physiology and performance, there has been increasing clarity in recent years over the reverse of this: the effect of training and performance on menstrual status and the interplay of menstrual status, dietary intake, and osteoporosis, referred to as the female triad (Yeager et al. 1993).

This review of the female athlete builds on existing reviews of the subject and relevant sections are divided into gender differences, variation throughout the menstrual cycle, and the effect of OCs.

Performance

Effect of gender

The best women athletes are capable of beating almost all except the very best men in their chosen event, but the best men can still outperform the best women. The women's World Records in running events have improved faster than those of males from 1950 until the current time. However, the common prediction that women will run faster than men, particularly over longer endurance events, is believed not to be accurate. Recent and more relevant prediction models identify that endurance running World Records are nearing their limit and consequently the gender difference of 8–14% over distances from 1500 to 42,000 m is unlikely to decrease further. Even at the longer distances, 100–200 km, there is no evidence for women covering the distance faster (Table 23.1). Although these gender differences are perceived as relatively small, Cheuvront et al. (2005), who provide a review of these data, point out that the models predict that women will

Table 23.1 Official records and world best performances recognized by the International Amateur Athletic Federation (IAAF) (May 2006).

Distance	Male	Female
100 m	9.77	10.49
200 m	19.32	21.34
400 m	43.18	47.60
800 m	1:41.11	1:53.28
1500 m	3:26.00	3:50.46
5000 m	12:37.35	14:24.68
10 000 m	26:17:53	29:31.78
20 km	55:48	1:03:26
Marathon	2:04:55	2:15:25
100 km	6:13.33	6:33.11

break the 4-min-mile barrier only in 2033 if at all, some 80 years after Roger Bannister achieved this feat.

One reason for the differences in endurance performance is almost certainly related to the lower $\dot{V}o_{2max}$ of females. When body size and the higher body fat content of women are taken into account the difference is reduced to around 5% and this is thought to be a result of the lower hemoglobin content in women (Nygaard & Hede 1987).

Sprinting too shows no indication that the best women can beat the best men. The principal difference in sprint performance is a result of differences in muscle cross-sectional area which is almost certainly because of the anabolic effect of testosterone. The evidence for testosterone as the anabolic agent derives from studies where testosterone or a synthetic analog have been administered to healthy males or hypogonadal older men and in these instances reutilization of intracellular amino acids increases, leading to enhanced net protein balance. The effect of administration of ovarian hormones on protein synthesis is not clear, although animal and *in vitro* studies suggest that estrogen inhibits muscle protein synthesis (Tipton 2001). In addition to a greater muscle mass, males have, on average, a greater percentage area occupied by type 2 fibers and this is likely to contribute to the greater ground forces exerted by men, although women's greater type 1 : 2 fiber area ratio might benefit them during eccentric contractions with longer cross-bridge cycle (and attachment) times (Sale 1999). Women are also more effective in combining eccentric with concentric contractions, being able to reutilize the energy absorbed in a preceding eccentric contraction more effectively than men (Sale 1999). As the difference in fiber composition is largely result of fiber size and not number, it is unclear if sprint and strength-trained women would still show larger type 1 fibers if compared with endurance-trained men. It is more likely that there is a continuum of fiber size reflecting the dominant usage and this would be consistent with data reporting that skeletal muscle adaptations to resistance exercise training are similar in males and females, with at least one study reporting no differences in myosin heavy-chain or in sarcoplasmic proteins (Tipton 2001).

In their review, Cheuvront *et al.* (2005) speculate as to the future and propose that there remains one way in which women could reduce the performance gap, and that is through the recent IOC medical commission recommendation which will allow athletes undergoing sexual reassignment surgery to compete in their reassigned sex category, whether reassigned after or before puberty. The implication of this decision is that if the surgery occurs after puberty, then these athletes could still have a significant advantage (i.e., more lean mass). Whether this inclusive policy will be abused will only be known in the future.

Although the gender differences offer material for an interesting debate, of more practical importance is whether the menstrual cycle and the administration of OCs affect performance.

Effect of the menstrual cycle

There appears little support for the concept that menstrual phase affects performance, body composition, skeletal muscle contractile characteristics, or cardiorespiratory factors including $\dot{V}o_{2max}$, in spite of anecdotal evidence to the contrary (Janse de Jonge 2003). An exception to this may be related to the recovery period between intermittent sprints, where an improvement in work completed has been demonstrated to occur in the luteal phase of the cycle: this observation is supported by an increase in oxygen consumption during recovery (Middleton & Wenger 2006) although no other reports support this difference in work capacity with intermittent sprints.

Effect of oral contraceptive administration

Using a longitudinal design, Casazza *et al.* (2002) found that 4 months of triphasic OC administration caused significant increases in body mass and fat mass and an 11% decrease in $\dot{V}o_{2max}$, which is greater than that reported for 10 months administration of a monophasic OC, where no difference or little difference in $\dot{V}o_{2max}$ has been found (Rickenlund *et al.* 2004). Anaerobic performance too appears to be negatively affected. When a triphasic OC is administered over three cycles, it is possible to detect reduced anaerobic performance when the hormone milieu is represented by high estrogen and high progesterone (pill days 16–18) as opposed to low levels of both hormones (pill days 26–28) (Redman & Weatherby 2004).

The mechanism behind this may be the attenuation of the catecholamine response to exercise while taking OC. This will potentially reduce the vasoconstriction to inactive tissues and reduce the mean arterial pressure in the active muscle. In addition, elevated levels of nitric oxide, a potent vasodilator, have been found. Both of these responses to OCs could limit peak exercise performance (Casazza et al. 2002). During high intensity exercise it could be that the high steroids restrict carbohydrate metabolism and the availability of glucose as a substrate (Redman & Weatherby 2004). However, direct evidence for the mechanism behind the reduced performance is not at present available.

Energy systems

Effect of gender

Considerable attention has been paid over the last 20 years to gender differences in fuel utilization during exercise. Although early problems with poorly controlled studies have now largely been addressed, there are still equivocal results relating to gender differences.

Fuels oxidized by the muscles for energy are protein, fat, and carbohydrate (CHO). Protein is of particular significance during prolonged exercise. Yet, as of 2006, there are only five studies that have investigated gender differences in amino acid use during endurance exercise and one of the studies had very small numbers. The conclusion of these studies is that the amino acid, leucine, is oxidized faster in males than in females and this may be related to a greater responsiveness to catecholamines in men. Administration of beta-blockers to men during exercise caused an upregulation of leucine oxidation, whereas in women it increased their reliance on fat. This was a carefully controlled study where the genders were matched for $\dot{V}o_{2max}$ and training history and might suggest that nutritional supplementation of amino acids and/or protein may be better justified in men than women (Lamont 2005).

Increased lipolysis, as indicated by a greater rate of glycerol appearance, is consistent in showing increased rates in females compared with men during moderate exercise of the same relative intensity (Blaak 2001; Mittendorfer et al. 2002). An alternative source of lipid, intramuscular triacylglycerol (IMTG) has been more difficult to determine because of the inherent error involved in its measurement. However, three studies (Mittendorfer et al. 2002; Roepstorff et al. 2002; Steffensen et al. 2002), the latter two both from the same laboratory, have now indicated an increased IMTG use in women. Conversely, a recent study (Zehnder et al. 2005), utilizing magnetic resonance spectroscopy (MRS), which allows a direct, non-invasive measure of IMTG from exactly the same location before and after exercise, concluded that male athletes depleted more IMTG than females. Although it might have been thought that this latter methodology would yield a definitive answer, the authors themselves acknowledge certain limitations including the possibility of a higher training status of the males compared to the females. This was reflected in the higher IMTG levels at rest in the males. As higher IMTG concentrations are directly associated with higher IMTG utilization, this may have confounded the data. This latter point illustrates the difficulty in comparing genders, as to match subjects on all the major variables that affect performance is virtually impossible.

Whether the increased lipolysis results in an increased whole-body fat oxidation is unclear. Until 2001, studies concluded that during submaximal exercise the respiratory exchange ratio (RER) was lower in women than in men, indicating women's increased reliance on lipid as a fuel, when the intensity is around the optimal for lipid utilization (i.e., 45–65% $\dot{V}o_{2max}$) (Tarnopolsky & Ruby 2001). However, subsequent studies using kinetic data have been unable to detect a difference (Ruby et al. 1997; Mittendorfer et al. 2002; Roepstorff et al. 2002) in whole-body lipid utilization. Stable isotopes, the necessary tools for kinetic studies, are expensive and as a consequence these studies have relatively small numbers in addition to the subject-matching problems already identified. A study recently published (Venables et al. 2004), although only using quantitative data from RER, investigated 157 men and 143 women and reported that the men had lower rates of fat oxidation and an earlier shift to using CHO as the dominant fuel.

Evidence for the source of the differing CHO utilization appears more robust, with biopsy, isotopic tracer, and MRS studies concluding that muscle glycogen utilization is greater for men than women. Tracer studies of glucose appearance, however, are more ambiguous with both a lower rate of appearance in women and no difference being reported (Tarnopolsky & Ruby 2001).

With little consistency in the effect of gender on substrate metabolism, there is little motivation to seek an underpinning mechanism, although suggestions include the attenuated catecholamine response of females during submaximal exercise. Elevated catecholamine levels would be expected to enhance both lipolysis and glycogenolysis, but this is unlikely to be the sole answer. Other potential causes include the influence of testosterone, but short-term administration to healthy active males had no influence on fuel utilization pathways (Braun et al. 2005). Finally, fiber composition differences between the genders, with a relatively greater fiber area of type I fibers in females, may also contribute to differences in fuel selection. Until there is clarity as to whether gender differences do exist, these options remain unexplored.

In practice, if assumptions are that females are smaller and have a lower $\dot{V}O_{2max}$, then to run at the same pace as males they would need to run at a higher percentage of their maximum which would raise the contribution from CHO thus minimizing the gender differences. However, if $\dot{V}O_{2max}$ is similar and both are running at the same percentage of their maximum, then the female will derive more energy from fat.

Effect of menstrual phase

Only in the last few years have stable isotopes been utilized to investigate differences in fuel use between follicular and luteal phases of the menstrual cycle. These studies have indicated no differences in the turnover rates of glycerol (Casazza et al. 2004) and free fatty acids (FFA) (Jacobs et al. 2005). An elegant experiment by Horton et al. (2006), using stable isotopes and human subjects, separated the effects of estrogen and progesterone by measuring in three phases of the cycle: early follicular, representing low estrogen and low progesterone; mid-follicular, representing elevated estrogen and low progesterone; and mid-luteal, representing elevated estrogen and elevated progesterone. These authors hypothesized that FFA and glycerol turnover would be greatest when estrogen was elevated and progesterone low. This was based on the potential inhibitory effect of estrogen on CHO utilization and the anti-estrogen affect of progesterone. However, their findings were unable to confirm their hypothesis and they concluded that there was no effect of the menstrual cycle on glycerol and FFA turnover (as reflected by palmitate flux) at rest or during moderate (50% $\dot{V}O_{2max}$) exercise.

Effect of oral contraceptive administration

The administration of exogenous hormones through triphasic OCs increases triacyglycerol mobilization. A longitudinal study associated the elevation in triacylglycerol mobilization with elevated circulating levels of cortisol, a lipolytic hormone, at rest and during exercise (Casazza et al. 2004). The same group (Jacobs et al. 2005) went on to identify that this increase in lipolytic rate was not matched by an increase in whole body or plasma FFA oxidation either at rest or during moderate exercise. Using a novel method for the determination of plasma and local FFA oxidation, the authors concluded that OC use increases both plasma-derived and total FFA re-esterification.

Investigations of glucose kinetics have used different models of investigation, but regardless of whether estradiol is given to amenoerrheic women (Ruby et al. 1997), to males (Carter et al. 2001), or through OC administration (Suh et al. 2003), the conclusion is that glucose flux decreases. As there is no change in whole-body CHO, this implies an increased use of skeletal muscle glycogen or lactate to compensate.

In summary, it would appear that gender comparisons are inherently difficult to interpret because of an inability to truly match subjects. From the studies that have been attempted, it can be concluded

Table 23.2 Gender differences in fuel utilization during exercise.

Fuel source	Comparison of male and female utilization pattern
Amino acid	Male > Female
Glycogen utilization	Male > Female
Fat utilization	Female > Male
Glucose flux	Male ≥ Female

that oxidation rates of amino acids and glycogen are greater in men, while lipolysis is higher in women (Table 23.2). The effect of menstrual cycle on fuel selection in humans would appear to be minimal, although on administration of OCs there is an increase in lipolysis. However, this does not result in increased fat oxidation but an increase in re-esterification from both plasma and the local skeletal muscle. OCs will also decrease glucose flux, which may be compensated by an increase in skeletal muscle glycogen or lactate.

Menstrual cycle disorders

The fact that physical activity, which is generally accepted as being beneficial for young and adult females, could have negative consequences for health and cause menstrual cycle disturbances was eventually accepted by those involved in sport in the 1970s. Since then, menstrual cycle disorders have been linked to disordered eating and osteoporosis. These three conditions represent different elements of an interlinked disease, although each can occur in isolation. This linking of the three conditions has been termed the female triad (Yeager *et al.* 1993).

The incidence of menstrual cycle disorders may be underestimated because disorders can occur that are asymptomatic. These conditions include "luteal phase defects," where the luteal phase does not produce sufficient progesterone to allow implantation of the fertilized egg. A more severe form of this is when the follicular development is so impaired that no ovulation occurs but there is some proliferation of the uterine lining. In both of these conditions, athletes may believe that they are menstruating "normally." Even accounting for this potential un-derestimation, the evidence is compelling that the incidence of oligomenorrhea (defined as menstrual cycles of longer than 35 days) is widespread: it has been reported to be 61% in rhythmic gymnasts 1 year after menarche and to be 21–40% in runners in the gynecologic age range of 5–30 years. Secondary amenorrhea (absence of menstrual cycle for 3 months) is variably reported to range from 2% to 31% in long-distance runners and appears to be related to both training distance and age, with higher mileage and younger age reporting higher figures. These figures are much higher than those reported for age-matched groups in sedentary women (9% for oligomenorrhea and 2–5% for amenorrhea; Redman & Loucks 2005).

These menstrual cycle disorders are caused by a disruption of the pulses of luteinizing hormone (LH) in the blood. It is these pulses of LH that dictate the release of the ovarian hormones and is the basis of ovarian function. Many variables can affect the ovarian axis, but for a number of years the higher incidence in athletes was linked to low body fat levels with primary amenorrhea (absence of menses in a girl by 15 years) being linked to a body fat of less than 17% and secondary amenorrhea similarly being linked to a critical value of 22% (Frisch & McArthur 1974). This hypothesis has now been modified and the more recent literature demonstrates unambiguously that energy availability is the key factor affecting the ovarian axis in athletes. This can be linked quantitatively with 5 days of an energy intake at ~125 kJ·kg FFM^{-1}·day^{-1} leading to disruptions of LH pulsatile activity (Redman & Loucks 2005) (Fig. 23.1). Some amenorrheic athletes report intakes as low as 67 kJ·kg FFM^{-1}·day^{-1} alongside exercise programs (Loucks & Nattiv 2005). The trigger of food deprivation is currently thought to be plasma glucose and/or leptin although the specific mechanism has yet to be elucidated (Wade & Jones 2004).

The consequence of the disturbed LH is low circulating estrogen, which profoundly affects bone mineral density. Numerous studies have consistently reported bone mineral densities in young athletes more normally associated with post-menopausal women (IOC Medical Commission 2005). In post-menopausal women, osteoporosis is associated with bone resorption pathology, but in young athletes

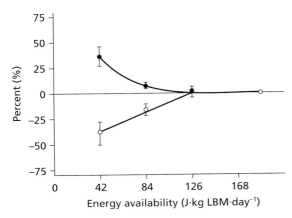

Fig. 23.1 Normalized incremental effects of restricted energy availability on luteinizing hormone (LH) pulse frequency (solid circles) and amplitude (open circles). Through normalization and repeated measures control, all of the normalized responses were exactly 0% and 100% at 182.2 and 41.8 kJ·kg^{-1}·LBM^{-1}·day^{-1}, respectively. Redrawn from Loucks and Thuma (2003).

suffering from osteoporosis the pathology appears to be manifested in low rates of bone formation (Redman & Loucks 2005). Recognizing this difference, the International Society for Clinical Densitometry (ISCD) in 2004 identified criteria for the diagnosis of osteoporosis in young athletes that are different from those for post-menopausal women. These criteria classify pre-menopausal women and adolescent girls who present with low bone densities, relative to their age, and possess one or more risk factors for fracture (e.g., hypogonadism, eating disorders, previous fractures) as osteoporotic. Although there is no direct relationship between the number of cycles per year and the maintenance of bone density, it is recommended that concerns be raised if an athlete has been amenorrheic for more than 6 months or has had numerous stress fractures. Specific clinical criteria for bone density measurement are presented in the IOC Position Stand (IOC Medical Commission 2005). A problem that may exist in the diagnosis is that exercise itself may mask osteoporosis in certain bones. For example, runners may have high bone density in the calcaneus but have low bone densities in the hip and spine while rowers can have average bone densities in the forearm but not in the hip. This suggests that the higher density of the peripheral

limbs is sport-specific (Nattrass & Drinkwater 1998) and should be considered in the estimation of the bone densities.

An additional consequence of the low estrogen in these athletes is the effect that this has on endothelial vasodilatation. In amenorrheic athletes, perfusion of skeletal muscle is reduced and oxidative metabolism is impaired (Harber *et al.* 1998), thus potentially affecting performance and recovery in these athletes.

Therapeutic intervention is recommended within the first year from the onset of symptoms, when the bone loss is most rapid, and should initially focus on a strategy to make changes in nutrition and training (IOC Medical Commission 2005). In order to avoid these clinical consequences, the focus must be on ensuring that athletes increase their energy intake to match any increase in energy expenditure. This mismatch of energy intake and energy expenditure can occur, at least acutely, in athletes within a range of body fat levels and is not peculiar to those with low body fat. The motivation not to increase energy intake occurs predominantly in sports where body image or leanness is, or is perceived as being, of benefit to performance. Eating disorders, however, represent a continuum, with minimal levels of eating disorders being subclinical. The IOC Medical Commission (2005) recommend that an athlete suspected of having an eating disorder should be referred to a dietitian, and if positively diagnosed should be considered by the coaching team to be "injured" and to receive treatment from a multidisciplinary team with the initiual goal of enhancing nutritional practices. Clear guidance on treatment regimens is provided in the IOC position stand (IOC Medical Commission 2005). If the athlete refuses treatment, training and competition should be withheld until they agree to participate. This, to a competitive athlete who overtly feels well may seem extremely harsh, but reflects the seriousness of the condition.

It is clear that early diagnosis is imperative and studies are now investigating whether it is possible to identify those athletes who are most susceptible. One such report that compared the susceptibility of elite athletes and non-athletes (Torstveit & Sundgot-Borgen 2005) identified some risk factors that make non-athletes more susceptible to the female triad than elite athletes. This report has led to an exchange of correspondence (Di-Pietro & Stachenfeld 2005), which perhaps can be summarized to say that significant work in the prevention of the athlete triad has yet to be conducted.

Energy balance

There are many published reports to show that when females increase their energy expenditure through an exercise program, they report lower dietary intakes than expected for their high activity level. This observation has been dismissed by some on account of errors arising because of defects in the methodology of the dietary intake measures. Some of these errors were eliminated in a recent short-term study (McLaughlin et al. 2006) where males and females were matched for percentage body fat and ad lib eating was measured when subjects were unaware that this was being monitored. This supported the early observations and indicated that differences did exist in the energy intake between genders in response to an 8-day exercise program, with no dietary compensation occurring in females whereas males increased their dietary intake to match the energy expenditure. This situation is not sustainable, however, and in the long term some other mechanisms must come into play.

In long-term training studies, females in general do not lose body fat and it may be that this represents some overcompensation for short-term energy deficits as some reports even suggest an increase in body fat. This gender difference is supported by cross-sectional studies indicating that there is no relationship between physical activity and body composition in females although this exists in males (Westerterp 1999). Although body mass reduction with exercise is related to initial body mass, even when subjects are matched for body fat this gender difference is still evident (Andersson et al. 1991) and may be related to the observation that with a similar percentage body fat women have approximately 50% more fat cells than men and within each fat cell there may be a minimum "plateau" to which the fat cell can reduce (Krotkiewski et al. 1983).

If females do not lose body mass and reports suggest that dietary intake is not increased, at least in the short term, then they may compensate by reducing their energy expenditure outside of the formal exercise. A major component of this is resting metabolic rate (RMR). However, this appears to be more dependent on the intensity of the exercise than any gender differences per se. Decreases in RMR are noted in response to too high an exercise intensity, yet in order to get an increase in RMR it must be at least 70% $\dot{V}_{O_{2max}}$. Other aspects of physical activity external to formal exercise include daily tasks, and although there are few long-term studies in humans, the available evidence suggests that compensation can occur in this component if the volume and/or intensity of the formal exercise is high. This may contribute differentially in each gender. Intuitively, however, this might be more of an individual response than a gender one (Westerterp 1999).

The distribution of the subcutaneous adipocytes differs between the genders, with the classic location of the adipose tissue in females within the gluteal–femoral region, whereas in men higher amounts lie around the abdominal area. This reflects differences in sensitivity to catecholamines, lipoprotein lipase, and insulin of the adipocytes in the two populations. Adipocytes from abdominal tissue are more sensitive to catecholamines than those from other adipose depots, but the difference is greater in females (Jensen et al. 1996). This differing regional sensitivity can be illustrated when epinephrine is infused into subjects: the leg FFA release is doubled in men but does not change in women, whereas the release was higher in women than men from the upper body region (Blaak 2001). Studies on obese men and women give some credence to the concept that the location of fat influences fat loss with exercise. It is possible to divide obese females into those with "apple-shaped" obesity (android) and "pear-shaped" obesity (gynoid). Android-shaped obesity females respond more like males in that they will tend to lose body fat with an exercise program whereas the gynoid-shaped obesity females do not decrease their fat and in some instances increase body fat with no change in lean body mass after physical training (Krotkiewski & Bjorntorp 1986). However, direct evidence is required before these regional differences in fat utilization can be linked to differing energy balance responses to exercise in athletes.

Menstrual cycle phase and oral contraceptive administration

Analyses of dietary records have consistently shown that energy intake is increased during the luteal phase of the menstrual cycle. It may be that this relates to the need to maintain energy balance as basal metabolic rate progressively increases throughout the menstrual cycle (Solomon *et al.* 1982). These changes in energy balance are not evident when the menstrual cycle is suppressed with administration of depot medroxyprogesterone nor is there any change in body weight (Pelkman *et al.* 2001). The lack of gain in body weight tends to be a consistent finding whether a monophasic or triphasic OC is used. This finding is disputed by Casazza *et al.* (2002) who reported increases in body fat and weight with a triphasic OC over four cycles, suggesting a shift in the energy balance equation. It would appear at this stage that any weight fluctuation during the menstrual cycle is variable. Therefore, there is little or no robust data that support the fact that a change in body weight arising from the menstrual cycle can affect performance.

Nutrition

Although the known prevalence of underreporting may call into question some of the reported data, there are some athletes who undoubtedly have low energy intakes. Athletes participating in sports where low body mass is an advantage to performance are constantly concerned with dietary restriction. This can lead to a negative energy balance, which may negate any positive outcomes for performance and also lead to negative consequences of inadequate nutrient intake, a higher risk of injury, and increased risk of illness.

Under weight maintenance conditions, the athletic female must achieve energy balance by consuming sufficient food energy to match expenditure. Although energy intakes of less than 7500 kJ are unlikely to meet their energy requirements, female athletes who eat more than 5000–6500 kJ, and include a variety of food groups, can achieve adequate intakes of most of the essential nutrients with the possible exception of iron. Women will lose on average 1.3 mg·day^{-1} iron during menstrual flow which is double that of men and may lead to women being more susceptible to iron deficiency anemia. Iron depletion occurs in three stages: iron depletion, iron deficient erythropoiesis, and iron deficient anemia. Iron depletion is identified through serum ferritin levels (<12 µg·L^{-1}). When iron stores are depleted, erythropoiesis is affected and consequently results in the second stage of iron deficient erythropoiesis, which will, after a few weeks, result in anemia, characterized by low hemoglobin levels <12 g·dL^{-1} in women and 13 g·dL^{-1} in men. As a preventive measure, screening of the early stage of iron deficiency through measurement of serum ferritin is recommended for athletes to avoid performance decrements arising from lowered hemoglobin. Iron depletion is relatively common (30%) in women although in exercising women this may be masked as inflammation arising from recent training can falsely elevate serum ferritin. Accepting this potential compounding factor, most studies would now suggest that the prevalence of anemia in athletes is no more than that of the general population, although few reports have studied both athletes and controls simultaneously. However, a small fall in hemoglobin is unlikely to have any functional consequences for a sedentary person. The early reports of low levels of hemoglobin did not take account of possible increases in plasma volume associated with endurance training (Harris 2000).

Ergogenic aids

A study on Canadian athletes indicated that 69% of athletes used some form of dietary supplement at the Atlanta Games, with this increasing to 74% at the Sydney Games (Huang *et al.* 2006). Vitamins were the most commonly used, with over 60% of men and women taking supplements. Creatine (14%) and amino acid (15%) use were also commonly used at both Games, with the predominant use in swimming and cycling. Potentially, there are a large number of ergogenic aids that may enhance performance, but only four are supported by robust evidence. These are CHO, creatine, bicarbonate, and caffeine. These will be described in more detail in Chapter 6.

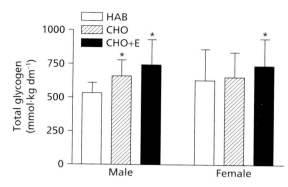

Fig. 23.2 Total muscle glycogen in response to habitual diet (Hab), high carbohydrate diet (CHO; isoenergenic but 75% CHO) and carbohydrate and additional energy (CHO + ~34% additional energy, the difference between men and women's habitual energy intake). * Significant increase compared to habitual diet ($P < 0.05$). Redrawn from Tarnopolsky *et al.* (2001).

Manipulation of CHO in the diet is possibly one of the most researched areas of nutritional ergogenic aids. Although early evidence suggested the existence of gender differences with respect to CHO loading practices, later evidence clarified the reason for this finding. In the initial studies, both males and females increased their CHO intake to 75% of total energy intake. However, because dietary intake of the female subjects was substantially less than that of the males, the absolute levels of CHO intake of the women were not sufficient to trigger glycogen supercompensation. A later study was able to clarify that women are capable of supercompensation when the absolute amount of CHO increase is similar to that of men (Fig. 23.2). The practical interpretation of this is that in order for women to be able to super-compensate they need to increase energy intake by about 30% in order to obtain the minimum amount of CHO intake (8 g·kg^{-1}·day^{-1}) to stimulate super-compensation (Tarnopolsky & Ruby 2001).

Caffeine is a potent ergogenic aid because of its lipolytic action and because of its actions on the central nervous system. Because there is an established difference in lipolysis between men and women, it might be expected that differences in the pharmacokinetics of caffeine would exist between the genders. However, McLean and Graham (2002) have shown that neither gender nor menstrual cycle has

an effect on the pharmacokinetics of caffeine, thus negating any need to differentiate between genders in prescriptions for caffeine use. However, on administration of OCs, caffeine elimination is impaired and there is an increase in caffeine residence time (Rowland & Tozer 1989, cited McLean & Graham 2002). This may have some implications for female athletes who choose to use caffeine in competition, as many athletes report sleeping difficulties after caffeine use.

No direct comparisons have been conducted in terms of gender differences with bicarbonate administration, with women appearing to benefit from similar doses to men (Bishop & Claudius 2005). Similarly, a meta-analysis of the effect of creatine supplementation on body weight and performance concluded that there was no effect of gender (Branch 2003).

Immunology and inflammation

Effect of gender

Most of the literature reporting that women suffer less muscle damage and pain than men has used serum creatine kinase levels as a marker of muscle damage, but this marker is questionable, with large variations occurring, particularly with severe exercise. Also, much of the evidence stems from animal models, where estrogen is believed to provide a protective effect against muscle damage (Clarkson & Hubal 2001).

Human muscle function studies in general would suggest that there is no gender difference or that women are more susceptible, with recent evidence, using quantified stimuli intensities with multidimensional and valid pain measures, confirming that there is no gender difference in delayed onset muscle pain (Dannecker *et al.* 2005).

Although these functional studies have not been able to conclude that there is a sex difference in the muscle damage response to exercise, a recent well-controlled study (Timmons *et al.* 2005) suggests that women respond to prolonged cycle exercise with a greater lymphocyte response, although this was only significant at $P = 0.07$. The lymphocyte increase with exercise is driven primarily by natural killer (NK) cells and may represent a compensatory response to the lower resting NK levels found in women than men. These authors suggest that the differing response is unlikely to be related to estrogen levels as no difference in lymphocyte levels was found across the menstrual cycle. However, throughout this review it is clear that often the differing estrogen levels across the menstrual cycle may not have provided sufficient power with the subject number investigated.

Effect of menstrual phase and oral contraceptive administration

No differences exist across the menstrual cycle phases, but women taking triphasic OCs are reported to have higher total leukocytes and neutrophils during quasi-luteal (when estradiol levels at their lowest) than during quasi-follicular phases and these luteal values were always greater than men (Timmons *et al.* 2005) (Fig. 23.3). This suggests that women are susceptible to a greater neutrophil mobilization, possibly correlating with greater muscle soreness, during this time. The cause of this greater response in the quasi-luteal phase is not elevated cortisol as this remains consistent throughout the cycle, nor does it reflect changes in the cytokine interleukin-6 (IL-6), which is thought to cause the increase in cortisol (Timmons *et al.* 2005).

There is some indication that women may recover more quickly after exercise than men when the functional decrease is severe and that women taking OC agents recover more slowly (Savage &

Clarkson 2002), but further investigations of neutrophil and cytokine changes over time may give some insight into these functional and creatine kinase observations.

Extreme environments

Thermoregulation

EFFECT OF GENDER

During exercise in the heat, the greatest heat loss mechanism is through sweating. Women have a greater number and density of heat-activated sweat glands than men (Bar-Or *et al.* 1968) and this potential capacity for enhanced heat loss is supplemented by a lower lean tissue mass generating heat and a larger body surface area : body mass ratio in women. These factors suggest that women should be able to withstand heat stress better than men. However, the dynamics of sweating may be different; women's sweat rate is generally lower than that of men, but a greater fraction of the sweat evaporates (59% vs. 52% of the total body water loss; Kaciuba-Uscilko & Grucza 2001). As it is the evaporation of the sweat that is effective in removing the heat, this may at least in part compensate for the reduced sweating rate. Except for quantitative differences in sweating, men and women seem to respond to deviations in core temperature in a similar manner when such factors as the subject's aerobic capacity, adiposity, body surface area, and body mass are controlled (Kaciuba-Uscilko & Grucza 2001). During realistic

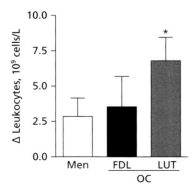
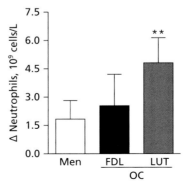

Fig. 23.3 Changes in leukocytes and neutrophils after endurance exercise in men and in women during two quasi-phases of the oral contraceptive pill cycle. Values are means ± SD. * Different from quasi-follicular and men. Redrawn from Timmons *et al.* (2005).

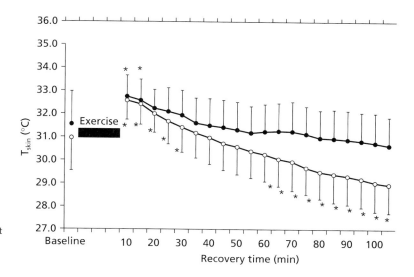

Fig. 23.4 Forearm skin temperature (T_{skin}) in men (open circles) and women (solid circles). Values are mean ± SD. * Indicates a gender effect ($P < 0.05$). Redrawn from Marchand *et al.* (2001).

performance, of course, these variables are not controlled but there is little or no evidence suggesting women are more vulnerable to heat than men. Indeed, the above evidence might suggest the opposite and Cheuvront & Haymes (2001) quote data from the Barcelona Olympic men and women's marathons that suggest that similar race completions were attained in spite of the heat and humidity being greater during the women's event.

One aspect that may differ between the sexes is heat flux during recovery from exercise, with women indicating higher heat flux up until 1 h post-exercise, resulting in lower core temperatures (Marchand *et al.* 2001). This is likely to be a result of their higher body surface area : mass ratio and may explain anecdotal reports of women feeling cold after exercise (Fig. 23.4).

The large surface area : body mass ratio may be a positive factor for women in the heat, but could make women more susceptible to core temperature variation in cold environments. The latter is countered in practice to some extent by the higher subcutaneous fat content of women leading to lower skin temperature (T_{skin}); when men and women are matched for body fat and body size and immersed in cold water there is no evidence to suggest that there is a sex effect (Tikuisis *et al.* 2000). There therefore seems to be little to differentiate the genders with reference to thermoregulation.

EFFECT OF MENSTRUAL PHASE AND ORAL CONTRACEPTIVE ADMINISTRATION

It is not clear whether the elevated core temperature associated with ovulation, reaching a peak in the mid-luteal phase of the menstrual cycle, makes females more at risk from heat stress at this time. Reports are controversial with the luteal phase recording both higher or no difference in heart rate, ratings of perceived exertion and core temperature, and with higher, lower, or no difference reported for skin temperature. There is no controversy around the fact that a higher threshold for sweating and higher gains for sweating rate have been reported, but this may represent the fact that few studies have investigated these variables. If any differences do exist, then they do not affect $\dot{V}_{O_{2max}}$, blood lactate concentration, or exercise performance, the last of which is perhaps most important with remaining contradictions relating to the intersubject variation in hormone levels (Kaciuba-Uscilko & Grucza 2001; Marsh & Jenkins 2002).

Administration of OC reduced phase differences in thermoregulatory function noted in a menstruating group of control women, although the increased rectal temperature for the onset of sweating was not affected. However, additional perturbations caused by estrogen administration may indirectly affect thermal tolerance; fluid retention may cause an increase in arginine vasopressin (AVP) and altered thirst responses (Kaciuba-Uscilko & Grucza 2001). However, this would not appear to result in the need to alter rehydration strategies after exercise-induced dehydration (Maughan *et al.* 1996).

Acclimation

Heat acclimation studies suggest that women respond similarly to men, except that that the sweating difference becomes more exaggerated (Avellini *et al.* 1980). In addition, a recent study conducted of women taking OCs indicated that exogenous reproductive hormones neither enhanced nor impaired the ability of women to complete 7–8 weeks of strenuous physical training and heat acclimation (Armstrong *et al.* 2005).

Altitude

The decrease in $\dot{V}o_{2max}$ with altitude is similar in males and females (Robergs *et al.* 1998), with gender contributing minimally to the interindividual variability (Fulco *et al.* 1998). Although women have greater effective ventilation relative to CO_2 than men and also a higher ratio in the luteal as opposed to the follicular menstrual phase, this does not manifest itself as differences in the response to rapidly ascending to 4300 m (Muza *et al.* 2001). It would appear that the variables that negatively affect the response of an individual to hypoxia are a lower lactate threshold and a larger lean body mass. In practice, therefore, assuming that females, in general, will have a smaller lean body mass, there would be no evidence to suggest that females will be more affected on exposure to altitude than males.

There is some indication that gender differences may exist on exposure to altitude when considering fuel utilization pathways. Specifically, CHO oxidation has been reported to increase during standard exercise in men exposed to acute and chronic altitude

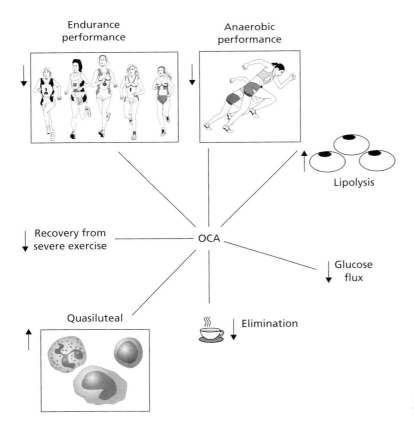

Fig. 23.5 Summary diagram of the effects of oral contraceptives.

when compared to sea level (Roberts *et al.* 1996) whereas women would appear to be more reliant on fat at altitude (Beidleman *et al.* 2002; Braun *et al.* 2005). These changes in metabolic response occur despite the absence of differences between genders in growth hormone, insulin, catecholamine, or cortisol levels (Sandoval & Matt 2002).

Conclusions

Much progress has been made in recent years with regard to the female triad and the message is now clear that those working with female athletes must be alert to energy deficits, whether in particularly lean or "normal" weight women. Gender comparisons will always prove difficult because of the inherent difficulties with subject matching, although it is clear that established differences in hemoglobin,

muscle mass, fat mass, and power will ensure that women will not be faster than men in the foreseeable future. Differences between phases of the menstrual cycle too are problematic because of the large interindividual differences in hormone levels and whether an individual athlete is affected by these hormonal changes is possibly more dependent on the context that the athlete finds themselves in rather than anything to do with menstrual phase. Perhaps the most productive way forward in trying to elucidate the effect of the sex steroids on female physiology is to use a model whereby exogenous steroids are administered in the form of OCs. This allows the investigation of the mechanistic effects of these hormones in addition to establishing whether they are deleterious to an athlete's performance. A summary diagram of known effects is given in Fig. 23.5.

References

Andersson, B., Xu, X.F., Rebuffe-Scrive, M., Terning, K., Krotkiewski, M. & Bjontorp, P. (1991) The effects of exercise training on body composition and metabolism on men and women. *International Journal of Obesity Related Metabolic Disorders* **15**, 75–81.

Armstrong, L.E., Maresh, C.M., Keith, N.R., *et al.* (2005) Heat acclimation and physical training adaptations of young women using different contraceptive hormones. *American Journal of Physiology* **288**, E868–E875.

Avellini, B.A., Kamon, E. & Krajewski, J.T. (1980) Physiological responses of physically fit men and women to acclimation to humid heat. *Journal of Applied Physiology* **49**, 254–261.

Bar-Or, O., Lundegren, H.M., Magnusson, L.I. & Buskirk, E.R. (1968) Distribution of heat activated sweat glands in obese and lean men and women. *Human Biology* **40**, 235–248.

Beidleman, B.A., Rock, P.B., Muza, S.R., *et al.* (2002) Substrate oxidation is altered in women during exercise upon acute altitude exposure. *Medicine and Science in Sports and Exercise* **34**, 430–437.

Bishop, D. & Claudius, B. (2005) Effects of induced metabolic alkalosis on prolonged intermittent: sprint performance. *Medicine and Science in Sports and Exercise* **37**, 759–767.

Blaak, E. (2001) Gender differences in fat metabolism. *Current Opinions in Clinical Nutrition and Metabolic Care* **4**, 499–502.

Branch, J.D. (2003) Effect of creatine supplementation on body composition and performance: a meta-analysis. *International Journal of Sport Nutrition and Exercise Metabolism* **13**, 198–226.

Braun, B., Gerson, L., Hagobian, T., Grow, D. & Chipkin, S.R. (2005) No effect of short-term testosterone manipulation on exercise substrate metabolism in men. *Journal of Applied Physiology* **99**, 1930–1937.

Capranica, L., Minganti, C., Billat, V., *et al.* (2005) Newspaper coverage of women's sports during the 2000 Sydney Olympic Games: Belgium, Denmark, France and Italy. *Research Quarterly in Exercise and Sport* **76**, 212–223.

Carter, S., McKenzie, S., Mourtzakis, M., Mahoney, D.J. & Tarnopolsky, M.A. (2001) Short term 17-β-oestradiol decreases glucose R_a but not whole body metabolism during endurance exercise. *Journal of Applied Physiology* **90**, 139–146.

Casazza, G.A., Jacobs, K.A., Suh, S., Miller, B.F., Horning, M.A. & Brooks, G.A. (2004) Menstrual cycle phase and oral contraceptive effects on triglyceride mobilisation during exercise. *Journal of Applied Physiology* **97**, 302–309.

Casazza, G.A., Suh, S., Miller, B.F., Navazio, F.M. & Brooks, G.A. (2002) Effects of oral contraceptives on peak exercise capacity. *Journal of Applied Physiology* **93**, 1698–1702.

Cheuvront, S.N., Carter, R. III, DeRuisseau, K.C. & Moffat, R.J. (2005) Running performance differences between men and women. An update. *Sports Medicine* **35**, 1017–1024.

Cheuvront, S.N. & Haymes, E.M. (2001) Thermoregulation and marathon running biological and environmental influences. *Sports Medicine* **31**, 743–762.

Clarkson, P.M. & Hubal, M.J. (2001) Are women less susceptible to exercise-induced muscle damage? *Current Opinions in Clinical Nutrition and Metabolic Care* **4**, 527–531.

Dannecker, E.A., Hausenblas, H.A., Kaminski, T.W. & Robinson, M.E. (2005) Sex differences in delayed onset muscle pain. *Clinical Journal of Pain* **21**, 120–126.

Janse de Jonge, X.A. (2003) Effects of the menstrual cycle on exercise performance. *Sports Medicine* **33**, 833–851.

Di-Pietro, L. & Stachenfeld, N. (2005) The female athlete triad revisited. *Medicine and Science in Sports and Exercise* **37**, 1643–1645.

Frisch, R.E. & McArthur, J.W. (1974) Menstrual cycles: fatness as a determinant of minimum weight for height necessary for their maintenance or onset. *Science* **185**, 949–951.

Fulco, C.S., Rock, P.B. & Cymerman, A. (1998) Maximal and submaximal exercise performance at altitude. *Aviation, Space and Environmental Medicine* **69**, 793–801.

Harber, V.J., Petersen, S.R. & Chilibeck, P.D. (1998) Thyroid hormone concentrations and muscle metabolism in amenorrhheic and eumenorrheic athletes. *Canadian Journal of Applied Physiology* **23**, 293–306.

Harris, S.S. (2000) Exercise-related anaemia. In: *Women in Sport. The Encyclopaedia of Sports Medicine* (Drinkwater, B.L., ed.) Blackwell Science, London: 311–320.

Horton, T.J., Miller, E.K. & Bourret, K. (2006) No effect of menstrual cycle phase on glycerol or palmitate kinetics during 90 min of moderate exercise. *Journal of Applied Physiology* **100**, 917–925.

Huang, S., Johnson, K. & Pipe, A. (2006) The use of dietary supplements and medications by Canadian athletes at the Atlanta and Sydney Olympic Games. *Clinical Journal of Sports Medicine* **16**, 27–33.

International Olympic Committee Medical Commission Working Group on Women in Sport (2005) Position stand on the female athlete triad. Available from URL: http://multimedia.olympic. org/pdf/en_report_917.pdf.

International Society for Clinical Densitometry (2004) International Society for Clinical Densitometry Position Development Conference 2004. Diagnosis of osteoporosis in men, premenopausal women and children. *Journal of Clinical Densitometry* **7**, 17–26.

Jacobs, K.A., Casazza, G.A., Suh, S., Horning, M.A. & Brooks, G.A. (2005) Fatty acid re-esterification but not oxidation is increased by oral contraceptive use in women. *Journal of Applied Physiology* **98**, 1720–1731.

Jensen, M.D., Cryer, P.E., Johnson, C.M. & Murray M.J. (1996) Effects of epinephrine on regional fatty acid and energy metabolism in men and women. *American Journal of Physiology* **270**, E259–E264.

Kaciuba-Uscilko, H. & Grucza, R. (2001) Gender differences in thermoregulation. *Current Opinion in Clinical Nutrition and Metabolic Care* **4**, 533–536.

Krotkiewski, M. & Bjorntorp, P. (1986) Muscle tissue in obesity with different distribution of adipose tissue. Effects of physical training. *International Journal of Obesity* **10**, 331–341.

Krotkiewski, M., Bjorntorp, P., Sjostrom, L. & Smith, U. (1983) Impact of obesity on

metabolism in men and women. *Journal of Clinical Laboratory Investigation* **72**, 1150–1162.

Lamont, L.S. (2005) Gender differences in amino acid use during endurance exercise. *Nutritional Reviews* **63**, 419–422.

Loucks, A.B. & Nattiv, A. (2005) Essay: The female athlete. *Lancet* **366**, 549–550.

Loucks, A.B. & Thuma, J.R. (2003) Luteinizing hormone pulsatility is disrupted at a threshold of energy availability in regularly menstruating women. *Journal of Clinical Endocrinology and Metabolism* **88**, 297–311.

Marsh, S.A. & Jenkins, D.G. (2002) Physiological responses to the menstrual cycle. *Sports Medicine* **32**, 601–614.

Marchand, I., Johnson, D., Montgomery, D., Brisson, G.R. & Perrault, H. (2001) Gender differences in temperature and vascular characteristics during exercise recovery. *Canadian Journal of Applied Physiology* **26**, 425–441.

Maughan, R.J., McArthur, M. & Shirreffs, S.M. (1996) Influence of menstrual status on fluid replacement after exercise induced dehydration in healthy young women. *British Journal of Sports Medicine* **30**, 41–47.

McLaughlin, R., Malkova, D. & Nimmo, M.A. (2006) Spontaneous activity responses to exercise in males and females. *European Journal of Clinical Nutrition* **60**, 1055–1061.

McLean, C. & Graham, T.E. (2002) Effects of exercise and thermal stress on caffeine pharmacokinetics in men and eumenorrheic women. *Journal of Applied Physiology* **93**, 1471–1478.

Middleton, L.E. & Wenger, H.A. (2006) Effects of menstrual phase on performance and recovery in intense intermittent activity. *European Journal of Applied Physiology* **96**, 53–58.

Mittendorpher, B., Horowitz, J.F. & Klein, S. (2002) Effect of gender on lipid kinetics during endurance exercise of moderate intensity in untrained subjects. *American Journal of Physiology* **283**, E58–E65.

Muza, S.R., Rock, P.B., Fulco, C.S., *et al.* (2001) Women at altitude: ventilatory acclimatization at 4300 m. *Journal of Applied Physiology* **91**, 1791–1799.

Nattrass, S.M. & Drinkwater, B.L. (1998) Does mechanical loading of peripheral skeletal sites affect prediction of axial BMD? *Bone* **23**, S315.

Nygaard, E. & Hede, K. (1987) Physiological profiles of the male and female. In: *Exercise Benefits, Limits and Adaptations* (MacLeod, D., Maughan, R., Nimmo, M., Reilly, T. & Williams, C.E., eds.) E. & F.N. Spon, London: 239–255.

Pelkman, C.L., Chow, M., Heinbach, R.A. & Rolls, B.J. (2001) Short-term effects of a progestational contraceptive drug on food intake, resting energy expenditure, and body weight in young women. *American Journal of Nutrition* **73**, 19–26.

Redman, L.M. & Loucks, A.B. (2005) Menstrual disorders in athletes. *Sports Medicine* **35**, 747–755.

Redman, L. & Weatherby, R.P. (2004) Measuring performance during the menstrual cycle: A model using oral contraceptives. *Medicine and Science in Sports and Exercise* **36**, 130–136.

Rickenlund, A., Carlstrom, K., Ekblom, B., Brismar, T.B., von Schoultz, B. & Hirschberg, A.L. (2004) Effects of oral contraceptives on body composition and physical performance in female athletes. *Journal of Clinical Endocrinology and Metabolism* **89**, 4364–4370.

Robergs, R.A., Quintana, R., Parker, D.L. & Frankel, C.C. (1998) Multiple variables explain the variability in the decrement in $\dot{V}o_{2max}$ during acute hypobaric hypoxia. *Medicine and Science in Sports and Exercise* **30**, 869–879.

Roberts, A.C., Butterfield, G.E., Cymerman, A., Reeves, J.T., Wolfel, E.E. & Brooks, G.A. (1996) Acclimatization to 4300 m altitude decreases reliance on fat as a substrate. *Journal of Applied Physiology* **81**, 1762–1771.

Roepstorff, C., Steffensen, C.H., Madsen, M., *et al.* (2002) Gender differences in substrate utilization during submaximal exercise in endurance-trained subjects. *American Journal of Physiology* **282**, E435–E447.

Ruby, B.C., Robergs, R.A., Waters, D.L., Burge, M., Mermier, C. & Stolarczyk, L. (1997) Effects of oestradiol on substrate turnover during exercise in amenorrheic females. *Medicine and Science in Sports and Exercise* **29**, 1160–1169.

Sale, D.G. (1999) Neuromuscular function. In: *Gender Differences in Metabolism: Practical and Nutritional Implications* (Tarnopolsky, M., ed.) CRC Press, Florida: 61–85.

Sandoval, D.A. & Matt, K.S. (2002) Gender differences in the endocrine and metabolic responses to hypoxic exercise. *Journal of Applied Physiology* **92**, 504–512.

Savage, K.J. & Clarkson, P.M. (2002) Oral contraceptive use and exercise induced muscle damage and recovery. *Contraception* **66**, 67–71.

Solomon, S.J., Kurzer, M.S. & Calloway, D.H. (1982) Menstrual cycle and basal metabolic rate in women. *American Journal of Clinical Nutrition* **36**, 611–616.

Steffensen, C.H., Roepstorff, C., Madsen, M. & Keins, B. (2002) Myocellular triacylglycerol breakdown in females but not in males during exercise. *American Journal of Physiology* **282**, E634–E642.

Suh, S.H., Casazza, G.A., Horning, M.A., Miller, B.F. & Brooks, G.A. (2003) Effects of oral contraceptives on glucose flux and substrate oxidation rates during rest and exercise. *Journal of Applied Physiology* **94**, 285–294.

Tarnopolsky, A. & Ruby, B.C. (2001) Sex differences in carbohydrate metabolism. *Current Opinions in Clinical Nutrition and Metabolic Care* **4**, 521–526.

Tarnopolsky, M.A. & Saris, W.H. (2001) Evaluation of gender differences in physiology: an introduction. *Current Opinions in Clinical Nutrition and Metabolic Care* **4**, 489–492.

Tarnopolsky, M.A., Zawada, C., Richmond, L.B., Carter, S., Shearer, J., Graham, T. *et al.* (2001) Gender differences in carbohydrate loading are related to energy intake. *Journal of Applied Physiology* **91**, 225–230.

Tikuisis, P., Jacobs, I., Moroz, D., Vallerand, A.L. & Martineau, L. (2000) Comparison of thermoregulatory responses between men and women immersed in cold water. *Journal of Applied Physiology* **89**, 1403–1411.

Timmons, B.W., Hamadeh, M.J., Devries, M.C. & Tarnopolsky, M.A. (2005) Influence of gender, menstrual phase, and oral contraceptive use on immunological changes in response to prolonged cycling. *Journal of Applied Physiology* **99**, 979–985.

Tipton, K.D. (2001) Gender differences in protein metabolism. *Current Opinions in Clinical Nutrition and Metabolic Care* **4**, 493–498.

Torstveit, M.K. & Sundgot-Borgen, J. (2005) The female athlete triad: are elite athletes at increased risk? *Medicine and Science in Sports and Exercise* **37**, 184–193.

Venables, M.C., Achten, J. & Jeukundrup, A.E. (2004) Determinants of fat oxidation during exercise in healthy men and women: a cross-sectional study. *Journal of Applied Physiology* **98**, 160–167.

Wade, G.N. & Jones, J.E. (2004) Neuroendocrinology of nutritional infertility. *American Journal of Physiology* **287**, R1277–R1296.

Westerterp, K. (1999) Nutritional implications of gender differences in metabolism: Energy metabolism, Human Studies. In: *Gender Differences in Metabolism Practical and Nutritional Implications* (Tarnopolsky, M., ed.) CRC Press, New York: 249–265.

Yeager, K.K., Agostini, R., Nattiv, A. & Drinkwater, B. (1993) The female athlete triad. *Medicine and Science in Sports and Exercise* **25**, 775–777.

Zehnder, M.M. I, Kreis, R., Saris, W., Boutellier, U. & Boesch, C. (2005) Gender-specific usage of intramyocellular lipids and g lycogen during exercise. *Medicine and Science in Sports and Exercise* **37**, 1517–1524.

Part 11

Exercise and Health

Chapter 24

Health Benefits of Exercise and Physical Fitness

MICHAEL J. LAMONTE, KARL F. KOZLOWSKI, AND FRANK CERNY

The preceding chapters have elegantly discussed a variety of structural and functional adaptations to exercise training and nutritional fortification that enhance physical performance in competitive sport settings. Indeed, recent advances in the scientific basis of athletic conditioning and sports medicine have resulted in marked improvements in performance records (Tipton 1997). The public's interest in exercise also has increased substantially in the past 50 years or so, to great extent because of its presumed health benefits. To this point, on the eve of the 1996 Olympiad in Atlanta, Georgia, while announcing release of the seminal US Surgeon General's report on Physical Activity and Health, Dr. David Satcher pointed out that few will ever achieve the level of athletic performance displayed by athletes competing in the Olympic Games, but that everyone can benefit from an active way of living (US Department of Health and Human Services 1996). In fact, human evolution has depended on a physically active lifestyle; hunting, gathering, fighting, fleeing, and surviving long enough to reproduce were essential elements of our ancestral past (Eaton *et al.* 1988). A sedentary way of life therefore is an unnatural aberration from our evolutionary constitution and should logically be unhealthy to our species. Because of the high prevalence of sedentary lifestyles and the strong association between physical inactivity and numerous adverse health outcomes (US Department of Health and Human Services 1996), population attributable

risks for physical inactivity are high and rival those of smoking, obesity, and other established risk factors as causes of decreased longevity (Hahn *et al.* 1990).

In this chapter, we briefly review current evidence on the health benefits of physical activity and physical fitness. Readers are referred elsewhere for more thorough reviews (Bouchard *et al.* 1994, 2007; Haskell *et al.* 2007; Kesaniemi *et al.* 2001; US Department of Health and Human Services 1996). To illustrate key points, we select individual studies that are cited frequently in consensus statements and systematic reviews, with an emphasis on studies published since 2000. When possible, we highlight streams of evidence from both observational and experimental studies. We also discuss relevant biologic mechanisms that may explain associations between activity, fitness, and specific health outcomes. We begin with a brief discussion of terminology, assessment methods, and paradigms that pertain to exercise.

Exercise terminology, assessment, and paradigms

An important distinction to make is that physical activity (PA) refers to a behavior, specifically body movement that occurs from skeletal muscle contraction and that results in increased energy expenditure above resting metabolic rate (US Department of Health and Human Services 1996). It now is accepted that activity-related energy expenditure, or the total *dose* of PA, is more important for health benefits than is the specific type of PA (e.g., walking, running, cycling, occupational activities; Haskell *et al.* 2007; LaMonte & Ainsworth 2001). Exercise, or "exercise

The Olympic Textbook of Science in Sport, 1st edition. Edited by R.J. Maughan. Published 2009 by Blackwell Publishing. ISBN: 978-1-4051-5638-7.

training," is a subcategory of PA that is systematically structured toward enhancing one or more components of physical fitness (US Department of Health and Human Services 1996). Physical fitness is a set of physiological attributes (e.g., cardiorespiratory fitness, body composition, muscular strength and endurance, flexibility, agility, balance) that may be enhanced through exercise training or through regular participation in PA (US Department of Health and Human Services 1996). Although it is plausible that enhancing each aspect of physical fitness may in some manner confer health benefits, the component of physical fitness that most often has been related with health outcomes is cardiorespiratory fitness (CRF). Determinants of CRF include age, sex, health status, and genetics; however, the principal modifiable determinant is habitual PA level. CRF responses to a standardized dose of aerobic exercise vary widely among individuals, and the observed heterogeneity is not random but rather aggregates in families through both genetic and environmental components (Bouchard & Rankinen 2001). Nevertheless, in most individuals and particularly among those who are sedentary, increases in PA result in increases in CRF, whereas CRF declines soon after cessation of PA (American College of Sports Medicine 1998). Thus, CRF can be used as an objective surrogate measure of recent PA patterns.

Physical activity assessment methods

PA is a complex multidimensional behavior that is difficult to assess in free-living populations. A gold standard measurement does not exist, so a variety of methods have been used to assess PA and these measurements have a broad range of accuracy, reproducibility, and feasibility (LaMonte & Ainsworth 2001). For example, self-administered questionnaires have relatively low cost and administrative burden and can be used to obtain a crude categorization of activity status (e.g., sedentary versus active) or to obtain more detailed descriptions of activities (e.g., type, duration, frequency) and their estimated energy cost (e.g., kcal·week^{-1}). Several issues must be considered when selecting a specific questionnaire and when generalizing associations between health outcomes and activity levels obtained therewith. These

include consideration of the purpose for assessing PA (e.g., global population surveillance versus quantification of energy expended in specific types of activity such as walking) and of the transportability of a questionnaire's component PA domains and items across population subgroups (e.g., elderly, race ethnic minorities, women). Response biases (e.g., recall bias, social desirability bias) limit the accuracy of self-reported PA assessments. Alternatively, direct monitoring of body movement and related energy expenditure can be performed using electronic motion sensors (e.g., accelerometers, pedometers), global positioning satellite technology, heart rate monitors, portable indirect calorimeters, or some combination thereof. Direct PA assessment is not influenced by response biases and some methods provide an accurate quantification of PA intensity. Thus, direct monitoring may improve the accuracy of free-living PA assessment compared with self-reported methods. However, lack of information on the type of activity being performed, potential changes in habitual PA behavior as a consequence of monitoring (e.g., reactivity), and the associated costs and administrative burden have precluded using direct monitoring in most large-scale studies on health outcomes.

Cardiorespiratory and muscular fitness assessment methods

In studies on health outcomes, methods of quantifying CRF have included the duration or the final estimated work-rate achieved during maximal and submaximal exercise testing, performance on the 6-min and 400-m walk tests, and in a few studies indirect calorimetry measures of maximal oxygen uptake. Because CRF is less prone to misclassification resulting from response biases or behavior reactivity, it may better reflect the adverse consequences of a sedentary lifestyle than do self-reported or directly monitored activity habits (Blair et al. 2001). This might be because CRF is a more reliable measure than is reported free-living PA and because CRF may better reflect the combined effects of genetics and behavior in determining an individual's health risk. Recent studies also have reported on the health benefits of enhancing skeletal muscle strength and endurance (Williams et al. 2007). Measures of muscular fitness that have been related with health outcomes have included isometric grip strength, isokinetic torque assessed at different joints, isotonic force of different muscle groups, and integrated tests of function such as the "up and go" test (Kraemer *et al.* 2005; Steffen *et al.* 2002).

Broadening the exercise paradigm

The US Surgeon General's report on the health benefits of PA promoted a broadening of the exercise paradigm from one that focused almost exclusively on enhancing physical fitness to one that includes both health and fitness domains (US Department of Health and Human Services 1996). Historically, under the exercise and fitness paradigm recommendations included relatively intense exercise and a more formal exercise prescription. Exercise benefits were thought to result through a threshold concept, which asserts that improvements in physical fitness and functioning can only occur after the exercise prescription level is achieved. The health and fitness paradigm derives from epidemiologic data that suggest an inverse dose–response curve between PA, fitness, and health outcomes. The dose–response curve generally is characterized by a steep reduction in health risk across lower and intermediate PA categories, followed by a more gradual decline and tapering off across the highest PA categories. Accordingly, even moderate amounts and intensities of PA may confer important health benefits among those who are sedentary and unfit.

A simple schematic of possible relationships among PA, fitness, and health is shown in Fig. 24.1. Factors such as genetics, the environment, and other health behaviors also likely influence these relationships.

In his J.B. Wolffe Memorial lecture, Dr. William Haskell (1994) further elaborated on the specificity of causal pathways between PA, fitness, and health, noting that some health outcomes may derive only when PA sufficiently enhances one or more domains of physical fitness, whereas other health outcomes occur only if the metabolic capacity of skeletal muscle is enhanced, irrespective of changes in maximal physical performance. The dose of PA or exercise training may be different for changes in various biologic factors (e.g., lipids, connective tissue, myofibrillar ATPase) that are required for improved health status compared with that required for enhanced physical performance (Haskell 1994; Kesaniemi *et al.* 2001).

How much physical activity is required for health benefits?

During the past decade, a critical mass of observational and experimental evidence has been marshalled into consensus recommendations on the type and amount of PA and exercise training required to achieve specific health and fitness outcomes (American College of Sports Medicine 1998; Haskell *et al.* 2007; Thompson *et al.* 2003; US Department of Health and Human Services 1996; Williams *et al.* 2007). In 2007, the American College of Sports Medicine and the American Heart Association jointly released updated recommendations on PA and health which advised adults to achieve a minimum of 30 min per day of moderate intensity (3–6 METs) PA on at least 5 days per week; or at least 20 min per day of vigorous intensity (more than 6 METs) activity on 3 or more days per week (Haskell *et al.* 2007). The targeted minimum volume of PA is about 8 MET-hours per week (approximately 1000 kcal·week^{-1}) in addition

Fig. 24.1 Possible causal relationships between physical activity, fitness, and health. Physical activity may have direct benefits on fitness which in turn affects health outcomes (a); or, physical activity may benefit health but may not significantly improve measures of fitness (b).

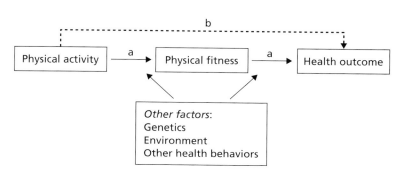

to routine activities of daily living. The targeted volume of energy expenditure can be achieved through a combination of moderate and vigorous intensity activities. Sedentary individuals should gradually increase their PA levels toward meeting the minimal recommended dose. Greater health benefits likely are conferred in individuals whose PA energy expenditure exceeds the minimum dose recommended above (Haskell *et al.* 2007). Recent clinical trial data indicate that recommended levels of moderate intensity exercise are a sufficient stimulus to improve CRF (Church *et al.* 2007; Duncan *et al.* 2005), and that exercise adherence is greater for moderate compared with high intensity exercise programs (Duncan *et al.* 2005; Dunn *et al.* 2005).

Energy expenditure for individual activities can be estimated by multiplying the frequency, duration, and absolute intensity (e.g., METs) of the activity; total energy expenditure is then estimated by summing the individual activities. Standardized energy costs in METs have been published for a variety of activity types (Ainsworth *et al.* 2000). An example that fulfills the required energy expenditure for health-related benefits might be 30 min brisk walking (moderate intensity) on 3 days, plus 20 min jogging (vigorous intensity) on another 1 day of the week. Given that brisk walking (3.5 miles·h^{-1} [5.6 km·h^{-1}] on level ground) is a 3.8 MET activity and that jogging (10 min·mile^{-1} [9.6 km·h^{-1}] on level ground) is a 10 MET activity, the weekly volume of combined moderate intensity (30 min × 3.8 METs × 3 days = 342 MET-min) and vigorous intensity (20 min × 10 METs × 1 day = 200 MET-min) physical activity would be 542 MET-min per week or 9 MET-hours per week.

What level of physical fitness benefits health?

Identifying a minimum threshold level of CRF or muscular fitness for health benefits is more difficult. Compared with PA, fewer reports are available on the association between CRF or muscular fitness and health outcomes. The lack of standardized assessment methods and of standardized reporting of CRF and muscular fitness data presents a major challenge to identifying a minimum level of each to recommend for health benefits. Several studies in adults with

and without existing disease have shown CRF levels of less than 5 METs typically are associated with substantially high risk of all-cause and cardiovascular mortality, whereas CRF levels of 10 METs or higher are associated with excellent survival (Franklin 2002). However, because the distribution of CRF differs by sex and declines disproportionately with advancing age (Fleg *et al.* 2005), the minimum level of CRF required for health benefits may be sex- and age-specific (Sui *et al.* 2007). At present, available data are insufficient to identify a minimum level of health-related muscular strength, power, or endurance.

Physical activity, fitness, and health outcomes

In the above sections we have clarified relevant terminology, briefly reviewed measurement issues, and overviewed current recommendations on the amount of PA required to benefit health. We now highlight selected findings from studies on PA, fitness, and health outcomes that support the current PA recommendations.

Mortality

Clear and strong evidence supports an inverse association between levels of PA or CRF and mortality from all-causes (Lee & Skerrett 2001), cardiovascular disease (Kohl 2001), and all cancers combined (Thune & Furberg 2001). These associations generally are graded, are seen in women and men and in older and younger individuals, and remain significant after accounting for differences in competing risk predictors. Most of the early studies on CRF and mortality endpoints were in middle-aged men (Kohl 2001; Lee & Skerrett 2001; Thune & Furberg 2001; US Department of Health and Human Services 1996). Recent studies have confirmed that the benefits of higher functional capacity also extend to women (Gulati *et al.* 2003; Mora *et al.* 2003) and to older populations (Messenger-Rapport *et al.* 2003; Spin *et al.* 2002). A comprehensive review of published studies indicated that the minimal dose of PA recommended for health benefits (e.g., approximately 8–10 MET-h·week^{-1}) is associated with a significant 20–30% lower risk of all-cause mortality (Lee & Skerrett 2001).

Benefits of PA and CRF in those with existing disease

Much of the earlier work on PA, CRF, and health outcomes was completed in samples of adults that were selected to be free of many chronic diseases or in patients with cardiovascular disease. Recent studies have expanded on earlier work to show that higher levels of PA and CRF also delay mortality in a variety of population subgroups that have increased mortality risk because of existing disease. These data are summarized in Table 24.1 and include studies in adults with diagnoses of diabetes mellitus (Hu et al. 2005; Wei et al. 2000), hypertension (Evenson et al. 2004; Fang et al. 2005), metabolic syndrome (Katzmarzyk et al. 2004), overweight and obesity (Church et al. 2005; Hu et al. 2004), cardiovascular disease (Garg et al. 2006; Myers et al. 2002), breast and colorectal cancers (Holmes et al. 2005; Meyerhardt et al. 2006), and in the frail elderly (Newman et al. 2006). Each of the above conditions is associated with premature mortality and it is clear that afflicted individuals who are physically active and fit have lower mortality risk than their less active and unfit peers. Thus, clinicians should be vigilant in promoting PA and enhancing CRF as a cornerstone strategy of chronic disease management.

PA intensity versus PA volume and mortality risk

Higher levels of energy expended in moderate and vigorous intensity activities each confer significant mortality risk reduction when considered in separate analyses (Haskell et al. 2007; Kesaniemi et al. 2001; US Department of Health and Human Services 1996). Given that a larger volume of energy expenditure is associated with lower mortality risk, and because for the same duration of activity vigorous PA results in a greater energy expended than does moderate PA, it is of interest to determine whether or not vigorous PA confers health benefits beyond those of moderate PA alone. A small number of recent studies have simultaneously examined the effect of different PA intensities on health risk while holding constant total energy expenditure (Lee et al. 1995; Manson et al. 1999, 2002). Significant and similar cardiovascular disease (CVD) risk reduction was seen

in walking activity and in vigorous PA when energy expenditure was held constant. For example, the multivariable adjusted risk of CVD was, on average, 14% and 6% lower ($P < 0.05$ each) for each 5 MET-hour increment of energy expenditure in walking and vigorous activity, respectively (Manson et al. 1999). In another study, at a similar total energy expenditure, vigorous but not non-vigorous PA was associated with all-cause mortality (Lee et al. 1995). Disentangling the associations of PA intensity and energy expenditure with health outcomes is difficult and remains an important research focus. Even if it becomes clear that for the same total dose of PA, vigorous intensity PA confers health benefits independent of those obtained through moderate intensity PA, adults should not be persuaded to disregard the substantial health benefits that clearly have been documented for moderate amounts and intensities of PA.

Muscular fitness and mortality risk

Muscular fitness recently has been examined as a mortality predictor in large epidemiologic studies. In a cohort of 44 452 US male health professionals, men who reported at least 30 min of resistance exercise per week had a 23% lower risk ($P < 0.05$) of cardiovascular events even after controlling for risk factors and overall PA level (Tanasescu et al. 2002). In anther study on 9105 adults, an overall muscular fitness index was computed from the sex-specific tertiles of scores on a 1 repetition maximum (1 RM) bench press, a 1 RM leg press, and the maximum number of bent-leg sit-ups performed in 1 min (FitzGerald et al. 2004). Age- and sex-adjusted relative risks of all-cause mortality for low, moderate, and high muscular fitness were 1.0, 0.56 (95% confidence interval [CI], 0.40–0.80), and 0.65 (95% CI, 0.42–0.99), respectively. Additional adjustment for CRF and other factors attenuated, but did not eliminate, the association between muscular fitness and mortality. The health benefits of greater muscular fitness also appear to be important in the elderly. In a study on 2292 adults 70–79 years of age, greater levels of grip strength assessed by isometric dynamometry and quadriceps strength assessed by isokinetic dynamometry were associated with significantly

Table 24.1 Prospective associations of physical activity (PA) or cardiorespiratory fitness (CRF) with mortality in adults with existing chronic diseases.

Existing disease & reference	Population and outcome	Follow-up (deaths)	Exposures	Main findings RR (95% CI)*
Diabetes Hu et al. (2005)	3708 Finnish adults, ages 25–74 yr, with physician-diagnosed diabetes mellitus Study outcome: all-cause and CVD mortality	≈ 19 yr (1423 deaths; 906 CVD)	PA from questionnaire (combined occupational, commuting, and leisure PA)	*All-cause mortality:* Low: RR = 1.00 (referent) Moderate: RR = 0.61 (0.51–0.73) High: RR = 0.55 (0.47–0.66) *CVD mortality:* Low: RR = 1.00 (referent) Moderate: RR = 0.57 (0.46–0.72) High: RR = 0.54 (0.43–0.67)
Wei et al. (2000)	1263 US men, mean age 50 yr, with physician diagnosed diabetes mellitus or FPG ≥ 126 mg/dL Study outcome: all-cause mortality	12 yr (180 deaths)	CRF from maximal treadmill exercise test (†see legend for CRF groups) PA from questionnaire (leisure PA)	*CRF:* Moderate / High: RR = 1.00 (referent) Low: RR = 2.10 (1.50–2.90) *PA:* Active: RR = 1.00 (referent) Inactive: RR = 1.70 (1.20–2.30)
Hypertension Fang et al. (2005)	4857 US adults, ages 25–74 yr, with physician diagnosed hypertension or resting BP ≥ 140/90 mmHg Study outcome: all-cause and CVD mortality	17 yr (2244 deaths; 1173 CVD)	PA from questionnaire (recreational & non-recreational)	*All-cause mortality:* Low: RR = 1.00 (referent) Moderate: RR = 0.88 (0.80–0.98) High: RR = 0.83 (0.72–0.95) *CVD mortality:* Low: RR = 1.00 (referent) Moderate: RR = 0.84 (0.73–0.97) High: RR = 0.80 (0.66–0.96)
Evenson et al. (2004)	5712 US adults, mean age ≈ 45 yr, with physician diagnosed hypertension or resting BP ≥ 140/90 mmHg Study outcome: all-cause and CVD mortality	25 yr (Men: 709 deaths; 278 CVD; Women: 516 deaths; 190 CVD)	CRF from maximal treadmill exercise test (quintiles of test duration)	Women *All-cause mortality* *Normotensive:* Quintile 5 (high CRF): RR = 1.00 (referent) Quintile 4: RR = 1.10 (0.70–1.90) Quintile 3: RR = 1.50 (0.90–2.40) Quintile 2: RR = 1.90 (1.20–3.10) Quintile 1 (low CRF): RR = 2.30 (1.40–3.60)

Hypertensive:
Quintile 5 (high CRF): RR = 1.90 (0.90–3.80)
Quintile 4: RR = 2.30 (1.30–4.10)
Quintile 3: RR = 2.50 (1.50–4.20)
Quintile 2: RR = 3.30 (2.00–5.40)
Quintile 1 (low CRF): RR = 3.20 (2.00–5.10)

In women, results were similar for CVD mortality.

In men, results were similar to those in women for all-cause mortality, but were variable for CVD mortality.

Metabolic syndrome
Katzmarzyk *et al.* (2004)

3757 US men ages 20–83 yr, who met ATP 3 criteria for metabolic syndrome (see legend)

Study outcome: all-cause and CVD mortality

8 yr (480 deaths; 161 CVD)

†CRF from maximal exercise treadmill testing

All-cause mortality:
Moderate/High: RR = 1.00 (referent)
Low: RR = 2.01 (1.38–2.93)

CVD mortality:
Moderate/High: RR = 1.00 (referent)
Low: RR = 2.25 (1.27–3.97)

Overweight/obesity
Hu F *et al.* (2004)

116 564 US women, ages 30–55 yr

Study outcome: all-cause mortality (similar findings reported for CVD and cancer mortality)

24 yr (10 282)

PA from questionnaire (leisure PA, hr/wk)

BMI from self-reported HT and WT

BMI <25.0 kg/m²
≥3.5 hr/wk: RR = 1.00 (referent)
1.0–3.4 hr/wk: RR = 1.18 (1.09–1.29)
<1.0 hr/wk: RR = 1.55 (1.42–1.70)

BMI 25.0–29.9 kg/m²
≥3.5 hr/wk: RR = 1.28 (1.12–1.46)
1.0–3.4 hr/wk: RR = 1.33 (1.20–1.47)
<1.0 hr/wk: RR = 1.64 (1.46–1.83)

BMI ≥30.0 kg/m²
≥3.5 hr/wk: RR = 1.91 (1.60–2.30)
1.0–3.4 hr/wk: RR = 2.05 (1.82–2.30)
<1.0 hr/wk: RR = 2.42 (2.14–2.73)

(Continued)

Table 24.1 (*cont'd*)

Existing disease & reference	Population and outcome	Follow-up (deaths)	Exposures	Main findings RR (95% CI)*
Church *et al.* (2005)	2316 US men, ages 21–99 yr, with diabetes by physician diagnosis or FPG ≥ 126 mg/dL Study outcome: CVD mortality (similar findings reported for all-cause mortality)	16 yr (179 CVD deaths)	†CRF from a maximal exercise test BMI from measured HT and WT	*BMI 18.5–24.9 kg/m²* High: RR = 1.0 (referent) Moderate: RR = 2.3 (1.2–4.6) Low: RR = 2.7 (1.3–5.7) *BMI 25.0–29.9 kg/m²* High: RR = 1.5 (0.7–3.4) Moderate: RR = 1.6 (0.9–3.2) Low: RR = 2.7 (1.4–5.1) *BMI ≥ 30.0 kg/m²* Moderate/high: RR = 2.3 (0.6–3.6) Low: RR = 2.8 (1.4–5.6)
CVD Garg *et al.* (2006)	460 US adults, mean age 72 yr, with clinical diagnosis of peripheral arterial disease Study outcome: all-cause mortality	5 yr (75 deaths)	PA from accelerometer (quartiles of PA units)	Quartile 4 (high PA): RR = 1.00 (referent) Quartile 3: RR = 1.34 (0.43–3.18) Quartile 2: RR = 2.66 (0.92–7.67) Quartile 1 (low PA): RR = 3.48 (1.23–9.87) Linear trend: P = 0.003
Myers *et al.* (2002)	3679 US men, mean age 62 yr, with diagnosed cardiovascular disease Study outcome: all-cause mortality	6 yr (968 deaths)	CRF from maximal treadmill exercise test (quintiles of METs)	*METs:* ≥ 10.7: RR = 1.00 (referent) 8.3–10.6: RR = 1.80 (1.40–2.20) 6.5–8.2: RR = 2.30 (1.70–2.80) 5.0–6.4: RR = 3.10 (2.40–3.70) 1.0–4.9: RR = 4.20 (3.30–5.20) RR approximated from Fig. 2 of Myers *et al.*

Breast cancer			
Holmes et al. (2005)	2987 US women with stages I, II, or III breast cancer Study outcome: all-cause mortality	8 yr (463 deaths)	PA from questionnaire (Leisure PA, MET–hr/wk)	*Met–hr/wk:* <3.0: RR = 1.00 (referent) 3.0–8.9: RR = 0.71 (0.56–0.89) 9.0–14.9: RR = 0.59 (0.41–0.84) 15.0–23.9: RR = 0.56 (0.41–0.77) ≥ 24.0: RR = 0.65 (0.48–0.88)
Colorectal cancer			
Meyerhardt et al. (2006)	573 US women, mean age 65 yr, with stage I, II, III colorectal cancer Study outcome: all-cause mortality	10 yr (71 deaths)	PA from questionnaire (Leisure PA, MET–hr/wk)	*MET–hr/wk:* <3.0: RR = 1.00 (referent) 3.0–8.9: RR = 0.77 (0.48–1.23) 9.0–17.9: RR = 0.50 (0.28–0.90) ≥ 18.0: RR = 0.43 (0.25–0.74)
Frail elderly			
Newman et al. (2006)	3075 US adults, ages 70–79 yr Study outcome: all-cause mortality and combined fatal/non-fatal CVD events	5 yr (351 deaths; 308 CVD events)	PA from a 400 m walk test (scored in minutes; slower test duration = lower PA/function)	*All-cause mortality:* RR = 1.29 (1.12–1.48) *CVD events:* RR = 1.20 (1.01–1.42) RR = risk of outcome per SD walk time (1 minute)

*In each study, the point and interval estimates of association were adjusted for age, sex (where applicable), and several other risk predictors. CVD, cardiovascular disease; PA, physical activity; CRF, cardiorespiratory fitness; RR, relative risk; CI, confidence interval; FPG, fasting plasma glucose; BP, blood pressure; HT, height; WT, weight; BMI, body mass index (WT [kg] ÷ HT² [m]); METs, metabolic equivalents (1 MET = 3.5 mL O₂/kg/min); MET–hr/wk, MET-hours per week of PA energy expenditure (see body of manuscript for computations).

ATP 3 = US National Cholesterol Education Program Adult Treatment Panel III; metabolic syndrome was defined as the presence of at least 3 of the following: waist circumference > 102 cm, resting BP ≥ 130/85 mmHg, fasting triglyceride ≥ 150 mg/dL, glucose ≥ 110 mg/dL, and high density lipoprotein cholesterol <40 mg/dL.

†CRF in this study was defined according to the age and sex standardized distribution of maximal exercise test duration: low CRF = lowest 20%, moderate CRF = middle 40%, and high CRF = upper 40%.

lower all-cause mortality risk, even after controlling for overall PA level and comorbid conditions (Newman *et al.* 2006). In fact, controlling for thigh muscle area or lean mass had little effect on the association between quadriceps strength and mortality which suggests that muscle quality may be more important than muscle quantity as a determinant of health outcomes. The limited available data suggest that muscular fitness may confer health benefits through mechanisms that are independent of PA or CRF and other aspects of body composition. Whether the protective effect is caused by maximum muscular strength per se, by regular participation in resistance exercises, or both is not known and should be examined in future studies.

Changes in PA or CRF and mortality risk

The vast majority of studies, including those reviewed above, have related a single assessment of PA or physical fitness with mortality risk. A stronger test for a causal relationship is to examine the association between changes in PA or fitness and the subsequent risk of death. Few studies have reported on this issue. Paffenbarger *et al.* (1993) reported on 10 269 men who completed PA questionnaires in 1962 or 1966 and again in 1977, and who were followed up for mortality during the subsequent 11 years. After accounting for differences in several health characteristics, initially sedentary men who took up PA of moderate or higher intensity had a 23% (95% CI, 4–42%) lower mortality risk than their peers who were sedentary across both PA assessments. Blair *et al.* (1995) examined mortality risk in 9777 men who had their CRF assessed by maximal treadmill exercise testing at two examinations separated by an average of 5 years, and who then were followed for an average of 5 additional years. After adjusting for changes in several risk factors, men initially classified has having low CRF who were reclassified as having moderate or higher CRF on the second treadmill test had a 64% lower mortality risk ($P < 0.05$) than men who were unfit at both examinations. These earlier studies on mortality risk reduction through changes in PA or CRF levels have been confirmed in other studies (Erikssen *et al.* 1998; Gregg *et al.* 2003; Talbot *et al.* 2007).

Non-fatal disease

The favorable effect of PA or fitness on mortality outcomes are complemented by benefits in reducing risk of non-fatal disease outcomes. We next briefly summarize studies that have related PA and fitness to the risk of selected non-fatal diseases that are highly prevalent among adults in the USA and other industrialized countries and that contribute substantially to the economic and mortality burden of chronic diseases worldwide.

Diabetes

One of the most consistently reported inverse associations between PA or CRF and non-fatal disease occurrence is for diabetes mellitus. The association has been reported in women and men, and generally remains significant after controlling for differences in fasting glucose, adiposity, nutrient intake, and family history of diabetes (LaMonte *et al.* 2005). Even in adults with impaired glucose tolerance ("pre-diabetes"), the age-adjusted rates of new onset diabetes mellitus were 19.0, 11.0, and 6.0 per 1000 person-years in men with low, moderate, and high CRF ($P < 0.001$), respectively (Wei *et al.* 1999). In this same study, each 1-MET increase in CRF between two separate maximal exercise tests was associated, on average, with a 28% lower risk ($P < 0.05$) of developing diabetes. In a recent study on post-menopausal women, diabetes risk across the upper four quintiles of reported PA was 12%, 26%, 20%, and 33% lower ($P = 0.002$) in Caucasian women, but was not related with PA in women from race-ethnic minority groups (Hsia *et al.* 2005). This disparate finding may reflect the problems associated with questionnaire-based PA assessment in women, particularly in racially diverse population samples (LaMonte & Ainsworth 2001).

Hypertension

The benefits of PA and CRF in lowering hypertension risk are reasonably well established (American College of Sports Medicine 1998; US Department of Health and Human Services 1996), although reported data are less consistent than for diabetes. Earlier studies were conducted mostly on middle-aged men and were based on self-reported PA levels. More recent studies have included measures of CRF (Barlow *et al.* 2006; Carnethon *et al.* 2003) and have been conducted in women (Barlow *et al.* 2006; Carnethon *et al.* 2003; Hu *et al.* 2004). Among women who were especially at risk for developing hypertension because of elevated resting blood pressure ("pre-hypertension"), the risk of future hypertension was 71% and 76% lower in those with moderate and high CRF, respectively, compared with those with low CRF ($P < 0.01$; Barlow *et al.* 2006). Initially sedentary men who reported being moderately or vigorously active on a second PA assessment had a 21% lower risk ($P < 0.05$) of developing hypertension than did men who were habitually sedentary (Paffenbarger & Lee 1997).

Metabolic syndrome

Higher PA and CRF also are associated with lower risk of developing multiple coexisting risk factors and diseases (Carnethon *et al.* 2003, 2004; Jurca *et al.* 2005; LaMonte *et al.* 2005). A recent study related CRF with the development of metabolic syndrome, defined as the presence of at least three out of five metabolic risk factors related to abnormalities in blood pressure control, body fat distribution, and carbohydrate and lipid metabolism (LaMonte *et al.* 2005). Across incremental tertiles of CRF, the risk of developing metabolic syndrome was 1.0 (referent), 0.74, and 0.47 ($P < 0.001$) in men, and was 1.0, 0.80, and 0.37 ($P < 0.01$) in women (LaMonte *et al.* 2005). Even in women and men who had two metabolic syndrome risk factors at baseline and thus were at high risk for transitioning to metabolic syndrome, higher CRF was associated with a 43–66% lower risk of developing the full metabolic syndrome during follow-up. A report in men from the same study also showed that higher muscular fitness was associated with lower risk of developing metabolic syndrome (Jurca *et al.* 2005). After adjusting for differences in age, adiposity, number of metabolic syndrome risk factors present at baseline, men in the highest quartile of muscular strength had a 34% lower risk ($P < 0.05$) of developing metabolic syndrome compared with men in the lowest quartile.

Further adjustment for CRF did not eliminate the significant inverse association between muscular strength and metabolic syndrome risk. Women and men who report maintaining regular PA over multiple assessments have a 51% lower risk ($P < 0.05$) of developing metabolic syndrome compared with their habitually sedentary peers (Carnethon *et al.* 2004).

Cardiovascular events

The majority of data on PA or CRF and cardiovascular risk have been from studies on mortality outcomes. A small number of recent studies have reported on the role of PA and CRF in preventing non-fatal CVD events among initially asymptomatic adults. Women and men with higher CRF levels had significantly lower risk of non-fatal CVD events including myocardial infarction and stroke (Sui *et al.* 2007). Among men with two or more major CVD risk factors and thus whom would be considered at high-risk for CVD events, rates of non-fatal CVD events were 50% lower in men with high compared with low CRF. These findings are consistent with another recent study on CRF and CVD events in Finnish men (Laukkanen *et al.* 2004).

Mental health

An emerging body of work beneficially links PA and physical fitness with mental health issues, including cognitive decline, depression, and anxiety disorders (Bouchard *et al.* 1994, 2007; Kesaniemi *et al.* 2001). Clinical trial data show that PA levels commensurate with public health recommendations confer similar, and in some instances even better effects than pharmacotherapy in managing clinically diagnosed anxiety disorder and depression (Blumenthal *et al.* 2007; Dunn *et al.* 2005). For example, Dunn *et al.* (2005) showed that among adults with clinical depression who were resistant to conventional pharmacotherapy, moderate intensity exercise training at a dose equivalent to that recommended for health benefits was associated with remission in 55% of those in the intervention group compared with only 11% in a non-exercise control group ($P < 0.05$). Evidence also is accumulating for beneficial effects of physical activity on risk of cognitive decline and dementia. A

2-year follow-up on 18 000 adult US nurses showed a 20% lower risk ($P < 0.05$) of cognitive decline among those in the highest compared with the lowest physical activity category (Weuve *et al.* 2004). In another study, the risk of clinical dementia was 93% greater ($P < 0.05$) in older men reporting the least compared with the most weekly walking distance (Abbott *et al.* 2004).

Weight management

There are major challenges to disentangling the complex multifactorial etiology of adiposity, PA, and health outcomes. Sedentary habits could be an antecedent or a consequence of obesity. It is difficult to know how much of the increased health risks seen in obese adults results from excessive body fat, physical inactivity, or both. Moderate and higher PA and CRF levels appear to lower mortality and morbidity risk in individuals with different levels of adiposity (Barlow *et al.* 2006; Church *et al.* 2005; Holmes *et al.* 2005; Hu *et al.* 2004; LaMonte *et al.* 2005; Lee *et al.* 1995; Manson *et al.* 1999, 2002; Wei *et al.* 1999). Less certain is whether or not recommended levels of PA are sufficient for weight management (Grundy *et al.* 1999; Kesaniemi *et al.* 2001; Saris *et al.* 2003). Aerobic PA alone produces only modest weight loss (e.g., 1–2 kg) compared to that seen with combined PA and diet intervention (Grundy *et al.* 1999; Saris *et al.* 2003), but increases in PA with or without overall weight loss have resulted in reductions in abdominal adiposity (Grundy *et al.* 1999). Both aerobic activities and resistance exercise are important in preserving lean body mass during periods of energy restriction and in maintaining weight loss thereafter (Grundy *et al.* 1999; Saris *et al.* 2003). Prospective studies show that maintaining moderate and higher PA and CRF levels during early adulthood attenuates weight gain and the transition from normal weight to overweight or obesity (Grundy *et al.* 1999; Saris *et al.* 2003). Some individuals may obtain important metabolic and health benefits from increased PA or CRF in the absence of weight loss, whereas in others both increased energy expenditure and weight loss or improved body composition may be required to improve health. Further research is needed to better understand issues pertaining to the type and amount of PA required to produce specific weight-related outcomes, the role of genetics in mediating exercise-related effects on body weight and composition, and the effects of PA and exercise on weight, body composition, and health outcomes at different points during the lifespan.

Biologic mechanisms for health benefits

Laboratory and clinical studies using animal and human models have documented a variety of acute and long-term structural and functional responses to PA that improve both physical performance and risk factors for chronic disease (Bouchard *et al.* 1994; Kesaniemi *et al.* 2001). Several of these responses are key mechanisms through which exercise training and PA are thought to reduce the risk of morbidity and mortality, particularly due to cardiovascular disease and cancer. An extensive review of these mechanisms is beyond the scope of this chapter. Established biologic pathways that mediate the beneficial effects of PA, CRF, and muscular fitness include improvements in blood pressure regulation, lipid and lipoprotein metabolism, insulin sensitivity and glycemic control, adiposity and fat distribution, lean body mass and bone mineral content, oxidative stress and immunologic reactivity, and cardiac oxygen demand and electrical stability (Bouchard *et al.* 1994, 2007; Kesaniemi *et al.* 2001). It also appears that PA and physical fitness may favorably influence novel biomarkers involved with intra- and intercellular signaling pathways, endothelial cell function, inflammation, thrombosis and thrombolysis, angiogenesis, and cellular apoptosis (Kasapis & Thompson 2005; Mora *et al.* 2006, 2007). A growing body of evidence also indicates that the human response to both acute and chronic PA is governed to some extent by the human genome (Rankinen *et al.* 2006). Additional research on these established and newly emerging pathways will further elucidate the biologic basis of the health benefits conferred by PA and physical fitness.

Hazards of physical activity and exercise

The net benefits of regular PA and enhanced physical fitness only can be realized after considering any risks that may result from being physically active.

During leisure and recreational activity, the most common risk is for musculoskeletal injuries, such as sprained ligaments, strained muscles, and overuse injuries (Haskell *et al.* 2007; Hootman *et al.* 2001; Thompson *et al.* 2003). Incidence of activity-related musculoskeletal injury is only slightly higher among adults who meet recommended PA levels (17.9 per 1000) compared with their sedentary peers (12.4 per 1000; Carlson *et al.* 2006). Injury risk is higher in those with a history of previous musculoskeletal injury and appears to be positively associated with the intensity of PA (Hootman 2001). The risk of exercise-related cardiovascular complications (e.g., cardiac arrest or myocardial infarction) is quite low, but is transiently increased particularly during vigorous PA (Haskell *et al.* 2007; Thompson *et al.* 2003). Cardiac events during exercise are most likely to occur in individuals with existing cardiovascular disease and in those who are sedentary and deconditioned. The hazards of PA and exercise can be reduced through sensible habits that include properly warming up before and cooling down after exertion, gradually increasing the volume and intensity of PA toward the dose recommended for health benefits, monitoring untoward sensations or responses during exercise, and when indicated, medical screening examinations (American College of Sports Medicine 1998; Haskell *et al.* 2007; Thompson *et al.* 2003). Overall, PA levels within the range recommended for health benefits have an acceptable risk : benefit ratio (Thompson *et al.* 2003).

Conclusions

Physical activity is not a fad, rather it is part of our evolutionary way of living – the kind for which our bodies are engineered and which facilitates proper function of our anatomy, biochemistry and physiology. Sedentary life habits result in maladaptive changes in our constitution and increase the likelihood of disease and premature death. Over the past couple of decades, a substantial amount of observational and experimental research has informed on developing practical exercise recommendations directed toward adults who are sedentary and have low physical fitness. A minimum weekly dose of 8 MET-hours of energy expended (approxiamtely 1000 kcal·week^{-1}) in moderate and vigorous intensity activities is sufficient for most adults to achieve healthy levels of CRF and to lower the mortality and morbidity associated with several diseases. It appears that many of the health benefits associated with PA and fitness are dose-dependent; thus, greater health benefits may accrue with PA levels above the minimum recommended dose. The health benefits of an active and fit way of life transcend gender, race, and age groups, are independent of other major risk factors, and are seen in apparently healthy adults and in those who have existing chronic diseases. Increases in muscular fitness also may influence health through different but related biologic pathways as those that mediate the benefits of aerobic activities.

There are about 70 million US adults (of a total population of about 300 million) who report being sedentary, and similar rates are seen in many other countries. Because of the large number at risk and because of the high relative risks for a variety of adverse health outcomes in sedentary individuals, the population health burden attributed to sedentary habits is substantial. Continued and increased attention to this problem should be given by those involved in healthcare, research, and public health. Additional research on how PA and physical fitness positively influence the population's health must be complemented by development of cost-effective interventions that employ efficacious and practical approaches to changing PA behavior, and by efforts to evaluate and enhance the role of environmental factors that determine individual and community PA habits. Fitness and good health are not destinations, but rather a lifelong journey. A major vehicle for travel along this journey is regular physical activity.

References

American College of Sports Medicine. (2004) Position stand. Exercise and hypertension. *Medicine and Science in Sports and Exercise* **36**, 533–553.

American College of Sports Medicine. (1998) Position Stand. The recommended quantity and quality of exercise for developing and maintaining cardiorespiratory and muscular fitness, and flexibility in healthy adults. *Medicine and Science in Sports and Exercise* **30**, 975–991.

US Department of Health and Human Services. (1996) *Physical activity and health: A report of the Surgeon General. Atlanta, GA.* US Department of Health and Human Services, Centers for Disease Control and Prevention, National Center for Chronic Disease Prevention and Health Promotion.

Abbott, R.D., White, L.R., Ross, G.W., Masaki, K.H., Curb, J.D. & Petrovitch, H. (2004) Walking and dementia in physically capable elderly men. *JAMA* **292**, 1447–1453.

Ainsworth, B.E., Haskell, W.L., Whitt, M.C., Irwin, M.L., Swartz, A.M., Strath, S.J., *et al.* (2000) Compendium of physical activities: an update of activity codes and MET intensities. *Medicine and Science in Sports and Exercise* **32**, S498–504.

Barlow, C.E., LaMonte, M.J., Fitzgerald, S.J., Kampert, J.B., Perrin, J.L. & Blair, S.N. (2006) Cardiorespiratory fitness is an independent predictor of hypertension incidence among initially normotensive healthy women. *American Journal of Epidemiology* **163**, 142–150.

Blair, S.N., Cheng, Y. & Holder, J.S. (2001) Is physical activity or physical fitness more important in defining health benefits? *Medicine and Science in Sports and Exercise* **33**, S379–399; discussion S419–320.

Blair, S.N., Kohl, H.W. 3rd, Barlow, C.E., Paffenbarger, R.S. Jr., Gibbons, L.W. & Macera, C.A. (1995) Changes in physical fitness and all-cause mortality: a prospective study of healthy and unhealthy men. *JAMA* **273**, 1093–1098.

Blumenthal, J.A., Babyak, M.A., Doraiswamy, P.M., Watkins, L., Hoffman, B.M., Barbour, K.A., *et al.* (2007) Exercise and pharmacotherapy in the treatment of major depressive disorder. *Psychosomatic Medicine* **69**, 587–596.

Bouchard, C., Blair, S.N. & Haskell, W.L. (2007) *Physical Activity and Health.* Human Kinetics, Champaign, IL.

Bouchard, C. & Rankinen, T. (2001) Individual differences in response to regular physical activity. *Medicine and Science in Sports and Exercise* **33**, S446–451; discussion S452–443.

Bouchard, C., Shephard, R.J. & Stephens, T. (1994) The Consensus Statement. In *Physical Activity, Fitness, and Health* (Bouchard, C., Shephard, R.J. & Stephens, T., eds.) Human Kinetics, Champaign, IL: 9–76.

Carlson, S.A., Hootman, J.M., Powell, K.E., Macera, C.A., Heath, G.W., Gilchrist, J., *et al.* (2006) Self-reported injury and physical activity levels: United States 2000 to 2002. *Annals of Epidemiology* **16**, 712–719.

Carnethon, M.R., Gidding, S.S., Nehgme, R., Sidney, S., Jacobs, D.R. Jr. & Liu, K. (2003) Cardiorespiratory fitness in young adulthood and the development of cardiovascular disease risk factors. *JAMA* **290**, 3092–3100.

Carnethon, M.R., Loria, C.M., Hill, J.O., Sidney, S., Savage, P.J. & Liu, K. (2004) Risk factors for the metabolic syndrome: the Coronary Artery Risk Development in Young Adults (CARDIA) study, 1985–2001. *Diabetes Care* **27**, 2707–2715.

Church, T.S., Earnest, C.P., Skinner, J.S. & Blair, S.N. (2007) Effects of different doses of physical activity on cardiorespiratory fitness among sedentary, overweight or obese postmenopausal women with elevated blood pressure: a randomized controlled trial. *JAMA* **297**, 2081–2091.

Church, T.S., LaMonte, M.J., Barlow, C.E. & Blair, S.N. (2005) Cardiorespiratory fitness and body mass index as predictors of cardiovascular disease mortality among men with diabetes. *Archives of Internal Medicine* **165**, 2114–2120.

Duncan, G.E., Anton, S.D., Sydeman, S.J., Newton, R.L. Jr., Corsica, J.A., Durning, P.E., *et al.* (2005) Prescribing exercise at varied levels of intensity and frequency: a randomized trial. *Archives of Internal Medicine* **165**, 2362–2369.

Dunn, A.L., Trivedi, M.H., Kampert, J.B., Clark, C.G. & Chambliss, H.O. (2005) Exercise treatment for depression: efficacy and dose response. *American Journal of Preventive Medicine* **28**, 1–8.

Eaton, S.B., Konner, M. & Shostak, M. (1988) Stone agers in the fast lane: chronic degenerative diseases in evolutionary perspective. *American Journal of Medicine* **84**, 739–749.

Eriks;sen, G., Liestol, K., Bjornholt, J., Thaulow, E., Sandvik, L. & Erikssen, J. (1998) Changes in physical fitness and changes in mortality. *Lancet* **352**, 759–762.

Evenson, K.R., Stevens, J., Thomas, R. & Cai, J. (2004) Effect of cardiorespiratory fitness on mortality among hypertensive and normotensive women and men. *Epidemiology* **15**, 565–572.

Fang, J., Wylie-Rosett, J. & Alderman, M.H. (2005) Exercise and cardiovascular outcomes by hypertensive status: NHANES I epidemiological follow-up study, 1971–1992. *American Journal of Hypertension* **18**, 751–758.

FitzGerald, S.J., Barlow, C.E., Kampert, J.B., Morrow, J.R Jr., Jackson, A.W. & Blair, S.N. (2004) Muscular fitness and all-cause mortality: a prospective study. *Journal of Physical Activity and Health* **1**, 7–18.

Fleg, J.L., Morrell, C.H., Bos, A.G., Brant, L.J., Talbot, L.A., Wright, J.G., *et al.* (2005) Accelerated longitudinal decline of aerobic capacity in healthy older adults. *Circulation* **112**, 674–682.

Franklin, B.A. (2002) Survival of the fittest: evidence for high-risk and cardioprotective fitness levels. *Current Sports Medicine Reports* **1**, 257–259.

Garg, P.K., Tian, L., Criqui, M.H., Liu, K., Ferrucci, L., Guralnik, J.M., *et al.* (2006) Physical activity during daily life and mortality in patients with peripheral arterial disease. *Circulation* **114**, 242–248.

Gregg, E.W., Cauley, J.A., Stone, K., Thompson, T.J., Bauer, D.C., Cummings, S.R., *et al.* (2003) Relationship of changes in physical activity and mortality among older women. *JAMA* **289**, 2379–2386.

Grundy, S.M., Blackburn, G., Higgins, M., Lauer, R., Perri, M.G. & Ryan, D. (1999) Physical activity in the prevention and treatment of obesity and its comorbidities: evidence report of independent panel to assess the role of physical activity in the treatment of obesity and its comorbidities. *Medicine and Science in Sports and Exercise* **31**, 1493–1500.

Gulati, M., Pandey, D.K., Arnsdorf, M.F., Lauderdale, D.S., Thisted, R.A.,

Wicklund, R.H., *et al.* (2003) Exercise capacity and the risk of death in women: the St James Women Take Heart Project. *Circulation* **108**, 1554–1559.

Hahn, R.A., Teutsch, S.M., Rothenberg, R.B. & Marks, J.S. (1990) Excess deaths from nine chronic diseases in the United States, 1986. *JAMA* **264**, 2654–2659.

Haskell, W.L. (1994) J.B. Wolffe Memorial Lecture. Health consequences of physical activity: understanding and challenges regarding dose-response. *Medicine and Science in Sports and Exercise* **26**, 649–660.

Haskell, W.L., Lee, I.M., Pate, R.R., Powell, K.E., Blair, S.N., Franklin, B.A., *et al.* (2007) Physical Activity and Public Health: Updated Recommendation for Adults from the American College of Sports Medicine and the American Heart Association. *Medicine and Science in Sports and Exercise* **39**, 1423–1434.

Holmes, M.D., Chen, W.Y., Feskanich, D., Kroenke, C.H. & Colditz, G.A. (2005) Physical activity and survival after breast cancer diagnosis. *JAMA* **293**, 2479–2486.

Hootman, J.M., Macera, C.A., Ainsworth, B.E., Martin, M., Addy, C.L. & Blair, S.N. (2001) Association among physical activity level, cardiorespiratory fitness, and risk of musculoskeletal injury. *American Journal of Epidemiology* **154**, 251–258.

Hsia, J., Wu, L., Allen, C., Oberman, A., Lawson, W.E., Torrens, J., *et al.* (2005) Physical activity and diabetes risk in postmenopausal women. *American Journal of Preventive Medicine* **28**, 19–25.

Hu, F.B., Willett, W.C., Li, T., Stampfer, M.J., Colditz, G.A. & Manson, J.E. (2004) Adiposity as compared with physical activity in predicting mortality among women. *New England Journal of Medicine* **351**, 2694–2703.

Hu, G., Barengo, N.C., Tuomilehto, J., Lakka, T.A., Nissinen, A. & Jousilahti, P. (2004) Relationship of physical activity and body mass index to the risk of hypertension: a prospective study in Finland. *Hypertension* **43**, 25–30.

Hu, G., Jousilahti, P., Barengo, N.C., Qiao, Q., Lakka, T.A. & Tuomilehto, J. (2005) Physical activity, cardiovascular risk factors, and mortality among Finnish adults with diabetes. *Diabetes Care* **28**, 799–805.

Jurca, R., LaMonte, M.J., Barlow, C.E., Kampert, J.B., Church, T.S. & Blair, S.N. (2005) Association of muscular strength with incidence of metabolic syndrome in

men. *Medicine and Science in Sports and Exercise* **37**, 1849–1855.

Kasapis, C. & Thompson, P.D. (2005) The effects of physical activity on serum C-reactive protein and inflammatory markers: a systematic review. *Journal of the American College of Cardiology* **45**, 1563–1569.

Katzmarzyk, P.T., Church, T.S. & Blair, S.N. (2004) Cardiorespiratory fitness attenuates the effects of the metabolic syndrome on all-cause and cardiovascular disease mortality in men. *Archives of Internal Medicine* **164**, 1092–1097.

Kesaniemi, Y.K., Danforth, E. Jr., Jensen, M.D., Kopelman, P.G., Lefebvre, P. & Reeder, B.A. (2001) Dose–response issues concerning physical activity and health: an evidence-based symposium. *Medicine and Science in Sports and Exercise* **33**, S351–358.

Kohl, H.W. 3rd. (2001) Physical activity and cardiovascular disease: evidence for a dose response. *Medicine and Science in Sports and Exercise* **33**, S472–483.

Kraemer, W.J., Fleck, S.J. & Ratamess, J. (2005) General principles of exercise testing and exercise prescription for muscle strength and endurance. In *Exercise Testing and Exercise Prescription for Special Cases.* (Skinner, J.S., ed.) Lippincott Williams & Wilkins, Philadelphia, PA: 38–53.

LaMonte, M.J. & Ainsworth, B.E. (2001) Quantifying energy expenditure and physical activity in the context of dose response. *Medicine and Science in Sports and Exercise* **33**, S370–378.

LaMonte, M.J., Barlow, C.E., Jurca, R., Kampert, J.B., Church, T.S. & Blair, S.N. (2005) Cardiorespiratory fitness is inversely associated with the incidence of metabolic syndrome: a prospective study of men and women. *Circulation* **112**, 505–512.

LaMonte, M.J., Blair, S.N. & Church, T.S. (2005) Physical activity and diabetes prevention. *Journal of Applied Physiology* **99**, 1205–1213.

Laukkanen, J.A., Kurl, S., Salonen, R., Rauramaa, R. & Salonen, J.T. (2004) The predictive value of cardiorespiratory fitness for cardiovascular events in men with various risk profiles: a prospective population-based cohort study. *European Heart Journal* **25**, 1428–1437.

Lee, I.M., Hsieh, C.C. & Paffenbarger, R.S. Jr. (1995) Exercise intensity and longevity in men. The Harvard Alumni Health Study. *JAMA* **273**, 1179–1184.

Lee, I.M. & Skerrett, P.J. (2001) Physical activity and all-cause mortality: what is the dose–response relation? *Medicine and Science in Sports and Exercise* **33**, S459–471.

Manson, J.E., Greenland, P., LaCroix, A.Z., Stefanick, M.L., Mouton, C.P., Oberman, A., *et al.* (2002) Walking compared with vigorous exercise for the prevention of cardiovascular events in women. *New England Journal of Medicine* **347**, 716–725.

Manson, J.E., Hu, F.B., Rich-Edwards, J.W., Colditz, G.A., Stampfer, M.J., Willett, W.C., *et al.* (1999) A prospective study of walking as compared with vigorous exercise in the prevention of coronary heart disease in women. *New England Journal of Medicine* **341**, 650–658.

Messenger-Rapport, B., Snader, C., Blackstone, E., Yu, D. & Lauer, M. (2003) Value of exercise capacity and heart rate recovery in older people. *Journal of the American Geriatric Association* **51**, 63–68.

Meyerhardt, J.A., Giovannucci, E.L., Holmes, M.D., Chan, A.T., Chan, J.A., Colditz, G.A., *et al.* (2006) Physical activity and survival after colorectal cancer diagnosis. *Journal of Clinical Oncology* **24**, 3527–3534.

Mora, S., Cook, N., Buring, J.E., Ridker, P.M. & Lee, I.M. (2007) Physical activity and reduced risk of cardiovascular events: potential mediating mechanisms. *Circulation* **116**, 2110–2118.

Mora, S., Lee, I.M., Buring, J.E. & Ridker, P.M. (2006) Association of physical activity and body mass index with novel and traditional cardiovascular biomarkers in women. *JAMA* **295**, 1412–1419.

Mora, S., Redberg, R.F., Cui, Y., Whiteman, M.K., Flaws, J.A., Sharrett, A.R., *et al.* (2003) Ability of exercise testing to predict cardiovascular and all-cause death in asymptomatic women: a 20-year follow-up of the lipid research clinics prevalence study. *JAMA* **290**, 1600–1607.

Myers, J., Prakash, M., Froelicher, V., Do, D., Partington, S. & Atwood, J.E. (2002) Exercise capacity and mortality among men referred for exercise testing. *New England Journal of Medicine* **346**, 793–801.

Newman, A.B., Kupelian, V., Visser, M., Simonsick, E.M., Goodpaster, B.H., Kritchevsky, S.B., *et al.* (2006) Strength, but not muscle mass, is associated with mortality in the health, aging and body composition study cohort. *Journals of Gerontology. Series A, Biological Sciences and Medical Sciences* **61**, 72–77.

Newman, A.B., Simonsick, E.M., Naydeck, B.L., Boudreau, R.M., Kritchevsky, S.B., Nevitt, M.C., *et al.* (2006) Association of long-distance corridor walk performance with mortality, cardiovascular disease, mobility limitation, and disability. *JAMA* **295**, 2018–2026.

Paffenbarger, R.S., Hyde, R.T., Wing, A.L., Lee, I.M., Jung, D.L. & Kampert, J.B. (1993) The association of changes in physical-activity level and other lifestyle characteristics with mortality among men. *New England Journal of Medicine* **328**, 538–545.

Paffenbarger, R.S. Jr. & Lee, I.M. (1997) Intensity of physical activity related to incidence of hypertension and all-cause mortality: an epidemiological view. *Blood Pressure Monitoring* **2**, 115–123.

Rankinen, T., Bray, M.S., Hagberg, J.M., Perusse, L., Roth, S.M., Wolfarth, B., *et al.* (2006) The human gene map for performance and health-related fitness phenotypes: the 2005 update. *Medicine and Science in Sports and Exercise* **38**, 1863–1888.

Saris, W.H., Blair, S.N., van Baak, M.A., Eaton, S.B., Davies, P.S., Di Pietro, L., *et al.* (2003) How much physical activity is enough to prevent unhealthy weight gain? Outcome of the IASO 1st Stock Conference and consensus statement. *Obesity Reviews* **4**, 101–114.

Spin, J.M., Prakash, M., Froelicher, V.F., Partington, S., Marcus, R., Do, D., *et al.* (2002) The prognostic value of exercise testing in elderly men. *American Journal of Medicine* **112**, 453–459.

Steffen, T.M., Hacker, T.A. & Mollinger, L. (2002) Age- and gender-related test performance in community-dwelling elderly people: Six-Minute Walk Test, Berg Balance Scale, Timed Up & Go Test, and gait speeds. *Physical Therapy* **82**, 128–137.

Sui, X., LaMonte, M.J. & Blair, S.N. (2007) Cardiorespiratory fitness as a predictor of nonfatal cardiovascular events in asymptomatic women and men. *American Journal of Epidemiology* **165**, 1413–1423.

Talbot, L.A., Morrell, C.H., Fleg, J.L. & Metter, E.J. (2007) Changes in leisure time physical activity and risk of all-cause mortality in men and women: The Baltimore Longitudinal Study of Aging. *Preventive Medicine* **45**, 169–176.

Tanasescu, M., Leitzmann, M.F., Rimm, E.B., Willett, W.C., Stampfer, M.J. and Hu, F.B. (2002) Exercise type and intensity in relation to coronary heart disease in men. *JAMA* **288**, 1994–2000.

Thompson, P.D., Buchner, D., Pina, I.L., Balady, G.J., Williams, M.A., Marcus, B.H., *et al.* (2003) Exercise and physical activity in the prevention and treatment of atherosclerotic cardiovascular disease: a statement from the Council on Clinical Cardiology (Subcommittee on Exercise, Rehabilitation, and Prevention) and the Council on Nutrition, Physical Activity, and Metabolism (Subcommittee on Physical Activity). *Circulation* **107**, 3109–3116.

Thune, I. & Furberg, A.S. (2001) Physical activity and cancer risk: dose–response and cancer, all sites and site-specific. *Medicine and Science in Sports and Exercise* **33**, S530–550.

Tipton, C.M. (1997) Sports medicine: a century of progress. *Journal of Nutrition* **127**, 878S–885S.

Wei, M., Gibbons, L.W., Kampert, J.B., Nichaman, M.Z. & Blair, S.N. (2000) Low cardiorespiratory fitness and physical inactivity as predictors of mortality in men with type 2 diabetes. *Annals of Internal Medicine* **132**, 605–611.

Wei, M., Gibbons, L.W., Mitchell, T.L., Kampert, J.B., Lee, C.D. & Blair, S.N. (1999) The association between cardiorespiratory fitness and impaired fasting glucose and type 2 diabetes mellitus in men. *Annals of Internal Medicine* **130**, 89–96.

Weuve, J., Kang, J.H., Manson, J.E., Breteler, M.M., Ware, J.H. & Grodstein, F. (2004) Physical activity, including walking, and cognitive function in older women. *JAMA* **292**, 1454–1461.

Williams, M.A., Haskell, W.L., Ades, P.A., Amsterdam, E.A., Bittner, V., Franklin, B.A., *et al.* (2007) Resistance exercise in individuals with and without cardiovascular disease: 2007 update: a scientific statement from the American Heart Association Council on Clinical Cardiology and Council on Nutrition, Physical Activity, and Metabolism. *Circulation* **116**, 572–584.

Index